Mitochondrial Medicine

Mitochondrial Medicine

Edited by

Salvatore DiMauro MD
Lucy G Moses Professor of Neurology
Department of Neurology
Columbia University Medical Center
New York, NY
USA

Michio Hirano MD
Associate Professor of Neurology
Department of Neurology
Columbia University Medical Center
New York, NY
USA

Eric A Schon PhD
Lewis P Rowland Professor of Neurology
Department of Neurology
Professor of Genetics and Development (in Neurology)
Department of Genetics and Development
Columbia University Medical Center
New York, NY
USA

CRC Press
Taylor & Francis Group
Boca Raton London New York

CRC Press is an imprint of the
Taylor & Francis Group, an **informa** business

First published 2006 by Informa Healthcare

Published 2019 by CRC Press
Taylor & Francis Group
6000 Broken Sound Parkway NW, Suite 300
Boca Raton, FL 33487-2742

ISBN 13: 978-0-367-44636-9 (pbk)
ISBN 13: 978-1-84214-288-2 (hbk)

Visit the Taylor & Francis Web site at
http://www.taylorandfrancis.com

and the CRC Press Web site at
http://www.crcpress.com

A CIP record for this book is available from the British Library.

Library of Congress Cataloging-in-Publication Data
Data available on application

Cover based on a design by Eduardo Bonilla MD and Pablo Abreu.

Dedication

This book, directed to practicing clinicians and clinical scientists, has been inspired by – and is dedicated to – Lewis P (Bud) Rowland in celebration of his 80th birthday. Throughout his career – most of it spent as chairman of the Department of Neurology at the University of Pennsylvania and of the Neurological Institute at Columbia University Medical Center (CUMC) – Bud Rowland has been a staunch and tireless advocate of clinical research, that is, research that starts at the bedside (with astute questions asked by inquiring clinicians), moves back to the lab (with appropriate experiments designed collaboratively by clinical and basic scientists) and, hopefully, returns to the patients in the form of rational therapeutic approaches.

The three editors, who have been working together on translational research in mitochondrial diseases for many years because of Bud Rowland's vision, encouragement, and support, offer this book to him as a token of their gratitude and affection. Although all three, as well as several other contributors to this book, work at CUMC, which hopefully provides uniformity of style and a minimum of overlap, other contributors represent institutions around the world. This international presence appropriately reflects both the worldwide interest in mitochondrial diseases and the worldwide recognition of Bud Rowland as a leader in neurological research.

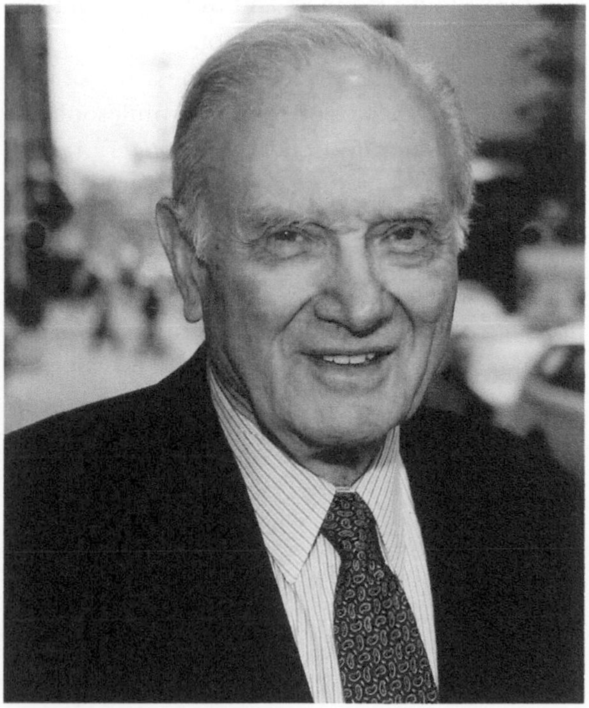

Lewis P (Bud) Rowland (photo courtesy of Kara Flannery)

However, Bud Rowland's mentoring goes well beyond neurology and clinical research, affecting, as it does, more general professional and personal values. The oldest of us (SDM) will never forget his first encounter with Dr Rowland, when, as a postdoctoral fellow freshly arrived in Philadelphia from the lofty halls of Italian academe, he participated in his first clinical rounds: to a resident asking him the reason for a patient's symptom, Bud answered 'I don't know: find out and tell us next week,' an admission never uttered by any departmental chairman in recent history at the 750-year-old University of Padua. True to this anecdote, Dr Rowland teaches by example and benevolent Socratic provocation. Despite his many honors and awards, he is totally unaffected and does not like affectation in others. He is simple and direct in his manners and in his writing style, which makes him a superb editor.

In many ways, he personifies the sense of duty and noble simplicity of the stoic philosophy. A reading of Marcus Aurelius' '*Meditations*'[1] reveals that numerous qualities extolled by the Roman emperor are typical of Bud Rowland. These include: 'good morals and the government of [one's] temper; simplicity in [one's] way of living; not to give credit to what is said by miracle-workers and jugglers; abstaining from rhetoric; no vainglory in those things that men call honors; readiness to listen to those who have anything to propose for the common weal; and readiness to give way without envy to those who possess any particular faculty.' (*Meditations*, Book I).

To continue with this praise would embarrass Dr Rowland, for whom, like for Marcus Aurelius, 'What then is worth being valued? To be received with clapping of hands? No. Neither must we value the clapping of tongues, for the praise that comes from the many is a clapping of tongues.' (*Meditations*, Book VI). Enough, then, with the clapping of our tongues, confident that Bud will – again in the words of Marcus Aurelius – 'receive from his friends what is meant to be an esteemed favor, without being humbled by it'.

SDM, MH, EAS

Reference

1. Marcus Aurelius. *Meditations*. Long G, Translator. Mineola, NY: Dover Publications, Inc., 1997.

Contents

List of Boxes ix
List of Contributors xi
Preface xiii
List of Abbreviations xv

Introduction: the birth of mitochondrial medicine 1
Rolf Luft

1. The mitochondrial respiratory chain and its disorders 7
   Salvatore DiMauro and Eric A Schon

2. Mitochondrial neurology I: encephalopathies 27
   Michio Hirano, Petra Kaufmann, Darryl De Vivo and Kurenai Tanji

3. Mitochondrial neurology II: myopathies and peripheral neuropathies 45
   Arthur P Hays, Maryam Oskoui, Kurenai Tanji, Petra Kaufmann and Eduardo Bonilla

4. Mitochondrial cardiology 75
   Jeffrey A Towbin

5. Mitochondrial ophthalmology 105
   Valerio Carelli, Piero Barboni and Alfredo A Sadun

6. Mitochondrial gastroenterology 143
   Laurence Bindoff

7. Mitochondrial otology 161
   Patrick F Chinnery and Timothy D Griffiths

8. Mitochondrial endocrinology 179
   Maria A Yialamas, Leif C Groop and Vamsi K Mootha

9. Mitochondrial nephrology 197
Agnès Rötig and Patrick Niaudet

10. Mitochondrial hematology and oncology 209
Norbert Gattermann and Stefanie Zanssen

11. Mitochondrial reproductive medicine 241
David R Thorburn

12. Mitochondrial psychiatry 261
Salvatore DiMauro, Michio Hirano, Petra Kaufmann and J John Mann

13. Mitochondrial dysfunction and neurodegenerative disorders 279
Kim Tieu and Serge Przedborski

14. Therapeutic approaches 309
Salvatore DiMauro and Eric A Schon

Appendix 329
Index 337

Boxes

Box 1.1 - What is the endosymbiotic hypothesis? 8

Box 1.2 - ATP and glycolysis 14

Box 1.3 - The Krebs cycle 19

Box 2.1 - Diagnosis of mtDNA mutations 31

Box 2.2 - The 'MELAS paradox' 36

Box 3.1 - Replication of mitochondrial DNA 48

Box 3.2 - Deleted and duplicated mtDNAs 57

Box 3.3 - ATP synthesis 62

Box 4.1 - tRNA hotspots 84

Box 5.1 - Cybrid technology 127

Box 6.1 - Mitochondrial nucleotide pools 150

Box 7.1 - Transcription of mitochondrial DNA 168

Box 7.2 - Translation of mitochondrial mRNAs 172

Box 8.1 - Microarray technology 186

Box 9.1 - Polarography 202

Box 11.1 - Why is there maternal inheritance? 243

Box 11.2 - Is Dolly a clone? 251

Box 12.1 - Mitochondrial DNA haplogroups 270

Box 13.1 - The biogenesis of iron-sulfur clusters 281

Box 13.2 - Mitochondrial fusion, fission, and movement 286

Box 13.3 - Mitochondrial protein importation 290

Box 14.1 - 'Mito mice' 310

Box 14.2 - Xenotopic expression 322

Contributors

Piero Barboni MD
Centro Oftalmologia Salus, Bologna, Italy

Laurence Bindoff MD
Institute of Clinical Medicine, Department of Neurology, University of Bergen, Haukeland University Hospital, Bergen, Norway

Eduardo Bonilla MD
Departments of Neurology and Pathology, Columbia University Medical Center New York, NY, USA

Valerio Carelli MD PhD
Department of Neurological Sciences, University of Bologna, Bologna, Italy

Patrick F Chinnery PhD MRCP MRCPath
Regional Neuroscience Centre, The Medical School, Newcastle upon Tyne, UK

Darryl C De Vivo MD
Department of Neurology, Columbia University Medical Center New York, NY, USA

Salvatore DiMauro MD
Departments of Neurology, and Genetics and Development, Columbia University Medical Center, New York, NY, USA

Norbert Gattermann MD
Department of Hematology, Oncology, and Clinical Immunology, Heinrich-Heine-University, Düsseldorf, Germany

Timothy D Griffiths DM FRCP
Regional Neuroscience Centre, The Medical School, Newcastle upon Tyne, UK

Leif C Groop MD PhD
Department of Endocrinology, Malmö University Hospital, Malmö, Sweden

Arthur P Hays MD
Department of Pathology, Columbia University Medical Center, New York, NY, USA

Michio Hirano MD
Department of Neurology, Columbia University Medical Center, New York, NY, USA

Petra Kaufmann MD
Department of Neurology, Columbia University Medical Center, New York, NY, USA

Rolf Luft MD PhD
Department of Endocrinology, Karolinska Hospital, Stockholm, Sweden

J John Mann MD
Department of Psychiatry, Columbia University Medical Center, New York, NY, USA

Vamsi Mootha MD
Department of Systems Biology, Harvard Medical School, Cambridge, and Department of Medicine, Massachusetts General Hospital, Boston MA, USA

Patrick Niaudet MD
INSERM U393, Hôpital Necker-Enfants Malades, Paris, France

Maryam Oskoui
Departments of Neurology, Columbia University Medical Center, New York, NY, USA

Serge Przedborski MD PhD
Department of Neurology and Pathology, Center for Neurobiology & Behavior, Columbia University Medical Center, New York, NY, USA

Agnès Rötig PhD
INSERM U393, Hôpital Necker-Enfants Malades, Paris, France

Alfredo A Sadun MD PhD
Department of Ophthalmology, Doheny Eye Institute, University of Southern California Los Angeles, CA, USA

Eric A Schon PhD
Departments of Genetics and Development and Neurology, Columbia University Medical Center, New York, NY, USA

Kurenai Tanji MD
Departments of Pathology and Neurology, Columbia University Medical Center, New York, NY, USA

David R Thorburn PhD
Murdoch Children's Research Institute, Royal Children's Hospital, Parkville, Victoria, Australia

Kim Tieu PhD
Department of Environmental Medicine & Center for Aging and Developmental Biology, University of Rochester, Rochester, NY, USA

Jeffrey A Towbin MD
Division of Pediatric Cardiology, Texas Children's Hospital, Baylor College of Medicine, Houston, TX, USA

Maria A Yialamas MD
Department of Medicine, Massachusetts General Hospital, Boston, MA, USA

Stephanie Zanssen MD PhD
Department of Neurology, Columbia University Medical Center, New York, NY, USA

Preface

Nowadays, mitochondrial dysfunction is included in the differential diagnosis of complicated disorders by most well informed clinicians. However, there are still two opposite attitudes, leading either to under-diagnosis (what is this confusing clinical presentation?) or to over-diagnosis (this clinical presentation is so confusing that it must be mitochondrial!). The multisystemic nature of most – but not all – mitochondrial diseases has been illustrated by innumerable articles and reviews and is generally appreciated by pediatricians and neurologists: by pediatricians, especially pediatric neurologists, because the energy crisis that accompanies mitochondrial dysfunction almost invariably affects the developing nervous system; by neurologists, because the extreme dependence of both central and peripheral nervous systems on oxidative metabolism makes these tissues especially vulnerable to mitochondrial dysfunction.

However, general practitioners and clinicians interested in medical specialties other than neurology are less aware of the impact of respiratory chain defects on the etiology and physiopathology of the diseases they study. It is, in part, to fill this gap that we have put together in a single book authoritative and – as much as the rapid progress in this field allows it – state-of-the art reviews of mitochondrial diseases in all major subspecialties of medicine.

A few disclaimers are in order. First, according to a generally accepted convention, we have limited the concept of mitochondrial disease to defects of the mitochondrial respiratory chain, the terminal energy-yielding pathway of mitochondrial metabolism and the only one under the dual control of nuclear DNA and mitochondrial DNA. An exception was made for defects of β-oxidation, which are frequent causes of peripheral neuropathies and cardiomyopathies and are therefore considered in the differential diagnosis of these disorders (Chapters 3 and 5).

Second, all three editors and several contributors work at the same institution, Columbia University Medical Center (CUMC). This degree of CUMC-centrism was intentional and aimed at maximizing uniformity of style while minimizing conceptual overlaps. Still, eight of the 14 chapters have been written by recognized experts from other institutions around the world.

Third, despite our efforts to limit them, there are several overlaps: this is practically inevitable when dealing with syndromes that involve multiple organs and systems. For example, MELAS, which typically affects the central and peripheral nervous systems, can also cause cardiomyopathy, diabetes mellitus, sensorineural hearing loss, and intestinal pseudo-obstruction, and is therefore considered in the chapters on central and peripheral neurology (Chapters 2 and 3), cardiology (Chapter 4), gastroenterology (Chapter 6), otology (Chapter 7), and endocrinology (Chapter 8). Clinical emphasis and pathogenic considerations obviously vary in different chapters, making repetitions not only inevitable, but, in fact, useful.

Fourth, not all subspecialties of medicine are covered. For instance, there is no chapter on dermatology because skin and hair diseases are either rarely associated with mitochondrial dysfunction or grossly overlooked. On the other hand, we have included a chapter on psychiatric disorders, which are rarely considered as typical manifestations of mitochondrial dysfunction, but are, in fact, not at all uncommon. We think that 'mitochondrial psychiatry' deserves more attention both for clinical and therapeutic reasons and because it offers a window on the pathogenetic mechanisms of affective and behavioral disorders.

An unusual feature of this book is the lack of an opening section consisting of several chapters devoted to mitochondrial basic science, including mitochondrial biogenesis, genetics, and bioenergetics. Basic concepts are summarized in Chapter 1, but the omission of an entire 'basic' section is intentional and motivated by the clinical slant of the book. However, we have devised a 'lighter' and – we hope – more clinically relevant way of highlighting basic concepts of mitochondrial biogenesis through 'inserts' peppered throughout the chapters. These scientific vignettes have been written by the more basic science-oriented of the three editors (EAS) and have been placed in close proximity to clinical questions to which they are directly relevant. The scientific value of the book is further enhanced by an appendix, also contributed by EAS, listing all known pathogenic mtDNA mutations (as of August 31st, 2005). It is intended as an identikit, which allows one not only to associate clinical capsules with known mutations, but also to check if a newly found mutation has already been described.

Unquestionably, the concept of mitochondrial disease – and arguably the more fundamental concept of organellar medicine – was introduced in 1962 with the description of a young Swedish woman, who suffered from non-thyroidal hypermetabolism due to loose coupling of muscle mitochondria. We are honored to have a personal rendition of how it all started by Professor Rolf Luft, who identified that first patient with mitochondrial dysfunction and, 22 years later, reviewing the stunning progress of the field opened by him, aptly coined the term 'mitochondrial medicine' that we have borrowed for the title of our book.

We hope that this book will achieve its scope, to review the clinical spectrum of mitochondrial diseases and – in the process – to attract medical students and residents to this fascinating and still rapidly progressing area of clinical research. We are grateful to our colleagues both at CUMC and elsewhere who have shared our enthusiasm for this endeavor by contributing chapters and graciously accepting our editorial suggestions. We are also grateful to our families for their understanding as our work on this book cut further into the time that we could devote to them.

SDM, MH, EAS

Abbreviations

AA	acetoacetate
AA-CoA	acetoacetyl-CoA
Aβ	amyloid ß peptide (Greek beta symbol)
ABAD	aβ-binding alcohol dehydrogenase
ABC	ATP-binding cassette
ACE	angiotensin-converting enzyme
ACT	acetoacetyl-CoA thiolase
AD	Alzheimer's disease
ADC	apparent diffusion coefficient
ADP	adenosine diphosphate
ADPEO	autosomal dominant progressive external ophthalmoplegia
AHS	Alpers-Huttenlocher syndrome
AID	aminoglycoside-induced deafness
AIDP	acute idiopathic demyelinating polyneuropathy
AISA	acquired idiopathic sideroblastic anemia
ALS	amyotrophic lateral sclerosis (Lou Gehrig disease)
AML	acute myeloid leukemia
ANT	adenine nucleotide translocator
AOA1	ataxia with oculomotor apraxia
APAF1	Apoptotic protease activating factor 1
APP	amyloid precursor protein
APTX	gene responsible for AOA 1
ARCO	autosomal recessive cardiopathy and ophthalmoplegia
ARPEO	autosomal recessive progressive external ophthalmoplegia
AS	Asperger syndrome
ASD	autistic spectrum disorder
ASD	atrial septal defect
ASH	asymmetric septal hypertrophy
ATP	adenosine triphosphate
ATP12	assembly factor for ATP synthase (complex V)
ATP7B	gene mutated in Wilson's disease
AZT	azidothymidine
Aβ	amyloid beta peptide
B17.2L	molecular chaperone of complex I
BCS1L	cytochrome *b–c* complex assembly protein (complex III)
BHB	D-β-hydroxybutyrate (Greek beta symbol)
BHD	Birt-Hogg-Dube syndrome
BMI	body mass index
BMR	basal metabolic rate
BNP	brain natriuretic peptide
BrdU	bromodeoxyuridine
BSN	bilateral striatal necrosis.
CACT	carnitine: acylcarnitine translocator
CADASIL	cerebral autosomal dominant arteriopathy with subcortical infacts and leukoencephalopathy
CEON	Cuban epidemic optic neuropathy
CGL	chronic granulocytic leukemia
CHF	congestive heart failure
CHO	choline
CIDP	chronic idiopathic demyelinating polyneuropathy
CK	creatine kinase

CMAP	compound motor action potential
$CMRO_2$	cerebral oxygen metabolic rate
CMT	Charcot-Marie-Tooth disease
CNS	central nervous system
CO	cytochrome *c* oxidase (also COX)
CoA	coenzyme A
CoQ10	coenzyme Q10
COX	cytochrome *c* oxidase (also CO)
CPEO	chronic progressive external ophthalmoplegia
CPT	carnitine palmitoyltransferase
CT	computerized tomography
CR	creatinine
CREB	cAMP-responsive element binding protein
CSF	cerebrospinal fluid
Cu-his	copper-histidine
CVS	chorionic villus sample
Cyt *b*	cytochrome *b*
DAG	diacylglycerol
DAPC	dystrophin-associated protein complex
DCA	dichloroacetate
DCM	dilated cardiomyopathy
DDP1	deafness/dystonia protein (mutated in Mohr-Tranebjaerg syndrome)
dGK	deoxyguanosine kinase
DGUOK	deoxyguanosine kinase
DHODH	dihydroorotate dehydrogenase
DIC	dicarboxylate carrier
DIDMOAD	diabetes insipidus, diabetes mellitus, optic atrophy, and deafness (Wolfram syndrome)
DKA	diabetic ketoacidosis
D-loop	displacement loop of mtDNA
DNA	deoxyribonucleic acid
DNM1	gene encoding dynamin-related protein
DOA	autosomal dominant optic atrophy
DRP-1	dynamin-related protein 1
DSM	*Diagnostic and Statistical Manual of Mental Disorders*
Dup-mtDNA	duplicated mtDNA
DWI	diffusion-weighted imaging
ECM	encephalomyopathy
ECM	extracellular matrix
EE	ethylmalonic encephalomyopathy
EEG	electroencephalography
EF-TU	mitochondrial elongation factor
EFE	endocardial fibroelastosis
EFG1	elongation factor G1
EGFR	epidermal growth factor receptor
EM	electron microscopy
EMG	electromyography
EOM	extraocular muscle
ERG	electroretinography
ERRα	estrogen related receptor alpha
EtBr	ethidium bromide
ETC	electron transport chain
ETF	electron-transfer flavoprotein
ETFDH	electron-transfer dehydrogenase
ETHE1	ethylmalonic encephalopathy 1
FA	Friedreich ataxia (also FRDA)
FAD	flavin adenine dinucleotide
FADH	reduced flavin adenine dinucleotide
FALS	familial ALS
FBSN	familial bilateral striatal necrosis
FH	fumarase
Fis1p	fission-related protein
FISH	fluorescence in situ hybridization
FLAIR	fluid-attenuated inversion recovery
FLCN	folliculin gene
FRDA	Friedreich ataxia (also FA)
FSE	fast spin echo
FSGS	focal segmental glomerular sclerosis
FSH	follicle-stimulating hormone
FTT	failure to thrive
Fzo1p	fuzzy onion protein 1

G4.5	gene encoding tafazzins (mutated in Barth syndrome) (also *TAZ*)
GABP	GA binding protein A
GAD	glutamic acid decarboxylase
GC/MS	gas chromatography/mass spectrometry
GDP	guanosine diphosphate
GH	growth hormone
GI	gastrointestinal tract (also GIT)
GRACILE	growth retardation, aminoaciduria, lactic acidosis, early death
GSH	glutathione
GTP	guanosine triphosphate
H&E	hematoxylin & eosin
HADD	hyperactivity attention deficit disorder
HBD	D-beta-hydroxybutyrate dehydrogenase
HCC	Hurtle cell carcinoma
HCM	hypertrophic cardiomyopathy
HD	Huntington's disease
HIF-1	hypoxia-inducible transcription factor
HLHS	hypoplastic left heart syndrome
HLRCC	hereditary leiomyoma and renal cell carcinoma
HNP	head neck paraganglioma
HPHI-3	HIFα-prolyl hydroxylase (also PDHI-3)
HRT	Heidelberg retina tomography
HSC	hematopoietic stem cell
HSP	hereditary spastic paraplegia
HSP	promoter of mtDNA heavy strand replication
HSP60	heat shock protein 60 (mitochondrial import chaperonin)
HVR	hypervariable region of mtDNA
IAPs	inhibitors of apoptosis proteins
ICARS	international cooperative ataxia scores
ICSI	intracytoplasmic sperm injection
IGF	insulin growth factor
IMS	intermembrane space
ISC	iron-sulfur cluster
IVF	in vitro fertilization
KIF5A	kinesin family member 5
KSS	Kearns-Sayre syndrome
L/P	lactate/pyruvate ratio
LAC	lactate
LARS2	gene encoding leucyl-tRNA synthetase
LCAD	long-chain acyl-CoA dehydrogenase
LCHAD	long-chain 3-hydroxyacyl-CoA dehydrogenase
LH	luteinizing hormone
LHON	Leber hereditary optic neuropathy
LOH	loss of heterozygosity
LRPPRC	leucine-rich pentatricopeptide repeat-containing protein
LS	Leigh syndrome
LSFC	Leigh syndrome, French Canadian type
LSP	promoter of mtDNA light strand replication
LVNC	left ventricular non-compaction
LVOTO	left ventricular outflow tract obstruction
MCAD	medium-chain acyl-CoA dehydrogenase
MCUL	multiple cutaneous and uterine leiomyoma
MDS	mtDNA depletion syndrome
MDS	myelodysplastic syndrome
Mdv1p	mitochondrial division protein
MELAS	mitochondrial encephalomyopathy, lactic acidosis, stroke-like episodes
MERRF	myoclonus epilepsy with ragged-red fibers
MFN1	mitofusin 1
MFN2	mitofusin 2
MIDD	maternally inherited diabetes and deafness
MILS	maternally inherited Leigh syndrome

MIM	mitochondrial inner membrane
MitoQ	mitoquinone
MLASA	mitochondrial myopathy lactic acidosis and sideroblastic anemia (also MSA)
MMPI	Minnesota Multiphasic Personality Inventory
MNGIE	mitochondrial neurogastrointestinal encephalomyopathy
MODY	maturity-onset diabetes of the young
MOM	mitochondrial outer membrane
MPO	myeloperoxidase
MPP	1 methyl-4-phenylpiridinium
MPTP	1 methyl-4-phenyl-1,2,3,6-tetrahydropyridine
MPTP	mitochondrial permeability transition pore (also PTP and PTPC)
MR	mental retardation
MRC	mitochondrial respiratory chain (also RC)
MRI	magnetic resonance imaging
MRPS16	mitochondrial ribosomal protein subunit 16
MRS	magnetic resonance spectroscopy
MSA	mitochondrial myopathy and sideroblastic anemia (also MLASA)
MSL	multiple symmetric lipomas
mtDNA	mitochondrial DNA
mtTFA	mitochondrial transcription factor A (also TFAM)
MTP	mitochondrial trifunctional protein
MTS	Mohr-Tranebjaerg syndrome
MTS	mitochondrial targeting signal
MyHC	myosin heavy chain
NAA	N-acetyl aspartate
NAD	nicotinamide adenine dinucleotide
NADH	reduced nicotinamide adenine dinucleotide
NADP	nicotinamide adenine dinucleotide phosphate
NADPH	reduced nicotinamide adenine dinucleotide phosphate
NARP	neuropathy, ataxia, retinitis pigmentosa
ND	NADH dehydrogenase (complex I)
nDNA	nuclear DNA
NDUF	NADH dehydrogenase-ubiquinone oxidoreductase (complex I)
NFL	nerve fiber layer
NIDDM	non insulin-dependent diabetes mellitus
NMDA	N-methyl-D-aspartate
NNH	Navajo neurohepatopathy
NO	nitric oxide
NOS	nitric oxide synthase
NRF1	nuclear respiratory factor 1
NRF2	nuclear respiratory factor 2
NRTI	nucleoside reverse transcriptase inhibitor
OCT	optical coherence tomography
OCT	3-oxoacid-CoA transferase
OCTN2	organic cation transporter gene for L-carnitine
O_H	origin of heavy strand replication of mtDNA
O_L	origin of light strand replication of mtDNA
OPA1	dynamin-related GTPase mutated in autosomal dominant optic atrophy
OXPHOS	oxidative phosphorylation
PAM	presequence translocase-associated motor
PARK6	gene encoding the parkin protein
PBL	peripheral blood leucocytes
PCr	creatine phosphate
PCR	polymerase chain reaction
PD	Parkinson's disease
PDGFβ	platelet-derived growth factor β
PDHC	pyruvate dehydrogenase complex
PDHI-3	HIFα-prolyl hydroxylase (also HPHI-3)

PEO	progressive external ophthalmoplegia
PEO1	gene encoding Twinkle
PEPSI	proton echo-planar spectroscopic imaging
PET	positron emission tomography
PGC1α	peroxisome proliferators-activated receptor γ coactivator 1
PGD	pre-implantation genetic diagnosis
PHA	phytohemoagglutinin
Pi	inorganic phospate
PINK1	PTEN-induced putative kinase 1
PKC	protein kinase C
PMB	papillo-macular bundle
PME	progressive myoclonic epilepsy
PN	peripheral neuropathy
POLG	polymerase γ
PPK	palmoplantar keratoderma
PS	Pearson syndrome
PS1	presenilin 1
PS2	presenilin 2
PTH	parathyroid hormone
PTP	permeability transition pore (also MPTP and PTPC)
PTPC	permeability transition pore complex (also PTP)
PUS1	pseudouridylation synthase
RAAS	renin-angiotensin aldosterone system
RARS	refractory anemia with ringed sideroblasts
RC	respiratory chain (also MRC)
rCBF	regional cerebral blood flow
RCMD-RS	refractory cytopenia with multilineage dysplasia and ringed sideroblasts
RFLP	restriction fragment length polymorphism
RGC	retinal ganglion cell
RNA	ribonucleic acid
RNAi	RNA interference
ROS	reactive oxygen species
RPE	retinal pigmented epithelium
RRF	ragged-red fibers
rRNA	ribosomal RNA
RTA	retinal thickness analyzer
RTPCR	reverse transcription PCR
SAM	sorting and assembly machinery
SANDO	sensory ataxic neuropathy, dysarthria and ophthalmoplegia
SCAD	short-chain acyl-CoA dehydrogenase
SCO	synthesis of cytochrome *c* oxidase
SDH	succinate dehydrogenase
SHOX	short stature homeobox protein
SIDS	sudden infant death syndrome
SMA	spinal muscular atrophy
SMN1	survival motor neuron gene (mutated in SMA)
SNAP	sensory nerve action potential
SNpc	substantia nigra pars compacta
SNHL	sensorineural hearing loss
SOD	superoxide dismutase
SOD1	Cu/Zn-superoxide dismutase
SOD2	Mn-superoxide dismutase
SPECT	single photon emission computed tomography
SPG7	spastic paraplegia 7 gene
SSVs	strongly SDH-reactive blood vessels
SUCLA	succinyl-CoA synthetase ligase
SURF1	surfeit gene 1
TAA	tobacco alcohol amblyopia
TAZ	tafazzin gene (also G4.5)
TFAM	transcription factor A (mitochondrial)
TIM	translocase of the inner membrane
TIMM8A	gene encoding DDP1, deafness-dystonia protein-1
TK2	thymidine kinase 2
TM	tropomyosin
Tn	troponin
TOM	translocase of the outer membrane
TP	thymidine phosphorylase
tRNA	transfer RNA
TSH	thyroid-stimulating hormone

TZDs	thiazolidinediones
Ugo1p	Ugo-related protein
UQ	ubiquinone
VEP	visual evoked potential
VF	ventricular fibrillation
VHL	von Hippel-Lindau tumor suppressor gene
VLCAD	very long-chain acyl-CoA dehydrogenase
VSD	ventricular septal defect
VT	ventricular tachycardia
WD	Wilson's disease
WFS1	gene encoding the protein wolframin. Mutated in Wolfram syndrome
WHO	World Health Organization
WPW	Wolff-Parkinson-White
wt-mtDNA	wild-type mtDNA

Introduction: the birth of mitochondrial medicine

'I was in the position to undertake the first studies of a cell organelle in humans in 1959–62. They were performed following observations made at the bedside of a patient with striking symptoms never encountered before. These clinical observations, first, led to an idea about the origin of the symptoms, and, second, to studies of this particular organelle, the mitochondrion.'[1]

This quote was the introduction to my 1994 review, '*The development of mitochondrial medicine*'. This was the first time the term 'mitochondrial medicine' was used – it is now a household expression in medicine and the title of this book. The studies referred to in this review were published in 1962[2] and mark the birth of mitochondrial medicine, and, in essence the birth of medicine involving subcellular particles.

The subject of these studies was a 30-year-old woman with symptoms since age 7, including: *profuse perspiration* combined with markedly increased fluid intake and normal urine volumes; *extremely high caloric intake* (about 3000 kcal per day) with a stable body weight of 38 kg at a body height of 159 cm. Laboratory studies showed a strikingly increased basal metabolic rate (BMR) of about +200%. Thyroid function measured by numerous tests was normal. Classical myxedema followed subtotal thyroidectomy and the administration of thyroid-depressing drugs, although the BMR was still +100%.

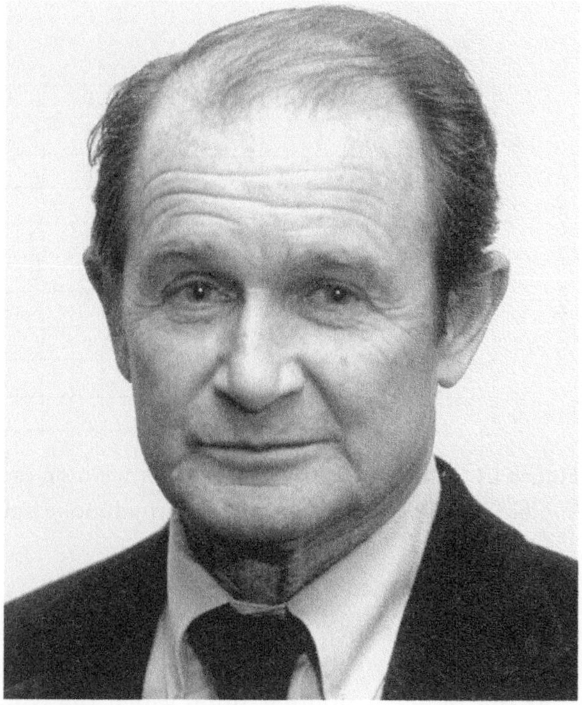

Rolf Luft

From the literature, it was evident that the mitochondrion is the site of cell respiration, that the uptake of oxygen by mitochondria is controlled by the components of ATP production (inorganic phosphate, Pi, and the phosphate acceptor, ADP), and that respiratory control allows the body to adjust oxygen consumption to actual energy need. Theoretically, the patient's

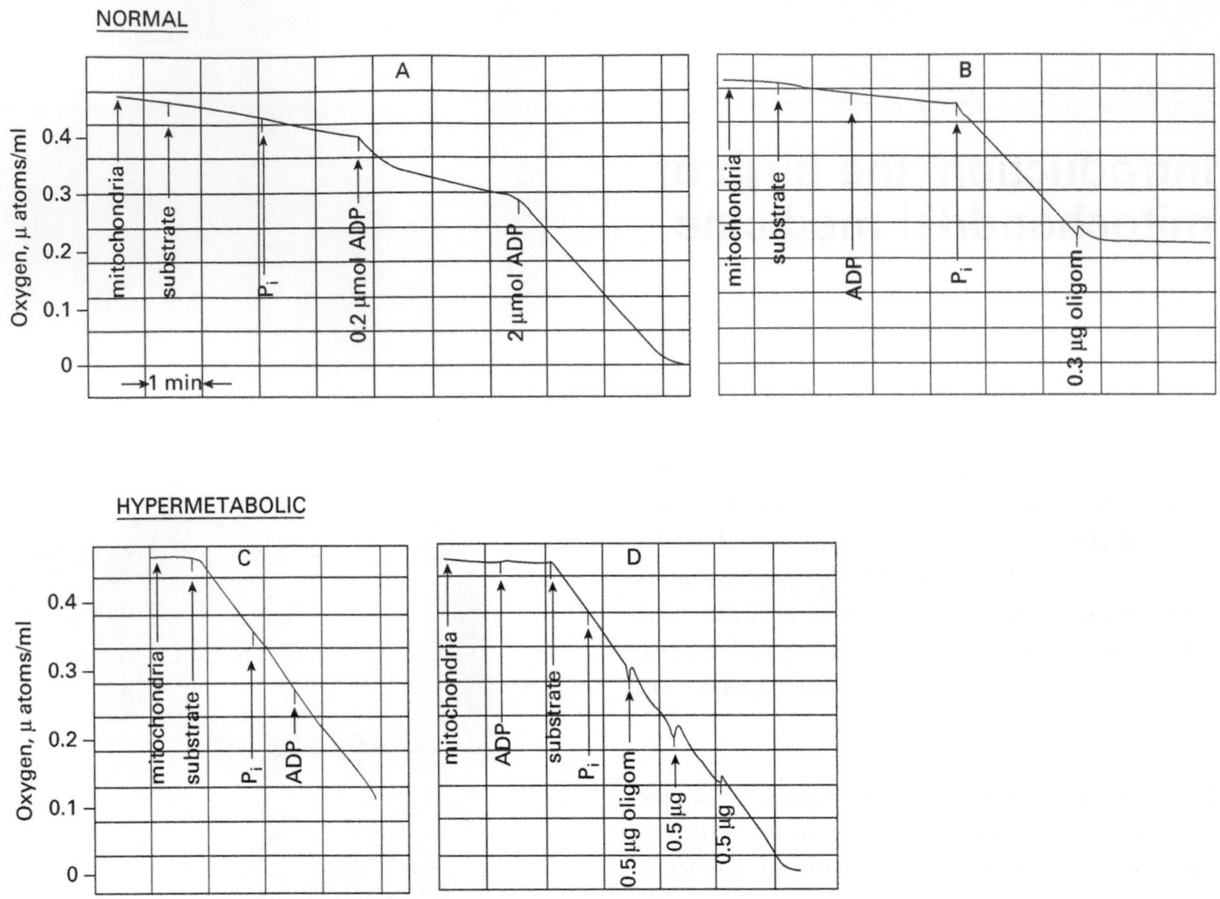

Figure I.1 Effect of Pi, ADP, and oligomycin on respiration of skeletal muscle mitochondria from a normal subject (A and B) and from the hypermetabolic patient (C and D)

condition might then be ascribed to a derangement of respiratory control in the mitochondrion.

At the time, all findings upon which the concept of oxidative phosphorylation was based were derived from studies of rat liver mitochondria. After developing similar techniques for isolated human muscle mitochondria, a series of studies were performed on isolated mitochondria from the patient's gracilis muscles. The main results of these studies are republished here in Figures I.1 and I.2. The data show a nearly maximal rate of respiration in the presence of substrate alone, i.e. without addition of ADP + Pi, but an almost normal phosphorylating efficiency (expressed as P/O ratio) on their addition. The mitochondria also exhibited high ATPase activity, which was only slightly stimulated by 2,4-dinitrophenol, a known uncoupler of respiration from phosphorylation. These were the features of 'loosely coupled' respiration – deficient respiratory control with partially maintained ability to synthesize ATP – and accounted for all her symptoms: the abnormal production of heat, which the body tried to relieve by increased perspiration, and the enormous caloric intake to compensate for the increased combustion. Electron microscopy of muscle revealed striking structural abnormalities with large accumulation of mitochondria of highly variable

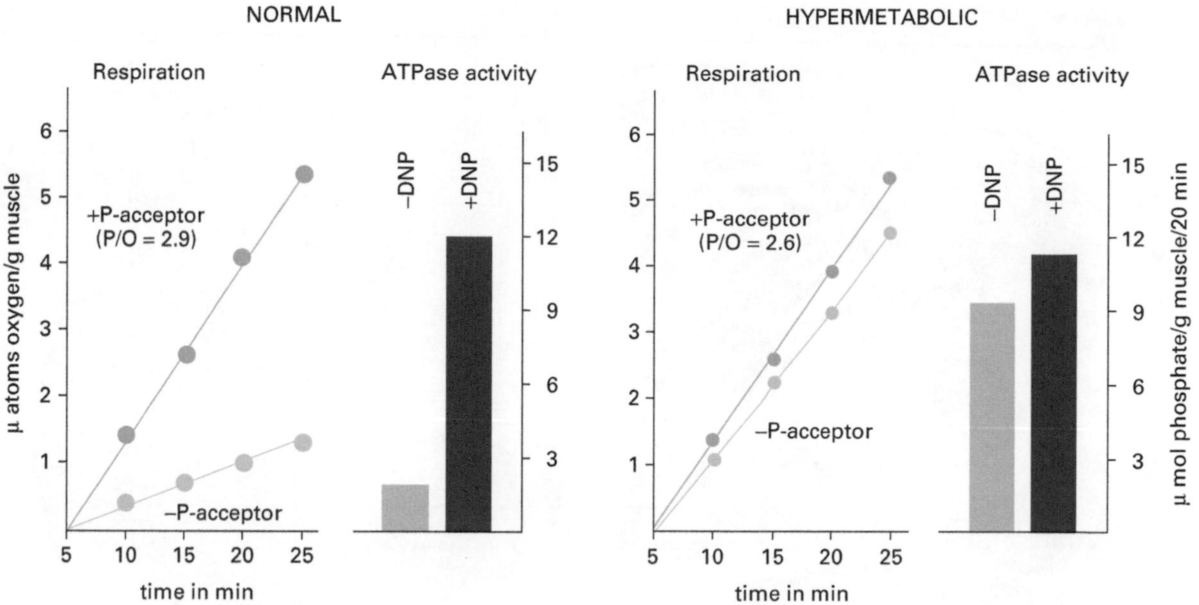

Figure I.2 Respiratory control, phosphorylation efficiency, and ATPase activity of isolated skeletal muscle mitochondria from a normal subject (left) and from the hypermetabolic patient (right). DNP, 2,4-dinitrophenol

size located in the perinuclear zone of the myocytes, and often containing paracrystalline inclusions (Figures I.3 and I.4).

This was the first demonstration of mitochondrial dysfunction in a human patient. This was also the first disease involving a subcellular organelle and demonstrated how studies of patients sometimes have to be extended to the basic sciences. As is well known, a major advance in our understanding of human mitochondria occurred several years later, when Peter Mitchell presented his chemiosmotic hypothesis of oxidative phosphorylation. However, with the identification of the first mitochondrial disease, the field of mitochondrial medicine was born. Over the next few years interesting observations were made. In 1963, Nass and Nass[3] showed in chick embryos the probable presence of DNA in mitochondria (mtDNA), a suggestion later confirmed by Schatz et al.[4] in yeast mitochondria. By 1981, the complete sequence of human mitochondrial DNA (mtDNA) was elucidated by Sanger and coworkers.[5] In 1988, a breakthrough in mitochondrial pathophysiology occurred with the reports by Holt, Harding and Morgan-Hughes[6] of the association of sporadic human mitochondrial myopathies with huge deletions of mtDNA and by Wallace et al.[7] of a point mutation in the mtDNA of patients with Leber's hereditary optic neuropathy. During the following years, hundreds of mtDNA mutations were found in multisystemic or tissue-specific syndromes. In 1995, nuclear mutations affecting respiratory chain complexes were identified,[8] opening a new avenue in mitochondrial medicine. Observations in the 1990s seemed to connect mitochondrial dysfunction with a large number of medical conditions, such as diabetes and its complications; neurodegenerative disorders such as Parkinson's disease; and the aging process per se. In general, these mitochondrial disorders must affect oxidative phosphorylation, its enzyme complexes, and their regulation through mtDNA and nuclear DNA, but the precise mechanisms have proven elusive. A fuller understanding of mitochondrial biology will also need to encompass the unique

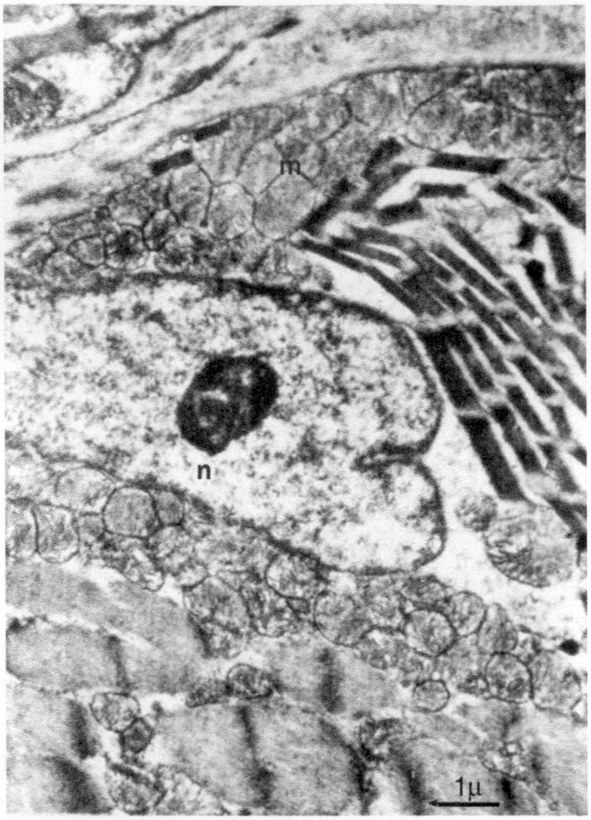

Figure I.3 Electron micrograph from a muscle fiber of the hypermetabolic patient. Cell nucleus (n) and a multitude of mitochondria (m) surrounding it. On the right is a bundle of dense cell inclusions (×4700)

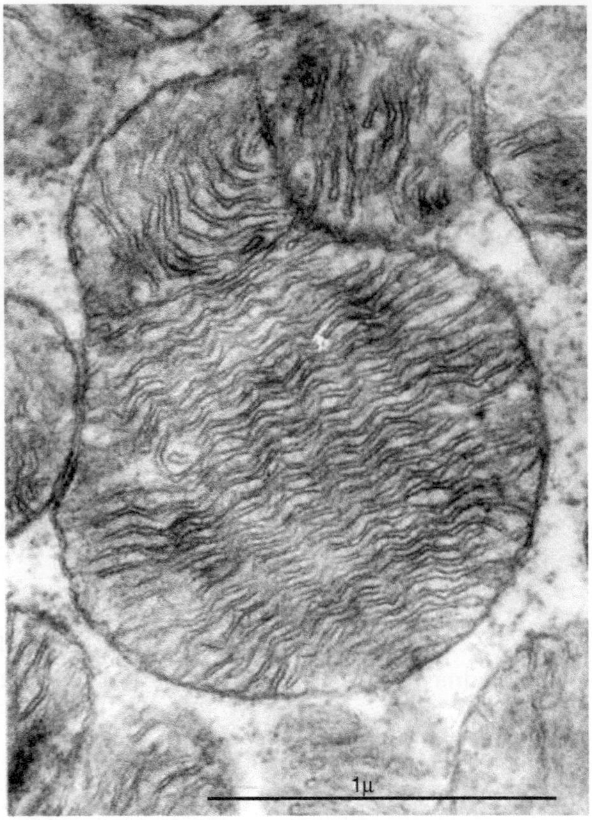

Figure I.4 Electron micrograph of a giant mitochondrion in a muscle fiber of the hypermetabolic patient (×4700)

genetics of mtDNA, including its high mutation rate and the basis for the accumulation of age-related mutations. Presumably because of the relatively poor mtDNA repair mechanisms, mtDNA damage persists in the cell and proliferates, eventually leading to a level of mutant DNA where oxidative phosphorylation declines. Understanding how these mutations lead to a spectrum of clinical findings is another important challenge.

We sought to provide a molecular explanation for the syndrome we studied – called Luft's disease. However, we were limited by the fact that there were no other individuals with this disorder in whom to confirm our hypotheses about the origin of the disease and the basis for the mitochondrial dysfunction. Although I was still interested in pursuing this work further, my coworker, Lars Ernster, a well-known specialist in the biochemistry of mitochondria, was not interested as long as I could not find more patients with this or other disorders of mitochondrial function. Thus, the etiology of this syndrome is still unknown. Many have wondered what happened to the patient. After a year in the hospital, she went home and was not seen by me afterwards. She committed suicide a few years later in a district hospital of her home town, and I was never able to find out if her condition had changed with time. Rumours were that she had increased in body weight. Members of her family refused to participate in further studies to elucidate a possible heretable basis of the disorder or its pathophysiology. Later, a second patient with exactly the same symptoms was reported by Haydar et al.[9] and DiMauro et al.[10] but they too were unable to provide a molecular basis for the findings. Despite the mystery that still surrounds the etiology of Luft's disease, the demonstration of human disease resulting from biochemical and morphological abnormalities of mitochondria opened the field of mitochondrial medicine, which has continued to grow from that time.

This is the story of how basic studies in a single patient provided a stimulus to what is now an active and growing field. It has been a privilege to follow this exciting chapter of medicine, including the discoveries in the basic sciences. I was privileged to witness how advances in many disciplines, including molecular biology and molecular genetics, have been used for the advancement of mitochondrial medicine and how studies in mitochondrial biochemistry and genetics have widened the field. Last, but not least, it is gratifying to know that more and more young scientists put their efforts into extending our knowledge of the role mitochondria play in a wide range of medical conditions.

Rolf Luft
Professor of Endocrinology
Karolinska Hospital
Stockholm, Sweden

References

1. Luft R. The development of mitochondrial medicine. *Proc Natl Acad Sci USA* 1994; **91**: 8731–8738.
2. Luft R, Ikkos D, Palmieri G et al. A case of severe hypermetabolism of nonthyroid origin with a defect in the maintenance of mitochondrial respiratory control: A correlated clinical, biochemical, and morphological study. *J Clin Invest* 1962; **41**: 1776–1804.
3. Nass S, Nass M. Intramitochondrial fibers with DNA characteristics. *J Cell Biol* 1963; **19**: 593–629.
4. Schatz G, Haslbrunner E, Tuppy H. Deoxyribonucleic acid associated with yeast mitochondria. *Biochem Biophys Res Commun* 1964; **15**: 127–132.
5. Anderson S, Bankier AT, Barrel BG et al. Sequence and organization of the human mitochondrial genome. *Nature* 1981; **290**: 457–465.
6. Holt IJ, Harding AE, Morgan Hughes JA. Deletions of muscle mitochondrial DNA in patients with mitochondrial myopathies. *Nature* 1988; **331**: 717–719.
7. Wallace DC, Singh G, Lott MT et al. Mitochondrial DNA mutation associated with Leber's hereditary optic neuropathy. *Science* 1988; **242**: 1427–1430.
8. Bourgeron T, Rustin P, Chretien D et al. Mutation of a nuclear succinate dehydrogenase gene results in mitochondrial respiratory chain deficiency. *Nature Genet* 1995; **11**: 144–149.
9. Haydar NA, Conn HL, Afifi A et al. Severe hypermetabolism with primary abnormality of skeletal muscle mitochondria. *Ann Int Med* 1971; **74**: 548–558.
10. DiMauro S, Bonilla E, Lee CP et al. Luft's disease. Further biochemical and ultrastructural studies of skeletal muscle in the second case. *J Neurol Sci* 1976; **27**: 217–232.

1

The mitochondrial respiratory chain and its disorders

Salvatore DiMauro and Eric A Schon

Introduction

This introductory chapter is meant to give the reader both some basic information about mitochondrial metabolism and a bird's eye view of mitochondrial diseases, in the hope of putting into better perspective the more specialized chapters that follow. Much of the text, some figures, and one table are reproduced from a review article published by us in the *New England Journal of Medicine* three years ago,[1] with kind permission from the publishers. Both text and Figure 1.2 have been updated, as required by the extremely fast pace of progress in this area of medicine.

More than a billion years ago, aerobic bacteria colonized primordial eukaryotic cells that lacked the ability to use oxygen metabolically (see Box 1.1). This symbiotic relationship became permanent, as the bacteria evolved into mitochondria, thus endowing the host cells with aerobic metabolism, a much more efficient way to produce energy than is anaerobic glycolysis. Structurally, mitochondria are composed of four compartments: the outer membrane, the inner membrane, the intermembrane space, and the matrix (the region inside the inner membrane). They perform numerous tasks, such as pyruvate oxidation, the Krebs cycle, and amino acid, fatty acid, and steroid metabolism, but arguably the most crucial is the generation of energy as adenine triphosphate, or ATP, via the electron transport chain/oxidative phosphorylation system (the 'respiratory chain') (Figure 1.1). Emphasis in this chapter and throughout the book will be on the respiratory chain because – by a widely accepted convention – the term 'mitochondrial diseases' is used restrictively to define disorders affecting this terminal pathway (the 'business end' of mitochondrial metabolism, where energy is generated).

The respiratory chain

The respiratory chain is located in the inner mitochondrial membrane, and consists of five multimeric protein complexes (Figure 1.2): NADH dehydrogenase-ubiquinone oxidoreductase (complex I; approximately 46 subunits); succinate dehydrogenase-ubiquinone oxidoreductase (complex II; 4 subunits); ubiquinone-cytochrome *c* oxidoreductase (complex III; 11 subunits); cytochrome *c* oxidase (complex IV; 13 subunits); and ATP synthase (complex V; approximately 16 subunits). The respiratory chain also requires two small electron carriers, ubiquinone (coenzyme Q10) and cytochrome *c*.

ATP synthesis involves two coordinated processes (Figure 1.2). First, electrons (actually hydrogen ions derived from NADH and $FADH_2$ in intermediary metabolism) are transported 'horizontally' from complexes I and II to coenzyme Q

Box 1.1 What is the endosymbiotic hypothesis?

The *endosymbiotic hypothesis* proposes that eukaryotes contain organelles – specifically, mitochondria and chloroplasts – that were derived from prokaryotic organisms that 'invaded' the proto-eukaryotic cell early in evolution.[1] The earliest champion of endosymbiosis was Constantin Mereschkowsky, who proposed, in 1905, that some cells were actually the product of the fusion of two different types of cells,[2] but it was Ivan Wallin, in 1927, who first proposed the idea that mitochondria are descended from endosymbiotic bacteria.[3] These and other early pioneers of the endosymbiotic theory were essentially forgotten until 1967, when Lynn Sagan (nee Margulis) revived and popularized it.[4]

In a nutshell, endosymbiosis arose when the early atmosphere of the Earth began to change from an environment high in hydrogen, ammonia, methane, and carbon dioxide to one rich in oxygen and nitrogen. Both (geo)chemical and biological processes were responsible for this change. The increase in oxygen – a toxic compound to most organisms – began about 2 billion years ago, more than a billion years after life arose.[5] However, the evolution of the electron transport (i.e. respiratory) chain, in which oxygen was the terminal electron acceptor and which was reduced by hydrogen to produce non-toxic H_2O, allowed bacteria not only to live in an oxygen-laden environment, but to positively thrive in it. This is because the protons that were pumped across the bacterial membrane by the respiratory chain (a process coupled to electron transfer) were used to produce ATP-based energy under aerobic conditions far more efficiently than could be produced under anaerobic conditions (e.g. glycolysis). It was therefore proposed that a prokaryote with the capacity for oxidative energy metabolism 'invaded' an aerobic proto-eukaryote dependent on glycolysis, ultimately to give rise to the modern eukaryote containing mitochondria and/or chloroplasts.

However, this scenario has a number of problems, not the least of which is the 'chicken-and-egg' problem of reconciling oxygen's toxicity with its requirement to drive electron transport and hence ATP synthesis. Also, bacteria don't export ATP, so how could the proto-eukaryotic host take advantage of the engulfed bacterium? Thus, there has been much debate regarding the exact nature and order of the endosymbiotic events, and the question as to which prokaryote was the primordial endosymbiont has generated even more controversy. A leading school of thought now proposes that mitochondria are derived from hydrogenosomes, organelles that synthesize ATP anaerobically in amitochondriate protists, producing H_2 (and CO_2) as a byproduct.[6] This anaerobic symbiont (a bacterium producing H_2 and CO_2) merged with its host (a bacterium generating methane from H_2 and CO_2), allowing the host to survive even when hydrogen was missing. The transfer of symbiont genes to the host nucleus[7] eventually allowed the host to respond to changing nutritional and environmental conditions (including a cytosolically localized glycolytic pathway). One of these adaptations eventually resulted in the aerobic mitochondria we see today.[1] Support for the hydrogenosome hypothesis came recently from the discovery that *Nyctotherus ovalis*, an anaerobic ciliate that thrives in the hindgut of cockroaches, has an *anaerobic* mitochondrion that produces hydrogen.[8]

References

1. Martin W, Hoffmeister M, Rotte C, Henze K. An overview of endosymbiotic models for the origins of eukaryotes, their ATP-producing organelles (mitochondria and hydrogenosomes), and their heterotrophic lifestyle. *Biol Chem* 2001; **382**: 1521–1539.
2. Mereschkowsky C. Uber natur und urschprung der chromatophoren in pflanzreiche. *Biol Centralbl* 1905; **25**: 593–604.
3. Wallin IE. *Symbionticism and the Origin of Species*. London: Ballière Tindall Cox; 1927.
4. Sagan L. On the origin of mitosing cells. *J Theor Biol* 1967; **14**: 255–274.
5. Kasting JF. Earth's early atmosphere. *Science* 1993; **259**: 920–926.
6. Martin W, Muller M. The hydrogen hypothesis for the first eukaryote. *Nature* 1998; **392**: 37–41.
7. Timmis JN, Ayliffe MA, Huang CY, Martin W. Endosymbiotic gene transfer: organelle genomes forge eukaryotic chromosomes. *Nat Rev Genet* 2004; **5**: 123–135.
8. Gray MW. The hydrogenosome's murky past. *Nature* 2005; **434**: 29–31.

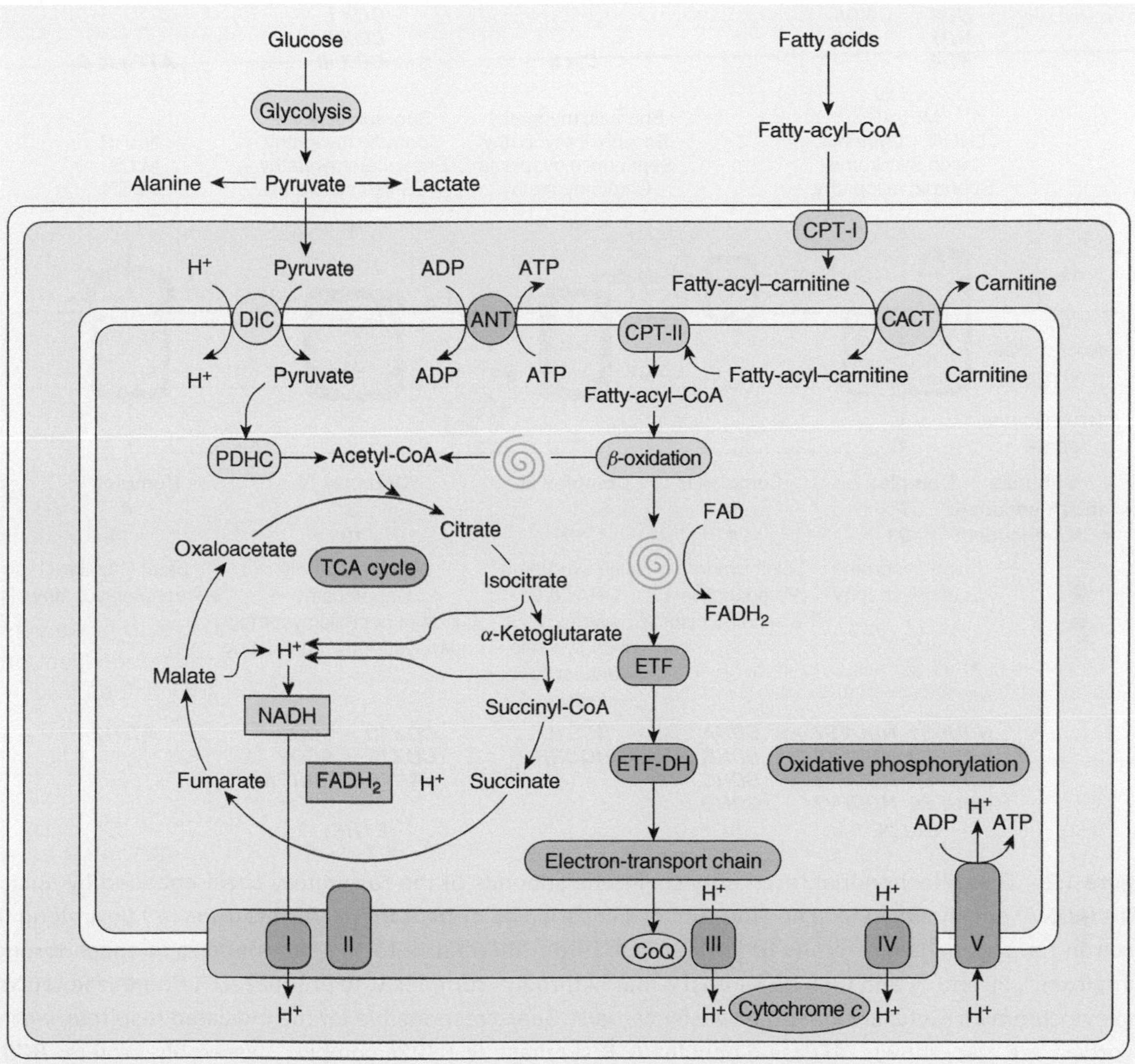

Figure 1.1 Selected metabolic pathways in mitochondria. The spirals represent the spiral of reactions of the β-oxidation pathway, resulting in the liberation of acetyl-coenzyme A (CoA) and the reduction of flavoprotein. ADP denotes adenosine diphosphate, ATP adenosine triphosphate, ANT adenine nucleotide translocator, CACT carnitine–acylcarnitine translocase, CoQ coenzyme Q, CPT carnitine palmitoyltransferase, DIC dicarboxylate carrier, ETF electron-transfer flavoprotein, ETFDH electron-transfer dehydrogenase, FAD flavin adenine dinucleotide, $FADH_2$ reduced FAD, NADH reduced nicotinamide adenine dinucleotide, PDHC pyruvate dehydrogenase complex, TCA tricarboxylic acid, I complex I, II complex II, III complex III, IV complex IV, and V complex V

to complex III to cytochrome *c* to complex IV, and ultimately to the final electron acceptor, molecular oxygen, thereby producing water. At the same time, protons are pumped 'vertically' across the mitochondrial inner membrane (i.e. from the matrix to the intermembrane space) by complexes I, III, and IV. ATP is generated by the influx of these protons back into the mitochondrial matrix through complex V (ATP synthase), the world's tiniest rotary motor.[2,3]

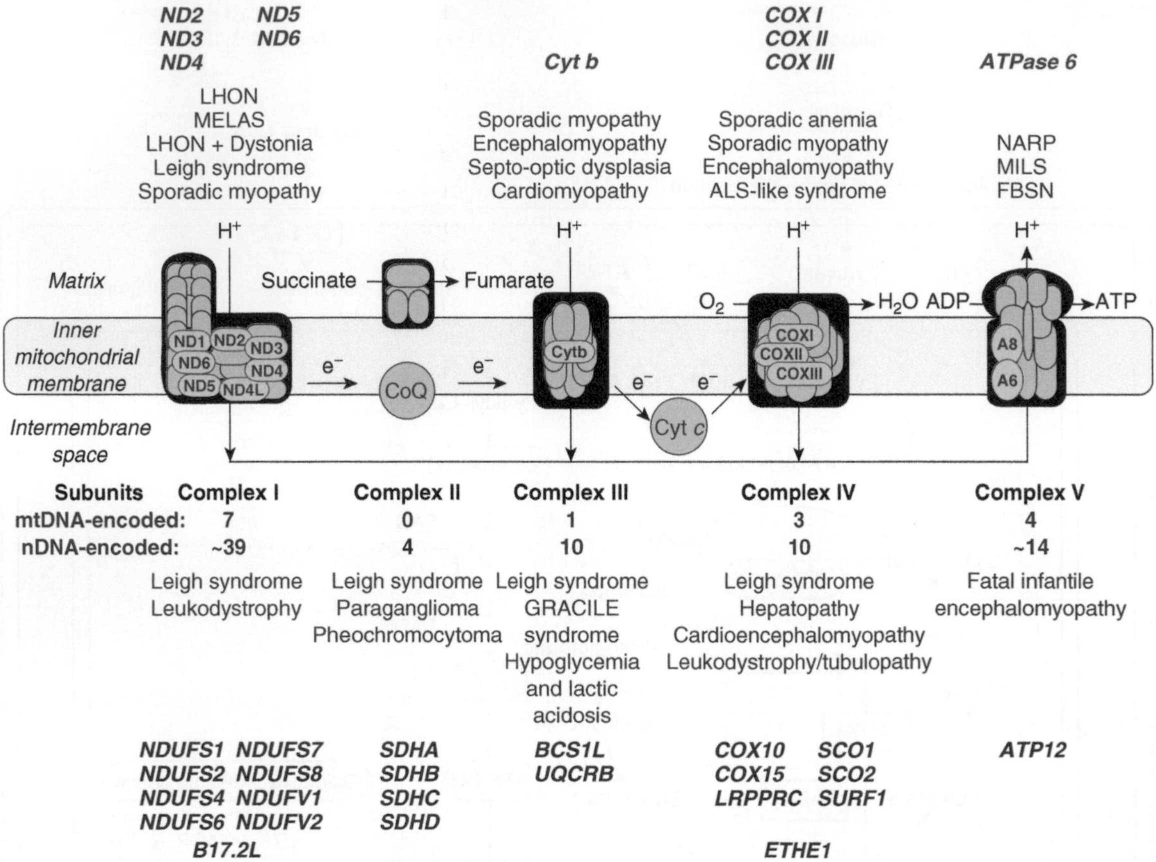

Figure 1.2 The mitochondrial respiratory chain. The subunits of the respiratory chain encoded by nuclear DNA (nDNA) are shown in blue and the subunits encoded by mtDNA in red. As electrons (e^-) flow along the electron transport chain, protons (H^+) are pumped from the matrix to the intermembrane space through complexes I, III, and IV and then back into the matrix through complex V, to produce ATP. Coenzyme Q (CoQ) and cytochrome *c* (Cyt*c*) are electron-transfer carriers. Genes responsible for the indicated respiratory-chain disorders are also shown. *ATPase 6* denotes ATP synthase 6; *B17.2L* complex I assembly protein; *BCS1L* cytochrome *b–c* complex assembly protein (complex III); *ETHE1* ethylmalonic encephalopathy protein; *NDUF* NADH dehydrogenase–ubiquinone oxidoreductase; *SCO* synthesis of cytochrome oxidase; *SDHA, SDHB, SDHC,* and *SDHD* succinate dehydrogenase subunits; *SURF1* surfeit gene 1; FBSN familial bilateral striatal necrosis; LHON Leber's hereditary optic neuropathy; *LRPPRC* leucine-rich pentatricopeptide repeat-containing protein; MELAS mitochondrial encephalomyopathy, lactic acidosis, and strokelike episodes; MILS maternally inherited Leigh's syndrome; NARP neuropathy, ataxia, and retinitis pigmentosa; GRACILE growth retardation, aminoaciduria, lactic acidosis, and early death; and ALS amyotrophic lateral sclerosis

Because of their bacterial origin, mitochondria are the only organelles of the cell, besides the nucleus, to contain their own DNA (called mtDNA), and their own machinery for synthesizing RNA and proteins. Each mitochondrion, of which there are hundreds or thousands per cell, contains approximately five mitochondrial genomes. Although crucially important, mtDNA has only 37 genes.

Thus, most gene products present in the organelle (~1200 in number) are nucleus-encoded and are imported from the cytoplasm.

Because many respiratory chain disorders involve brain and skeletal muscle, they are also known as 'mitochondrial encephalomyopathies.' The fact that the respiratory chain is under dual genetic control makes this group of disorders particularly fascinating, because they involve both mendelian and mitochondrial genetics. Moreover, contrary to common belief, these diseases are not all that rare. In fact, with an estimated prevalence of 1 in 5000, they are amongst the most common inborn errors of metabolism.[4]

The genetic classification of the primary mitochondrial diseases distinguishes disorders due to defects in mtDNA, which are inherited according to the rules of mitochondrial genetics, and those due to defects in nDNA, which are transmitted by mendelian inheritance. Since the discovery of the first pathogenic mutations in human mitochondrial DNA (mtDNA) in 1988,[5,6] the role of mitochondria in human disease has exceeded all expectations.

Mitochondrial genetics

Human mtDNA, a wonderful example of genetic economy, is a 16 569-bp (base pair) double-stranded circular molecule containing 37 genes (Figure 1.3). Of these, 24 are needed for mtDNA translation (two ribosomal RNAs (rRNAs) and 22 transfer RNAs (tRNAs)), and 13 encode subunits of the respiratory chain: seven subunits of complex I (ND1, 2, 3, 4, 4L, 5, and 6 (ND stands for NADH dehydrogenase)), one subunit of complex III (cytochrome *b*, or cyt *b*), three subunits of cytochome *c* oxidase (COX I, II, and III), and two subunits of ATP synthase (A6 and A8). Mitochondrial genetics differs from mendelian genetics in three major aspects:

- *Maternal inheritance*. As a general rule, all mitochondria (and all mtDNAs) in the zygote derive from the ovum. Therefore, a mother carrying an mtDNA mutation passes it on to all her children, but only her daughters will transmit it to their progeny. Recent evidence of paternal transmission of mtDNA in skeletal muscle (but not in other tissues) in a patient with a mitochondrial myopathy[7] seems to be the proverbial exception that confirms the rule.[8–10]
- *Heteroplasmy/threshold effect*. In contrast to nuclear genes, each usually expressed from one maternal and one paternal allele, there are thousands of mtDNA molecules in each cell. As a rule, pathogenic mutations of mtDNA are present in some but not all genomes, such that cells and tissues will harbor two populations of mtDNA, normal (wild-type) and mutant, a situation known as *heteroplasmy*. Heteroplasmy can also exist at the organellar level, such that a single mitochondrion can harbor both normal and mutated mtDNAs. In normal subjects, all mtDNAs are identical, a situation called *homoplasmy*. Not surprisingly, a minimum critical number of mutant mtDNAs must be present before oxidative dysfunction occurs and clinical signs become apparent: this is the *threshold effect*. Also not surprisingly, the pathogenic threshold will be lower in tissues that are highly dependent on oxidative metabolism, such as brain, heart, skeletal muscle, retina, renal tubules, and endocrine tissue, which will, therefore, be especially vulnerable to the effects of pathogenic mtDNA mutations.
- *Mitotic segregation*. Because the redistribution of organelles at the time of cell division is a stochastic process, the proportion of mutant mtDNAs in daughter cells can shift; if and when the pathogenic threshold in a previously unaffected tissue is surpassed, the phenotype can also change. This explains the age-related, and even tissue-related, variability of clinical features frequently observed in mtDNA-related disorders.

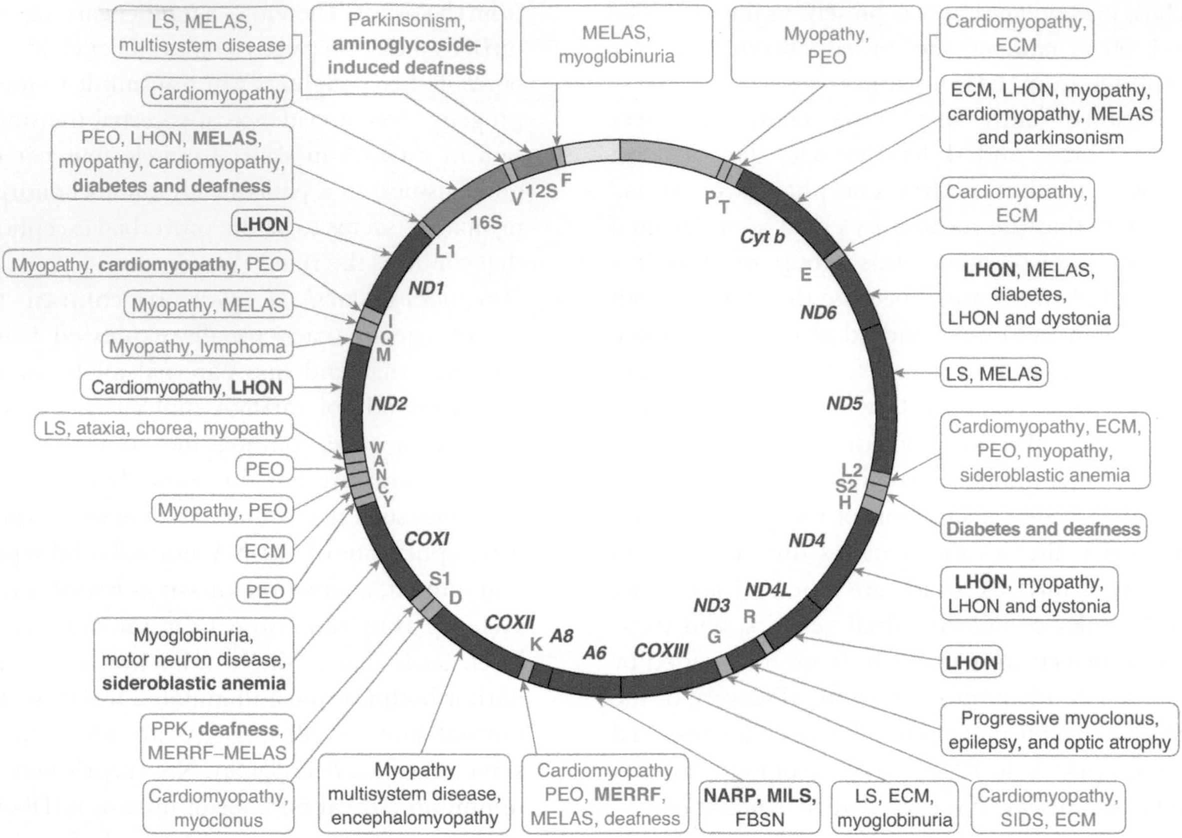

Figure 1.3 Mutations in the human mitochondrial genome that are known to cause disease. The map of the 16,569 bp mtDNA shows differently colored areas representing the protein-coding genes for the seven subunits of complex I (ND), the three subunits of cytochrome c oxidase (CO), cytochrome *b* (cyt b), and the two subunits of ATP synthase (A6 and A8), the 12S and 16S rRNAs (12S, 16S), and the 22 tRNAs identified by one-letter codes for the corresponding amino acids. Disorders that are frequently or prominently associated with mutations in a particular gene are shown in bold. Diseases due to mutations that impair mitochondrial protein synthesis are shown in blue. Diseases due to mutations in protein-coding genes are shown in red. ECM denotes encephalomyopathy; FBSN familial bilateral striatal necrosis; LHON Leber's hereditary optic neuropathy; LS Leigh's syndrome; MELAS mitochondrial encephalomyopathy, lactic acidosis, and strokelike episodes; MERRF myoclonic epilepsy with ragged-red fibers; MILS maternally inherited Leigh's syndrome; NARP neuropathy, ataxia, and retinitis pigmentosa; PEO progressive external ophthalmoplegia; PPK palmoplantar keratoderma; and SIDS sudden infant death syndrome

Disorders due to defects in mtDNA

The small mitochondrial genome has turned out to be a veritable Pandora's box of pathogenic mutations that are associated with a wide variety of clinical syndromes, as illustrated by the 'morbidity map' of mtDNA (Figure 1.3). The circle is peppered with mutations, although a few hotspots stand out, such as the $tRNA^{Leu(UUR)}$, $tRNA^{Lys}$, and cyt *b* genes. In contrast, relatively few mutations have been described in the rRNA genes, and these are found in the 12S rRNA. Not illustrated in the morbidity map are the hundreds of different large-scale deletions associated with disease, each removing anywhere from 2 to 10 kilobases (kb), and invariably deleting tRNA genes.

Although clinically distinct, most (but by no means all) mtDNA-related diseases share a number of features, including lactic acidosis and massive mitochondrial proliferation in muscle (resulting in ragged-red fibers, or RRF). In muscle biopsies, the mutated mtDNAs accumulate preferentially in RRF, and RRF are typically negative for COX activity (see Chapter 3).

There are two major types of mtDNA mutations: those that affect mitochondrial protein synthesis as a whole (mutations in tRNA or rRNA genes, or giant deletions) and those that affect specific proteins of the respiratory chain. Although one might have expected a straightforward relationship between the site of the mutation and the clinical phenotype, no such obvious genotype–phenotype correlation exists, even within a single gene. For example, mutations in the $tRNA^{Leu(UUR)}$ gene are associated most frequently with mitochondrial encephalomyopathy, lactic acidosis, and stroke-like episodes (MELAS) syndrome, but cause other syndromes as well. Conversely, mutations in different genes can cause the same syndrome; MELAS, again, is a prime example (Figure 1.3). There are exceptions, of course: save one case,[11] all patients with the myoclonus epilepsy with RRF (MERRF) syndrome have mutations in the $tRNA^{Lys}$ gene;[12] all patients with Leber hereditary optic neuropathy (LHON) have mutations in ND genes;[13] and most mutations in the cyt *b* gene cause exercise intolerance.[14]

Because mitochondria and mtDNAs are ubiquitous, every tissue in the body can be affected by mtDNA mutations, which is why mitochondrial diseases are often multisystemic, as illustrated in Table 1.1. Included in the table are the most common mtDNA-related syndromes, known by acronyms: Kearns–Sayre syndrome (KSS), progressive external ophthalmoplegia (PEO), Pearson syndrome (PS), MERRF, MELAS, neuropathy, ataxia, retinitis pigmentosa (NARP), maternally inherited Leigh syndrome (MILS), and LHON. Certain constellations of symptoms and signs (Table 1.1) are characteristic of these syndromes, and the diagnosis in typical patients is relatively easy. On the other hand, due to heteroplasmy and the threshold effect, different tissues harboring the same mtDNA mutation may be affected to different degrees, thus explaining the frequent occurrence of oligosymptomatic or asymptomatic individuals within a single family. Selective involvement of specific organs can also occur, presumably due to skewed heteroplasmy (i.e. disproportionately high levels of the mutation in a given tissue). Thus, we have come to recognize mitochondrial diabetes, mitochondrial cardiomyopathies, mitochondrial myopathies, and mitochondrial deafness. These and other mitochondrial disorders belonging to different medical specialties are discussed in the chapters that follow.

While most mtDNA-related diseases are maternally inherited, there are exceptions. Most notably, the generation of giant deletions (Δ-mtDNAs) is almost always a sporadic event, likely occurring in oogenesis or early embryogenesis. Oocytes from normal women contain about 150000 mtDNA molecules, of which some may harbor deletions.[15] A 'bottleneck' exists between ovum and embryo, such that only a minority of maternal mtDNAs repopulates the fetus (see Chapter 11). Thus, on rare occasions one such partially deleted mtDNA (or, depending upon when in oogenesis the deletion occurred, its replicated progeny) may slip through. The few mutated mtDNAs present in the blastocyst can then enter all three germ layers and result in KSS (a multisystem disorder), segregate to the hematopoietic lineage and cause PS, or segregate to muscle and cause PEO (Table 1.1). In all three cases, the deletion is 'single,' i.e. all mutated mtDNAs in the patient are identical, because they are a clonal expansion of the original deleted molecule. Mutations in protein-coding genes often also occur spontaneously in myogenic stem cells, presumably after germ-layer differentiation, and result in isolated

Box 1.2 ATP and glycolysis

Adenosine triphosphate, or ATP (Figure B1.2.1), is the common bioenergetic currency of the cell. The so-called 'high-energy' bond between the second (β) and the third (γ) phosphate groups of ATP is a source of energy for a vast number of biochemical reactions in the cell, in a reaction in which ATP is converted to ADP (adenosine diphosphate) + free phosphate (Pi) + energy (ATP + H_2O = ADP + Pi + Δ).

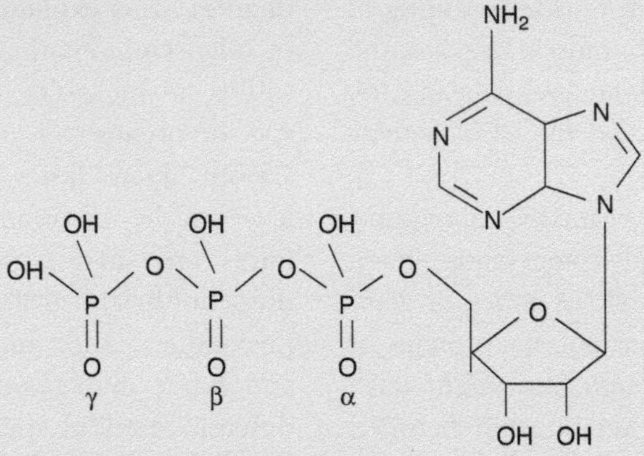

Figure B1.2.1 The structure of ATP. The three phosphate groups are denoted as α, β, and γ

ATP must be synthesized continuously, and in massive amounts, for the cell and the organism to survive. It is generated from ADP and free phosphate, or Pi, in one of three ways: (1) as a reaction by-product from various cellular processes; (2) from ATP-forming reactions in glycolysis in the cytosol; and (3) from ATP synthesis in oxidative phosphorylation in the mitochondria. ATP is produced 'de novo' from the food we eat via the latter two processes. We will focus here on glycolysis.

Glycolysis (Figure B1.2.2) is an anaerobic process that converts glucose into lactic acid, with the concomitant production of ATP; almost a dozen enzymes are involved. Glycolysis proceeds in two stages. In the first, *'ATP-priming,'* stage, glucose, a six-carbon sugar is converted into two molecules of glyceraldehyde-3-phosphate, a three-carbon molecule. Importantly, two molecules of ATP are *consumed* in this stage, not produced. In the second stage, the two molecules of glyceraldehyde-3-phosphate are converted to two molecules of lactic acid (another three-carbon molecule), with the production of four molecules of ATP, for a net synthesis of two ATPs per molecule of glucose consumed (i.e. 4 – 2 = 2). Because glycolytic ATP is generated from ADP as part of specific reactions in the pathway, the reaction to form ATP is called *substrate level phosphorylation.*

The generation of lactic acid from pyruvic acid is highly favored under anaerobic conditions, which is why lactate increases in our muscles when we exercise so strongly that we create an 'oxygen debt.'

Under aerobic conditions, however, glycolysis still operates (although no oxygen is required for any of the glycolytic reactions), but rather than producing lactate, the penultimate reaction product – pyruvic acid – is transported into the mitochondria to be oxidized further in the tricarboxylic acid cycle (Box 1.3).

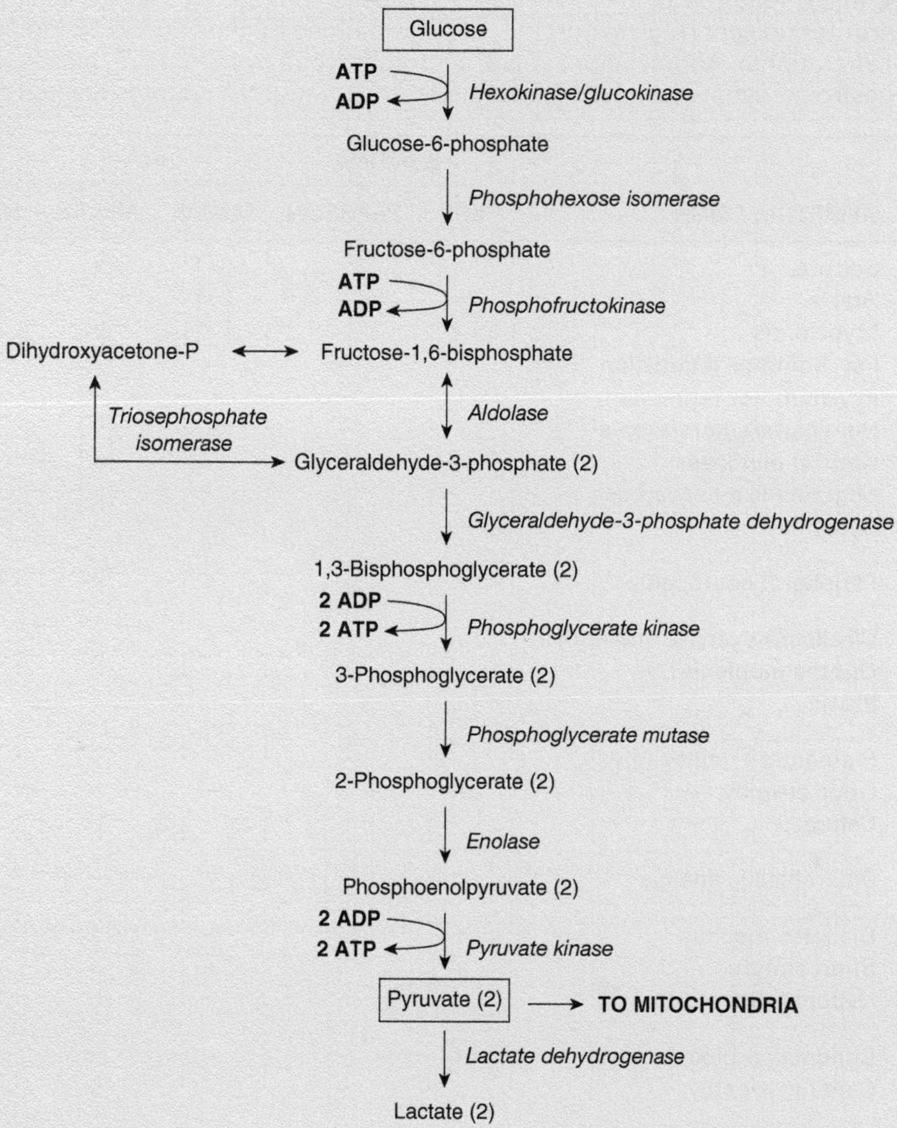

Figure B1.2.2 Glycolysis

myopathies.[14] Interestingly, 13 of the 18 known mutations in the cyt *b* gene fall into this category.

The pathogenesis of these disorders is still unclear, although it is generally accepted that impaired ATP production plays a central role. This concept has been borne out by numerous studies using cytoplasmic hybrid ('cybrid') cell cultures, that is, established human cell lines that are first depleted of their own mtDNA and then repopulated with patient mitochondria containing mutated genomes (see Box 5.1).[16]

The extraordinary variability of clinical presentations can largely be attributed to the peculiar rules of mitochondrial genetics, especially heteroplasmy and the threshold effect. For example, different mutational loads readily explain the different

Table 1.1 Clinical features of mtDNA-related diseases. Boxes highlight typical features of specific syndromes (except Leigh syndrome, which is defined by the neuroradiological or neuropathological alterations). Abbreviations: CNS, central nervous system; PNS, peripheral nervous system; GI, gastrointestinal system; ENT, ear-nose-throat. Δ-mtDNA denotes deleted mtDNA.

		Δ-mtDNA		tRNA		ATPase	
TISSUE	**SYMPTOM / SIGN**	**KSS**	**PEARSON**	**MERRF**	**MELAS**	**NARP**	**MILS**
CNS	Seizures	–	–	[+]	+	–	+
	Ataxia	+	–	[+]	+	[+]	±
	Myoclonus	–	–	[+]	±	–	–
	Psychomotor retardation	–	–	–	–	–	+
	Psychomotor regression	+	–	±	+	–	–
	Hemiparesis/hemianopia	–	–	–	[+]	–	–
	Cortical blindness	–	–	–	[+]	–	–
	Migraine-like headaches	–	–	–	[+]	–	–
	Dystonia	–	–	–	+	–	+
PNS	Peripheral neuropathy	±	–	±	±	[+]	–
Muscle	Weakness/exercise intolerance	+	–	+	+	+	+
	Ophthalmoplegia	+	±	–	–	–	–
	Ptosis	[+]	–	–	–	–	–
Eye	Pigmentary retinopathy	[+]	–	–	–	+	±
	Optic atrophy	–	–	–	–	±	±
	Cataracts	–	–	–	–	–	–
Blood	Sideroblastic anemia	±	[+]	–	–	–	–
Endocrine	Diabetes mellitus	±	–	–	±	–	–
	Short stature	+	–	+	+	–	–
	Hypoparathyroidism	±	–	–	–	–	–
Heart	Conduction block	[+]	–	–	±	–	–
	Cardiomyopathy	±	–	–	±	–	±
GI	Exocrine pancreatic dysfunction	±	[+]	–	–	–	–
	Intestinal pseudo-obstruction	–	–	–	–	–	–
ENT	Sensorineural hearing loss	–	–	+	+	±	–
Kidney	Fanconi syndrome	±	±	–	±	–	–
Laboratory	Lactic acidosis	+	+	+	+	–	±
	Muscle biopsy: RRF	+	±	+	+	–	–
Inheritance	Maternal	–	–	+	+	+	+
	Sporadic	+	+	–	–	–	–

severities of NARP and MILS, two encephalomyopathies caused by the same genetic defect in the *ATPase 6* gene.[17] What is difficult to explain is the distinct 'tissue proclivity' shown by seemingly similar mutations, especially in the brain: for example, the stroke-like episodes in MELAS, the myoclonus in MERRF, and the pigmentary retinopathy in KSS. Conversely, many patients with mitochondrial diabetes evince symptoms even though they harbor relatively low proportions of mutated mtDNA in blood, implying that the pathogenetic mechanism goes beyond mere energy deficit (see Chapter 8). Even more puzzling, mutations that are present ubiquitously in patients often have tissue-specific effects (e.g. deafness due to mutations in 12S rRNA, cardiopathy due to mutations in $tRNA^{Ile}$, and optic atrophy due to mutations in ND genes). The generation of animal models harboring mtDNA mutations ('mito-mice')[18,19] may provide some answers to these pathogenic riddle (see Box 14.1).

Respiratory chain disorders due to defects in nuclear DNA

In recent years, interest has shifted towards mendelian genetics in mitochondrial disease. This shift is understandable, not only because most of the 75-plus respiratory chain proteins are encoded by nDNA (Figure 1.3), but also because proper assembly and function of respiratory chain complexes requires approximately 60 additional ('ancillary') nucleus-encoded proteins, mutations of which can cause mitochondrial disease,[20] in a sort of 'murder by proxy.'

Mutations in structural components of the respiratory chain

These have been found thus far only for complexes I[21,22] and II,[23–26] and have been generally associated with severe neurological disorders of childhood, such as Leigh syndrome (LS) or leukodystrophy.[20] Interestingly, however, mutations in complex II have also been associated with tumors, namely paragangliomas and pheochromocytomas (see Chapter 10). Although its genetic basis remains unknown and is likely to be heterogeneous, coenzyme Q10 (CoQ10) deficiency is also emerging as an important cause of autosomal recessive mitochondrial diseases, ranging from severe infantile encephalomyopathy,[27–29] to predominantly myopathic forms (with or without recurrent myoglobinuria),[30–33] to predominantly encephalopathic presentations (with ataxia and cerebellar atrophy).[34–37]

Mutations in 'ancillary' proteins of the respiratory chain

No pathogenic mutations have been identified in any nDNA-encoded subunits of complexes III, IV, or V, but defects in all but complex II[38–45] have been related to mutations in ancillary proteins required for assembly or insertion of cofactors. Interestingly, although COX deficiency is generalized in disorders due to mutations in genes for assembly proteins, both the enzyme defect and the symptomatology are more severe in certain tissues: thus, mutations in *SURF1* affect predominantly the brain and cause Leigh syndrome;[46–48] mutations in *SCO2*[49] or *COX15*[50] cause infantile cardiomyopathy in addition to brain disease, and mutations in *COX10*,[51,52] *SCO1*[53] and *LRPPRC*[54] affect liver and kidney preferentially. While pathogenic mutations may still be discovered in structural subunits of complexes III–V, it is also possible that they may not be compatible with life, because, contrary to complexes I and II, which operate 'in parallel' (thus allowing for metabolic compensation), complexes III and IV are 'in series,' while complex V is the sole site of oxidative phosphorylation[55] (Figure 1.2). This concept would apply only to the 'all-or-none' type of mendelian inheritance, as mutations in mtDNA-encoded components of complexes III–V do indeed occur (see above), but are incompletely expressed because of heteroplasmy.

Defects in intergenomic signaling

In the course of evolution, mitochondria lost their original independence, and mtDNA is now the slave of nuclear DNA, depending, as it does, on numerous nucleus-encoded factors for its integrity and replication.[56] Mutations in these factors cause diseases that affect mtDNA quantity, quality, or function, and that are inherited as mendelian traits. These disorders can be divided – for now – into two major groups: (i) abnormalities of mtDNA replication or maintenance, resulting in mtDNA depletion, multiple deletions, or a combination of the two conditions; and (ii) defects of mtDNA translation.

Alterations of mtDNA replication or maintenance

The quantitative alteration is exemplified by abnormal reductions in the number of mtDNA molecules (both per cell and per organelle).[57,58] The qualitative alteration is exemplified by multiple deletions (in contrast to the single species of deleted mtDNAs present in sporadic KSS, PEO, and PS).[56]

Ophthalmoplegia is the clinical hallmark of multiple mtDNA deletions, but both the autosomal dominant (ADPEO) and recessive (ARPEO) forms include other manifestations.[59] Families with ADPEO often show proximal limb weakness, peripheral neuropathy, sensorineural hearing loss, cataracts, endocrine dysfunction, and severe depression.[60,61] There are two major presentations of ARPEO, one associated with cardiomyopathy (autosomal recessive cardiomyopathy and ophthalmoplegia, or ARCO[62]), and the other with peripheral neuropathy, gastrointestinal dysmotility, and leukoencephalopathy (mitochondrial neurogastrointestinal encephalomyopathy, or MNGIE[63]).

Since 1999, the molecular bases of defects of intergenomic communication have begun to be unraveled. Interestingly, both the quantitative and qualitative defects may result from impaired regulation of mitochondrial genomic integrity. Such impairment can be direct (e.g. in proteins required for mtDNA replication and maintenance) or indirect (e.g. in proteins required to maintain nucleotide pools in mitochondria). For example, some families with ADPEO have mutations in the mitochondrial adenine nucleotide translocator 1[64] (ANT1), while others have mutations in Twinkle, a mitochondrial protein similar to bacteriophage T7 primase/helicase.[65] Mutations in the mitochondrial-specific DNA polymerase γ have been associated with both dominant and recessive multiple deletion disorders,[66,67] and with Alpers syndrome, an autosomal recessive infantile hepatocerebral syndrome.[68–70] The molecular basis of ARCO remains unknown, but MNGIE is clearly due to loss of function in thymidine phosphorylase (TP), resulting in markedly increased levels of thymidine and deoxyuridine in the blood of patients.[71,72] Notably, TP is not a mitochondrially targeted protein, and yet it appears to affect selectively mitochondrial nucleotide pools required for maintaining mtDNA integrity and abundance. This concept is bolstered by the pathogenicity of the ANT1 mutations and by recent findings that mutations in mitochondrial thymidine kinase (TK2),[73,74] deoxyguanosine kinase (dGK),[75,76] and in the ADP-forming succinyl- CoA synthetase (SUCLA2)[77] are associated with the myopathic and hepatocerebral forms of mtDNA depletion. Knowledge of these mutations makes prenatal diagnosis feasible for some families with the infantile mtDNA depletion syndromes, and may offer new approaches to therapeutic intervention (e.g. lowering blood thymidine levels in patients with MNGIE[72]).

Defects of mtDNA translation

The first patients with defects of mtDNA translation have only recently been described and it is to be expected that this group of disorders will expand rapidly.

Two siblings died in infancy of hepatocerebral syndrome, but – contrary to infants with mutations in *DGUOK* or *POLG* – they had no evidence of mtDNA depletion.[78] However, biochemical analyses of fibroblasts and skeletal muscle showed combined

Box 1.3 The Krebs cycle

Under aerobic conditions, cytosolic pyruvic acid derived from glycolysis is transported into mitochondria (via the malate–aspartate shuttle). Once inside the organelle, pyruvate is oxidized completely to produce CO_2 and (ultimately) H_2O. The oxidation takes place in the Krebs cycle, named in honor of the great biochemist Hans Krebs; it is also known as the tricarboxylic acid (TCA) or citric acid cycle.

The TCA cycle is the central pathway for the aerobic oxidation of *all* fuels, not just carbohydrates, but also proteins and lipids. This can be accomplished because the carbon atoms in all three types of molecules are eventually converted to the key TCA intermediate coenzyme A (CoA), a complex molecule consisting of a derivative of ATP, pantothenic acid, and a β-mercaptoethylamine (Figure B1.3.1). The SH group of the β-mercaptoethylamine binds to an acetyl group, forming the thioester acetyl-CoA (A stands for acetyl) (Figure B1.3.1). Thus, carbon atoms from all sources, once they become incorporated into acetyl groups, can enter the TCA cycle.

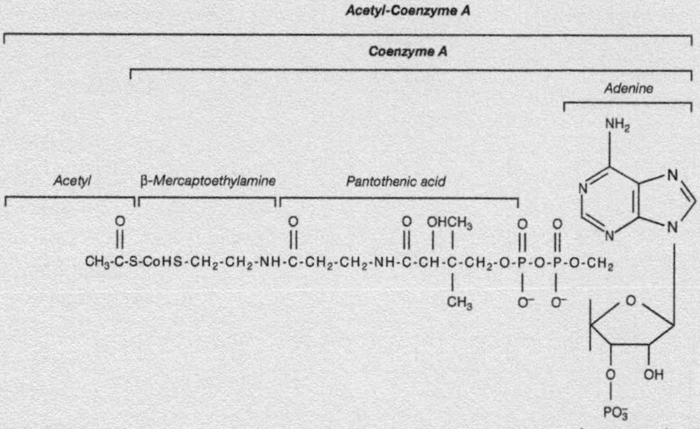

Figure B1.3.1 CoA and acetyl-CoA

In the case of pyruvate, the *pyruvate dehydrogenase complex (PDHC)* transfers CoA to pyruvate to form acetyl-CoA plus CO_2; in the process, the co-factor NAD^+ (nicotinamide adenine dinucleotide) is reduced to NADH. NAD^+ and NADH (Figure B1.3.2) are important molecules because they are central players in moving 'reducing equivalents' (i.e. H^+ ions) throughout the cell.

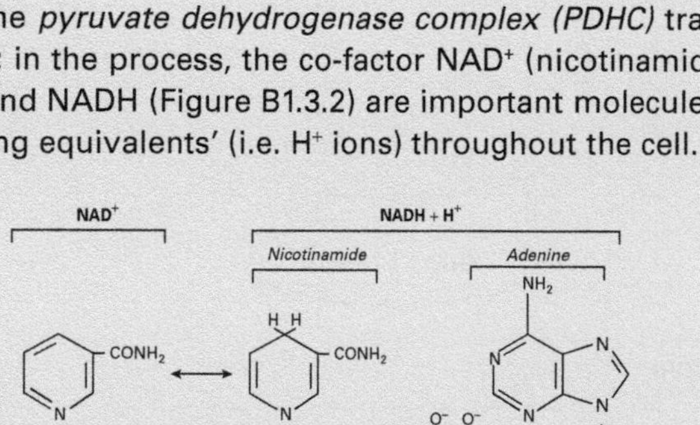

Figure B1.3.2 Pyramidine nucleotides. Shown are NAD^+ and NADH. The arrow shows where phosphoric acid is esterified to produce $NADP^+$ and NADPH

(Continued)

Box 1.3 (Continued)

Once acetyl-CoA is made, it can be oxidized in the TCA cycle (Figure B1.3.3). The cycle is a series of enzymatic reactions that form a true cycle: oxaloacetate (in the presence of acetyl-CoA) → citrate → *cis*-aconitate → isocitrate → oxalosuccinate → α-ketoglutarate → succinyl-CoA → succinate → fumarate → malate and finally back to oxaloacetate.

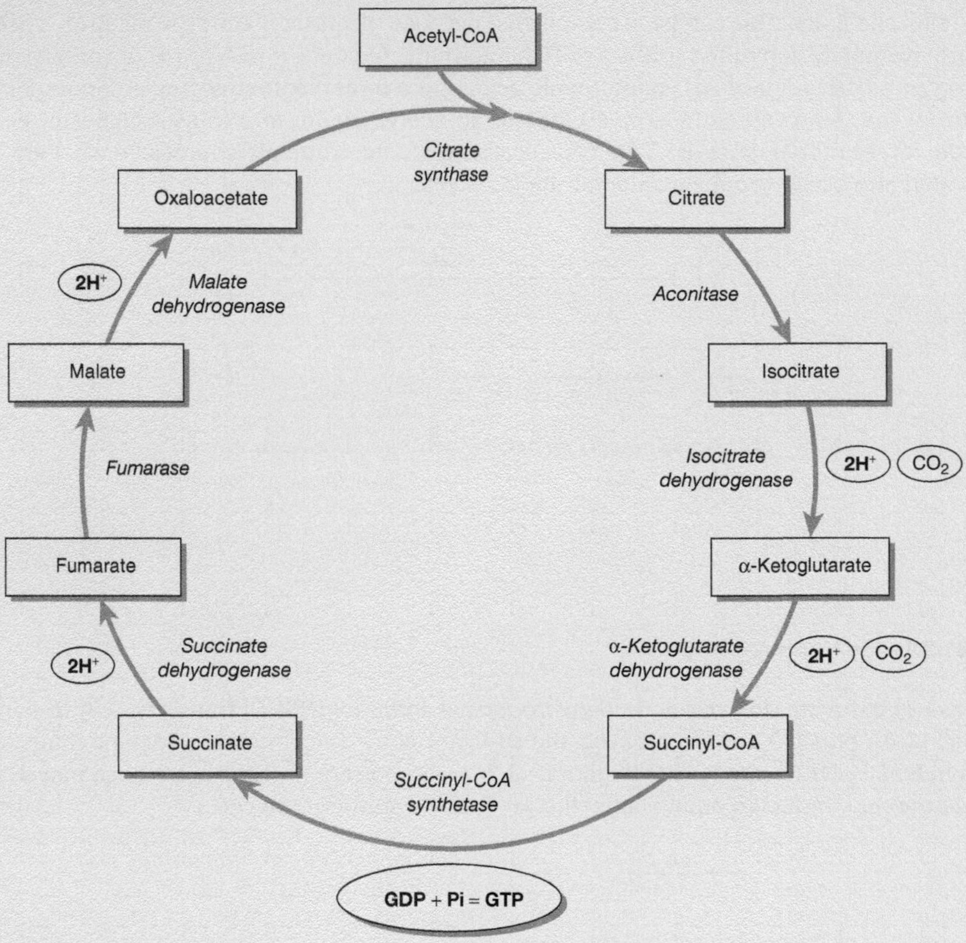

Figure B1.3.3 The TCA cycle

During one turn of the cycle, two molecules of CO_2 are produced, as are eight protons (as NADH + H^+) and one molecule of guanosine triphosphate, or GTP (another reaction entailing substrate level phosphorylation). The GTP can also be converted to ATP by nucleoside diphosphokinase.

$$GTP + ADP = GDP + ATP$$

Of the three carbons in pyruvate, one is oxidized to CO_2 in the 'priming' reaction to make acetyl CoA, and the other two are oxidized from acetyl-CoA to CO_2 in the TCA cycle. Since there are actually two molecules of pyruvate formed per molecule of glucose, the oxidation of glucose requires two 'turns' of the cycle.

defects of respiratory chain complexes containing mtDNA-encoded subunits, and blue-native polyacrylamide gel electrophoresis of fibroblasts showed low levels of all complexes except complex II. The defective gene (*EFG1*), identified through microcell-mediated chromosome transfer and microsatellite mapping, encodes one of four elongation factors required in humans – together with two initiation factors and one termination factor – for the synthesis of mtDNA-encoded proteins.[78]

A newborn girl with dysmorphic features, hypotonia, limb edema, increased liver transaminases, and intractable lactic acidosis, died at age 3 days.[79] Multiple respiratory chain defects (sparing complex II) were detected in liver, muscle, and cultured skin fibroblasts. Defective mitochondrial translation was shown in fibroblasts by in vitro pulse labeling. Because the level of 12S rRNA was reduced, a defect of one of the associated mitochondrial ribosomal small subunit proteins was suspected, which led to the identification of a pathogenic point mutation in the gene encoding mitochondrial ribosomal protein subunit 16 (*MRPS16*).[79]

Defective pseudouridylation of mitochondrial tRNA genes has been associated with the autosomal recessive syndrome of mitochondrial myopathy and sideroblastic anemia (MLASA).[80] Linkage analysis, homozygosity testing, and direct sequencing of six candidate genes revealed a homozygous missense mutation in the gene *PUS1* (which encodes the mitochondrial enzyme pseudouridine synthase 1) in all affected individuals from two pedigrees.[80]

Defects of the membrane lipid milieu

Except for cytochrome *c*, which is located in the intermembrane space, all other components of the respiratory chain are embedded in the lipid milieu of the inner mitochondrial membrane, which is predominantly composed of cardiolipin. Cardiolipin is not merely a scaffold; rather, it is an integral part of some respiratory chain components and is indispensable for their proper function.[81] It stands to reason, therefore, that defects in cardiolipin would cause respiratory chain dysfunction and mitochondrial disease. This novel pathogenic concept is exemplified by an X-linked disorder, Barth syndrome, characterized by mitochondrial myopathy, cardiomyopathy, growth retardation, and leukopenia.[82] The gene that is mutated in Barth syndrome, *G4.5*,[83] encodes a family of acyl-CoA synthetases ('tafazzins') that must play an important role in cardiolipin synthesis, because cardiolipin levels are markedly decreased in skeletal and cardiac muscle and in platelets from these patients.[84–86]

Disorders with suspected or indirect respiratory chain involvement

Indirect involvement of mitochondria has been documented or suggested in many conditions, including normal aging, late-onset neurodegenerative diseases, and cancer, although the precise role of mitochondrial dysfunction in these conditions remains controversial (see Chapters 10 and 13).

Defects of mitochondrial protein importation

Cytosolic proteins destined for mitochondria have mitochondrial targeting signals (MTSs) that enable them to be routed to the appropriate compartment within the organelle, where they are then refolded to an active configuration.[87] While a number of mutations in MTSs have been found (interestingly, none affecting components of the respiratory chain), few errors in the highly complex importation machinery itself are known. Defects of the general protein importation machinery may be rare because they would affect such a wide array of proteins as to be lethal.[88] However, at least one such defect has been identified, deafness-dystonia syndrome (Mohr–Tranebjaerg syndrome), an X-linked recessive disorder characterized by progressive sensorineural deafness, dystonia, cortical blindness, and psychiatric symptoms (see Chapter 7).[89] It is due to mutations in *TIMM8A*, encoding deafness/dystonia protein (DDP1), a component of the mitochondrial protein import machinery located in the intermembrane space. Recently, an autosomal dominant form of hereditary spastic paraplegia (HSP) has been associated with mutations in the mitochondrial import chaperonin HSP60.[90]

Defects in mitochondrial motility, fission, and fusion

Mitochondria are not static organelles; they move within the cell on microtubular rails propelled by motor proteins, usually GTPases, called kinesins.[91] Also, in non-muscle cells, mitochondria fuse and split, often forming tubular networks and favoring distribution of the organelles at areas of high-energy demand.[92]

The first defect of mitochondrial motility has only recently been identified in a family with autosomal dominant hereditary spastic paraplegia and mutations in a gene (*KIF5A*) encoding one of the kinesins.[93]

The machinery for mitochondrial fission in mammals involves several proteins acting together, especially a GTPase known as dynamin-related protein 1 (DRP-1).[93] Thus far – but probably not for long – no defect of mitochondrial fission has been associated with disease.

Mitochondrial fusion also requires several proteins, including two outer membrane GTPases, mitofusin 1 (MFN 1) and mitofusin 2 (MFN 2), and a dynamin-related GTPase, OPA-1, which is located in the inner mitochondrial membrane.[92] Two diseases have been associated with defects of mitochondrial fusion, autosomal dominant optic atrophy and Charcot–Marie–Tooth type 2A. Autosomal dominant optic atrophy, the mendelian counterpart of LHON and a common cause of blindness in young adults (see Chapter 5) is due to mutations in the *OPA1* gene.[94,95] Charcot–Marie–Tooth 2A, an autosomal dominant axonal variant of this genetically heterogeneous polyneuropathy, is due to mutations in the *MFN2* gene.[96,97]

Neurodegenerative diseases

There are a few neurodegenerative disorders that are due to mutations in proteins targeted to the mitochondria but whose pathogeneses have not yet been defined. These include Friedreich's ataxia (FA), at least one form of HSP, Wilson's disease (WD), familial Parkinson's Disease (PD), and familial ALS (FALS).

Mitochondrial dysfunction is invoked as a final common pathogenic mechanism both in aging and in the most common late-onset neurodegenerative disorders, including Alzheimer's disease (AD), sporadic amyotrophic lateral sclerosis (ALS), Huntington's disease (HD), progressive supranuclear palsy (PSP), and sporadic Parkinson's disease (PD). The role of mitochondrial dysfunction – controversial as it is – in all of these disorders is discussed in Chapter 13.

The concept of mitochondrial disease was introduced more than 40 years ago, when Luft and coworkers (see Introduction) described a young woman with severe non-thyroidal hypermetabolism due to loose coupling of oxidation and phosphorylation in muscle mitochondria. Only one other patient with Luft syndrome has been identified, making this arguably the rarest human disease ever described. Although caution is needed in discriminating primary from secondary mitochondrial involvement, nowadays mitochondrial dysfunction needs to be taken into account by every medical subspecialty, justifying the term 'mitochondrial medicine' introduced by Luft and used as the title of this book.

Acknowledgments

Part of the work described here was supported by NIH grants NS11766, NS28828, NS39854, and HD32062, by grants from the Muscular Dystrophy Association, and by the Marriott Mitochondrial Disorders Research Fund (MMDRF).

References

1. DiMauro S, Schon EA. Mitochondrial respiratory-chain diseases. *New Engl J Med* 2003; **348**: 2656–2668.
2. Elston T, Wang H, Oster G. Energy transduction in ATP synthase. *Nature* 1998; **391**: 510–513.
3. Noji H, Yoshida Y. The rotary machine of the cell, ATP synthase. *J Biol Chem* 2001; **276**: 1665–1668.
4. Schaefer AM, Taylor RW, Turnbull DM, Chinnery PF. The epidemiology of mitochondrial disorders – past, present and future. *Biochim Biophys Acta* 2004; **1659**: 115–120.
5. Holt IJ, Harding AE, Morgan Hughes JA. Deletions of muscle mitochondrial DNA in patients with mitochondrial myopathies. *Nature* 1988; **331**: 717–719.
6. Wallace DC, Singh G, Lott MT et al. Mitochondrial DNA mutation associated with Leber's hereditary optic neuropathy. *Science* 1988; **242**: 1427–1430.
7. Schwartz M, Vissing J. Paternal inheritance of mitochondrial DNA. *New Engl J Med* 2002; **347**: 576–580.
8. Taylor RW, McDonnell MT, Blakely EL et al. Genotypes from patients indicate no paternal mitochondrial contribution. *Ann Neurol* 2003; **54**: 521–524.
9. Filosto M, Mancuso M, Vives-Bauza C et al. Lack of paternal inheritance of muscle mitochondrial DNA in sporadic mitochondrial myopathies. *Ann Neurol* 2003; **54**: 524–526.
10. Schwartz F, Vissing J. No evidence of paternal inheritance of mtDNA in patients with sporadic mtDNA mutations. *J Neurol Sci* 2004; **218**: 99–101.
11. Mancuso M, Filosto M, Mootha VK et al. A novel mitochondrial DNA tRNAPhe mutation causes MERRF syndrome. *Neurology* 2004; **62**: 2119–2121.
12. DiMauro S, Hirano M, Kaufmann P et al. Clinical features and genetics of myoclonic epilepsy with ragged red fibers. In: Fahn S, Frucht SJ, eds. *Myoclonus and Paroxysmal Dyskinesia*. Philadelphia: Lippincott Williams & Wilkins, 2002: 217–229.
13. Carelli V. Leber's hereditary optic neuropathy. In: Schapira AHV, DiMauro S, eds. *Mitochondrial Disorders in Neurology 2*. Boston: Butterworth-Heinemann, 2002: 115–142.
14. Andreu AL, Hanna MG, Reichmann H et al. Exercise intolerance due to mutations in the cytochrome *b* gene of mitochondrial DNA. *New Engl J Med* 1999; **341**: 1037–1044.
15. Chen X, Prosser R, Simonetti S et al. Rearranged mitochondrial genomes are present in human oocytes. *Am J Hum Genet* 1995; **57**: 239–247.
16. King MP, Attardi G. Human cells lacking mtDNA: repopulation with exogenous mitochondria by complementation. *Science* 1989; **246**: 500–503.
17. Tatuch Y, Christodoulou J, Feigenbaum A et al. Heteroplasmic mtDNA mutation (T>G) at 8993 can cause Leigh disease when the percentage of abnormal mtDNA is high. *Am J Hum Genet* 1992; **50**: 852–858.
18. Inoue K, Nakada K, Ogura A et al. Generation of mice with mitochondrial dysfunction by introducing mouse mtDNA carrying a deletion into zygotes. *Nature Genet* 2000; **26**: 176–181.
19. Sligh JE, Levy SE, Waymire KG et al. Maternal germ-line transmission of mutant mtDNAs from embryonic stem cell-derived chimeric mice. *Proc Natl Acad Sci USA* 2000; **97**: 14461–14466.
20. Shoubridge EA. Nuclear genetic defects of oxidative phosphorylation. *Hum Mol Genet* 2001; **10**: 2277–2284.
21. Ugalde C, Janssen RJRJ, van den Heuvel LP et al. Differences in assembly or stability of complex I and other mitochondrial OXPHOS complexes in inherited complex I deficiency. *Hum Molec Gen* 2004; **13**: 659–667.
22. Kirby DM, Salemi R, Sugiana C et al. *NUFS6* mutations are a novel cause of lethal neonatal mitochondrial complex I deficiency. *J Clin Invest* 2004; **114**: 837–845.
23. Bourgeron T, Rustin P, Chretien D et al. Mutation of a nuclear succinate dehydrogenase gene results in mitochondrial respiratory chain deficiency. *Nature Genet* 1995; **11**: 144–149.
24. Parfait B, Chretien D, Rotig A et al. Compound heterozygous mutation in the flavoprotein gene of the respiratory chain complex II in a patient with Leigh syndrome. *Hum Genet* 2000; **106**: 236–243.
25. Birch-Machin MA, Taylor RW, Cochran B et al. Late-onset optic atrophy, ataxia, and myopathy associated with a mutation of a complex II gene. *Ann Neurol* 2000; **48**: 330–335.
26. Rustin P, Rotig A. Inborn errors of complex II – Unusual human mitochondrial diseases. *Biochim Biophys Acta* 2002; **1553**: 117–122.

27. Rotig A, Appelkvist E-L, Geromel V et al. Quinone-responsive multiple respiratory-chain dysfunction due to widespread coenzyme Q10 deficiency. *Lancet* 2000; **356**: 391–395.
28. Rahman S, Hargreaves I, Clayton P, Heales S. Neonatal presentation of coenzyme Q10 deficiency. *J Pediatr* 2001; **139**: 456–458.
29. Salviati L, Sacconi S, Murer L et al. Infantile encephalomyopathy and nephropathy with CoQ10 deficiency: a CoQ10-responsive condition. *Neurology* 2005; **65**: 606–608.
30. Ogasahara S, Engel AG, Frens D, Mack D. Muscle coenzyme Q deficiency in familial mitochondrial encephalomyopathy. *Proc Natl Acad Sci USA* 1989; **86**: 2379–2382.
31. Sobreira C, Hirano M, Shanske S et al. Mitochondrial encephalomyopathy with coenzyme Q10 deficiency. *Neurology* 1997; **48**: 1238–1243.
32. Di Giovanni S, Mirabella M, Spinazzola A et al. Coenzyme Q10 reverses pathological phenotype and reduces apoptosis in familial CoQ10 deficiency. *Neurology* 2001; **57**: 515–518.
33. Lalani S, Vladutiu GD, Plunkett K et al. Isolated mitochondrial myopathy associated with muscle coenzyme Q10 deficiency. *Arch Neurol* 2005; **62**: 317–320.
34. Musumeci O, Naini A, Slonim AE et al. Familial cerebellar ataxia with muscle coenzyme Q10 deficiency. *Neurology* 2001; **56**: 849–855.
35. Lamperti C, Naini A, Hirano M et al. Cerebellar ataxia and coenzyme Q10 deficiency. *Neurology* 2003; **60**: 1206–1208.
36. Gironi M, Lamperti C, Nemni R et al. Late-onset cerebellar ataxia with hypogonadism and muscle coenzyme Q10 deficiency. *Neurology* 2004; **62**: 818–820.
37. Quinzii C, Kattah AG, Naini A et al. Coenzyme Q deficiency and cerebellar ataxia associated with an *aprataxin* mutation. *Neurology* 2005; **64**: 539–541.
38. de Lonlay P, Valnot I, Barrientos A et al. A mutant mitochondrial respiratory chain assembly protein causes complex III deficiency in patients with tubulopathy, encephalopathy and liver failure. *Nature Genet* 2001; **29**: 57–60.
39. De Meirleir L, Seneca S, Damis E et al. Clinical and diagnostic characteristics of complex III deficiency due to mutations in the *BCS1L* gene. *Am J Med Genet* 2003; **121**: 126–131.
40. Visapaa I, Fellman V, Vesa J et al. GRACILE syndrome, a lethal metabolic disorder with iron overload, is caused by a point mutation in *BCS1L*. *Am J Hum Genet* 2002; **71**: 863–876.
41. Fellman V. The GRACILE syndrome, a neonatal lethal metabolic disorder with iron overload. *Blood Cells Mol Dis* 2002; **29**: 444–450.
42. Shoubridge EA. Cytochrome *c* oxidase deficiency. *Am J Med Genet* 2001; **106**: 46–52.
43. Zeviani M, Pandolfo M. Nuclear gene mutations in mitochondrial disorders. In: Holt I, ed. *Genetics of Mitochondrial Diseases*. Oxford: Oxford University Press, 2003: 181–205.
44. De Meirleir L, Seneca S, Kissens W et al. Respiratory chain complex V deficiency due to a mutation in the assembly gene ATP12. *J Med Genet* 2004; **41**: 120–124.
45. Ogilvie I, Kennaway NG, Shoubridge EA. A molecular chaperone for mitochondrial complex I assembly is mutated in a progressive encephalopathy. *J Clin Invest* 2005; **115**: 2784–2792.
46. Zhu Z, Yao J, Johns T et al. SURF1, encoding a factor involved in the biogenesis of cytochrome *c* oxidase, is mutated in Leigh syndrome. *Nature Genet* 1998; **20**: 337–343.
47. Tiranti V, Hoertnagel K, Carrozzo R et al. Mutations of SURF-1 in Leigh disease associated with cytochrome c oxidase deficiency. *Am J Hum Genet* 1998; **63**: 1609–1621.
48. Pequignot MO, Dey R, Zeviani M et al. Mutations in the *SURF1* gene associated with Leigh syndrome and cytochrome *c* oxidase deficiency. *Hum Mut* 2001; **17**: 374–381.
49. Papadopoulou LC, Sue CM, Davidson MM et al. Fatal infantile cardioencephalomyopathy with COX deficiency and mutations in *SCO2*, a COX assembly gene. *Nature Genet* 1999; **23**: 333–337.
50. Antonicka H, Mattman A, Carlson CG et al. Mutations in *COX15* produce a defect in the mitochondrial heme biosynthetic pathway, causing early-onset fatal hypertrophic cardiomyopathy. *Am J Hum Genet* 2003; **72**: 101–14.
51. Valnot I, von Kleist-Retzow J-C, Barrientos A et al. A mutation in the human heme-A: farnesyltransferase gene (COX 10) causes cytochrome *c* oxidase deficiency. *Hum Mol Genet* 2000; **9**: 1245–1249.

52. Antonicka H, Leary SC, Guercin G-H et al. Mutations in *COX10* result in a defect in mitochondrial heme A biosynthesis and account for multiple, early-onset clinical phenotypes associated with isolated COX deficiency. *Hum Mol Genet* 2003; **12**: 2693–2702.
53. Valnot I, Osmond S, Gigarel N et al. Mutations of the *SCO1* gene in mitochondrial cytochrome c oxidase deficiency with neonatal-onset hepatic failure and encephalopathy. *Am J Hum Genet* 2000; **67**: 1104–1109.
54. Mootha VK, Lepage P, Miller K et al. Identification of a gene causing human cytochrome *c* oxidase deficiency by integrative genomics. *Proc Natl Acad Sci USA* 2003; **100**: 605–610.
55. Sue CM, Schon EA. Mitochondrial respiratory chain diseases and mutations in nuclear DNA: A promising start? *Brain Pathol* 2000; **10**: 442–450.
56. Hirano M, Marti R, Ferreira-Barros C, et al. Defects of intergenomic communication: autosomal disorders that cause multiple deletions and depletion of mitochondrial DNA. *Cell Develop Biol* 2001; **12**: 417–427.
57. Moraes CT, Shanske S, Tritschler HJ et al. MtDNA depletion with variable tissue expression: A novel genetic abnormality in mitochondrial diseases. *Am J Hum Genet* 1991; **48**: 492–501.
58. Hirano M, Marti RA, Vila MR, Nishigaki Y. mtDNA maintenance and stability genes: MNGIE and mtDNA depletion syndromes. In: Koehler CM, Bauer MF, eds. *Mitochondrial Function and Biogenesis*. Berlin: Verlag, 2004: 177–200.
59. Hirano M, DiMauro S. *ANT1, Twinkle, POLG*, and *TP*: New genes open our eyes to ophthalmoplegia. *Neurology* 2001; **57**: 2163–2165.
60. Servidei S, Zeviani M, Manfredi G et al. Dominantly inherited mitochondrial myopathy with multiple deletions of mitochondrial DNA: clinical, morphologic, and biochemical studies. *Neurology* 1991; **41**: 1053–1059.
61. Suomalainen A, Majander A, Wallin M et al. Autosomal dominant progressive external ophthalmoplegia with multiple deletions of mtDNA: Clinical, biochemical, and molecular genetic features of the 10q-linked disease. *Neurology* 1997; **48**: 1244–1253.
62. Bohlega S, Tanji K, Santorelli FM et al. Multiple mitochondrial DNA deletions associated with autosomal recessive ophthalmoplegia and severe cardiomyopathy. *Neurology* 1996; **46**: 1329–1334.
63. Nishino I, Spinazzola A, Papadimitriou A et al. Mitochondrial neurogastrointestinal encephalomyopathy: an autosomal recessive disorder due to thymidine phosphorylase mutations. *Ann Neurol* 2000; **47**: 792–800.
64. Kaukonen J, Juselius JK, Tiranti V et al. Role of adenine nucleotide translocator 1 in mtDNA maintenance. *Science* 2000; **289**: 782–785.
65. Spelbrink JN, Li F-Y, Tiranti V et al. Human mitochondrial DNA deletions associated with mutations in the gene encoding Twinkle, a phage T7 gene 4-like protein localized in mitochondria. *Nature Genet* 2001; **28**: 223–231.
66. Van Goethem G, Dermaut B, Lofgren A et al. Mutation of *POLG* is associated with progressive external ophthalmoplegia characterized by mtDNA deletions. *Nature Genet* 2001; **28**: 211–212.
67. Lamantea E, Tiranti V, Bordoni A et al. Mutations of mitochondrial DNA polymerase γA are a frequent cause of autosomal dominant or recessive progressive external ophthalmoplegia. *Ann Neurol* 2002; **52**: 211–219.
68. Naviaux RK, Nguyen KV. *POLG* mutations associated with Alpers' syndrome and mitochondrial DNA depletion. *Ann Neurol* 2004; **55**: 706–712.
69. Ferrari G, Lamantea E, Donati A et al. Infantile hepatocerebral syndromes associated with mutations in the mitochondrial DNA polymerase-γA. *Brain* 2005; **128**: 723–731.
70. Davidzon G, Mancuso M, Ferraris S et al. *POLG* mutations and Alpers syndrome. *Ann Neurol* 2005; **57**: 921–924.
71. Nishino I, Spinazzola A, Hirano M. Thymidine phosphorylase gene mutations in MNGIE, a human mitochondrial disorder. *Science* 1999; **283**: 689–692.
72. Spinazzola A, Marti R, Nishino I et al. Altered thymidine metabolism due to defects of thymidine phosphorylase. *J Biol Chem* 2002; **277**: 4128–4132.
73. Saada A, Shaag A, Mandel H et al. Mutant mitochondrial thymidine kinase in mitochondrial DNA depletion myopathy. *Nature Genet* 2001; **29**: 342–344.
74. Mancuso M, Salviati L, Sacconi S et al. Mitochondrial DNA depletion. Mutations in thymidine kinase

gene with myopathy and SMA. *Neurology* 2002; **59**: 1197–1202.

75. Mandel H, Szargel R, Labay V et al. The deoxyguanosine kinase gene is mutated in individuals with depleted hepatocerebral mitochondrial DNA. *Nature Genet* 2001; **29**: 337–341.
76. Salviati L, Sacconi S, Mancuso M et al. Mitochondrial DNA depletion and *dGK* gene mutations. *Ann Neurol* 2002; **52**: 311–317.
77. Elpeleg O, Miller C, Hershkovitz E et al. Deficiency of the ADP-forming succinyl-CoA synthase activity is associated with encephalomyopathy and mitochondrial DNA depletion. *Am J Hum Genet* 2005; **76**: 1081–1086.
78. Coenen MJH, Antonicka H, Ugalde C et al. Mutant mitochondrial elongation factor G1 and combined oxidative phosphorylation deficiency. *New Engl J Med* 2004; **351**: 2080–2086.
79. Miller C, Saada A, Shaul N et al. Defective mitochondrial translation caused by a ribosomal protein (MRPS16) mutation. *Ann Neurol* 2004; **56**: 734–738.
80. Bykhovskaya Y, Casas KA, Mengesha E et al. Missense mutation in pseudouridine synthase 1 (*PUS1*) causes mitochondrial myopathy and sideroblastic anemia (MLASA). *Am J Hum Genet* 2004;**74**: 1303–1308.
81. Schlame M, Rua D, Greenberg ML. The biosynthesis and functional role of cardiolipin. *Progr Lipid Res* 2000; **39**: 257–288.
82. Barth PG, Wanders RJA, Vreken P et al. X-linked cardioskeletal myopathy and neutropenia (Barth syndrome) (MIM 30260). *J Inher Metab Dis* 1999; **22**: 555–567.
83. Bione S, D'Adamo P, Maestrini E et al. A novel X-linked gene, G4.5, is responsible for Barth syndrome. *Nature Genet* 1996; **12**: 385–389.
84. Vreken P, Valianpour F, Nijtmans LG et al. Defective remodeling of cardiolipin and phosphatidylglycerol in Barth syndrome. *Biochem Biophys Res Comm* 2000; **279**: 378–382.
85. Schlame M, Towbin JA, Heerdt PM et al. Deficiency of tetralinoleoyl-cardiolipin in Barth syndrome. *Ann Neurol* 2002; **51**: 634–637.
86. Schlame M, Kelley RI, Feigenbaum A et al. Phospholipid abnormalities in children with Barth syndrome. *J Am Coll Cardiol* 2003; **42**: 1994–1999.
87. Okamoto K, Brinker A, Paschen SA et al. The protein import motor of mitochondria: a targeted molecular ratchet driving unfolding and translocation. *EMBO J* 2002; **21**: 3659–3671.
88. Fenton WA. Mitochondrial protein transport – A system in search of mutations. *Am J Hum Genet* 1995; **57**: 235–238.
89. Roesch K, Curran SP, Tranebjaerg L, Koehler CM. Human deafness dystonia syndrome is caused by a defect in assembly of the DDP1/TIMM8a-TIMM13 complex. *Hum Mol Genet* 2002; **11**: 477–486.
90. Hansen JJ, Durr A, Cournu-Rebeix I et al. Hereditary spastic paraplegia SPG13 is associated with a mutation in the gene encoding the mitochondrial chaperonin Hsp60. *Am J Hum Genet* 2002; **70**(5): 1328–1332.
91. Boldogh IR, Yang HC, Nowakowski WD et al. Arp2/3 complex and actin dynamics are required for actin-based mitochondrial motility in yeast. *Proc Natl Acad Sci USA* 2001; **98**: 3162–3167.
92. Bossy-Wetzel E, Barsoum MJ, Godzik A et al. Mitochondrial fission in apoptosis, neurodegeneration and aging. *Curr Opin Cell Biol* 2003; **15**: 706–716.
93. Fichera M, Lo Giudice M, Falco M et al. Evidence of kinesin heavy chain (*KIF5A*) involvement in pure hereditary spastic paraplegia. *Neurology* 2004; **63**: 1108–1110.
94. Delettre C, Lenaers G, Griffoin J-M et al. Nuclear gene *OPA1*, encoding a mitochondrial dynamin-related protein, is mutated in dominant optic atrophy. *Nature Genet* 2000; **26**: 207–210.
95. Alexander C, Votruba M, Pesch UEA et al. OPA1, encoding a dynamin-related GTPase, is mutated in autosomal dominant optic atrophy linked to chromosome 3q28. *Nature Genet* 2000; **26**: 211–215.
96. Zuchner S, Mersiyanova IV, Muglia M et al. Mutations in the mitochondrial GTPase mitofusin 2 cause Charcot–Marie–Tooth neuropathy type 2A. *Nature Genet* 2004; **36**: 449–451.
97. Kijima K, Numakura C, Izumino H et al. Mitochondrial GTPase mitofusin 2 mutation in Charcot–Marie–Tooth neuropathy type 2A. *Hum Genet* 2005; **116**: 23–27.

2

Mitochondrial neurology I: encephalopathies

Michio Hirano, Petra Kaufmann, Darryl De Vivo, and Kurenai Tanji

Introduction

The central nervous system (CNS) is metabolically very active and is therefore particularly vulnerable to defects of the mitochondrial respiratory chain. Given the functional complexity of the CNS, it is not surprising that bioenergetic defects in the brain and spinal cord produce diverse clinical manifestations, including dementia, seizures, myoclonus, and ataxia. The variability of CNS lesions is partially age-related. For example, in infants and young children, deep gray matter structures (basal ganglia and brainstem nuclei) are vulnerable to mitochondrial dysfunction, which manifests clinically as Leigh syndrome (LS) characterized by psychomotor regression. In contrast, juvenile or adult-onset mitochondrial diseases affecting the CNS often present with cortical dysfunction manifesting as dementia, epilepsy, myoclonus, stroke-like episodes, ataxia, or migraine headaches.

Examples of childhood-onset mitochondrial encephalomyopathies include: mitochondrial encephalomyopathy, lactic acidosis, and stroke-like episodes (MELAS); myoclonus epilepsy ragged-red fibers (MERRF); Kearns–Sayre syndrome (KSS characterized by ptosis, ophthalmoplegia, retinitis pigmentosa, heart block, and ataxia); and neuropathy, ataxia, retinitis pigmentosa (NARP). In this chapter, we highlight the most salient CNS manifestations of common mitochondrial diseases. Sensorineural hearing loss and ocular dysfunction are also very common features of mitochondrial diseases but are reviewed in separate chapters.

Leigh syndrome

Subacute necrotizing encephalomyelopathy was described in 1951 by Dr. Denis Leigh, who reported a 6.5-month-old infant presenting with developmental regression that progressed quickly and led to death 6 weeks later.[1] At autopsy, Dr. Leigh observed multiple symmetric foci of spongy degeneration with microvascular proliferation in the brainstem tegmentum, thalami, cerebellum, posterior columns of the spinal cord, and optic nerves (Figure 2.1). He astutely noted that the neuropathological alterations resembled those of Wernicke syndrome but spared the mamillary bodies, a consistent feature that distinguishes the two disorders.

Since the original report, hundreds of LS cases have reinforced the importance of the condition and confirmed its pathological signature. The clinical presentations are heterogeneous, due to variations in age-at-onset, rates of progression, frequency of epilepsy, and presence or absence of pigmentary retinopathy. The onset is often acute and may coincide with a febrile illness or may follow a seizure. Most LS patients present in infancy with psychomotor regression while some present in childhood or adolescence. Adult-onset

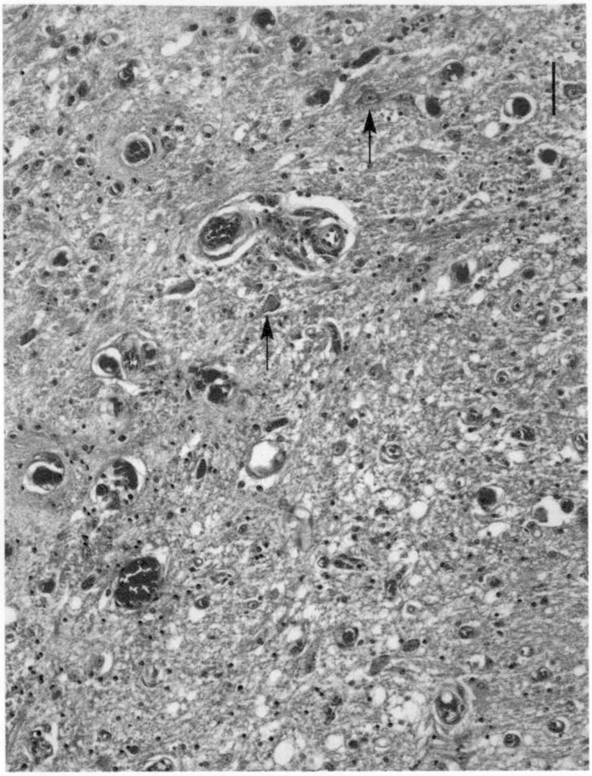

Figure 2.1 Leigh syndrome (LS). Section of the pontine tegmentum stained with hematoxylin and eosin (H&E) reveals a focus of spongy degeneration with microvascular proliferation. The black arrows denote surviving neurons. Bar = 100 μM

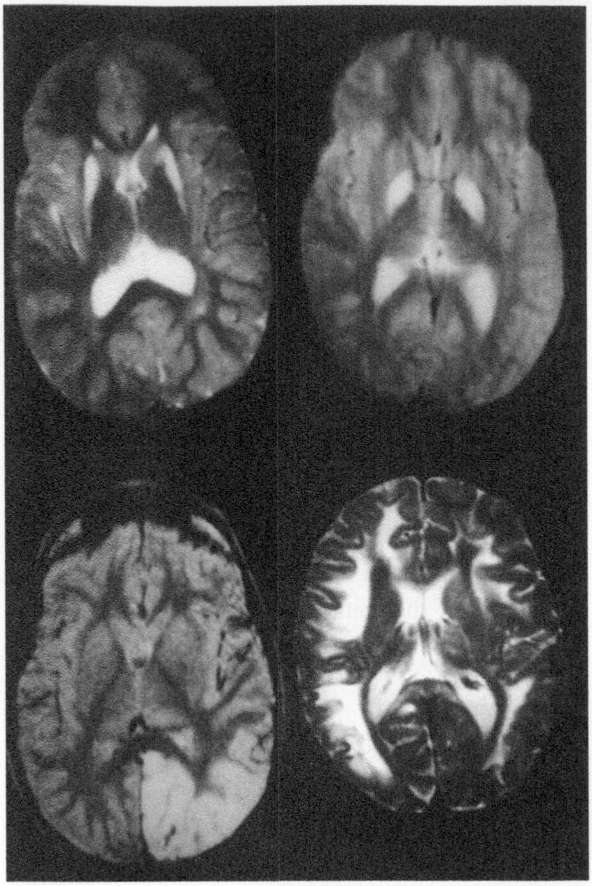

Figure 2.2 Brain T2-weighted magnetic resonance imaging (MRI) scans of patients with LS (upper images), mitochondrial encephalomyopathy, lactic acidosis, and stroke-like episodes (MELAS) (lower left image), and mitochondrial neurogastrointestinal encephalomyopathy (MNGIE) (lower right image). Brain MRIs of LS patients reveal increased T2-weighted signal in the putamen (upper left image) and in posterior lenticular nuclei (upper right image). MRI of a MELAS patient reveals an acute lesion in the left occipital lobe primarily affecting the cortex (lower left panel). MRI of a MNGIE patient demonstrates diffuse increased T2-signal in the white matter (lower right panel)

LS is uncommon. In infants with LS, besides developmental regression, generalized hypotonia, feeding problems, progressive vision loss due to optic neuropathy or pigmentary retinopathy, progressive external ophthalmoplegia, hearing loss, nystagmus, ataxia, and seizures are typical manifestations. In addition, failure to thrive, dysarthria, vomiting, and diarrhea are common manifestations. Respiratory dysfunction is often prominent and frequently causes death. Most infantile-onset LS patients die before age 2 years. In older infants or young children, LS may begin with ataxia, dystonia, or intellectual decline.

The clinical diagnosis of LS is usually made by brain magnetic resonance imaging (MRI) scans, which reveal increased signals in the basal ganglia and brainstem on T2-weighted or FLAIR images (Figure 2.2). The lesions are typically symmetric and commonly affect the putamen, globus pallidus,

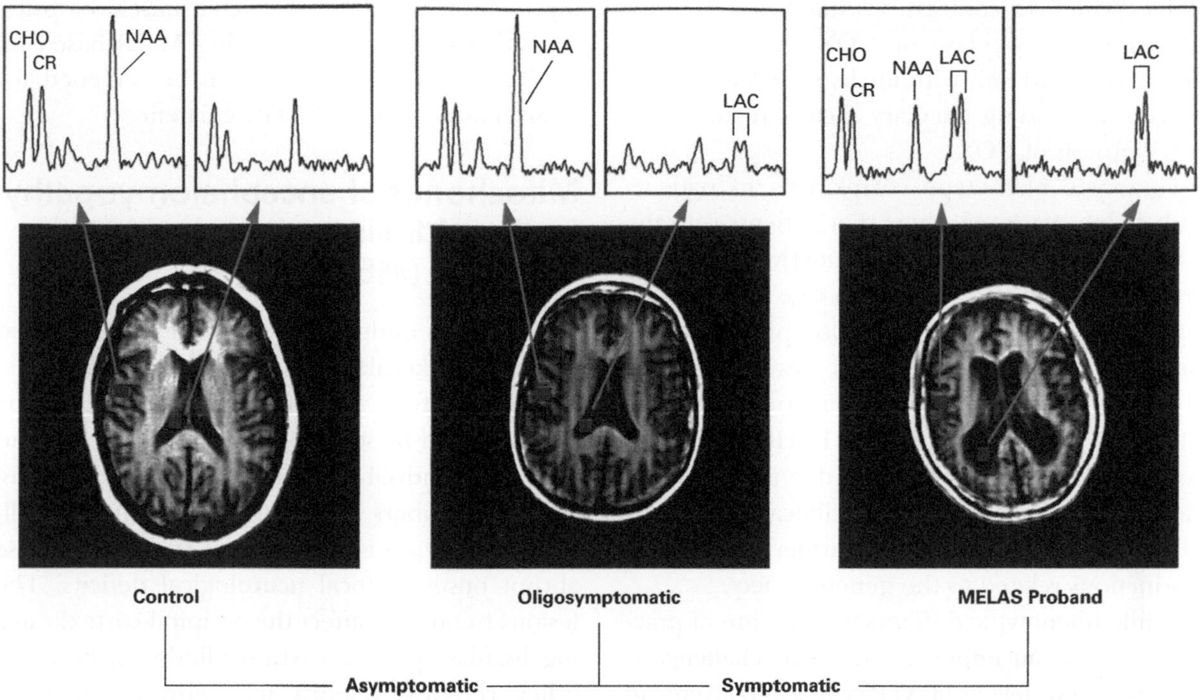

Figure 2.3 Brain magnetic resonance spectroscopy (MRS) of a control (left), oligosymptomatic individual with the MELAS A3243G mitochondrial DNA (mtDNA) mutation (center), and MELAS patient (right). In ventricular cerebrospinal fluid, lactate doublet peaks are undetectable in a control, mildly elevated in an oligosymptomatic individual, and highly elevated in a MELAS patient. In addition, there is mild cerebral atrophy in the oligosymptomatic brain and severe atrophy in the MELAS brain. CHO, choline; CR, creatine; NAA, N-acetyl-L-aspartate: LAC; lactate.

caudate, thalami, substantia nigra, inferior olivary nuclei, periaqueductal gray matter, and brainstem tegmentum. Magnetic resonance spectroscopy (MRS) scans reveal decreased *N*-acetylaspartate and increased lactate in the affected brain regions (Figure 2.3).

The notion that LS is due to inherited mitochondrial dysfunction originated with a report of two siblings with lactic acidosis and consanguineous parents.[2] Deficiency of pyruvate carboxylase was the first biochemical defect linked pathogenically to LS.[3] We now know that the biochemical causes of LS are heterogeneous and include defects of pyruvate dehydrogenase complex (PDHC), and mitochondrial respiratory chain complexes I, II, IV, and V.[4–8] The inheritance pattern depends on the specific defective gene, but may be autosomal recessive, X-linked recessive, or maternal. Although the specific causes of LS are biochemically and genetically diverse, the unifying metabolic defect in all patients is impaired adenosine triphosphate (ATP) synthesis.

Among the mitochondrial DNA (mtDNA) defects that cause Leigh syndrome, the T8993G point mutation in the ATP synthase gene is particularly common.[9] This mutation was originally described in patients with neuropathy, ataxia, and retinitis pigmentosa (NARP), but later found to also cause maternally inherited LS (MILS). Curiously, autosomal recessive LS due to deficiency of complex I or II has been associated only with mutation in genes encoding structural polypeptides. In contrast, LS due to complex IV (cytochrome *c* oxidase or COX) deficiency has been associated only with nuclear DNA mutations in genes encoding ancillary factors required for the synthesis of COX.

Genotype–phenotype correlations in patients with Leigh syndrome show that patients with the T8993G NARP mutation frequently (40%) have retinitis pigmentosa, which is a clue to the molecular diagnosis, because retinitis pigmentosa is rarely – if ever – seen in other forms of LS.[8] In addition, seizures are more common in patients with the NARP mutation or PDHC deficiency compared to children with LS due to COX deficiency.[8] It is likely that careful clinical evaluations of LS patients will reveal further phenotypic distinctions related to the genetic defect.

While phenotypic differences in LS are of practical interest, an important scientific challenge is to define how defects of ATP synthesis converge to produce the characteristic brain pathology. Some investigators have proposed that the selective involvement of the basal ganglia in LS is due to excitotoxicity and death of neurons with impaired mitochondrial energy metabolism.[10,11] Although deep gray matter structures of the central nervous system are prominently affected in LS, early brain lesions show vascular proliferation with 'spongy degeneration' characterized by vacuolization of neuropil, activated microglia, and reactive astrocytes, suggesting that the vascular changes precede neuronal death.[12]

To identify the molecular genetic cause of Leigh syndrome in patients, blood lactate and pyruvate may provide helpful preliminary clues. Defects of the mitochondrial respiratory chain and oxidative phosphorylation typically elevate lactate out of proportion to pyruvate (lactate:pyruvate ratio >20:1). By contrast, a defect of PDHC may be suspected when pyruvate and lactate are similarly increased. PDHC deficiency can be determined in cultured fibroblasts. Defects of the mitochondrial respiratory chain are better identified by biochemical analyses of skeletal muscle biopsies. In patients suspected of having MILS based on family history, blood DNA can be screened for point mutations in the ATPase 6 gene.

Mitochondrial encephalomyopathy lactic acidosis and stroke-like episodes (MELAS)

MELAS is a multisystem disorder characterized by: (1) stroke-like episodes at a young age, typically before age 40; (2) encephalopathy characterized by seizures, dementia, or both; and (3) mitochondrial myopathy with lactic acidosis, ragged-red fibers, or both.[13,14] The clinical hallmark of MELAS is stroke-like episodes that cause abrupt onset of focal neurological deficits. The lesions frequently affect the occipital cortex, causing hemianopsia or cortical blindness; however, other cerebral regions may also be affected. Additional features seen in many MELAS patients include basal ganglia calcifications, myoclonus, ataxia, episodic coma, optic nerve atrophy, pigmentary retinopathy, hearing loss, short stature, cardiomyopathy, electrocardiographic evidence of pre-excitation, cardiac conduction block, ophthalmoplegia, diabetes mellitus, gastrointestinal dysmotility, and nephropathy.

Almost all of the reported cases of MELAS have had a mitochondrial DNA point mutation (Box 2.1), therefore, maternal relatives are likely to harbor the same mutation. There are relatively few families in which more than one member has the full-fledged MELAS syndrome; more often maternally related individuals are oligosymptomatic and manifest only some features of MELAS.[14] The MELAS point mutation may also be found in asymptomatic family members.

Although superficially similar to garden-variety thrombotic or embolic strokes, the stroke-like episodes in MELAS are atypical because they affect young people and are often triggered by febrile illnesses, migraine-like headaches, and

Box 2.1 Diagnosis of mtDNA mutations

The diagnosis of mutations in mtDNA is relatively straightforward.[1]

Point mutations of mtDNA

Point mutations are diagnosed by polymerase chain reaction (PCR) of the mtDNA region of interest, followed by restriction fragment length polymorphism (RFLP) analysis. For example, with the mutation at position 3243 in the $tRNA^{Leu(UUR)}$ gene most commonly associated with MELAS, the A-to-G mutation converts the sequence in the region from 5′-**A**GCC-3′ to 5′-**G**GCC-3′. GGCC is the recognition sequence for the restriction enzyme *Hae*III, meaning that the mutation creates a new *Hae*III site that is absent in normal subjects. A PCR performed with primers flanking the $tRNA^{Leu(UUR)}$ gene generates a fragment that can be digested with *Hae*III to yield the fragmentation pattern diagnostic of the mutation (Figure B2.1.1)The proportion of mutated molecules can be determined by quantitating the amount of normal and mutation-derived fragments.

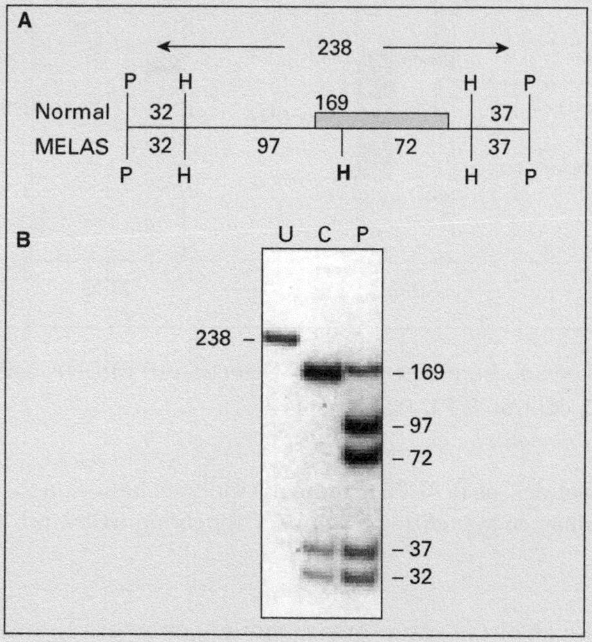

Figure B2.1.1 Example of PCR/RFLP to detect the MELAS-3243 mutation. **A.** The mutation creates a new *Hae*III site (H) within the $tRNA^{Leu(UUR)}$ gene (box). PCR amplification with primers (P) yields a 238-bp fragment, which, when cleaved with *Hae*III, cuts the 169-bp *Hae*III–*Hae*III fragment found in normal mtDNA into two fragments of 97 bp and 72 bp. **B.** The RFLP pattern can be visualized by electrophoresing the digestion products (in this case, radiolabeled) through a polyacrylamide gel

Large-scale deletions of mtDNA

In the case of mtDNA deletions, such as those found in KSS and ADPEO, diagnosis is confirmed using a Southern blot. Total DNA is digested with a restriction enzyme that cleaves mtDNA only once

(Continued)

Box 2.1 (Continued)

(e.g. *Pvu*II or *Bam*HI), thereby linearizing it. When subjected to Southern blotting (i.e. electrophoresis through an agarose gel followed by transfer of the digested fragments to nitrocellulose or nylon), and hybridization of the immobilized fragments with a suitable probe (in this case labeled mtDNA), two patterns are observed. In DNA isolated from normal subjects a single fragment of 16.6 kb, corresponding to the linearized full-length mtDNA, is observed. In KSS patients, however, beside the full-length fragment, a second, smaller band is observed, migrating below the full-length band (Figure B2.1.2). This is the partially deleted mtDNA. By digesting with an appropriate battery of enzymes, the site of the deletion can be mapped. In the case of the ~5-kb 'common deletion,' the deleted band is observed at ~11.5 kb on the blot. The two bands can be quantitated (e.g. by densitometry) to yield the percentage of mutation.

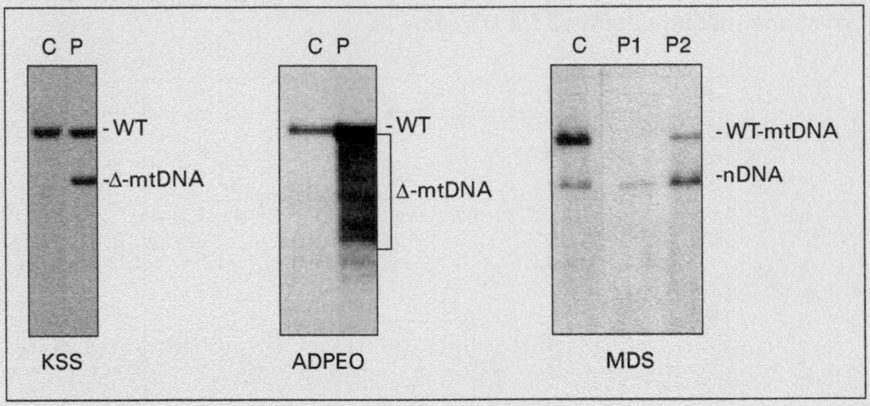

Figure B2.1.2 Example of Southern blot analysis. Detection of mtDNA deletions (KSS and ADPEO) and depletions (MDS). C, control, P, P1, P2, patients

In the case of multiple deletions, as in ADPEO, there are multiple bands on the gel, sometimes so many that they appear as a 'smear' of hybridizing fragments appearing below the 16.6-kb normal fragment.

Depletion of mtDNA

The ultimate deletion is loss of the entire mitochondrial genome: i.e. mtDNA depletion syndrome (MDS). Diagnosis in this case also involves a Southern blot, but requires a slight modification to allow for quantitation of the degree of depletion: two probes are used, one to visualize the wt-mtDNA and the other to visualize nuclear DNA. The nDNA is used as an internal control to normalize for the amount of total DNA loaded, and the ratio of mtDNA:nDNA in control vs the MDS patient is used to determine the % depletion in the patient. Typically, the nDNA probe is the nuclear gene encoding the 18S ribosomal RNA (rDNA), which is present at about 400 copies/cell; since mtDNA is about 1% of total DNA, the multi-copy rDNA signal comes up rapidly enough to allow it to be visualized with an intensity similar to that of the mtDNA signal.

References

1. Schon EA, Naini A, Shanske S. Identification of mutations in mtDNA from patients suffering mitochondrial diseases. *Methods Mol Biol* 2002; **197**: 55–74.

seizures. MRI scans of acute stroke-like events in MELAS reveal lesions with increased signal on T2-weighted or on fluid attenuation inversion recovery (FLAIR) images. The lesions do not conform to the territories of large cerebral arteries, but rather affect the cortex and subadjacent white matter with sparing of deeper white matter[15] (Figure 2.4). Acute MELAS brain lesions may fluctuate, migrate, or even disappear. Calcification of the basal ganglia is frequently observed.[16] Cerebral angiograms in MELAS patients have confirmed absence of large-vessel pathology by demonstrating normal results, increased caliber of arteries, veins, or capillary blush with early venous filling.[14] The acute stroke-like lesions appear as high signals on diffusion-weighted imaging (DWI) with normal or increased apparent diffusion coefficient (ADC) values suggesting vasogenic edema.[17–20] By contrast, acute ischemic strokes show increased DWI signal with decreased ADC values, indicative of cytotoxic edema.

Quantitative cerebral blood flow studies by xenon CT have revealed normal or increased blood flow in acute lesions and in unaffected brain tissue, suggesting that the stroke-like events are not due to focal ischemia.[21,22] Single photon emission computed tomography (SPECT) studies have generally revealed decreased tracer accumulation in acute and subacute lesions, possibly due to loss of metabolically active cells.[23–26] Interestingly, SPECT scans showed focal increased tracer in two MELAS patients studied three and six days prior to the appearance of brain CT lucencies in the same regions, indicating that localized increased blood flow preceded the stroke-like events. Similarly, a PET study of a patient six days before a stroke-like episode showed increased regional cerebral blood flow in the frontal lobe, where MRI then revealed a new lesion.[27] The focally increased blood flow prior to an acute stroke-like episode may reflect localized response to increased lactate, focal increased metabolism, or altered vasoregulation. Some studies of MELAS patients have shown decreased cerebral blood flow reactivity to carbon dioxide or acetazolamide in the setting of cerebral hyperemia, suggesting loss of vascular autoregulation;[21,28] however, other studies have demonstrated normal vasoreactivity to acetazolamide loading.[29,30]

Reflecting defects of the mitochondrial respiratory chain, PET studies of MELAS patients have demonstrated decreased cerebral oxygen metabolic rates ($rCMRO_2$) both focally and globally.[27,30] In addition, cerebral PET studies of patients with mitochondrial encephalopathies have revealed decreased oxygen consumption relative to glucose utilization, further confirming the impairment of oxidative phosphorylation.[30,31] MRS studies have revealed elevated lactate in MELAS brains, indicating a compensatory increase in anaerobic glycolysis.[32,33] We have observed that the levels of ventricular lactate correlated directly with the severity of the neurological impairment in MELAS (Figure 2.3).[33] Phosphorus MRS studies have shown decreased levels of high-energy phosphate compounds in the brains of patients with mitochondrial encephalomyopathies.[34]

Taken together, neuroradiological studies in MELAS have revealed that the atypical stroke-like episodes may not be due to acute ischemia, but rather related to metabolic dysfunction with decreased oxidative phosphorylation, increased lactic acid, and presumably, diminished ATP synthesis. Cerebral hyperemia has been observed both focally and globally and may be triggered by increased lactate, neuronal hyperexcitability, or altered vasoreactivity. The role, if any, of altered cerebrovascular autoregulation in MELAS remains uncertain.

Although at least 15 distinct mitochondrial DNA (mtDNA) mutations have been associated with MELAS, about 80% of patients have the A3243G $tRNA^{Leu(UUR)}$ gene mutation.[35,36] Most MELAS mutations are in tRNA genes, but some are in polypeptide-coding genes, including subunit III of cytochrome *c* oxidase (COX) and subunits 1, 5, and 6 of complex I. Interestingly, the G13513A mutation in subunit 5 of complex I (ND5) is a common cause of overlap syndromes between

MELAS, Leber hereditary optic neuropathy, and Leigh syndrome. It is not clear why mutations in such diverse mtDNA-encoded genes produce the MELAS phenotype. In the case of the A3243G MELAS mutation, the altered tRNA fails to undergo proper post-translational modification, namely, addition of a taurine to the anticodon uridine wobble-base, leading to impaired mitochondrial protein synthesis.[37]

To diagnose MELAS, neuroimaging studies and measurement of blood lactate are useful screening tests. The diagnosis can be confirmed by screening blood DNA for the common MELAS mutations. In cases without a common MELAS point mutation, muscle biopsy can be diagnostic by demonstrating ragged-red fibers, biochemical defects of the respiratory chain, or both. These, in turn, provide clues for further molecular genetic studies to identify the causative mutation.

Neuropathological studies of MELAS brain have revealed multifocal necrosis predominantly in the cerebral cortex and subcortical white matter, but also in the cerebellum, thalamus, and basal ganglia (Figure 2.4).[38,39] The lesions resemble areas of infarction, but do not conform to the territories of large cerebral vessels. Spongiform degeneration in the cortex, proliferation of capillaries, and some neuronal loss are invariably present. Abnormal and excessive mitochondria have been observed in smooth muscle and endothelial cells of small arterioles (less than 250 μm in diameter) and capillaries of MELAS brains.[40] Epithelial cells of the choroid plexus have also revealed morphologically abnormal and excessive mitochondria.[39,41] The changes in the cerebral blood vessels and choroid plexus may contribute to the breakdown of the blood–brain barrier, which has been demonstrated by the presence of fibrinogen in the frontal cortex of MELAS patients[39] and by neuroradiological studies showing evidence of vasogenic edema.

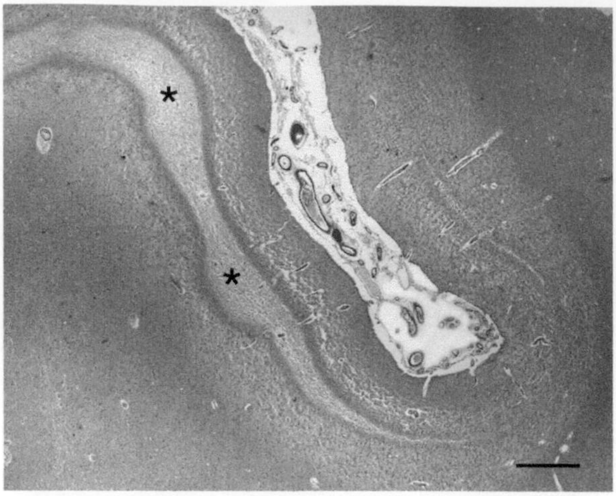

Figure 2.4 MELAS. Section of the occipital cortex stained with H&E illustrates an infarct (black asterisks). The lesion affects deep layers of the cortex. Bar=4 μm

Treatment of MELAS has been focused on symptomatic management of seizures, diabetes mellitus, and other medical complications. Some clinicians advocate aggressive control of epilepsy in MELAS because the increased metabolic stress of seizures may precipitate stroke-like events. Because levels of ventricular lactate correlated with severity of symptoms in patients with the MELAS A3243G mutation, dichloroacetate (DCA) therapy had been suggested for the treatment of MELAS. Several reports of open-label treatment suggested that DCA might be beneficial; however, in a double-blind, randomized, placebo-controlled trial of MELAS patients with the A3243G mtDNA mutation, we found no treatment benefit and the trial was terminated early due to peripheral nerve toxicity.[42] The observation of altered cerebral vasodilatation in MELAS prompted Koga and colleagues to administer L-arginine, a nitric oxide precursor, to stimulate vasodilation in this disorder (see Box 2.2).[43,44] In preliminary open-label studies, intravenous L-arginine shortly after the onset of stroke-like episodes appeared to improve outcomes, while oral administration during interictal phases seemed to decrease the frequency and severity of stroke-like events.[43,44] While promising, these findings need to be confirmed in controlled clinical trials.

Myoclonus epilepsy and ragged-red fibers (MERRF)

MERRF is a multisystem mitochondrial disorder defined by: myoclonus, generalized epilepsy, ataxia, and ragged-red fibers in the muscle biopsy. Onset is usually in childhood, but adult-onset has been described. Besides the defining criteria, other common clinical manifestations include impaired hearing, dementia, axonal peripheral neuropathy, short stature, exercise intolerance, and lactic acidosis. The following manifestations have been reported in fewer than half of the MERRF patients: optic nerve atrophy, cardiomyopathy, electrocardiographic pre-excitation syndrome, pigmentary retinopathy, pyramidal tract signs, ophthalmoparesis, pes cavus, and multiple lipomatosis.

MERRF has been associated with at least six different point mutations of mitochondrial DNA, however, about 80% of MERRF patients harbor an A-to-G transition mutation at nucleotide 8344 of the $tRNA^{Lys}$ gene.[45] A second point mutation was found in $tRNA^{Lys}$ at nucleotide 8356 (T8356C) in a pedigree with typical MERRF,[46] and in another with a MERRF–MELAS overlap syndrome.[47] Two additional mutations in $tRNA^{Lys}$ have been identified in MERRF patients, one at nucleotide 8363[48] and the other at nucleotide 8361.[49] Thus, the mitochondrial $tRNA^{Lys}$ gene is a hotspot for mutations causing MERRF. A mutation in $tRNA^{Phe}$ was identified in one family with MERRF[50] and a single patient was found to have multiple mitochondrial DNA deletions.[51] MtDNA point mutations at nucleotide 7512 in $tRNA^{Ser(UCN)}$ and at nucleotide 12147 in $tRNA^{His}$ have also been associated with MERRF and MELAS overlap syndromes.[52,53] A single patient with a point mutation in $tRNA^{Leu(UUR)}$ had a MERRF and Kearns–Sayre overlap syndrome.[54]

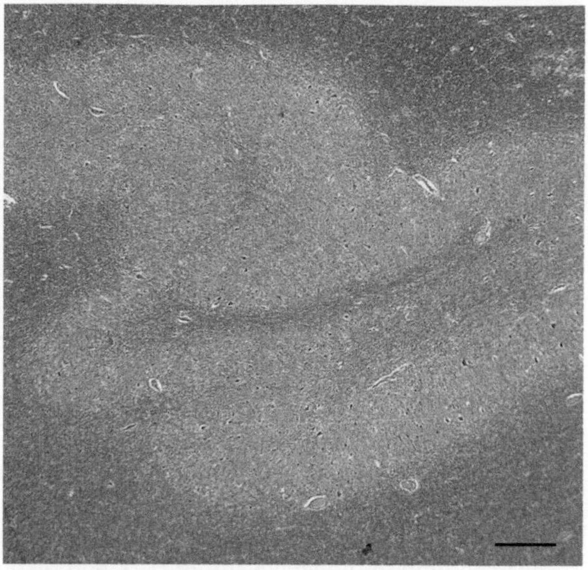

Figure 2.5 Myclonus epilepsy with ragged-red fibers (MERRF). Section of the dentate nucleus stained with H&E illustrates loss of multipolar neurons. Bar = 6 μm

In patients suspected of having MERRF, screening blood DNA for mtDNA mutations can confirm the diagnosis. As with MELAS, absence of a common mtDNA mutation does not exclude the diagnosis of MERRF. Therefore, in patients who fulfill clinical criteria for MERRF but lack one of the typical mtDNA mutations, muscle biopsy may be warranted to confirm the diagnosis.

Neuropathological studies have revealed multisystemic degeneration with selective neuronal loss, astrocytosis, and degeneration of myelinated tracts.[55] In MERRF, paucity of neurons is most prominent in the cerebellum, brainstem, and spinal cord.[38] In the cerebellum, neuronal loss is consistently seen in the dentate nucleus (Figure 2.5), is milder in Purkinje cells, and is rare in the granular layer.[55] The cerebellar lesions probably account for the prominent ataxia in MERRF. The inferior olivary nucleus is the most severely affected region in the brainstem, while the red nucleus and substantia

Box 2.2 The 'MELAS paradox'

The high morbidity and mortality of MELAS is due in large part to its angiopathic nature, which is almost unique in mitochondrial diseases. In mtDNA disorders associated with ragged-red fibers, the RRFs are typically negative for cytochrome *c* oxidase (COX) activity. In MELAS, however, the RRFs are typically COX-positive, even though COX activity in MELAS cells and cybrids is reduced by about 70%. There is also mitochondrial proliferation in the blood vessels – called 'strongly succinate dehydrogenase-positive vessels,' or SSVs – and these, too, are COX-positive. On the other hand, patients with MERRF also have RRFs and SSVs, but both the RRFs and the SSVs in that disorder are COX-negative. In spite of the greater degree of respiratory impairment in MERRF as compared to MELAS, it is MELAS, and not MERRF, that has the greater morbidity and mortality. Shouldn't it be the other way around?

Ironically, it may be the very presence of COX activity in SSVs that is killing the patient. In particular, Naini et al. have proposed that total COX activity in the vasculature of MELAS patients is increased above normal levels, and that this increase is harmful, due to alterations in circulating levels of nitric oxide (NO).[1] NO plays an important role in controlling vascular smooth muscle tone. Interestingly, NO can bind to the active site of COX and displace heme-bound oxygen. Thus, the higher morbidity observed in MELAS as compared to MERRF could be due to a shortage of NO required for vasodilation, due to a 'titration effect' by elevated amounts of COX in MELAS blood vessels.

But if the MELAS mutation impairs protein synthesis and reduces COX activity, how can COX activity be elevated over normal? This seeming paradox can be resolved by noting that even though overall COX activity in muscle is reduced on a relative basis (e.g. COX activity normalized to citrate synthase (CS) activity), it is not reduced on an absolute basis (COX activity per cell).[1] Furthermore, when one considers only the SSVs (and RRFs), the COX activity is actually increased over normals. For example, even though COX activity per mitochondrion is only about 1/3 that of normal mitochondria, if there is an ~10-fold increase in mitochondrial mass in an SSV, the absolute amount of COX activity in that SSV would be elevated approximately three-fold over normal.

Thus, in the normal situation, when the body senses a need for NO-induced vasodilation, it occurs normally. The same is true for MERRF patients, because they have COX-negative SSVs and COX-normal 'non-SSVs' (in those cells the mutation is below the threshold for dysfunction), thus allowing for sufficient circulating NO to induce vasodilation. In MELAS, however, vasodilation is inhibited or retarded, owing to the presence of elevated COX levels in both SSVs and in 'non-SSVs' that reduce the concentration of circulating NO. The failure to vasodilate at the appropriate time or place may precipitate the stroke-like episodes that are a hallmark of MELAS.

The 'NO titration' hypothesis implies that elevating NO levels should be therapeutically helpful in MELAS, using compounds such as L-arginine,[1] nitroglycerin[1,2] or even Nicorandil,[1] a potassium channel blocker used for the control of heart arrhythmias. In fact, Koga and colleagues studied the effects of L-arginine on the acute phase of strokes in MELAS patients and found a marked improvement in most symptoms.[2]

References

1. Naini A, Kaufmann P, Shanske S et al. Hypocitrullinemia in patients with MELAS: an insight into the 'MELAS paradox'. *J Neurol Sci* 2005; **229–230**: 187–193.
2. Koga Y, Akita Y, Nishioka J et al. L-arginine improves the symptoms of strokelike episodes in MELAS. *Neurology* 2005; **64**: 710–712.

nigra are involved to a lesser extent.[55] In the spinal cord, degeneration of the posterior columns is usually prominent and there are significant reductions of neurons in Clark's nucleus and milder loss in the anterior and posterior horns.

The cerebral cortex appears to be particularly vulnerable in MERRF, as suggested by the high frequency of dementia, myoclonus, and epilepsy. Giant somatosensory evoked potentials indicate abnormal cortical excitability, which may account for the cortical reflex myoclonus in MERRF.[56,57] PET studies have revealed decreased cerebral glucose metabolism and oxygen consumption with normal cerebral blood flows, indicating decreased baseline oxidative phosphorylation.[58] However, it is unclear whether the metabolic changes are the result or the cause of cerebral dysfunction.

Kearns–Sayre syndrome (KSS)

In 1958, Kearns and Sayre reported two patients with the clinical triad of 'retinitis pigmentosa, external ophthalmoplegia, and complete heart block'.[59] Thus, KSS was the first multisystem mitochondrial disorder to be defined clinically. The predominant clinical features are found in the central nervous system, skeletal muscle, and heart and the syndrome has been defined by Dr. Lewis P. Rowland by the obligatory triad of: (1) onset before age 20; (2) pigmentary retinopathy; and (3) progressive external ophthalmoplegia.[60] In addition, at least one of the following must be present: (1) cardiac conduction block; (2) cerebrospinal fluid protein greater than 100 mg/dL; (3) cerebellar ataxia. Other clinical manifestations seen in the majority of KSS patients include short stature, hearing loss, impaired intellect (mental retardation, dementia, or both), and limb weakness. Neuropsychological testing of 15 patients revealed specific cognitive defects, particularly visual construction, attention, and abstraction/flexibility, suggesting dysfunction of parieto-occipital lobes and prefrontal cortex.[61] Endocrinopathies that have been reported include diabetes mellitus, hypoparathyroidism, irregular menses, and growth hormone deficiency.[62]

Onset is usually in childhood, with insidious ptosis, ophthalmoparesis, or both. The extraocular movement defects sometimes cause blurred or double vision. Weakness of the orbicularis oculi can lead to corneal ulcerations and in one patient caused corneal perforation.[63] Symptoms sometimes appear at the time of, or shortly after, a febrile illness. The disease progresses over years. If the cardiac conduction defect becomes complete heart block, and a pacemaker is not inserted in time, the patient may die at a young age. Dysphagia is not uncommon; in one study of 12 patients, nine had documented cricopharyngeal achalasia (incomplete opening of the upper esophageal sphincter during the pharyngeal phase of swallowing).[64] Pearson syndrome (sideroblastic anemia with pancreatic exocrine insufficiency) can precede Kearns–Sayre syndrome.[65] This form of anemia can be fatal in infancy, and has been associated with the same mitochondrial DNA defect seen in KSS.

Large-scale deletions of mitochondrial DNA have been found in over 90% of KSS patients.[66] Large-scale duplications of mitochondrial DNA have been found in some patients.[66] Because mtDNA deletions are typically undetectable in blood of KSS patients, muscle biopsy is required to identify the pathogenic mutation.

The central nervous system shows spongiform changes predominantly in the white matter, including neuronal degeneration, gliosis, and demyelination (Figure 2.6).[38,68] Mineral deposits of calcium and iron have been noted in and around blood vessels in the basal ganglia and thalamus. Vascular proliferation has also been described, but without a consistent topographic pattern. Histological studies have revealed mitochondrial abnormalities in the cerebellar dentate

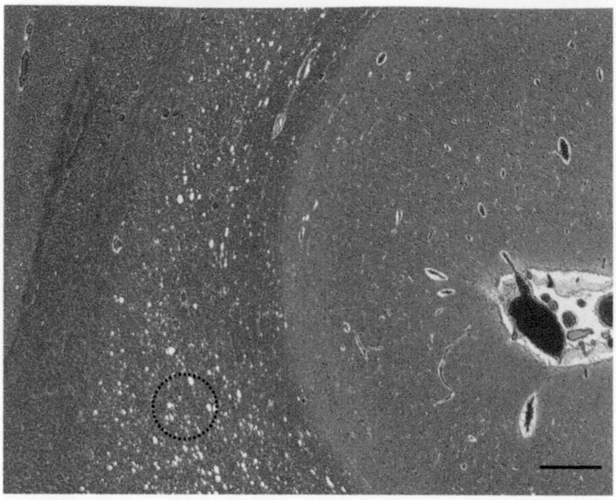

Figure 2.6 Kearns–Sayre syndrome (KSS). Section of the frontal cortex stained with H&E illustrates spongy degeneration (dotted circle) confined to white matter. Bar = 8 µm

nucleus, loss of Purkinje cells, spongiform degeneration of the cerebellar white matter, and disconnection of Purkinje cells at the dentate nucleus; these abnormalities may contribute to the cerebellar ataxia of KSS.[69,70]

Neuropathy ataxia retinitis pigmentosa (NARP)

NARP is a maternally transmitted multisystem disorder of young adult life, defined by the combination of sensory neuropathy, ataxia, seizures, dementia, and retinitis pigmentosa. Lactic acid in blood may be normal or slightly elevated, and muscle biopsies do not show RRF.

The most common molecular defect is a point mutation (T8993G) in the gene that encodes ATPase 6.[9] When this mutation approaches homoplasmic levels, onset is in infancy, and the clinical and neuropathologic features are those of Leigh syndrome (maternally inherited Leigh syndrome (MILS)).[8] A different mutation at the very same nucleotide (T8993C) causes a phenotype similar to MILS but generally milder. Both mutations can be identified in blood of patients.

Mitochondrial neurogastrointestinal encephalomyopathy (MNGIE)

Mitochondrial neurogastrointestinal encephalomyopathy (MNGIE) is an autosomal recessive multisystem disease, which is clinically recognizable by the combination of ptosis, ophthalmoplegia, peripheral neuropathy, severe gastrointestinal dysmotility leading to cachexia, and leukoencephalopathy evident on brain MRI.[71,72] The average age at onset is 19 years but can vary from infancy to 43 years. The disease is progressive and gastrointestinal manifestations lead to death, on average, at age 37 (range 18–58 years).[72]

MNGIE is caused by loss-of-function mutations in the gene encoding thymidine phosphorylase (TP),[73] a cytosolic enzyme that degrades the nucleosides thymidine and deoxyuridine. In MNGIE patients, TP activity in buffy coat is less than 10% of normal control means.[73] Loss of TP leads to dramatic elevations of thymidine and deoxyuridine in plasma of patients.[74] The diagnosis of MNGIE is confirmed by biochemical tests showing TP deficiency in buffy coat or elevated plasma thymidine and deoxyuridine. It has been hypothesized that accumulations of thymidine and deoxyuridine in MNGIE lead to depletion, multiple deletions, and site-specific point mutations of mtDNA, which cause mitochondrial respiratory chain defects;[75,76] therefore, MNGIE is a disease caused by mitochondrial nucleotide pool imbalances (see Box 6.1).

Although brain MRIs of MNGIE patients shows dramatically increased T2-weighted and FLAIR signals in the white matter (Figure 2.2),[77] patients generally do not show overt cognitive dysfunction; however, two patients developed psychosis in the terminal stage of the disease (M. Hirano, personal observation). The leukoencephalopathy in

MNGIE appears to be due to impairment of the blood–brain barrier and edema rather than to demyelination, thus accounting for the lack of clinical encephalopathy.[78]

Alpers syndrome

Alpers or Alpers–Huttenlocher syndrome was first reported by Bernard Alpers, who described a previously healthy 3-month-old girl who developed intractable seizures, blindness, and became stuporous before dying at age 4 months.[79] Neuropathology revealed widespread degeneration of the cortex and basal ganglia. Huttenlocher and colleagues described the pathological findings in the liver, which included microvesicular steatosis, proliferation of bile ducts, and cirrhosis.[80] Clinically, Alpers syndrome is characterized by autosomal recessive inheritance, normal early development, episodic neurodegeneration with psychomotor regression, seizures that become intractable, and hepatopathy. The occipital lobe is frequently affected, leading to cortical blindness. Onset is usually in infancy or childhood, but can extend to 25 years.

Ultrastructurally abnormal mitochondria in cerebral neurons suggested that the disease might be a mitochondrial encephalopathy[81] and this was confirmed by the identification of depletion of mtDNA associated with pathogenic mutations in mitochondrial DNA polymerase γ (POLG).[82]

Hepatocerebral syndrome with mtDNA depletion

Hepatocerebral syndrome with mtDNA depletion is clinically and etiologically similar to Alpers syndrome. The disorder was originally described in three large Druze kindreds whose affected children presented before age 6 month with severe hepatopathy, failure to thrive, hypoglycemia, psychomotor delay, oscillating nystagmus, and elevated blood lactate.[83] Most died before age 1 year. Histology of the liver revealed 'oncocytic transformation', i.e. marked proliferation of morphologically abnormal mitochondria, with microvesicular steatosis, cholestasis, and focal cytoplasmic biliary necrosis.[84] Liver samples revealed deficiencies of mitochondrial respiratory chain complexes containing mtDNA-encoded subunits (complexes I, III, and IV) and depletion of mtDNA (5–39% of control mean value).[83,84]

Mutations in the deoxyguanosine kinase gene (*DGUOK*) were identified as the cause of hepatocerebral syndrome with mtDNA depletion.[83] Deoxyguanosine kinase is located in the mitochondrial matrix, and is responsible for the phosphorylation of purine nucleosides that are required for mtDNA replication. Although a significant cause of mtDNA depletion, mutations in deoxyguanosine kinase were identified in only three of 21 (14%) patients with mtDNA depletion in liver indicating that additional genes can cause hepatic mtDNA depletion.[85]

Encephalomyopathy with mtDNA depletion

In a small consanguineous family with autosomal recessive encephalomyopathy and mtDNA depletion, a pathogenic mutation was identified in *SUCLA2*, a gene encoding the β-subunit of the ADP-forming succinyl-CoA synthetase ligase.[86] Although this is an enzyme of the Krebs cycle, it also appears to form a complex with the mitochondrial nucleotide diphosphate kinase.[86] Thus, the *SUCLA2* mutation may impair the penultimate step in the mitochondrial dNT salvage pathway and cause mtDNA depletion.

Coenzyme Q10 deficiency

Coenzyme Q10 (CoQ10) is a small lipophilic molecule located in the inner mitochondrial membrane and composed of a quinone group and a poly-isoprenoid tail. CoQ10 transfers reducing equivalents from complexes I and II to complex III. Deficiency of CoQ10 in skeletal muscle has been associated with three major phenotypes. A predominantly myopathic form is characterized by the triad of recurrent myoglobinuria, ragged-red fibers, and encephalopathy with seizures, ataxia, or mild mental retardation.[87] A more common ataxic form presents with cerebellar ataxia and atrophy with variable involvement of the peripheral nerves, muscle, and other CNS functions.[88,89] The third variant is a rare infantile encephalomyopathy with nephropathy.[90] It is important for clinicians to recognize patients with CoQ10 deficiency because the syndrome responds dramatically to CoQ10 supplementation (400–3000 mg daily in adult patients).

Deficiency of CoQ10 has been presumed to be due to defects in CoQ10 biosynthesis; however, in one family with four affected members (three siblings and a cousin), a stop-codon mutation in the aprataxin gene (*APTX*) was identified.[91] Aprataxin is thought to be involved in single-strand DNA break repair and mutations in the gene cause ataxia with oculomotor apraxia 1 (AOA1), an autosomal recessive disorder.[92,93] The relationship of aprataxin mutations to CoQ10 deficiency is unclear, but CoQ10 supplementation in the three siblings with aprataxin mutations was associated with dramatic improvement; all went from being wheelchair-bound to being able to walk a few steps. In addition, after initiating CoQ10 supplementation, seizures in the affected sister disappeared and she was able to discontinue her anti-epileptic drug. In two siblings of consanguineous parents with the infantile form of CoQ10 deficiency, we identified a homozygous missense mutation in the *COQ2* gene, which encodes para-hydroxybenzoate:polyprenyl transferase, a vital enzyme required for CoQ10 biosynthesis.[94,95]

Conclusions

Frequent and heterogeneous involvement of the central nervous system is often the predominant clinical manifestation in mitochondrial diseases. The encephalopathy in Leigh and Alpers syndromes, stroke-like episodes in MELAS, myoclonic epilepsy in MERRF, and ataxia in Kearns–Sayre syndrome, NARP and coenzyme Q10 deficiency are often clinically debilitating. Mitochondrial respiratory chain enzymes and oxidative phosphorylation are impaired in all of these disorders and therefore defective ATP synthesis appears to be the pathogenic common denominator. If so, why should defects of ATP production cause diverse phenotypes?

Pathological, biochemical, and molecular genetic studies have shed some light on the pathogenic similarities and differences in mitochondrial encephalopathies. For example, Leigh syndrome predominantly affects deep gray matter structures, basal ganglia, periaqueductal gray matter and bulbar nuclei in the brainstem while MELAS is associated with cortical lesions. The divergent topologies of the lesions may be related to age-specific vulnerabilities of the brain; however, this explanation begs the questions as to why deep gray matter structures in infants with Leigh syndrome and cerebral cortex in children with MELAS are differentially vulnerable to bioenergetic defects. Excitoxicity may contribute to the neuronal degeneration in both disorders. This notion is supported by the clinical observation that acute cerebral lesions are often temporally associated with seizures.

Curiously, in both Leigh syndrome and MELAS, cerebral microvascular changes have been observed before neuronal degeneration ensues, suggesting that vasculopathy could contribute to the pathogenesis of these disorders. In addition to microvascular proliferation, breakdown of the blood–brain barrier has been seen in MELAS and neuroimaging studies have revealed vasogenic edema in acute stroke-like episodes and focal and generalized cerebral hyperemia. Breakdown of the blood–brain barrier has also been observed in KSS and MNGIE. It is not yet clear whether the vascular changes are deleterious by allowing lactate and other potentially toxic metabolites to permeate the brain or are compensatory phenomena in response to the metabolic abnormalities. Clearly, better characterization of CNS lesions in mitochondrial medicine will be important to understand these complex diseases and to develop much-needed therapies.

References

1. Leigh D. Subacute necrotizing encephalomyelopathy in an infant. *J Neurol Neurosurg Psychiatry* 1951; **14**: 216–221.
2. Worsley HE, Brookfield RW, Elwood JS et al. Lactic acidosis with necrotizing encephalopathy in two sibs. *Arch Dis Child* 1965; **40**: 492–501.
3. Hommes FA, Polman HA, Reerink JD. Leigh's encephalomyelopathy: an inborn error of gluconeogenesis. *Arch Dis Child* 1968; **43**: 423–426.
4. Bourgeron T, Rustin P, Chretien D et al. Mutation of a nuclear succinate dehydrogenase gene results in mitochondrial respiratory chain deficiency. *Nature Genet* 1995; **11**: 144–149.
5. Ugalde C, Janssen RJ, van den Heuvel LP et al. Differences in assembly or stability of complex I and other mitochondrial OXPHOS complexes in inherited complex I deficiency. *Hum Mol Genet* 2004; **13**: 659–667.
6. Tiranti V, Hoertnagel K, Carrozzo R et al. Mutations of SURF-1 in Leigh disease associated with cytochrome *c* oxidase deficiency. *Am J Hum Genet* 1998; **63**: 1609–1621.
7. Zhu S, Yao J, Johns T et al. *SURF1*, encoding a factor involved in the biogenesis of cytochrome *c* oxidase, is mutated in Leigh syndrome. *Nat Genet* 1998; **20**: 337–343.
8. Santorelli FM, Shanske S, Macaya A et al. The mutation at nt 8993 of mitochondrial DNA is a common cause of Leigh syndrome. *Ann Neurol* 1993; **34**: 827–834.
9. Holt IJ, Harding AE, Petty RK et al. A new mitochondrial disease associated with mitochondrial DNA heteroplasmy. *Am J Hum Genet* 1990; **46**: 428–433.
10. Beal MF. Does impairment of energy metabolism result in excitotoxic neuronal death in neurodegenerative illnesses? *Ann Neurol* 1992; **31**: 119–130.
11. Macaya A, Munell F, Burke RE et al. Disorders of movement in Leigh syndrome. *Neuropediatrics* 1993; **24**: 60–67.
12. Cavanagh JB, Harding BN. Pathogenic factors underlying the lesions in Leigh's disease. Tissue responses to cellular energy deprivation and their clinico-pathological consequences. *Brain* 1994; **117**(Pt 6): 1357–1376.
13. Pavlakis SG, Phillips PC, DiMauro S et al. Mitochondrial myopathy, encephalopathy, lactic acidosis, and strokelike episodes: a distinctive clinical syndrome. *Ann Neurol* 1984; **16**: 481–488.
14. Hirano M, Pavlakis S. Mitochondrial myopathy, encephalopathy, lactic acidosis, and strokelike episodes (MELAS): current concepts. *J Child Neurol* 1994; **9**: 4–13.
15. Matthews PM, Tampieri D, Berkovic SF et al. Magnetic resonance imaging shows specific abnormalities in the MELAS syndrome. *Neurology* 1991; **41**: 1043–1046.
16. Sue CM, Crimmins DS, Soo YS et al. Neuroradiological features of six kindreds with MELAS $tRNA^{Leu}$ A2343G point mutation: implications for pathogenesis. *J Neurol Neurosurg Psychiatry* 1998; **65**: 233–240.
17. Yoneda M, Maeda M, Kimura H et al. Vasogenic edema on MELAS: a serial study with diffusion-weighted MR imaging. *Neurology* 1999; **53**: 2182–2184.
18. Ohshita T, Oka M, Imon Y et al. Serial diffusion-weighted imaging in MELAS. *Neuroradiology* 2000; **42**: 651–656.
19. Oppenheim C, Galanaud D, Samson Y et al. Can diffusion weighted magnetic resonance imaging help differentiate stroke from stroke-like events in MELAS? *J Neurol Neurosurg Psychiatry* 2000; **69**: 248–250.
20. Kolb SJ, Costello F, Lee AG et al. Distinguishing ischemic stroke from the stroke-like lesions of MELAS using apparent diffusion coefficient mapping. *J Neurol Sci* 2003; **216**: 11–15.
21. Morita K, Ono S, Fukunaga M et al. Increased accumulation of N-isopropyl-p-(^{123}I)-iodoamphetamine in two cases with mitochondrial encephalomyopathy with lactic acidosis and strokelike episodes (MELAS). *Neuroradiology* 1989; **31**: 358–361.
22. Ooiwa Y, Uematsu Y, Terada T et al. Cerebral blood flow in mitochondrial myopathy, encephalopathy,

lactic acidosis, and strokelike episodes. *Stroke* 1993; **24**: 304–309.
23. Satoh M, Ishikawa N, Yoshizawa T et al. N-isopropyl-p-[^{123}I]iodoamphetamine SPECT in MELAS syndrome: comparison with CT and MR imaging. *J Comput Assist Tomogr* 1991; **15**: 77–82.
24. Seyama K, Suzuki K, Mizuno Y et al. Mitochondrial encephalomyopathy with lactic acidosis and stroke-like episodes with special reference to the mechanism of cerebral manifestations. *Acta Neurol Scand* 1989; **80**: 561–568.
25. Watanabe Y, Hashikawa K, Moriwaki H et al. SPECT findings in mitochondrial encephalomyopathy. *J Nucl Med* 1998; **39**: 961–964.
26. Gropen T, Prohovnik I, Tatemichi T et al. Cerebral hyperemia in MELAS. *Stroke* 1994; **25**: 1873–1876.
27. Takahashi S, Tohgi H, Yonezawa H et al. Cerebral blood flow and oxygen metabolism before and after a stroke-like episode in patients with mitochondrial myopathy, encephalopathy, lactic acidosis and stroke-like episodes (MELAS). *J Neurol Sci* 1998; **158**: 58–64.
28. Clark JM, Marks MP, Adalsteinsson E et al. MELAS: Clinical and pathologic correlations with MRI, xenon/CT, and MR spectroscopy. *Neurology* 1996; **46**: 223–227.
29. Molnar MJ, Valikovics A, Molnar S et al. Cerebral blood flow and glucose metabolism in mitochondrial disorders. *Neurology* 2000; **55**: 544–548.
30. Nariai T, Ohno K, Ohta Y et al. Discordance between cerebral oxygen and glucose metabolism, and hemodynamics in a mitochondrial encephalomyopathy, lactic acidosis, and strokelike episode patient. *J Neuroimaging* 2001; **11**: 325–329.
31. Frackowiak RS, Herold S, Petty RK et al. The cerebral metabolism of glucose and oxygen measured with positron tomography in patients with mitochondrial diseases. *Brain* 1988; **111**(Pt 5): 1009–1024.
32. Dubeau F, De Stefano N, Zifkin BG et al. Oxidative phosphorylation defect in the brains of carriers of the $tRNA^{Leu(UUR)}$ A3243G mutation in a MELAS pedigree. *Ann Neurol* 2000; **47**: 179–185.
33. Kaufmann P, Shungu DC, Sano MC et al. Cerebral lactic acidosis correlates with neurological impairment in MELAS. *Neurology* 2004; **62**: 1297–1302.
34. Eleff SM, Barker PB, Brandband SJ et al. Phosphorus magnetic resonance spectroscopy of patients with mitochondrial cytopathies demonstrated decreased levels of brain phosphocreatine. *Ann Neurol* 1990; **27**: 626–630.
35. Goto Y, Nonaka I, Horai S. A mutation in the $tRNA^{Leu(UUR)}$ gene associated with the MELAS subgroup of mitochondrial encephalomyopathies. *Nature* 1990; **348**: 651–653.
36. Hirano M. MELAS. In: Gilman S, ed. Medlink Neurology. Vol. 2004. San Diego: Medlink Corporation, 2004.
37. Yasukawa T, Suzuki T, Ueda T et al. Modification defect at anticodon wobble nucleotide of mitochondrial $tRNAs^{Leu(UUR)}$ with pathogenic mutations of mitochondrial myopathy, encephalopathy, lactic acidosis, and stroke-like episodes. *J Biol Chem* 2000; **275**: 4251–4257.
38. Sparaco M, Bonilla E, DiMauro S et al. Neuropathology of mitochondrial encephalomyopathies due to mitochondrial DNA defects. *J Neuropath Exp Neurol* 1993; **52**: 1–10.
39. Tanji K, Kunimatsu T, Vu TH et al. Neuropathological features of mitochondrial disorders. *Semin Cell Dev Biol* 2001; **12**: 429–439.
40. Ohama E, Ohara S, Ikuta F et al. Mitochondrial angiopathy in cerebral blood vessels of mitochondrial encephalomyopathy. *Acta Neuropath* 1987; **74**: 226–233.
41. Ohama E, Ikuta F. Involvement of choroid plexus in mitochondrial encephalomyopathy (MELAS). *Acta Neuropath* 1987; **75**: 1–7.
42. Kaufmann P, Engelstad K, Wei Y et al. A randomized placebo-controlled trial of dichloroacetate in MELAS. Toxicity overshadows possible benefit. *Neurology* 2006; in press.
43. Koga Y, Akita Y, Nishioka J et al. L-arginine improves the symptoms of strokelike episodes in MELAS. *Neurology* 2005; **64**: 710–712.
44. Koga Y, Ishibashi M, Ueki I et al. Effects of L-arginine on the acute phase of strokes in three patients with MELAS. *Neurology* 2002; **58**: 827–828.
45. Shoffner JM, Lott MT, Lezza AMS et al. Myoclonic epilepsy and ragged-red fiber disease (MERRF) is associated with a mitochondrial DNA tRNALys mutation. *Cell* 1990; **61**: 931–937.
46. Silvestri G, Moraes CT, Shanske S et al. A new mtDNA mutation in the $tRNA^{Lys}$ gene associated with myoclonic epilepsy and ragged-red fibers (MERRF). *Am J Hum Genet* 1992; **51**: 1213–1217.
47. Zeviani M, Muntoni F, Savarese N et al. A MERRF/MELAS overlap syndrome with a new point

mutation in the mitochondrial DNA $tRNA^{Lys}$ gene. *Eur J Hum Genet* 1993; **1**: 80–87.
48. Ozawa M, Nishino I, Horai S et al. Myoclonus epilepsy associated with ragged-red fibers: a G-to-A mutation at nucleotide pair 8363 in mitochondrial $tRNA^{Lys}$ in two families. *Muscle Nerve* 1997; **20**: 271–278.
49. Rossmanith W, Raffelsberger T, Roka J et al. The expanding mutational spectrum of MERRF substitution G8361A in the mitochondrial $tRNA^{Lys}$ gene. *Ann Neurol* 2003; **54**: 820–823.
50. Mancuso M, Filosto M, Mootha VK et al. A novel mitochondrial $tRNA^{Phe}$ mutation causes MERRF syndrome. *Neurology* 2004; **62**: 2119–2121.
51. Blumenthal DT, Shanske S, Schochet SS et al. Myoclonus epilepsy with ragged red fibers and multiple mtDNA deletions. *Neurology* 1998; **50**: 524–525.
52. Nakamura M, Nakano S, Goto Y et al. A novel point mutation in the mitochondrial $tRNA^{Ser(UCN)}$ gene detected in a family with MERRF/MELAS overlap syndrome. *Biochem Biophys Res Commun* 1995; **214**: 86–93.
53. Melone MA, Tessa A, Petrini S et al. Revelation of a new mitochondrial DNA mutation (G12147A) in a MELAS/MERRF phenotype. *Arch Neurol* 2004; **61**: 269–272.
54. Nishigaki Y, Tadesse S, Bonilla E et al. A novel mitochondrial $tRNA^{Leu(UUR)}$ mutation in a patient with features of MERRF and Kearns-Sayre syndrome. *Neuromuscul Disord* 2003; **13**: 334–340.
55. Fukuhara N. MERRF: A clinicopathological study. Relationship between myoclonus epilepsies and mitochondrial myopathies. *Rev Neurol* 1991; **147**: 476–479.
56. Thompson PD, Hammans SR, Harding AE. Cortical reflex myoclonus in patients with the mitochondrial DNA transfer RNA^{Lys}(8344) (MERRF) mutation. *J Neurol* 1994; **241**: 335–340.
57. So N, Berkovic S, Andermann F et al. Myoclonus epilepsy and ragged-red fibres (MERRF). *Brain* 1989; **112**: 1261–1276.
58. Berkovic SF, Carpenter S, Evans A et al. Myoclonus epilepsy and ragged-red fibres (MERRF): a clinical, pathological, biochemical, magnetic resonance spectrographic and positron emission tomographic study. *Brain* 1989; **112**: 1231–1260.
59. Kearns TP, Sayre GP. Retinitis pigmentosa, external ophthalmoplegia, and complete heart block. *Arch Ophthal* 1958; **60**: 280–289.
60. Rowland LP, Hays AP, DiMauro S et al. Diverse clinical disorders associated with morphological abnormalities of mitochondria. In: Cerri C, Scarlato G, eds. *Mitochondrial Pathology in Muscle Diseases*. Padua: Piccin Editore, 1983: 141–158.
61. Bosbach S, Kornblum C, Schroder R et al. Executive and visuospatial deficits in patients with chronic progressive external ophthalmoplegia and Kearns-Sayre syndrome. *Brain* 2003; **126**: 1231–1240.
62. Quade A, Zierz S, Klingmüller D. Endocrine abnormalities in mitochondrial myopathy. *Clin Investig* 1992; **70**: 396–402.
63. Schmitz K, Lins H, Behrens-Baumann W. Bilateral spontaneous corneal perforation associated with complete external ophthalmoplegia in mitochondrial myopathy (Kearns-Sayre syndrome). *Cornea* 2003; **22**: 267–270.
64. Kornblum C, Broicher R, Walther E et al. Cricopharyngeal achalasia is a common cause of dysphagia in patients with mtDNA deletions. *Neurology* 2001; **56**: 1409–1412.
65. Pearson HA, Lobel JS, Kocoshis SA et al. A new syndrome of refractory sideroblastic anemia with vacuolization of marrow precursors and exocrine pancreatic dysfunction. *J Pediatr* 1979; **95**: 976–984.
66. Moraes CT, DiMauro S, Zeviani M et al. Mitochondrial DNA deletions in progressive external ophthalmoplegia and Kearns-Sayre syndrome. *N Engl J Med* 1989; **320**: 1293–1299.
67. Poulton J, Deadman ME, Gardiner RM. Duplications of mitochondrial DNA in mitochondrial myopathy. *Lancet* 1989; **1**: 236–240.
68. Oldfors A, Fyhr IM, Holme E et al. Neuropathology in Kearns-Sayre syndrome. *Acta Neuropath* 1990; **80**: 541–546.
69. Tanji K, Vu TH, Schon EA et al. Kearns-Sayre syndrome: unusual pattern of expression of subunits of the respiratory chain in the cerebellar system. *Ann Neurol* 1999; **45**: 377–383.
70. Tanji K, DiMauro S, Bonilla E. Disconnection of cerebellar Purkinje cells in Kearns-Sayre syndrome. *J Neurol Sci* 1999; **166**: 64–70.
71. Hirano M, Silvestri G, Blake D et al. Mitochondrial neurogastrointestinal encephalomyopathy (MNGIE): Clinical, biochemical and genetic features of an autosomal recessive mitochondrial disorder. *Neurology* 1994; **44**: 721–727.
72. Hirano M, Nishigaki Y, Marti R. Mitochondrial neurogastrointestinal encephalomyopathy

(MNGIE): a disease of two genomes. *Neurologist* 2004; **10**: 8–17.
73. Nishino I, Spinazzola A, Hirano M. Thymidine phosphorylase gene mutations in MNGIE, a human mitochondrial disorder. *Science* 1999; **283**: 689–692.
74. Spinazzola A, Marti R, Nishino I et al. Altered thymidine metabolism due to defects of thymidine phosphorylase. *J Biol Chem* 2002; **277**: 4128–4133.
75. Nishigaki Y, Marti R, Copeland WC et al. Site-specific somatic mitochondrial DNA point mutations in patients with thymidine phosphorylase deficiency. *J Clin Invest* 2003; **111**: 1913–1921.
76. Nishigaki Y, Marti R, Hirano M. ND5 is a hot-spot for multiple atypical mitochondrial DNA deletions in mitochondrial neurogastrointestinal encephalomyopathy. *Hum Mol Genet* 2004; **13**: 91–101.
77. Millar WS, Lignelli A, Hirano M. MRI of five patients with mitochondrial neurogastrointestinal encephalomyopathy. *Am J Roentgenol* 2004; **182**: 1537–1541.
78. Szigeti K, Sule N, Adesina AM et al. Increased blood-brain barrier permeability with thymidine phosphorylase deficiency. *Ann Neurol* 2004; **56**: 881–886.
79. Alpers BJ. Diffuse progressive degeneration of the grey matter of the cerebrum. *Arch Neurol Psychiatry* 1931; **25**: 469–505.
80. Huttenlocher PR, Solitare GB, Adams G. Infantile diffuse cerebral degeneration with hepatic cirrhosis. *Arch Neurol* 1976; **33**: 186–192.
81. Sandbank U, Lerman P. Progressive cerebral poliodystrophy – Alpers' disease. Disorganized giant neuronal mitochondria on electron microscopy. *J Neurol Neurosurg Psychiatry* 1972; **35**: 749–755.
82. Naviaux RK, Nguyen KV. POLG mutations associated with Alpers' syndrome and mitochondrial DNA depletion. *Ann Neurol* 2004; **55**: 706–712.
83. Mandel H, Szargel R, Labay V et al. The deoxyguanosine kinase gene is mutated in individuals with depleted hepatocerebral mitochondrial DNA. *Nat Genet* 2001; **29**: 337–341.
84. Mandel H, Hartman C, Berkowitz D et al. The hepatic mitochondrial DNA depletion syndrome: ultrastructural changes in liver biopsies. *Hepatology* 2001; **34**: 776–784.
85. Salviati L, Sacconi S, Mancuso M et al. Mitochondrial DNA depletion and dGK gene mutations. *Ann Neurol* 2002; **52**: 311–317.
86. Elpeleg O, Miller C, Hershkovitz E et al. Deficiency of the ADP-forming succinyl-CoA synthatase activity is associated with encephalomyopathy and mitochondrial DNA depletion. *Am J Hum Genet* 2005; **76**: 1081–1086.
87. Ogasahara S, Engel AG, Frens D et al. Muscle coenzyme Q deficiency in familial mitochondrial encephalomyopathy. *Proc Natl Acad Sci USA* 1989; **86**: 2379–2382.
88. Lamperti C, Naini A, Hirano M et al. Cerebellar ataxia and coenzyme Q10 deficiency. *Neurology* 2003; **60**: 1206–1208.
89. Musumeci O, Naini A, Slonim AE et al. Familial cerebellar ataxia with muscle coenzyme Q10 deficiency. *Neurology* 2001; **56**: 849–855.
90. Rötig A, Appelkvist EL, Geromel V et al. Quinone-responsive multiple respiratory-chain dysfunction due to widespread coenzyme Q10 deficiency. *Lancet* 2000; **356**: 391–395.
91. Quinzii CM, Kattah AG, Naini A et al. Coenzyme Q deficiency and cerebellar ataxia associated with an aprataxin mutation. *Neurology* 2005; **64**: 539–541.
92. Date H, Onodera O, Tanaka H et al. Early-onset ataxia with ocular motor apraxia and hypoalbuminemia is caused by mutations in a new HIT superfamily gene. *Nat Genet* 2001; **29**: 184–188.
93. Moreira MC, Barbot C, Tachi N et al. The gene mutated in ataxia-ocular apraxia 1 encodes the new HIT/Zn-finger protein aprataxin. *Nat Genet* 2001; **29**: 189–193.
94. Salviati L, Sacconi S, Murer L et al. Infantile encephalomyopathy and nephropathy with CoQ10 deficiency: a CoQ10-responsive condition. *Neurology* 2005; **65**: 605–608.
95. Quinzii C, Naini AB, Salviati L et al. A mutation in para-hydroxybenzoate:polyprenyl transferase (CoQ2) causes primary coenzyme Q10 deficiency. *Am J Hum Genet* 2006; in press.

3

Mitochondrial neurology II: myopathies and peripheral neuropathies

Arthur P Hays, Maryam Oskoui, Kurenai Tanji, Petra Kaufmann, and Eduardo Bonilla

Introduction

Mitochondrial disorders result from dysfunction of the mitochondrial oxidative phosphorylation (OXPHOS) system, which is composed of the four enzyme complexes (complexes I–IV) of the electron transport respiratory chain, and of ATP synthase (complex V), which uses the proton gradient generated by the electron transport chain to produce ATP (see Chapter 1). As all organs in the body rely on ATP generated by OXPHOS for their normal function, impairment of this system can affect any organ system, making the diagnosis and classification of respiratory chain disorders particularly challenging. Patients can present with a wide variety of symptoms and signs that often do not fit into neat or preconceived clinical phenotypes.

Both the nuclear and mitochondrial genomes are necessary for assembly of the respiratory chain. Of the more than 80 structural subunits in the five enzyme complexes, 13 are encoded by the mitochondrial genome (mtDNA) and are essential for function. In addition to the structural components, a large and still incompletely characterized set of nuclear-encoded proteins is necessary for the proper assembly and maintenance of the complexes. Thus, mitochondrial disorders can be sporadic or transmitted by any mode of inheritance: maternal, autosomal dominant, autosomal recessive, or X-linked.

Tissues with high basal energy requirements are especially vulnerable to the energy failure that occurs in mitochondrial diseases. Therefore, muscle and peripheral nerves are frequently affected. This chapter reviews the main clinical phenotypes, the typical pathological changes, and the molecular lesions of those mitochondrial disorders that affect, at least to some degree, peripheral nerves or muscles. Table 3.1 summarizes the neuromuscular involvement in common mitochondrial disorders.

Mitochondrial myopathies

Structural alterations of mitochondria in skeletal muscle

In normal human muscle, mitochondria are localized under the sarcolemma and in the intermyofibrillar space, where they abut the I-band. The hallmark mitochondrial pathology in muscle of many, but not all patients are the ragged-red fibers (RRFs), which are typically detected with the modified Gomori trichrome stain (Figure 3.1A). However, the succinate dehydrogenase (SDH) stain, which produces a dark blue appearance of the fibers (Figure 3.1B), is the most sensitive and

Table 3.1 Neuromuscular involvement in common mitochondrial disorders

Syndrome	Key features	Neuropathy	Myopathy
NARP	Neuropathy, ataxia, retinitis pigmentosa	Axonal Sensory > Motor	Uncommon
MNGIE	GI dysmotility, cachexia, PEO, leukoencephalopathy, neuropathy	Demyelinating > Axonal Sensory > Motor	Common
SANDO	Sensory ataxia, dysarthria, PEO	Axonal Sensory ganglionopathy	Often subclinical
MSL	Lipomas, ataxia, neuropathy, deafness	Axonal > Demyelinating Sensory > Motor	Common
MELAS	Stroke-like events, migraine, vomiting	Axonal > Demyelinating Sensory > Motor	Common
KSS	Pigmentary retinopathy, PEO, cardiac conduction block, ataxia	Axonal Sensory > Motor	Common
LEIGH syndrome	Brainstem dysfunction, regression, lactic acidosis	Demyelinating Sensory = motor	Common
MERRF	Myoclonus, epilepsy, ataxia, lipomas, deafness, short stature	Axonal Sensory > Motor	Common
MTP	Typically presents in infancy with multi-organ involvement, but late-onset disease with predominantly neuromuscular symptoms has been described	Axonal Sensory = Motor	Limb-girdle myopathy, myoglobinuria
NNH	Presents in infancy with Reye-like syndrome	Demyelinating Sensory	Occasionally elevated CK, myopathy not described

NARP: neuropathy, ataxia, and retinitis pigmentosa; MNGIE: mitochondrial neurogastrointestinal encephalomyopathy; SANDO: sensory ataxic neuropathy, dysarthria, and ophthalmoparesis; MSL: multiple symmetric lipomas; MELAS: mitochondrial encephalomyopathy, lactic acidosis, and stroke-like episodes; KSS: Kearns–Sayre syndrome; MERRF: myoclonus epilepsy with ragged-red fibers; PEO: progressive external ophthalmoplegia; MTP: mitochondrial trifunctional protein deficiency; NNH: Navajo neurohepatopathy.

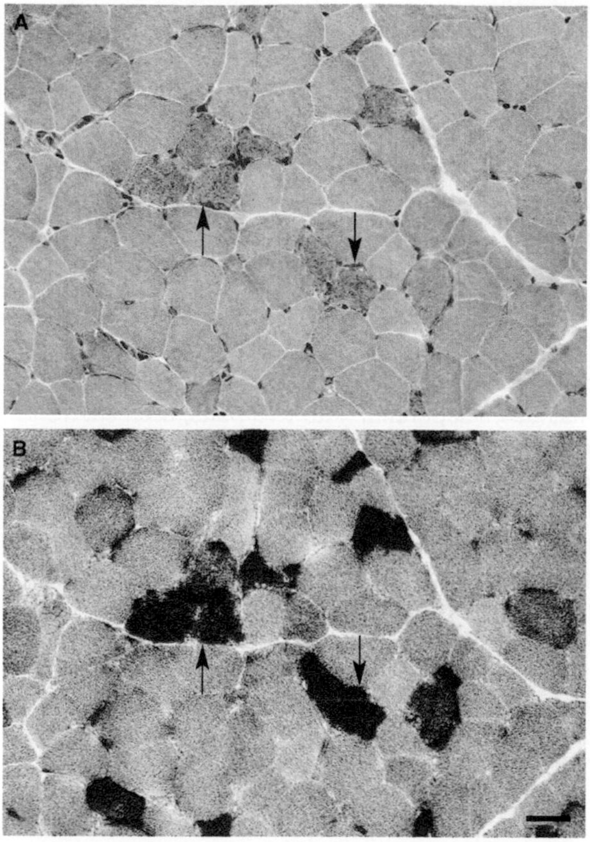

Figure 3.1 Ragged-red fibers (RRF). Histochemical stains for (**A**) modified Gomori trichrome and (**B**) succinate dehydrogenase (SDH) on serial muscle sections from a patient with mitochondrial myopathy. The trichrome stain shows reddish collections of subsarcolemmal mitochondria (black arrows) and the SDH stain shows bluish collections of mitochondria (black arrows) in RRF. Bar = 50 μm

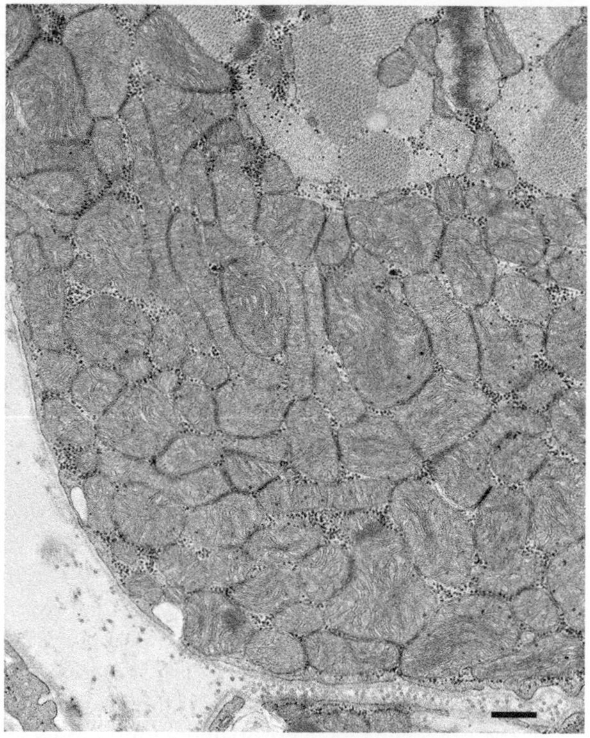

Figure 3.2 Electron micrograph of a subsarcolemmal collection of mitochondria in a ragged-red fiber (RRF) from a patient with mitochondrial myopathy. The mitochondria show variation in size and abnormal orientation of the cristae. Bar = 0.5 μm

precise method to identify these segmental accumulations of mitochondria. The appearance of the RRF is due to the proliferation of subsarcolemmal and intermyofibrillar abnormal mitochondria. (see Figure 3.2)

RRFS can account for 2% to 70% of all fibers, and the pathology is segmental; all fibers are affected at multiple locations throughout their length.[1] The segmental nature of the SDH alteration is an indicator of the underlying distribution of mtDNA mutations: thus, from a genetic point of view, the muscle fibers in these patients are linear mosaics.[2,3]

When examined by electron microscopy, the following alterations are commonly seen in RRF segments. First, enlarged mitochondria (up to 10 μm in diameter) occur in clusters or scattered among organelles of normal size (Figure 3.2). Occasionally, greatly elongated cylindrical mitochondria span several sarcomeres and show knots or loops. Second, abnormal cristae may be increased in number and irregularly oriented,

Box 3.1 Replication of mitochondrial DNA

In circular bacterial genomes, there is a single 'origin' of replication, with the synthesis of daughter-strand DNA (from the 'top' and 'bottom' strands of the parental DNA) beginning bi-directionally from the origin. RNA polymerase synthesizes short RNAs used to 'prime' DNA replication, and DNA polymerase extends the newly forming daughter DNA from those primers, using the parental strands as the template. Replication proceeds simultaneously in opposite directions: counterclockwise from the 'bottom strand' and clockwise from the 'top strand,' and ends with the creation of a pair of catenated circles (each circle is a double helix containing one 'old' parental strand and one 'new' daughter strand), which are then separated (i.e. de-catenated) into two free-standing circles by the action of an enzyme called topoisomerase II.

In the classic 'strand asymmetric' model described by David Clayton[1] (Figure B3.1.1A), human mtDNA also has a single origin of replication, but the origin has been 'separated' into two parts, each controlling synthesis of one of the two daughter DNA strands, called 'heavy' and 'light,' based on their mobility in alkali cesium gradients. Synthesis of the H-strand, by mitochondrial DNA polymerase γ, begins at the 'origin of heavy-strand replication' (O_H), which is located at '12-o'clock' on the circle, and proceeds in a clockwise direction. As with bacterial DNA, an RNA primer initiates DNA synthesis. This RNA (and a short stretch of extended DNA) hybridizes to the opposite L-strand, and displaces a portion of the H-strand in the region containing O_H, thereby exposing the so-called 'D-loop' (D is for 'displacement'). As the polymerase (and the displaced DNA) passes '8 o'clock,' synthesis of the L-strand begins, at the 'origin of light-strand replication' (O_L). The two oppositely growing strands continue until they both have completed their respective circles, forming a catenated pair of rings which are then decatenated by topo II. The process takes a surprisingly long time – about two hours.

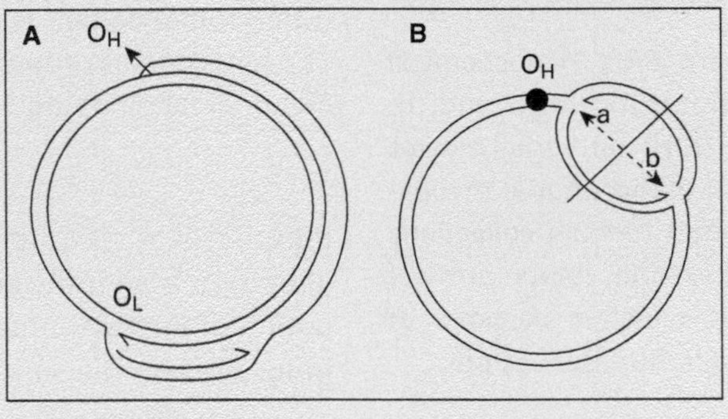

Figure B3.1.1 mtDNA replication (**A**) Clayton 'strand-asymmetric' model. (**B**) Holt 'strand-symmetric' model. Adapted from reference 2, with permission

Ian Holt has challenged this model, and has proposed an alternate, 'strand symmetric' model[2] (Figure B3.1.1B). In this model, there are multiple origins of replication on both strands, and the H- and L-strands are replicated simultaneously and bi-directionally from multiple replication 'eyes.'

In either model, if something goes wrong with mtDNA replication, pathology may ensue. For example, mutations in DNA polymerase γ can cause both autosomally inherited PEO associated with multiple mtDNA deletions[3] and mtDNA depletion syndrome.[4]

(Continued)

References

1. Clayton DA. Replication of animal mitochondrial DNA. *Cell* 1982; **28**: 693–705.
2. Bowmaker M, Yang MY, Yasukawa T et al. Mammalian mitochondrial DNA replicates bidirectionally from an initiation zone. *J Biol Chem* 2003; **278**: 50961–50969.
3. Lamantea E, Tiranti V, Bordoni A et al. Mutations of mitochondrial DNA polymerase γA are a frequent cause of autosomal dominant or recessive progressive external ophthalmoplegia. *Ann Neurol* 2002; **52**: 211–219.
4. Naviaux RK, Nguyen KV. POLG mutations associated with Alpers' syndrome and mitochondrial DNA depletion. *Ann Neurol* 2004; **55**: 706–712.

often forming honeycomb patterns or concentric whorls. Third, mitochondria may contain abnormal inclusions, including crystalline structures, globular bodies, myeloid bodies (Figure 3.3). There may also be enlargement and proliferation of mitochondrial granules.[4]

RRFs are usually negative for cytochrome *c* oxidase (COX) or have much reduced COX activity relative to the increased mitochondrial volume as seen by the SDH stain. The mitochondrial proliferation that results in RRFs is presumably an attempt by the muscle fiber to compensate for the respiratory chain defect. However, the signals that trigger segmental up-regulation of mitochondrial biogenesis in this setting are unknown (see Chapter 10). As a rule, RRFs are nearly always present in patients with mitochondrial DNA translation defects, whereas they are less abundant and sometimes absent in patients with defects in mtDNA protein-coding genes.

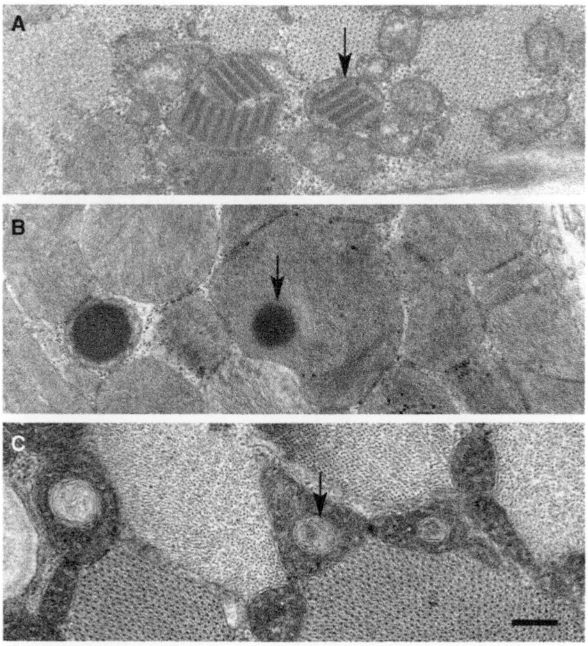

Figure 3.3 Electron microscopic illustrations of mitochondrial inclusions. The upper micrograph (**A**) shows paracrystalline inclusions in subsarcolemmal mitochondria (arrow). The middle micrograph (**B**) illustrates mitochondria with globular inclusions (arrow). The lower micrograph (**C**) shows myeloid inclusions in intermyofibrillar mitochondria (arrow). Bar = 0.5 μm

Molecular genetics, prototypes, and pathogenesis

mtDNA mutations

These have been classified into three main categories: large-scale rearrangements, point mutations in tRNAs or rRNAs, and point mutations in protein-coding genes. The first two types of molecular lesion impair mitochondrial protein translation in toto, producing multiple deficiencies in the enzymatic activities of the respiratory chain complexes, while mutations in protein-coding genes lead to specific deficiencies in respiratory chain complexes.

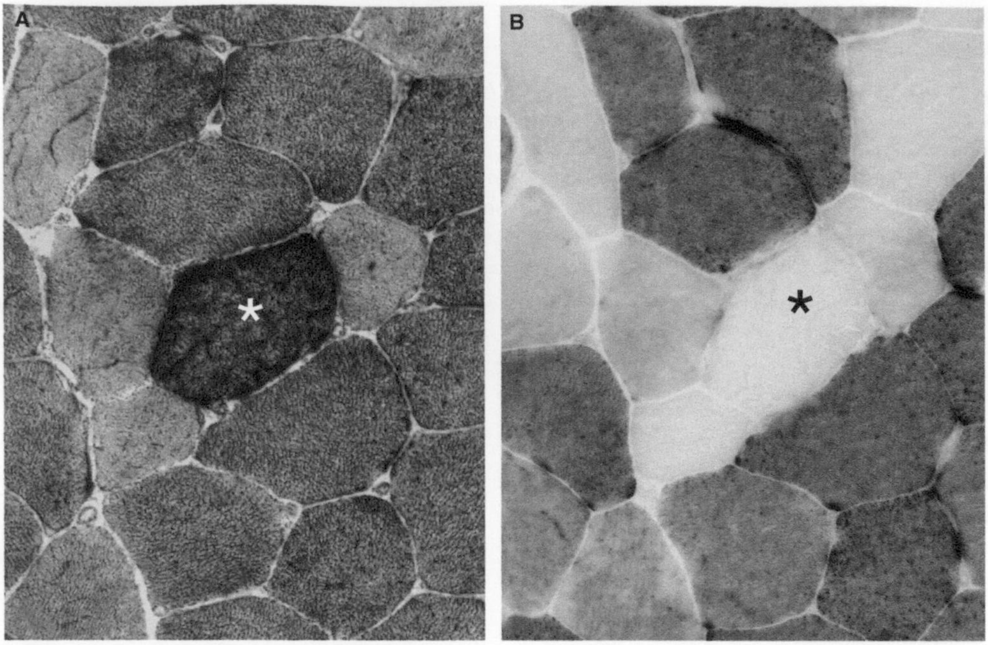

Figure 3.4 Kearns–Sayre syndrome (KSS). Serial muscle sections stained for (**A**) succinate dehydrogenase (SDH) and (**B**) cytochrome *c* oxidase (COX) activities. The SDH stain shows one RRF (white asterisk) and several normal fibers, the same fibers on the serial section (black asterisk) show lack of COX activity. Bar = 50 μm

LARGE-SCALE REARRANGEMENTS IN mtDNA

Large-scale rearrangements in mtDNA can take one of two forms: deletions (Δ-mtDNAs), which remove multiple tRNAs and protein-coding genes,[5] or duplications, which are dimers of Δ-mtDNAs and wild-type molecules (see Box 3.2).[6] Most patients with Δ-mtDNAs present as sporadic cases, although there are rare reports of germline transmission.[7] Maternally transmitted duplications are not pathogenic by themselves, but they can give rise to Δ-mtDNAs by mechanisms that remain unclear.[8] The mechanisms by which Δ-mtDNAs are generated are also unknown, although slip replication and recombination have been suggested.[9] All patients with large-scale Δ-mtDNAs are heteroplasmic and the disease phenotype depends on the load and distribution of mutations inherited at birth. The Δ-mtDNAs result from clonal expansion of a mutation that likely arises during oogenesis. In all reported cases, the same deletion is found in all affected tissues to varying degrees.

The most common and mildest phenotype caused by Δ-mtDNAs is a myopathy with progressive external ophthalmoplegia (PEO), ptosis and proximal limb weakness, usually slowly progressive and compatible with a normal lifespan. A much more severe phenotype is Kearns–Sayre syndrome (KSS), a devastating multisystemic disease of early onset (before age 20), characterized by PEO, pigmentary degeneration of the retina, and at least one of the following: cardiac conduction block, cerebrospinal fluid protein concentration greater than 100 mg/dL, and cerebellar ataxia. Additional features include diabetes mellitus, short stature, hearing loss, and dementia (see Chapter 2). The most severe phenotype is Pearson syndrome (PS), a predominantly hematological and almost invariably fatal disease of infancy, with sideroblastic anemia and exocrine pancreas dysfunction (see Chapter 10). Interestingly, the few children that outlive PS go on to develop KSS later in life.

Muscle biopsies from patients with large-scale Δ-mtDNAs always show the characteristic RRF pathology (Figure 3.4A). In situ hybridization studies using mtDNA probes within or outside the deletion have demonstrated that RRF segments contain large accumulations of Δ-mtDNAs and their transcripts (indicating that the mutation does not impair transcription) (see Boxes 7.1 and 7.2).[2,10] The relative proportion of wild-type mtDNAs is reduced in the RRF segments, which stain negative for COX (Figure 3.4B). Immunohistochemistry shows that polypeptides encoded by mtDNA – even those encoded by genes outside the deletion – are not detectable, suggesting that translation of mtDNA-encoded genes is virtually absent in these RRF segments.[3]

The pathogenesis of Δ-mtDNAs is well established, most clearly from cybrid (transmitochondrial cytoplasmic hybrid) experiments. In these cybrid cell lines, there was decreased oxygen consumption and decreased mitochondrial protein synthesis.[11]

rRNA MUTATIONS

The majority of mutations in rRNA genes have been associated with aminoglycoside-induced non-syndromic deafness[12] and cardiomyopathy,[13] These mutations will not be discussed further in this chapter.

tRNA MUTATIONS

Mutations in tRNA genes are the most common molecular causes of mitochondrial myopathies (Table 3.2 and Appendix). More than 60 different mutations have been reported, the majority manifesting a neuromuscular or cardiac phenotype.[14] The mutations are almost always heteroplasmic, nearly always associated with RRFs, and displaying a threshold effect in muscle. Here, we will discuss the two most common tRNA mutations and the neuromuscular aspects of the clinical syndromes they cause.

MITOCHONDRIAL ENCEPHALOMYOPATHY, LACTIC ACIDOSIS AND STROKE-LIKE EPISODES (MELAS) The clinical hallmarks of this syndrome are the stroke-like episodes with hemiparesis or hemianopia, almost invariably occurring before age 40, and often in childhood. Common additional findings include lactic acidosis, focal or generalized seizures, recurrent migraine-like headaches and vomiting, and dementia. The course is one of gradual deterioration. MELAS patients often have oligosymptomatic and asymptomatic maternal relatives.

RRFs are found on muscle biopsy. In contrast to those seen in most other tRNA point mutations and in large-scale Δ-mtDNAs, they are often positive for COX activity, even though the COX activity is usually reduced relative to the mitochondrial proliferation indicated by the SDH stain (Figure 3.5). Blood vessels in MELAS also show hyper-reactivity both for SDH and for COX. These so-called 'strongly SDH-reactive blood vessels' (SSVs) show that mitochondrial proliferation occurs not only in skeletal muscle but also in smooth muscles, pericytes, and endothelial cells of arterial walls.[15]

MELAS has been associated with at least fifteen different point mutations, four of which are located in the same gene, $tRNA^{Leu(UUR)}$, the most common being the A3243G transition, which is found in 80% of cases.[14] This mutation is also an important cause of PEO.[16]

The pathogenesis of the A3243G mutation is well established, at least in cybrid cell lines (Box 5.1). The altered tRNA fails to undergo proper postranscriptional modification: there is no addition of a taurine to the anticodon uridine wobble-base, leading to impaired mitochondrial protein synthesis.[17]

MYOCLONIC EPILEPSY AND RAGGED-RED FIBERS (MERRF) MERRF is characterized by myoclonus, generalized seizures, ataxia, and myopathy with RRFs. Less consistent clinical features include cardiomyopathy, dementia, neuropathy, multiple symmetrical lipomatosis, and short stature (see Chapter 2). The myoclonic jerks occur at rest and worsen during movement (action myoclonus). Onset is usually in childhood, but adult onset has also been described. As noted for MELAS, maternal family members in MERRF may be oligosymptomatic or asymptomatic.

Muscle biopsy reveals COX-negative RRFs and SSVs, but unlike MELAS, the SSVs in MERRF are COX-negative.

About 80% of the MERRF patients harbor an A8344G mutation in the $tRNA^{Lys}$ gene and a smaller percentage of these patients have a T8356C mutation in the same gene.[18,19]

Cultured myotubes harboring the A8344G mutation show no biochemical defect until the proportion of mutant mtDNAs exceeds 85%. There is a good correlation between the extent of the translation defect and the lysine content of different mtDNA-encoded polypeptides.[20,21] The mutation causes a defective aminoacylation of the $tRNA^{Lys}$, resulting in premature translation termination.[21]

MUTATIONS IN mtDNA PROTEIN CODING GENES

Mutations in mtDNA protein coding genes have been associated with muscle disease (Table 3.2). Here, we will discuss the most common neuromuscular phenotypes.

COMPLEX I MUTATIONS The first mutation to be reported was the G11778G transition in ND4 associated with Leber hereditary optic neuropathy (LHON).[22] Two additional mutations (G3460A and T14484C), also in complex I subunits, have been associated with this disorder and these three mutations account for most LHON cases. In most patients, pathology is confined to the optic nerve; in particular, there are no RRFs in muscle biopsies (see Chapter 5 for further details).

Isolated myopathy characterized by exercise intolerance, myalgia, lactic acidosis, complex I deficiency and COX-positive RRF on muscle biopsies has been observed in three sporadic patients: one had a nonsense mutation in the ND4 gene,[23] the second had an intragenic inversion in the ND1 gene,[24] and the third had a 2-bp deletion in the ND2 gene.[25] The third patient became a 'cause célèbre' when it was found that his muscle mtDNA was mostly of paternal origin. Although this situation does not negate the general rule that mtDNA is transmitted maternally, it raises the interesting possibility that tissue-specific paternal mtDNA inheritance might somehow favor mutagenesis.[25]

In addition, increasing numbers of ND5 gene mutations have been associated with multisystemic disorders such as MELAS[26] and with various overlap syndromes, including MELAS and LS,[27] MELAS and MERRF,[28] MELAS and LHON[29] and even MELAS, LS, and LHON.[30] Muscle biopsies from these patients invariably show more or less severe isolated complex I deficiency and morphological studies may show either COX-positive RRFs or COX-positive SSVs in some but not all patients.

ATP6 GENE MUTATIONS A mutation in the ATP6 gene (T8993G) was first reported in a syndrome of neuropathy, ataxia, and retinitis pigmentosa (NARP).[31] Onset is infancy or early childhood. Myopathy is rare, and muscle pathology does not show RRFs. This disorder is described in Chapter 2 and later in this chapter.

CYTOCHROME *B* (CYT *B*) MUTATIONS To date, 14 patients with mutations in the Cyt *b* gene have been reported, and ten of them had isolated myopathy. This myopathy is remarkably stereotypical,[32] with exercise intolerance and myalgia, sometimes accompanied by myoglobinuria (4/14). There is lactic acidosis and muscle biopsy shows COX-positive RRF, but no SSVs have been noted.[32] However, one patient with a Cyt *b* mutation had a predominantly central nervous system

Table 3.2 mtDNA point mutations with predominant myopathy

Gene	Base change	Clinical features	Family history	Reference
$tRNA^{Leu(UUR)}$	3250C	Respiratory/SIDS	+	(138)
$tRNA^{Leu(UUR)}$	A3302G	Respiratory	+	(139)
$tRNA^{Leu(UUR)}$	A3288G	Respiratory	+	(140)
$tRNA^{Pro}$	G15990A	Myopathy	–	(141)
$tRNA^{Phe}$	T618C	Respiratory	+	(142)
$tRNA^{Trp}$	G5521A	Ptosis	+	(143)
$tRNA^{Met}$	U4409C	Dystrophy	–	(144)
$tRNA^{Leu(CUN)}$	A12320G	Ptosis	–	(145)
$tRNA^{Leu(CUN)}$	G12276A	PEO	+	(146)
$tRNA^{Glu}$	T14709C	Myopathy, variable age of onset	–	(147)
$tRNA^{ASN}$	G5698A	PEO	–	(148)
$tRNA^{Ser(UCN)}$	A7480G	Deafness, dementia, ataxia	–	(149)
$tRNA^{Phe}$	T582C	Myopathy	–	(150)
$tRNA^{Ala}$	G5650A	Myopathy	–	(151)
$tRNA^{Leu(UUR)}$	A33280G	Myopathy and cardiomyopathy	–	(152)
$tRNA^{Leu(CUN)}$	G12315A	PEO, ptosis	–	(153)
$tRNA^{Ile}$	A4267G	Myopathy, ataxia, hearing loss	–	(154)
$tRNA^{Glut}$	T14687C	Retinopathy, myopathy, respiratory failure	–	(155)
$tRNA^{Leu(CUN)}$	G12334A	Exercise intolerance	–	(156)
$tRNA^{Cys}$	A5814G	Myopathy, cardiomyopathy	–	(157)
$tRNA^{Leu(UUR)}$	T3273C	Ptosis, exercise intolerance, PEO	–	(158)
$tRNA^{Leu(UUR)}$	T3291C	Mild myopathy	–	(159)
$tRNA^{Leu(UUR)}$	C3303T	Cardiomyopathy, myopathy	–	(160)
ND4	G11832A	Exercise intolerance	–	(23)
ND1	7-nt inversion	Exercise intolerance/ weakness	–	(24)
Cyt *b*	G15615A	Exercise intolerance	–	(161)
Cyt *b*	G15244A	Exercise intolerance/weakness	–	(162)
Cyt *b*	G15762A	Exercise intolerance/weakness	–	(163)
Cyt *b*	G15059A	Exercise intolerance weakness/myoglobinuria	–	(164)

(Continued)

Table 3.2 *(Continued)*

Gene	Base change	Clinical features	Family history	Reference
Cyt *b*	24-bp deletion	Exercise intolerance weakness/myoglobinuria	–	(32)
Cyt *b*	G14846A	Exercise intolerance/ weakness	–	(32)
Cyt *b*	G15168A	Exercise intolerance	–	(32)
Cyt *b*	G15084A	Exercise intolerance	–	(32)
Cyt *b*	G15723A	Exercise intolerance	–	(32)
Cyt *b*	T15800T	Exercise intolerance	–	(165)
COX I	G5920A	Exercise intolerance/ myoglobinuria	–	(36)
COX II	T7671A	Exercise intolerance/ weakness	–	(166)
COX III	15-bp deletion	Exercise intolerance/ myoglobinuria	–	(167)
COX I	G6708A	Exercise intolerance weakness/myoglobinuria	–	(168)
COX II	T7989C	Myoglobinuria, fatigue, weakness, bowel dysmotility, paroxysmal orthostatic tachycardia syndrome	–	(169)

presentation, described as juvenile Parkinson/MELAS overlap syndrome,[33] and two others had severe hypertrophic cardiomyopathy.[34] Most mutations were within or close to the functionally important ubiquinone-binding sites of Cyt *b*,[32] suggesting that they were likely to impair mitochondrial energy production.

In all patients with isolated myopathy so studied, the mutant mtDNA was absent in blood and fibroblasts. This is consistent with the muscle-specific clinical phenotype, the sporadic nature of the disorder, and the lack of transmission to the next generation. These features have led to the suggestion that the mutations in these patients arose in muscle progenitor cells, after differentiation of the primary germ layers.[32]

COX SUBUNIT MUTATIONS Mutations in each of the three mtDNA-encoded COX subunits can cause tissue-specific disorders such as myopathy (COX I and COX II)[35,36], sideroblastic anemia (COX I),[37] multisystemic disorders such as MELAS (COX III),[38] an ALS-like condition (COX I),[39] and encephalomyopathies (COX I and COX III).[40,41]

Although muscle biopsies from these patients usually show RRFs, these were not seen in two cases.[35,40] The histochemical 'signature' of these mutations is not the presence of RRFs but the striking numbers of COX negative or 'white' fibers that are not RRFs. So far, there is only one exception to this rule, proving, once again, that there are no 'dogmas' in muscle pathology. This

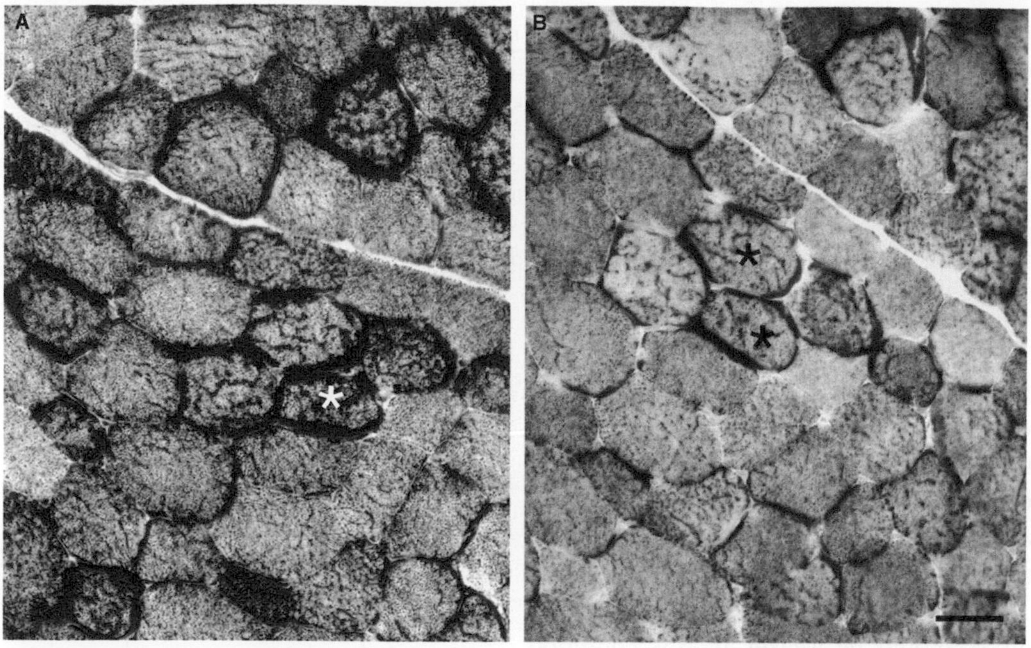

Figure 3.5 Mitochondrial encephalomyopathy, lactic acidosis and stroke-like episodes (MELAS). Serial muscle sections stained for (**A**) succinate dehydrogenase (SDH) and (**B**) cytochrome *c* oxidase (COX) activities. The SDH stain shows RRFs (white asterisks) and the same fibers on the section (asterisks) show COX activity. Bar = 50 μm

11-year-old boy with recurrent strokes and lactic acidosis, a typical MELAS syndrome, harbored a pathogenic missense mutation (T9957C) in the COX III gene.[38] Muscle biopsy showed a few RRFs, no histochemical evidence of COX deficiency, and numerous SSVs that reacted strongly for COX, a characteristic feature of MELAS-3243 mutation. Surprisingly, COX activity was biochemically normal in muscle extracts.

When studied by immunohistochemistry, COX-negative fibers from patients with mutations in mtDNA COX genes typically show lack or marked reduction of mtDNA-encoded COX I and COX II but normal expression of the mtDNA-encoded ND1 and of the nDNA-encoded COX IV.[36,42] These observations suggest that mutations in mtDNA COX genes have distinct immunohistochemical patterns, which differ from those observed in muscle from patients with Δ-mtDNA or with point mutations in tRNA genes (see above). These distinctive patterns are helpful not only in indicating the diagnosis of isolated COX deficiency but also in directing sequence analyses towards the mtDNA COX genes.[42]

Nuclear gene mutations (nuclear–mitochondrial communication disorders)

This is a particularly interesting group of disorders because the primary genetic defect is in the nDNA, but the consequences of the nuclear mutation are either quantitative (mtDNA depletion) or qualitative (multiple Δ-mtDNAs) defects of mtDNA. This is because, in the course of evolution, the symbiotic protobacteria that evolved into mitochondria have lost much of their autonomy and have become increasingly dependent on the host cell's genome, which encodes the factors controlling mtDNA replication, transcription and translation.

mtDNA DEPLETION SYNDROMES (MDS)

MDS are usually inherited as autosomal recessive traits but they can also be acquired (e.g. drug-induced). The autosomal recessive forms (arMDS) fall into two major groups, one dominated by myopathy, the other by hepatopathy, although both presentations often involve other tissues, including brain, kidney and heart.[43] The myopathic form can be apparent at birth (congenital myopathy) and cause respiratory failure fatal within months, or develop at about one year of age and progress more slowly, often simulating muscular dystrophy. The differential diagnosis from muscular dystrophy is made more difficult by the fact that MDS are associated with persistant and markedly elevated serum creatine kinase (CK) values. It is not clear why the CK is elevated and why muscle should be weaker in this condition than in other mitochondrial disorders. However, electron microscopic studies have shown focal defects of the muscle plasma membrane, similar to those observed in Duchenne muscular dystrophy.[44]

In the congenital myopathic form of MDS, muscle biopsy shows RRFs and diffuse COX deficiency. In the childhood form, initial biopsies may show only non-specific changes, while samples taken later show RRFs and COX-negative fibers. Biochemical studies show combined defects of respiratory chain complexes containing mtDNA-encoded subunits. The diagnosis is established by densitometry of Southern blots or by real-time PCR comparing the relative concentrations of mtDNA and nDNA.

To date, mutations in four nuclear genes have been identified in patients with MDS: changes in the deoxyguanosine kinase (*dGK* or *DGUOK*) and *POLG* genes have been associated with the hepatic[45] or hepatocerebral forms[45,46] and mutations in the thymidine kinase 2 (*TK2*) and succinyl-CoA synthetase ligase 2 (*SUCLA2*) genes have been associated with the myopathic and encephalomyopathic form.[47,48] After the identification of the *dGK* and *TK2* genes, we screened two large series of patients with predominantly hepatic or predominantly muscular symptoms, and found that three of 21 hepatic patients had *dGK* mutations[49] and four of 20 myopathic patients had *TK2* mutations.[49] These data indicated that other genes must be involved, as confirmed by recent reports.[48] It is noteworthy that one of two siblings with a homozygous I22M mutation in *TK2* had a syndrome mimicking spinal muscular atrophy (SMA) type I. We had previously described another child with the SMA phenotype and mtDNA depletion.[50] It is, therefore, important to consider mitochondrial dysfunction in all children with clinical features of SMA but without mutations in the survival motor neuron gene (*SMN1*).

There are also examples of drug-induced or secondary MDS, such as the iatrogenic mitochondrial myopathy observed in patients with AIDS treated with zidovudine, a nucleoside analog that probably interferes with both viral and mtDNA replication.[51,52]

MULTIPLE Δ-mtDNAs

Syndromes associated with multiple Δ-mtDNAs affect predominantly muscle and usually present as PEO or – much less frequently – as isolated proximal muscle weakness. They can be inherited as autosomal dominant or recessive traits.

Autosomal dominant PEO (adPEO), not unlike the sporadic form of PEO due to single Δ-mtDNAs mentioned earlier, is also a relatively benign condition with onset in adolescence or young adult life and slow progression. Bilateral ptosis, PEO, and proximal weakness dominate the clinical picture. Multisystemic involvement can also occur, with dysphagia, dysphonia, neuropathy, hearing loss, cataracts and, in some families, severe depression.[53,54] Muscle biopsy usually shows RRFs and COX-negative fibers, and biochemical analysis shows combined respiratory chain defects. Southern blot of total DNA isolated from muscle reveals multiple Δ-mtDNAs. Within the past 5 years, mutations in three genes have been associated

Box 3.2 Deleted and duplicated mtDNAs

In any one patient with sporadic KSS, PEO, or Pearson syndrome, there is only a single type of partially deleted mtDNA molecule (Δ-mtDNA). This observation implies that the population of rearranged mtDNA molecules in these patients is a clonal expansion of a single spontaneous deletion event that occurred early in oogenesis or embryogenesis. However, this does *not* mean that these patients harbor only deleted mtDNAs, for one simple reason: mtDNAs can undergo recombination, in which the Δ-mtDNA can recombine with a wild-type mtDNA (wt-mtDNA) to give a partially duplicated molecule (dup-mtDNA). Conversely, duplicated mtDNAs can rearrange spontaneously to give a wt-mtDNA plus a Δ-mtDNA.[1] As a rule, only Δ-mtDNAs are pathogenic, because they remove essential tRNA genes,[2] whereas dup-mtDNAs, which contain more than the entire complement of tRNA genes, behave essentially like wt-mtDNAs.[1]

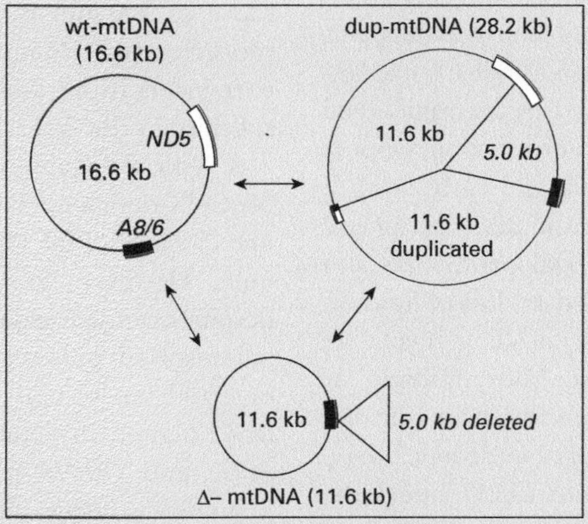

Figure B3.2.1 Relationship between deletions and duplications of mtDNA. The 'common deletion' is shown.

Importantly, the dup-mtDNAs and Δ-mtDNAs present in any one patient are related structurally: the partially duplicated molecule is essentially a tandem duplication of wt-mtDNA in which the material missing in the analogous Δ-mtDNA has been removed. In other words, the duplicated molecule is a wt-mtDNA into which the Δ-mtDNA has been inserted. In the case of the 'common deletion' of 4977 bp, shown in Figure B3.2.1, the Δ-mtDNA is 11 592 bp long (i.e. 16 569 – 4977) and the dup-mtDNA is 28 161 bp long (i.e. 16 569 + 16 569 – 4977, equivalent to 16 569 + 11 592). It is quite likely that many KSS patients who were thought to have only deletions actually contain both deletions and duplications in their cells, and perhaps other related rearrangements, such as deletion dimers, as well.

References

1. Tang Y, Manfredi G, Hirano M, Schon EA. Maintenance of human rearranged mitochondrial DNAs in long-term cultured transmitochondrial cell lines. *Mol Biol Cell* 2000; **11**: 2349–2358.
2. Nakase H, Moraes CT, Rizzuto R et al. Transcription and translation of deleted mitochondrial genomes in Kearns–Sayre syndrome: implications for pathogenesis. *Am J Hum Genet* 1990; **46**: 418–427.

with adPEO: adenine nucleotide translocator 1 (*ANT1*),[55] a helicase, (*PEO1* or *C10orf2*, formerly known as *Twinkle*),[56] and polymerase gamma (*POLG*).[57] However, it is already clear that mutations in these genes do not explain all cases of adPEO, and other genes remain to be identified.

Autosomal recessive PEO (arPEO) is more often multisystemic than adPEO, as illustrated by two syndromes: autosomal recessive cardiomyopathy and ophthalmoplegia (ARCO), and mitochondrial neurogastrointestinal encephalomyopathy (MNGIE). ARCO was reported in six patients from two unrelated Arab families, who presented with childhood-onset PEO, facial and proximal limb weakness, and severe cardiomyopathy requiring cardiac transplantation.[58] MNGIE is dominated by gastrointestinal symptoms (intestinal pseudo-obstruction, chronic diarrhea) leading to cachexia and early death.[59] Additional signs include ptosis, PEO, peripheral neuropathy, and leukoencephalopathy (see also Chapter 2). MNGIE is caused by loss-of-function mutations in the gene (*TP*) encoding thymidine phosphorylase, which cause both multiple Δ-mtDNAs and mtDNA depletion by altering the homeostasis of the mitochondrial nucleotide pool.[60] Interestingly, some families with arPEO without the characteristics of ARCO or MNGIE had mutations in *POLG*.[55,61] Thus, *POLG* mutations have to be considered in both adPEO and arPEO, as well as in the hepatocerebral syndrome (Alpers syndrome) with mtDNA depletion, as mentioned above.

Nuclear gene mutations causing isolated respiratory chain complex deficiencies

Recent research on mitochondrial diseases has uncovered an increasing number of disorders that are caused by mutations in nuclear genes encoding subunits of OXPHOS complexes or ancillary proteins that are essential for the biosynthesis of specific cofactors or for assembly of the complexes. Interestingly, mutations in nuclear genes encoding subunits ('direct hits') are known only for complexes I and II whereas defects in complex III, complex IV, or complex V are caused by mutations in assembly proteins or biosynthetic factors ('indirect hits' – for review, see reference 62). A detailed description of the literature of these disorders is beyond the scope of this chapter. We will focus on complex IV and discuss three pediatric syndromes associated with COX deficiency: LS, and the fatal and the benign COX-deficient myopathies of infancy.

COX-DEFICIENT LS

COX deficiency is arguably the most common cause of LS and is inherited as an autosomal recessive trait.[62] In most LS patients, COX activity is reduced in all tissues, with little or no tissue specifity in the severity of the defect.[63]

A logical hypothesis for the molecular basis of COX-deficient LS postulated mutations in one or more of the ten nDNA-encoded COX subunits. However, no such mutations were found despite extensive sequence studies.[64,65] This riddle was resolved only recently, when mutations were detected in several COX-assembly genes: the *SURF1* gene in patients with typical LS,[66,67] the *SCO2* and *COX15* genes in patients with fatal infantile cardioencephalomyopathy,[68] and in *SCO1* and *COX10* genes in patients with other multisystem disorders.[62]

Muscle histochemistry in patients with mutations in *SURF1* or *SCO2* genes shows only minor histological changes and no typical RRF. The histochemical pattern of COX-deficient LS is that of a generalized and diffuse reduction – not a total absence – of COX, affecting equally type I and type II fibers, intrafusal fibers of the muscle spindles, and the arterial walls.[42] In comparative studies, this histochemical pattern was more severe in patients with *SCO2* mutations than in patients with *SURF1* mutations. Although the number of patients with *SCO2* mutations was small, this difference was borne out by biochemical studies.[69]

Immunohistochemical studies in patients with *SURF1* mutations show similarly decreased staining for the mtDNA-encoded COX II and the nDNA-encoded COX IV and COX VIIa subunits.[63] In contrast, patients with *SCO2* mutations show a more severe reduction in the mtDNA-encoded COX I and COX II subunits than in the nDNA-encoded COX IV and COX VIa subunits.[68,69] This difference may relate to the fact that both COX I and COX II contain copper and all known *SCO*-like proteins bind copper.[70] The difference also suggests that the pathogenic mechanisms differ in the two disorders.

COX-DEFICIENT MYOPATHIES OF INFANCY

Two myopathic variants of COX deficiency, apparently transmitted as autosomal recessive traits, are presumably due to mutations in muscle-specific and developmentally regulated COX subunits or COX-assembly proteins,[71] although the molecular defects remain elusive in both conditions.

The fatal infantile myopathy causes respiratory insufficiency and death before 1 year of age. Heart, liver and brain are spared, but kidney is often affected, and patients may suffer from the DeToni–Fanconi syndrome.[72] Muscle biopsy shows RRFs and diffuse lack of COX stain in muscle fibers, but normal reaction in intramuscular blood vessels and in muscle spindles. Electrophoresis of the defective enzyme after immunoprecipitation failed to show any alteration in subunit pattern,[73] but immunohistochemistry with antibodies against individual subunits showed a selective defect of COX VIIa in four patients.[74]

The benign infantile myopathy also causes severe weakness early in life, often requiring assisted ventilation, but symptoms improve spontaneously and these children are usually normal by 2 or 3 years of age.[75,76] Muscle biopsies taken in the neonatal period show no RRFs but diffuse absence of COX stain, except for blood vessels and spindles. However, biopsies taken at later times show RRFs and increasing numbers of COX-positive fibers until the histochemistry returns to normal. Paradoxically, immunohistochemistry shows lack of both COX II and COX VIIa,[74] although the genes of both subunits harbored no mutations (M Hirano, unpublished observations).

Peripheral neuropathy in mitochondrial disorders

Manifestations of central nervous system injury dominate the clinical picture of most mitochondrial disorders and often overshadow peripheral nerve involvement, which is, however, increasingly recognized. In some mitochondrial syndromes, such as NARP, MNGIE, and SANDO (see list of acronyms (in Table 3.1)) peripheral neuropathy (PN) is a defining feature. In others, overt or subclinical PN has been described in some but not all patients. In most of these patients, PN is part of a multisystem disorder involving both central and peripheral nervous systems, although occasionally it can be the presenting symptom (see Table 3.1).[77]

Clinical features of neuropathies in mitochondrial disease

Clinically, most patients have mild chronic sensorimotor PN, most commonly a distal predominantly sensory PN, with reduced or absent deep tendon reflexes. There are also reports of painful paresthesias, pes cavus, and palpable nerves.[78–80] Some cases have exacerbations, mimicking acute inflammatory demyelinating polyneuropathy (AIDP) or chronic inflammatory demyelinating polyneuropathy (CIDP).[81,82]

Electrophysiological findings

Electrophysiological studies are mostly consistent with predominantly axonal PN, with decreased sensory and motor amplitudes and relatively preserved conduction velocities.[80,83] Less common are reports of pure demyelinating PN with temporal dispersion, prolonged distal latencies, slowed conduction velocities, and absent F waves.[84]

Asymmetrical slowing of conduction along nerves and conduction block can also be seen, mimicking acquired immuno-mediated demyelinating neuropathies. An electromyography (EMG) can show signs of chronic denervation, especially in distal muscles, together with myopathic features, especially in proximal muscles if – as is often the case – there is an associated myopathy.[85]

Nerve biopsy findings

Sural nerve biopsies of affected patients show loss of large and small myelinated fibers, sometimes with thinly myelinated fibers and demyelinated axons. Onion bulb-like formation can also be seen.[86] Abnormal and enlarged mitochondria, some with paracrystalline inclusions, have been reported in Schwann cell cytoplasm, axons, and in endothelial and smooth muscle cells of endoneurial and epineurial arterioles (Figure 3.6).[87,88]

Pathogenesis

The pathogenesis of PN in mitochondrial disease is incompletely understood. The wide spectrum of structural involvement in mitochondrial neuropathies may be due to the variety of biochemical abnormalities, or to the variable heteroplasmy of mtDNA mutations in axons, Schwann cells, and other structures in the peripheral nervous system.

In diseases with primary axonal involvement, a reduction in cellular energy may impair axonal transport. This mechanism is involved in moving organelles and macromolecules to the distal axon, using an ATP-driven microtubule-associated molecular motor.[89] This in turn can lead to depletion of essential macromolecules in the distal axon and subsequent degeneration.

In primary demyelinating neuropathy, abnormal mitochondria in the Schwann cells, capillary endothelial cells, or smooth muscle cells of the endoneurial and epineurial arterioles may lead to dysfunction of the myelin sheath.[90] However, some changes may be non-specific, as abnormal mitochondria have been documented in Schwann cells from 9% of patients with unselected peripheral neuropathies.[88]

Patients with mitochondrial disorders may also have higher susceptibility to develop PN from concurrent risk factors. Because of the often multisystemic nature of mitochondrial diseases, they have a higher incidence of diabetes mellitus, hypothyroidism, and malnutrition from gastrointestinal dysmotility. In addition, certain medications used to treat mitochondrial diseases, such as dichloroacetate may in themselves cause PN (see Chapter 14).

Mitochondrial syndromes associated with peripheral neuropathy

Neuropathy as a defining feature

NARP

This syndrome was first described in 1990 by Holt et al. as a maternally inherited disorder with developmental delay, retinitis pigmentosa, dementia, seizures, ataxia, and PN. Sequence analysis in this pedigree showed a heteroplasmic missense mutation (T8993G) in the mitochondrial ATP synthase subunit 6 gene.[31] The result of the T8993G mutation is a leucine to arginine substitution within the proton channel of the F_0 segment of Complex V (see Box 3.3), which impairs ATP synthesis.[91]

Patients with heteroplasmy between 70% and 90% show a typical NARP phenotype. Patients with more than 90% mutant mtDNAs usually present with maternally inherited Leigh's syndrome (MILS).[92,93] This disorder, historically called subacute necrotizing encephalomyelopathy, is characterized by hypotonia, failure to thrive, seizures, respiratory dysfunction, and ataxia. On T2-weighted MRI images, bilateral hyperintense signals can be observed in the basal ganglia, cerebellum or brainstem (see Chapter 12 for further details).

Clinically, NARP patients may have a history of delayed early motor development. On

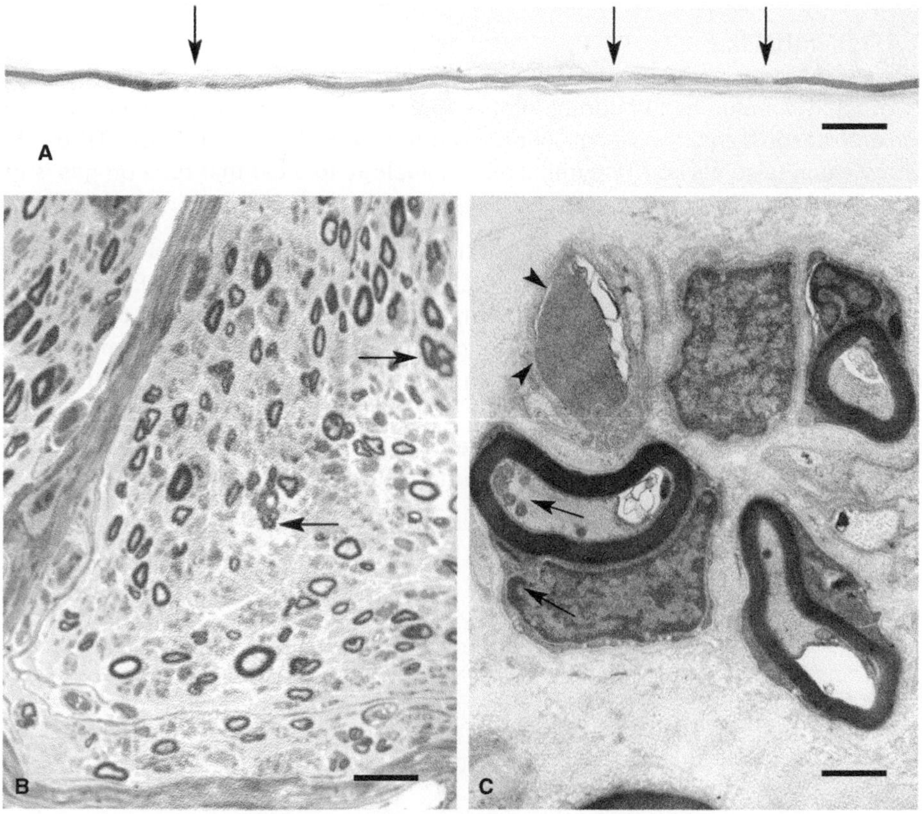

Figure 3.6 Sural nerve biopsy from a 41-year-old man with mitochondrial neurogastrointestinal encephalomyopathy (MNGIE) illustrating mixed pathological features of a myelinopathy and an axonopathy. (**A**) A teased myelinated fiber shows a short internode with a thin myelin sheath as indicated by the two nodes of Ranvier (arrow) on the right side. This segmental remyelination was accompanied by segmental demyelination in about one third of the myelinated fibers suggesting a neuropathy with a demyelinating process. Osmium tetroxide, bar = 100 μm. (**B**) A transverse semithin section of the nerve shows a mild loss of myelinated fibers and a few scattered small clusters of myelinated fibers (arrows) implying an axonopathy. These clusters are thought to be a regenerative response to axonal degeneration. There are also a few thinly myelinated fibers but no well-formed onion bulbs. Toluidine blue, bar = 20 μm. (**C**) Electron microscopy. An unmyelinated fiber shows an abnormal axon (arrowheads) suggesting degeneration. A few of the mitochondria display clusters (arrows) and enlargement (not shown) in axons and Schwann cells, These alterations are not specific for primary disorders of mitochondria. No paracrystalline inclusions or bizarre arrangement of cristae were observed within mitochondria. Bar = 1.0 μm

examination, there can be both proximal and distal neurogenic weakness, with absent ankle reflexes and loss of vibratory sensation. Neurophysiological studies are consistent with a sensorimotor axonal polyneuropathy. Muscle biopsy does not show RRFs.[94]

MNGIE

This disorder has been known by its current acronym since 1987 (when the M stood for 'myo' rather than 'mitochondrial')[95] but has been described with different acronyms: polyneuropathy,

Box 3.3 ATP synthesis

The proton gradient created by the pumping of H^+ ions from the matrix to the intermembrane space by the electron transport chain is the 'gasoline' used to power the synthesis of ATP by complex V of the respiratory chain (also called ATP synthase). The analogy to a car that runs on gas is quite apt, as ATP synthase is the world's tiniest motor.

ATP synthase is a marvel of engineering. It is a tiny rotary motor that couples the proton gradient generated by the electron transport chain to the synthesis of ATP from ADP and inorganic phosphate (called 'rotary catalysis'). It is a lollipop-shaped structure composed of two subcomplexes, called F_o and F_1. The F_o portion (the lollipop's 'stick') is embedded in the inner membrane and conducts protons from the intermembrane space to the matrix; it is composed of at least seven subunits (nucleus-encoded subunits a, b, c, e, and f, and mtDNA-encoded subunits A6 and A8). The F_1 portion (the lollipop's 'candy') protrudes into the matrix and uses the rotary motion of a cylinder of c subunits in F_o to convert ADP to ATP; it is composed of six subunits, all nucleus-enoded (α, β, γ, δ, ε, and OSCP).

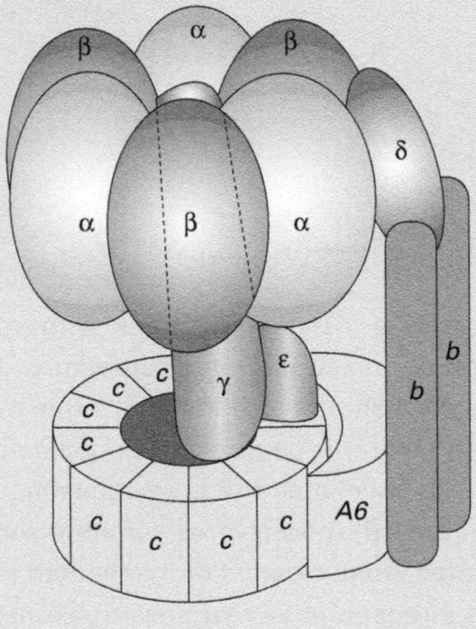

Figure B3.3.1 ATP synthase. Figure, with modification, courtesy of Boris Feniouk, http://www.biologie.uni-osnabrueck.de/biophysik/Feniouk/Gallery.html

How does this machine work? In brief, a cylinder of c subunits, connected to a central stalk (the γ subunit), acts as a rotor that is driven by the passage of protons through subunit A6, which is located on the side of the cylinder. Subunit A6, together with subunits b and 'OSCP', is part of the stator (see Figure B.3.3.1). The γ subunit acts as a cam which, when rotating, causes conformational changes in a trimer of α-β subunits in F_1 (arranged in a circle, like six orange slices) that allow for successive cycles of binding of ADP, reaction with inorganic phosphate to generate ATP, and release of the bound ATP.[1,2] The motor turns at more than 400 RPM, generating three ATPs per revolution.

What is going on at the molecular level? It appears that as protons flow through the A6 subunit in F_o, a specific aspartate residue on one of the ten c subunits is converted from the deprotonated form

(COO$^-$) to the protonated form (COOH).[3] Through a complex series of movements involving the protonated Asp residue on the c subunit and an arginine residue on the A6 subunit, the c subunit advances about 36° around the center of the cylinder. Once the proton is expelled into the matrix, the Asp residue is once again deprotonated, 're-setting' the orientation of the c subunit to its original conformation. The next proton to enter A6 starts the cycle anew, but on the next c-subunit in the cylinder, which has now moved into place opposite A6 (much like bullets in a revolver after firing).

The reaction to make ATP from ADP is reversible (i.e. complex V acts as both a synthase and a hydrolase), under the control of subunit ε, which acts as a unidirectional ratchet that can selectively switch off ATP hydrolysis depending on whether or not ε contacts the α-β dimer.

References

1. Abrahams JP, Leslie AG, Lutter R, Walker JE. Structure at 2.8Å resolution of F1-ATPase from bovine heart mitochondria. *Nature* 1994; **370**: 621–628.
2. Boyer PD. The ATP synthase – a splendid molecular machine. *Annu Rev Biochem* 1997; **66**: 717–749.
3. Rastogi VK, Girvin ME. Structural changes linked to proton translocation by subunit c of the ATP synthase. *Nature* 1999; **402**: 263–268.

ophthalmoplegia, leukoencephalopathy, and intestinal pseudo-obstruction (POLIP); oculogastrointestinal muscular dystrophy (OGIMD); and mitochondrial encephalomyopathy with sensorimotor neuropathy, ophthalmoplegia, and pseudo-obstruction (MEPOP).[96] It is an autosomal recessive disorder associated with multiple deletions and depletion of mtDNA, caused by a mutation in the thymidine phosphorylase gene (*TP*) on chromosome 22. The defining clinical features are severe gastrointestinal dysmotility, cachexia, ophthalmoparesis, peripheral neuropathy and leukoencephalopathy. Other characteristic features include ptosis, short stature, diverticulosis, hearing loss, and elevated cerebrospinal fluid protein. Gastrointestinal dysmotility is the most debilitating and often the presenting symptom.[59]

All MNGIE patients have mild to moderate peripheral sensorimotor polyneuropathy. In a minority of patients, the polyneuropathy is the presenting feature or dominates the clinical course.[97] In general, the neuropathy presents with stocking-glove sensory loss and areflexia of the lower extremities, and lesser involvement of the upper extremities. Nerve conduction studies show evidence of demyelination in most patients, with mixed demyelinating and axonal features in a third of them. Muscle biopsies show group atrophy, fiber type grouping, and target fibers, reflecting neurogenic abnormalities, as well as RRFs. On nerve biopsy, there is loss of myelinated fibers, segmental demyelination and segmental remyelination (Figure 3.6). Occasional onion bulb formation is observed. On electron microscopy, abnormal mitochondria have been described in Schwann cells.[98] The segmental nerve involvement has been attributed to uneven expression of the nuclear defect, resulting in patchy areas of mtDNA deletions and depletion.[97] Rare cases of MNGIE present with prominent demyelinating polyneuropathy mimicking CIDP or with Charcot– Marie–Tooth-like symptoms and bilateral pes cavus.[82,98] The multisystem involvement is a clue to the diagnosis.

SENSORY ATAXIC NEUROPATHY, DYSARTHRIA, AND OPHTHALMOPARESIS (SANDO)

The triad of symptoms that characterizes SANDO was originally described in 1997 in patients with sporadic severe sensory ataxic neuropathy as the presenting and predominant feature.[99] Since then, several other patients have been described. The cardinal features of SANDO include sensory ataxic neuropathy, dysarthria, and chronic external ophthalmoplegia. Associated features include ptosis, migraine, depression, and RRFs on muscle biopsy.[100] The neuropathy can precede other manifestations by several years. Multiple mtDNA deletions are present in affected tissue. Autosomal recessive inheritance was first suggested in 2003 by Van Goethem et al. who described compound heterozygous *POLG* missense mutations in SANDO. The *POLG* gene encodes a mitochondrial DNA polymerase involved in mtDNA replication and base excision repair.[100] The report of a heterozygous mutation in *PEO1* (formerly called *C10orf2* or *Twinkle*) in German siblings suggests that autosomal dominant inheritance is also possible.[101]

The clinical features of this sensory ataxic neuropathy include loss of vibratory and position sense in the distal lower extremities, mildly diminished pinprick and temperature sensation, areflexia, and sensory ataxic gait. Nerve conduction studies show absent sensory responses in both upper and lower extremities, with relatively preserved motor responses and conduction velocities. EMG is consistent with mild chronic reinnervation.[102] Sural nerve biopsies show loss of large and small myelinated axons, with regenerative clusters and endoneurial fibrosis. No onion bulb formation has been described. This is a presumed sensory ganglionopathy with degeneration of sensory axons. No abnormal mitochondria have been described on sural nerve biopsies, but no postmortem examination of the dorsal root ganglia is available.[100]

CHARCOT–MARIE–TOOTH TYPE 2A (CMT 2A)

Mitochondria move on microtubular rails and are propelled by motor proteins, usually GTPases, called kinesins. Mutations in the gene *MNF2* encoding one such motor protein, mitofusin 2, have been associated with an autosomal dominant variant of CMT, CMT2A.[103]

MULTIPLE SYMMETRIC LIPOMATOSIS (MSL)

This disorder, also known as Madelung's disease, is characterized by multiple non-encapsulated lipomas around the neck and shoulder girdle region. Up to 86% of patients have a predominantly axonal sensorimotor neuropathy, and over 50% also have central nervous system involvement.[104] Associated clinical features include cerebellar ataxia, hearing loss, optic atrophy, pyramidal signs and proximal myopathy. Clinical signs of neuropathy are usually mild, involving diminished vibratory and position sense and blunted deep tendon reflexes. Nerve conduction studies show markedly reduced amplitudes with slightly reduced conduction velocities, favoring a predominantly axonal neuropathy. EMG of proximal muscles may show myopathic units, while distal muscles often show a mild chronic neurogenic pattern.[105]

Muscle biopsies have shown RRFs, with COX-negative, SDH-positive fibers. Sural nerve biopsies have documented a predominantly axonal neuropathy, with loss of large myelinated axons.[106] Occasional circular arrays of Schwann cells arranged in an onion-bulb-like fashion have been reported.[105] Electron microscopy has shown loss of myelinated fibers; surviving myelinated fibers are sometimes surrounded by small onion bulbs. Furthermore, abnormal enlarged mitochondria with amorphous matrix have been documented in both axons and Schwann cells.[105] This syndrome is associated either with multiple mtDNA deletions or with the A8344G point mutation in the $tRNA^{Lys}$ gene of mtDNA, which also causes MERFF.[107]

NAVAJO NEUROHEPATOPATHY (NNH)

NNH is an autosomal recessive disorder affecting children from the Navajo Reservation in the Southwest of the United States, where the incidence is estimated at 1 per 1600 live births.[108] Diagnosis requires that four of the following seven criteria be present: (1) sensory neuropathy; (2) motor neuropathy; (3) corneal anesthesia, ulcers, or scarring; (4) liver disease; (5) documented metabolic or immunologic derangement; (6) central nervous system demyelination; and (7) positive family history of NNH.[109] Mean age at onset is 13 months, and most patients do not survive beyond the first decade of life. Affected children present with either Reye-like syndrome or severe progressive sensorimotor PN. Infants are hypotonic, weak, hyporeflexic, with delayed gross motor function. Laboratory studies show elevated liver enzymes and lactate; occasionally, serum CK can be up to ten times higher than normal.[110] Sural nerve biopsies are nearly devoid of large- and small-caliber myelinated fibers. Unmyelinated axons show signs of degeneration and regeneration.[111] Ultrastructural mitochondrial abnormalities in liver biopsies have shown ringed cristae, swelling and loss of cristae, and pleomorphic mitochondrial contours.[108] Molecular and biochemical studies in liver have shown mtDNA depletion and mitochondrial dysfunction. It has been suggested that mtDNA depletion is caused by a defect of a nDNA-encoded protein involved in mtDNA replication,[110] but the putative mutant gene remains to be identified.

Neuropathy as a frequently reported feature

MELAS

MELAS is a multisystem disorder characterized clinically by stroke-like episodes, encephalopathy with seizures or dementia, mitochondrial myopathy, migrainous headaches and recurrent vomiting (see above and Chapter 2). Other associated features include short stature, hearing loss, diabetes mellitus, and peripheral neuropathy.[112] The incidence of neuropathy in these patients is estimated at 22%.[90] Patients have sensory greater than motor distal PN with diminished or absent deep tendon reflexes and decreased vibration sense. Electrophysiological studies are consistent with axonal or mixed axonal and demyelinating polyneuropathy, but purely demyelinating neuropathy has also been reported.[79]

MERRF

MERRF is a multisystem disorder characterized by myoclonus, generalized epilepsy, ataxia and RRF on muscle biopsy (see Chapter 2).[113] The clinical phenotype is described earlier in this chapter.

PN is common in MERRF patients and often presents as mild sensorimotor PN, which can be subclinical.[114] Nerve conduction studies may show decreased amplitudes of compound muscle action potentials (CMAPs) or sensory nerve action potentials (SNAPs), indicating axonal involvement. EMG often shows a myopathic process in proximal muscles. Sural nerve biopsy has shown reduction of large myelinated fibers, consistent with primary axonal degeneration.[78]

LEIGH SYNDROME (SUBACUTE NECROTIZING ENCEPHALOMYELOPATHY)

Leigh syndrome (LS) is a neurodegenerative disorder of infancy or early childhood characterized by developmental regression, brainstem dysfunction and lactic acidosis (see Chapter 2).[115] Multiple foci of bilateral spongy degeneration were noted in the brainstem, basal ganglia, thalamus, and spinal cord in the original description and are the pathological hallmark of the syndrome. LS can result from several different metabolic defects affecting the pyruvate dehydrogenase complex, pyruvate carboxylase, complex I, complex II, COX, complex V, or biotinidase.[116–118] Mutations in both nuclear and mitochondrial genomes have been implicated. Two missense mutations in the same nucleotide (T8993G or T8993C) of the ATPase 6 gene of mtDNA have been associated with NARP at lower percentages of heteroplasmy and with maternally inherited Leigh syndrome (MILS) at higher mutation loads.[94]

PN presented in several patients with LS as a chronic demyelinating neuropathy, characterized clinically by hyporeflexia or areflexia and by slowed nerve conduction velocities on neurophysiological testing.[119,120] Rarely, patients present with acute demyelinating polyneuropathy.[121,122] Results of sural nerve biopsies have shown primary demyelination and remyelination, with some loss of both myelinated and unmyelinated axons.[123] Abnormal enlarged mitochondria with rounded cristae have been decribed in Schwann cells, but not in axons.[124] No onion bulb formation has been noted.

LHON (LEBER HEREDITARY OPTIC NEUROPATHY)

Patients with LHON are young adults, who present with acute or subacute, painless, central loss of vision that results in a permanent central scotoma and loss of sight (see Chapter 5). Several point mutations in three genes encoding complex I subunits are commonly implicated, G11778A, G3460A, and T14484C. Other neurological abnormalities have been reported in up to 59% of patients, including postural tremor, dystonia, and PN.[124] PN is rare, accounting for 11% of patients in one series.[125] Pathological findings in the sural nerve have shown signs of axonal degeneration and demyelination.[126]

mtDNA DELETION SYNDROMES: KSS, PS, PEO

Mitochondrial single-deletion syndromes are associated with three main phenotypes that are usually sporadic: Kearns–Sayre syndrome (KSS), Pearson syndrome (PS), and progressive external ophthalmoplegia (PEO). The clinical phenotypes of these disorders are described earlier in this chapter and in Chapters 3 and 10. Proximal myopathy is common in patients with KSS and PEO, with muscle biopsy showing RRFs and COX-negative fibers. PN has been rarely reported, and in such cases the PN is often subclinical, but axonal degeneration has been observed in sural nerve biopsy.[127]

LONG CHAIN 3 HYDROXYACYL-CoA DEHYDROGENASE DEFICIENCY AND MTP

Although these are not defects of the respiratory chain, we will describe them briefly here because PN (like cardiomyopathy, see Chapter 4) is an important clinical feature. The mitochondrial trifunctional protein (MTP) is involved in three steps of the β-oxidation of long-chain fatty acids (see Figure 1.1 in Chapter 1). As the name implies, this protein complex contains three enzyme activities, long-chain enoyl-CoA hydratase, long-chain 3-hydroxyacyl-CoA dehydrogenase (LCHAD), and long-chain thiolase. In some patients, all three enzyme activities are deficient; in others, there is isolated deficiency of LCHAD activity, with normal hydratase activity and moderately decreased thiolase activity. Both MTP and LCHAD deficiency typically present in early infancy with hypotonia, hypoketotic hypoglycemia, hepatomegaly with lipid storage, hepatic encephalopathy, cardiomyopathy, pigmentary retinopathy, and early high mortality.[128] A milder, less-frequent presentation with progressive sensorimotor polyneuropathy, limb girdle myopathy and myoglobinuria has been reported in adolescents or young adults.[129–131]

Electrophysiological studies have suggested progressive sensorimotor axonopathy with secondary demyelination. On sural nerve biopsy, there is axonal degeneration with normal myelin and no lipid deposit. The diagnosis is suggested by 3-hydroxy dicarboxylic aciduria and by an abnormal acylcarnitine profile, and is confirmed by enzyme measurement in cultured skin fibroblasts. General management involves dietary measures to avoid prolonged fasting and replacement of long-chain triglycerides with medium-chain fatty acids. There are anecdotal reports of improvement of the PN with prednisone or docosahexaenoic acid (cod liver oil).[129,132]

PARKINSONISM, DEAFNESS AND NEUROPATHY

A point mutation (T1095C) in the mitochondrial 12S rRNA gene has been associated with levodopa-responsive parkinsonism, deafness and axonal, predominantly sensory neuropathy.[133] Maternal relatives of this Italian proband had adult-onset bilateral sensorineural deafness or parkinsonism. Nerve conduction studies of the proband showed low or absent sensory amplitudes with normal motor conduction velocities. EMG showed evidence of chronic denervation. Another point mutation in the 12S rRNA gene (A1555G) has been associated with maternally inherited sensorineural deafness and levodopa-responsive parkinsonism without neuropathy.[134]

Treatment

There is no specific treatment for PN in mitochondrial disorders. Symptomatic treatment follows the same guidelines used for neuropathies of other etiologies.[135] Patients with mitochondrial disease and peripheral neuropathy should be evaluated for any contributing factors (e.g. diabetes mellitus, thyroid disease, chronic alcohol overuse) as these are potentially treatable. Sensory neuropathies associated with pain, discomfort and dysesthesias often respond to pharmacotherapy with gabapentin, carbamazepine, amitryptiline, or tramadol. In addition to pharmacotherapy, proper footcare and appropriate socks and shoes can help avoid complications. When motor neuropathies result in distal weakness, orthoses can often improve gait and decrease the risk of falling. Night splints for passive stretching may be useful in preventing contractures. A regular program of physical therapy can help maintain range of motion and improve gait safety. Although there is insufficient evidence of any beneficial effect on muscle and nerve symptoms, some advocate the use of antioxidant supplementation in mitochondrial disease (e.g. coenzyme Q10, L-carnitine, or alpha-lipoic acid) (see Chapter 14). There is a thiamine-responsive form of LS associated with pyruvate dehydrogenase E1α deficiency, which is transmitted by X-linked inheritance.[136,137] A trial of thiamine is warranted in these patients. Patients with MTP or LCHAD deficiency benefit from dietary management as mentioned above.

Unfortunately, one of the experimental medications that had been suggested for the treatment of MELAS, dichloroacetate (DCA), caused peripheral neuropathy in most patients. The results of a randomized clinical trial of DCA in MELAS suggest that any possible benefit is overshadowed by peripheral neurotoxicity.[170]

Conclusion

Mitochondrial disorders characteristically involve multiple systems, with a predilection for tissues with high energy requirements, such as muscle, nerve, and brain. New phenotypes and genotypes have emerged in recent years and continue to be discovered. It is important to recognize neuromuscular involvement in these patients, who are also at risk for motor or sensory impairment through other mechanisms.

References

1. DiMauro S, Schotland DL, Bonilla E et al. Progressive ophthalmoplegia, glycogen storage, and abnormal mitochondria. *Arch Neurol* 1973; **29**: 170–179.
2. Shoubridge EA, Karpati G, Hastings KE. Deletion mutants are functionally dominant over wild-type mitochondrial genomes in skeletal muscle fiber segments in mitochondrial disease. *Cell* 1990; **62**: 43–49.
3. Moraes CT, Ricci E, Petruzzella V et al. Molecular analysis of the muscle pathology associated with mitochondrial DNA deletions. *Nat Genet* 1992; **1**: 359–367.
4. DiMauro S, Bonilla E, Zeviani M et al. Mitochondrial myopathies. *Ann Neurol* 1985; **17**: 521–538.
5. Moraes CT, DiMauro S, Zeviani M et al. Mitochondrial DNA deletions in progressive external ophthalmoplegia and Kearns-Sayre syndrome. *N Engl J Med* 1989; **320**: 1293–1299.
6. Poulton J, Deadman ME, Bindoff L et al. Families of mtDNA re-arrangements can be detected in patients with mtDNA deletions: duplications may be a transient intermediate form. *Hum Mol Genet* 1993; **2**: 23–30.
7. Shanske S, Tang Y, Hirano M et al. Identical mitochondrial DNA deletion in a woman with ocular myopathy and in her son with Pearson syndrome. *Am J Hum Genet* 2002; **71**: 679–683.
8. Rotig A, Bessis JL, Romero N et al. Maternally inherited duplication of the mitochondrial genome

in a syndrome of proximal tubulopathy, diabetes mellitus, and cerebellar ataxia. *Am J Hum Genet* 1992; **50**: 364–370.
9. Mita S, Rizzuto R, Moraes CT, et al. Recombination via flanking direct repeats is a major cause of large-scale deletions of human mitochondrial DNA. *Nucleic Acids Res* 1990; **18**: 561–567.
10. Mita S, Schmidt B, Schon EA, et al. Detection of 'deleted' mitochondrial genomes in cytochrome-*c* oxidase-deficient muscle fibers of a patient with Kearns-Sayre syndrome. *Proc Natl Acad Sci USA* 1989; **86**: 9509–9513.
11. Hayashi J, Ohta S, Kikuchi A et al. Introduction of disease-related mitochondrial DNA deletions into HeLa cells lacking mitochondrial DNA results in mitochondrial dysfunction. *Proc Natl Acad Sci USA* 1991; **88**: 10614–10618.
12. Prezant TR, Agapian JV, Bohlman MC et al. Mitochondrial ribosomal RNA mutation associated with both antibiotic-induced and non-syndromic deafness. *Nat Genet* 1993; **4**: 289–294.
13. Arbustini E, Diegoli M, Fasani R et al. Mitochondrial DNA mutations and mitochondrial abnormalities in dilated cardiomyopathy. *Am J Pathol* 1998; **153**: 1501–1510.
14. DiMauro S, Schon EA. Mitochondrial respiratory-chain diseases. *N Engl J Med* 2003; **348**: 2656–2668.
15. Hasegawa H, Matsuoka T, Goto Y et al. Strongly succinate dehydrogenase-reactive blood vessels in muscles from patients with mitochondrial myopathy, encephalopathy, lactic acidosis, and stroke-like episodes. *Ann Neurol* 1991; **29**: 601–605.
16. Moraes CT, Ciacci F, Silvestri G et al. Atypical clinical presentations associated with the MELAS mutation at position 3243 of human mitochondrial DNA. *Neuromuscul Disord* 1993; **3**: 43–50.
17. Yasukawa T, Suzuki T, Ueda T et al. Modification defect at anticodon wobble nucleotide of mitochondrial $tRNAs^{Leu(UUR)}$ with pathogenic mutations of mitochondrial myopathy, encephalopathy, lactic acidosis, and stroke-like episodes. *J Biol Chem* 2000; **275**: 4251–4257.
18. Shoffner JM, Lott MT, Lezza AM et al. Myoclonic epilepsy and ragged-red fiber disease (MERRF) is associated with a mitochondrial DNA $tRNA^{Lys}$ mutation. *Cell* 1990; **61**: 931–937.
19. Silvestri G, Moraes CT, Shanske S et al. A new mtDNA mutation in the $tRNA^{Lys}$ gene associated with myoclonic epilepsy and ragged-red fibers (MERRF). *Am J Hum Genet* 1992; **51**: 1213–1217.
20. Boulet L, Karpati G, Shoubridge EA. Distribution and threshold expression of the $tRNA^{Lys}$ mutation in skeletal muscle of patients with myoclonic epilepsy and ragged-red fibers (MERRF). *Am J Hum Genet* 1992; **51**: 1187–1200.
21. Enriquez JA, Chomyn A, Attardi G. MtDNA mutation in MERRF syndrome causes defective aminoacylation of tRNA and premature translation termination. *Nat Genet* 1995; **10**: 47–55.
22. Wallace DC, Singh G, Lott MT et al. Mitochondrial DNA mutation associated with Leber's hereditary optic neuropathy. *Science* 1988; **242**: 1427–1430.
23. Andreu AL, Tanji K, Bruno C et al. Exercise intolerance due to a nonsense mutation in the mtDNA ND4 gene. *Ann Neurol* 1999; **45**: 820–823.
24. Musumeci O, Andreu AL, Shanske S et al. Intragenic inversion of mtDNA: a new type of pathogenic mutation in a patient with mitochondrial myopathy. *Am J Hum Genet* 2000; **66**: 1900–1904.
25. Schwartz M, Vissing J. Paternal inheritance of mitochondrial DNA. *N Engl J Med* 2002; **347**: 576–580.
26. Santorelli FM, Tanji K, Kulikova R et al. Identification of a novel mutation in the mtDNA ND5 gene associated with MELAS. *Biochem Biophys Res Commun* 1997; **238**: 326–328.
27. Crimi M, Galbiati S, Moroni I et al. A missense mutation in the mitochondrial *ND5* gene associated with a Leigh-MELAS overlap syndrome. *Neurology* 2003; **60**: 1857–1861.
28. Naini AB, Lu J, Kaufmann P et al. Novel mitochondrial DNA *ND5* mutation in a patient with clinical features of MELAS and MERRF. *Arch Neurol* 2005; **62**: 473–476.
29. Pulkes T, Eunson L, Patterson V et al. The mitochondrial DNA G13513A transition in *ND5* is associated with a LHON/MELAS overlap syndrome and may be a frequent cause of MELAS. *Ann Neurol* 1999; **46**: 916–919.
30. Liolitsa D, Rahman S, Benton S et al. Is the mitochondrial complex I *ND5* gene a hot-spot for MELAS causing mutations? *Ann Neurol* 2003; **53**: 128–132.
31. Holt IJ, Harding AE, Petty RK et al. A new mitochondrial disease associated with mitochondrial DNA heteroplasmy. *Am J Hum Genet* 1990; **46**: 428–433.

32. Andreu AL, Hanna MG, Reichmann H et al. Exercise intolerance due to mutations in the cytochrome *b* gene of mitochondrial DNA. *N Engl J Med* 1999; **341**: 1037–1044.
33. De Coo IF, Renier WO, Ruitenbeek W et al. A 4-base pair deletion in the mitochondrial cytochrome *b* gene associated with parkinsonism/MELAS overlap syndrome. *Ann Neurol* 1999; **45**: 130–133.
34. Andreu AL, Checcarelli N, Iwata S et al. A missense mutation in the mitochondrial cytochrome *b* gene in a revisited case with histiocytoid cardiomyopathy. *Pediatr Res* 2000; **48**: 311–314.
35. Hanna MG, Nelson IP, Rahman S et al. Cytochrome *c* oxidase deficiency associated with the first stop-codon point mutation in human mtDNA. *Am J Hum Genet* 1998; **63**: 29–36.
36. Karadimas CL, Greenstein P, Sue CM et al. Recurrent myoglobinuria due to a nonsense mutation in the *COX I* gene of mitochondrial DNA. *Neurology* 2000; **55**: 644–649.
37. Gattermann N, Retzlaff S, Wang YL et al. Heteroplasmic point mutations of mitochondrial DNA affecting subunit I of cytochrome *c* oxidase in two patients with acquired idiopathic sideroblastic anemia. *Blood* 1997; **90**: 4961–4972.
38. Manfredi G, Schon EA, Moraes CT et al. A new mutation associated with MELAS is located in a mitochondrial DNA polypeptide-coding gene. *Neuromuscul Disord* 1995; **5**: 391–398.
39. Comi GP, Bordoni A, Salani S et al. Cytochrome *c* oxidase subunit I microdeletion in a patient with motor neuron disease. *Ann Neurol* 1998; **43**: 110–116.
40. Bruno C, Martinuzzi A, Tang Y et al. A stop-codon mutation in the human mtDNA cytochrome *c* oxidase I gene disrupts the functional structure of complex IV. *Am J Hum Genet* 1999; **65**: 611–620.
41. Clark KM, Taylor RW, Johnson MA et al. An mtDNA mutation in the initiation codon of the cytochrome *c* oxidase subunit II gene results in lower levels of the protein and a mitochondrial encephalomyopathy. *Am J Hum Genet* 1999; **64**: 1330–1339.
42. Tanji K, Bonilla E. Neuropathologic aspects of cytochrome *c* oxidase deficiency. *Brain Pathol* 2000; **10**: 422–430.
43. Vu TH, Sciacco M, Tanji K et al. Clinical manifestations of mitochondrial DNA depletion. *Neurology* 1998; **50**: 1783–1790.
44. Bonilla E, Tanji K. Ultrastructural alterations in encephalomyopathies of mitochondrial origin. *Biofactors* 1998; **7**: 231–236.
45. Mandel H, Szargel R, Labay V et al. The deoxyguanosine kinase gene is mutated in individuals with depleted hepatocerebral mitochondrial DNA. *Nat Genet* 2001; **29**: 337–341.
46. Naviaux RK, Nguyen KV. POLG mutations associated with Alpers' syndrome and mitochondrial DNA mutations. *Ann Neurol* 2004; **55**: 706–712.
47. Saada A, Shaag A, Mandel H et al. Mutant mitochondrial thymidine kinase in mitochondrial DNA depletion myopathy. *Nat Genet* 2001; **29**: 342–344.
48. Elpeleg O, Miller C, Hershkovitz E et al. Deficiency of the ADP-forming succinyl-CoA synthase activity is associated with encephalomyopathy and mitochondrial DNA depletion. *Am J Hum Genet* 2005; **76**: 1081–1086.
49. Mancuso M, Salviati L, Sacconi S et al. Mitochondrial DNA depletion: mutations in thymidine kinase gene with myopathy and SMA. *Neurology* 2002; **59**: 1197–1202.
50. Pons R, Andreetta F, Wang CH et al. Mitochondrial myopathy simulating spinal muscular atrophy. *Pediatr Neurol* 1996; **15**: 153–158.
51. Dalakas MC, Illa I, Pezeshkpour GH et al. Mitochondrial myopathy caused by long-term zidovudine therapy. *N Engl J Med* 1990; **322**: 1098–1105.
52. Arnaudo E, Dalakas M, Shanske S et al. Depletion of muscle mitochondrial DNA in AIDS patients with zidovudine-induced myopathy. *Lancet* 1991; **337**: 508–510.
53. Servidei S, Zeviani M, Manfredi G et al. Dominantly inherited mitochondrial myopathy with multiple deletions of mitochondrial DNA: clinical, morphologic, and biochemical studies. *Neurology* 1991; **41**: 1053–1059.
54. Suomalainen A, Majander A, Haltia M et al. Multiple deletions of mitochondrial DNA in several tissues of a patient with severe retarded depression and familial progressive external ophthalmoplegia. *J Clin Invest* 1992; **90**: 61–66.
55. Kaukonen J, Juselius JK, Tiranti V et al. Role of adenine nucleotide translocator 1 in mtDNA maintenance. *Science* 2000; **289**: 782–785.
56. Spelbrink JN, Li FY, Tiranti V et al. Human mitochondrial DNA deletions associated with

mutations in the gene encoding Twinkle, a phage T7 gene 4-like protein localized in mitochondria. *Nat Genet* 2001; **28**: 223–231.
57. Van Goethem G, Dermaut B, Lofgren A et al. Mutation of *POLG* is associated with progressive external ophthalmoplegia characterized by mtDNA deletions. *Nat Genet* 2001; **28**: 211–212.
58. Bohlega S, Tanji K, Santorelli FM et al. Multiple mitochondrial DNA deletions associated with autosomal recessive ophthalmoplegia and severe cardiomyopathy. *Neurology* 1996; **46**: 1329–1334.
59. Nishino I, Spinazzola A, Papadimitriou A et al. Mitochondrial neurogastrointestinal encephalomyopathy: an autosomal recessive disorder due to thymidine phosphorylase mutations. *Ann Neurol* 2000; **47**: 792–800.
60. Nishino I, Spinazzola A, Hirano M. Thymidine phosphorylase gene mutations in MNGIE, a human mitochondrial disorder. *Science* 1999; **283**: 689–692.
61. Lamantea E, Tiranti V, Bordoni A et al. Mutations of mitochondrial DNA polymerase γ A are a frequent cause of autosomal dominant or recessive progressive external ophthalmoplegia. *Ann Neurol* 2002; **52**: 211–219.
62. Shoubridge EA. Nuclear genetic defects of oxidative phosphorylation. *Hum Mol Genet* 2001; **10**: 2277–2284.
63. Lombes A, Nakase H, Tritschler HJ et al. Biochemical and molecular analysis of cytochrome *c* oxidase deficiency in Leigh's syndrome. *Neurology* 1991; **41**: 491–498.
64. Adams PL, Lightowlers RN, Turnbull DM. Molecular analysis of cytochrome *c* oxidase deficiency in Leigh's syndrome. *Ann Neurol* 1997; **41**: 268–270.
65. Jaksch M, Hofmann S, Kleinle S et al. A systematic mutation screen of 10 nuclear and 25 mitochondrial candidate genes in 21 patients with cytochrome c oxidase (COX) deficiency shows $tRNA^{Ser(UCN)}$ mutations in a subgroup with syndromal encephalopathy. *J Med Genet* 1998; **35**: 895–900.
66. Zhu Z, Yao J, Johns T et al. *SURF1*, encoding a factor involved in the biogenesis of cytochrome *c* oxidase, is mutated in Leigh syndrome. *Nat Genet* 1998; **20**: 337–343.
67. Tiranti V, Hoertnagel K, Carrozzo R et al. Mutations of *SURF-1* in Leigh disease associated with cytochrome c oxidase deficiency. *Am J Hum Genet* 1998; **63**: 1609–1621.
68. Papadopoulou LC, Sue CM, Davidson MM et al. Fatal infantile cardioencephalomyopathy with COX deficiency and mutations in *SCO2*, a COX assembly gene. *Nat Genet* 1999; **23**: 333–337.
69. Sue CM, Karadimas C, Checcarelli N et al. Differential features of patients with mutations in two COX assembly genes, *SURF-1* and *SCO2*. *Ann Neurol* 2000; **47**: 589–595.
70. Glerum DM, Shtanko A, Tzagoloff A. *SCO1* and *SCO2* act as high copy suppressors of a mitochondrial copper recruitment defect in *Saccharomyces cerevisiae*. *J Biol Chem* 1996; **271**: 20531–20535.
71. DiMauro S, Bonilla E, Mancuso M et al. Mitochondrial myopathies. *Basic Appl Myol* 2003; **13**: 145–155.
72. DiMauro S, Mendell JR, Sahenk Z et al. Fatal infantile mitochondrial myopathy and renal dysfunction due to cytochrome-*c*-oxidase deficiency. *Neurology* 1980; **30**: 795–804.
73. Bresolin N, Zeviani M, Bonilla E et al. Fatal infantile cytochrome *c* oxidase deficiency: decrease of immunologically detectable enzyme in muscle. *Neurology* 1985; **35**: 802–812.
74. Tritschler HJ, Bonilla E, Lombes A et al. Differential diagnosis of fatal and benign cytochrome *c* oxidase-deficient myopathies of infancy: an immunohistochemical approach. *Neurology* 1991; **41**: 300–305.
75. DiMauro S, Nicholson JF, Hays AP et al. Benign infantile mitochondrial myopathy due to reversible cytochrome *c* oxidase deficiency. *Ann Neurol* 1983; **14**: 226–234.
76. Zeviani M, Peterson P, Servidei S et al. Benign reversible muscle cytochrome *c* oxidase deficiency: a second case. *Neurology* 1987; **37**: 64–67.
77. Bouillot S, Martin-Negrier ML, Vital A et al. Peripheral neuropathy associated with mitochondrial disorders: 8 cases and review of the literature. *J Peripher Nerv Syst* 2002; **7**: 213–220.
78. Chu CC, Huang CC, Fang W et al. Peripheral neuropathy in mitochondrial encephalomyopathies. *Eur Neurol* 1997; **37**: 110–115.
79. Rusanen H, Majamaa K, Tolonen U et al. Demyelinating polyneuropathy in a patient with the $tRNA^{Leu(UUR)}$ mutation at base pair 3243 of the mitochondrial DNA. *Neurology* 1995; **45**: 1188–1192.

80. Peyronnard JM, Charron L, Bellavance A, Marchand L. Neuropathy and mitochondrial myopathy. *Ann Neurol* 1980; **7**: 262–268.
81. Hara H, Wakayama Y, Kouno Y et al. Acute peripheral neuropathy, rhabdomyolysis, and severe lactic acidosis associated with 3243 A to G mitochondrial DNA mutation. *J Neurol Neurosurg Psychiatry* 1994; **57**: 1545–1546.
82. Bedlack RS, Vu T, Hammans S et al. MNGIE neuropathy: five cases mimicking chronic inflammatory demyelinating polyneuropathy. *Muscle Nerve* 2004; **29**: 364–368.
83. Yiannikas C, McLeod JG, Pollard JD, Baverstock J. Peripheral neuropathy associated with mitochondrial myopathy. *Ann Neurol* 1986; **20**: 249–257.
84. Fang W. Polyneuropathy in the mtDNA base pair 3243 point mutation. *Neurology* 1996; **46**: 1494–1495.
85. Girlanda P, Toscano A, Nicolosi C et al. Electrophysiological study of neuromuscular system involvement in mitochondrial cytopathy. *Clin Neurophysiol* 1999; **110**: 1284–1289.
86. Sladky JT. Histopathological features of peripheral nerve and muscle in mitochondrial disease. *Semin Neurol* 2001; **21**: 293–301.
87. Molnar M, Neudecker S, Schroder JM. Increase of mitochondria in vasa nervorum of cases with mitochondrial myopathy, Kearns-Sayre syndrome, progressive external ophthalmoplegia and MELAS. *Neuropathol Appl Neurobiol* 1995; **21**: 432–439.
88. Schroder JM, Sommer C. Mitochondrial abnormalities in human sural nerves: fine structural evaluation of cases with mitochondrial myopathy, hereditary and non-hereditary neuropathies, and review of the literature. *Acta Neuropathol* (Berl) 1991; **82**: 471–482.
89. Vallee RB, Bloom GS. Mechanisms of fast and slow axonal transport. *Annu Rev Neurosci* 1991; **14**: 59–92.
90. Karppa M, Syrjala P, Tolonen U, Majamaa K. Peripheral neuropathy in patients with the 3243A→G mutation in mitochondrial DNA. *J Neurol* 2003; **250**: 216–221.
91. Tatuch Y, Robinson BH. The mitochondrial DNA mutation at 8993 associated with NARP slows the rate of ATP synthesis in isolated lymphoblast mitochondria. *Biochem Biophys Res Commun* 1993; **192**: 124–128.
92. Tatuch Y, Christodoulou J, Feigenbaum A et al. Heteroplasmic mtDNA mutation (T→G) at 8993 can cause Leigh disease when the percentage of abnormal mtDNA is high. *Am J Hum Genet* 1992; **50**: 852–858.
93. Santorelli FM, Shanske S, Macaya A et al. The mutation at nt 8993 of mitochondrial DNA is a common cause of Leigh's syndrome. *Ann Neurol* 1993; **34**: 827–834.
94. Santorelli FM, Tanji K, Shanske S, DiMauro S. Heterogeneous clinical presentation of the mtDNA NARP/T8993G mutation. *Neurology* 1997; **49**: 270–273.
95. Bardosi A, Creutzfeldt W, DiMauro S et al. Myo-, neuro-, gastrointestinal encephalopathy (MNGIE syndrome) due to partial deficiency of cytochrome-*c*-oxidase. A new mitochondrial multisystem disorder. *Acta Neuropathol* (Berl) 1987; **74**: 248–258.
96. Hirano M, Silvestri G, Blake DM et al. Mitochondrial neurogastrointestinal encephalomyopathy (MNGIE): clinical, biochemical, and genetic features of an autosomal recessive mitochondrial disorder. *Neurology* 1994; **44**: 721–727.
97. Hirano M, Marti R, Spinazzola A et al. Thymidine phosphorylase deficiency causes MNGIE: an autosomal recessive mitochondrial disorder. *Nucleosides Nucleotides Nucleic Acids* 2004; **23**: 1217–1225.
98. Said G, Lacroix C, Plante-Bordeneuve V et al. Clinicopathological aspects of the neuropathy of neurogastrointestinal encephalomyopathy (MNGIE) in four patients including two with a Charcot-Marie-Tooth presentation. *J Neurol* 2005; **252**: 655–662.
99. Fadic R, Russell JA, Vedanarayanan VV et al. Sensory ataxic neuropathy as the presenting feature of a novel mitochondrial disease. *Neurology* 1997; **49**: 239–245.
100. Van Goethem G, Luoma P, Rantamaki M et al. *POLG* mutations in neurodegenerative disorders with ataxia but no muscle involvement. *Neurology* 2004; **63**: 1251–1257.
101. Hudson G, Deschauer M, Busse K et al. Sensory ataxic neuropathy due to a novel C10orf2 mutation with probable germline mosaicism. *Neurology* 2005; **64**: 371–373.
102. Okun MS, Bhatti MT. SANDO: another presentation of mitochondrial disease. *Am J Ophthalmol* 2004; **137**: 951–953.

103. Zuchner S, Mersiyanova IV, Muglia M et al. Mutations in the mitochondrial GTPase mitofusin 2 cause Charcot-Marie-Tooth neuropathy type 2A. *Nature Genet* 2004; **36**: 449–451.
104. Naumann M, Schalke B, Klopstock T et al. Neurological multisystem manifestation in multiple symmetric lipomatosis: a clinical and electrophysiological study. *Muscle Nerve* 1995; **18**: 693–698.
105. Naumann M, Kiefer R, Toyka KV et al. Mitochondrial dysfunction with myoclonus epilepsy and ragged-red fibers point mutation in nerve, muscle, and adipose tissue of a patient with multiple symmetric lipomatosis. *Muscle Nerve* 1997; **20**: 833–839.
106. Pollock M, Nicholson GI, Nukada H et al. Neuropathy in multiple symmetric lipomatosis. Madelung's disease. *Brain* 1988; **111**(Pt 5): 1157–1171.
107. Calabresi PA, Silvestri G, DiMauro S, Griggs RC. Ekbom's syndrome: lipomas, ataxia, and neuropathy with MERRF. *Muscle Nerve* 1994; **17**: 943–945.
108. Holve S, Hu D, Shub M et al. Liver disease in Navajo neuropathy. *J Pediatr* 1999; **135**: 482–493.
109. Singleton R, Helgerson SD, Snyder RD et al. Neuropathy in Navajo children: clinical and epidemiologic features. *Neurology* 1990; **40**: 363–367.
110. Vu TH, Tanji K, Holve SA et al. Navajo neurohepatopathy: a mitochondrial DNA depletion syndrome? *Hepatology* 2001; **34**: 116–120.
111. Appenzeller O, Kornfeld M, Snyder R. Acromutilating, paralyzing neuropathy with corneal ulceration in Navajo children. *Arch Neurol* 1976; **33**: 733–738.
112. Hirano M, Ricci E, Koenigsberger MR et al. MELAS: an original case and clinical criteria for diagnosis. *Neuromuscul Disord* 1992; **2**: 125–135.
113. Fukuhara N, Tokiguchi S, Shirakawa K, Tsubaki T. Myoclonus epilepsy associated with ragged-red fibres (mitochondrial abnormalities): disease entity or a syndrome? Light- and electron-microscopic studies of two cases and review of literature. *J Neurol Sci* 1980; **47**: 117–133.
114. Mizusawa H, Ohkoshi N, Watanabe M, Kanazawa I. Peripheral neuropathy of mitochondrial myopathies. *Rev Neurol* (Paris) 1991; **147**: 501–507.
115. Leigh D. Subacute necrotizing encephalomyelopathy in an infant. *J Neurochem* 1951; **14**: 216–221.
116. Vazquez-Memije ME, Shanske S, Santorelli FM et al. Comparative biochemical studies in fibroblasts from patients with different forms of Leigh syndrome. *J Inherit Metab Dis* 1996; **19**: 43–50.
117. Rahman S, Blok RB, Dahl HH et al. Leigh syndrome: clinical features and biochemical and DNA abnormalities. *Ann Neurol* 1996; **39**: 343–351.
118. Bruno C, Biancheri R, Garavaglia B et al. A novel mutation in the *SURF1* gene in a child with Leigh disease, peripheral neuropathy, and cytochrome-*c* oxidase deficiency. *J Child Neurol* 2002; **17**: 233–236.
119. Chabrol B, Mancini J, Benelli C et al. Leigh syndrome: pyruvate dehydrogenase defect. A case with peripheral neuropathy. *J Child Neurol* 1994; **9**: 52–55.
120. Grunnet ML, Zalneraitis EL, Russman BS, Barwick MC. Juvenile Leigh's encephalomyelopathy with peripheral neuropathy, myopathy, and cardiomyopathy. *J Child Neurol* 1991; **6**: 159–163.
121. Stickler DE, Carney PR, Valenstein ER. Juvenile-onset Leigh syndrome with an acute polyneuropathy at presentation. *J Child Neurol* 2003; **18**: 574–576.
122. Coker SB. Leigh disease presenting as Guillain-Barre syndrome. *Pediatr Neurol* 1993; **9**: 61–63.
123. Goebel HH, Bardosi A, Friede RL et al. Sural nerve biopsy studies in Leigh's subacute necrotizing encephalomyelopathy. *Muscle Nerve* 1986; **9**: 165–173.
124. Santoro L, Carrozzo R, Malandrini A et al. A novel SURF1 mutation results in Leigh syndrome with peripheral neuropathy caused by cytochrome *c* oxidase deficiency. *Neuromuscul Disord* 2000; **10**: 450–453.
125. Nikoskelainen EK, Marttila RJ, Huoponen K et al. Leber's 'plus': neurological abnormalities in patients with Leber's hereditary optic neuropathy. *J Neurol Neurosurg Psychiatry* 1995; **59**: 160–164.
126. Pages M, Pages AM. Leber's disease with spastic paraplegia and peripheral neuropathy. Case report with nerve biopsy study. *Eur Neurol* 1983; **22**: 181–185.
127. Zanssen S, Molnar M, Buse G, Schroder JM. Mitochondrial cytochrome *b* gene deletion in Kearns-Sayre syndrome associated with a subclinical type of peripheral neuropathy. *Clin Neuropathol* 1998; **17**: 291–296.
128. den Boer ME, Dionisi-Vici C, Chakrapani A et al. Mitochondrial trifunctional protein deficiency: a

severe fatty acid oxidation disorder with cardiac and neurologic involvement. *J Pediatr* 2003; **142**: 684–689.

129. Tein I, Vajsar J, MacMillan L, Sherwood WG. Long-chain L-3-hydroxyacyl-coenzyme A dehydrogenase deficiency neuropathy: response to cod liver oil. *Neurology* 1999; **52**: 640–643.
130. Bertini E, Dionisi-Vici C, Garavaglia B et al. Peripheral sensory-motor polyneuropathy, pigmentary retinopathy, and fatal cardiomyopathy in long-chain 3-hydroxy-acyl-CoA dehydrogenase deficiency. *Eur J Pediatr* 1992; **151**: 121–126.
131. Spiekerkoetter U, Bennett MJ, Ben-Zeev B et al. Peripheral neuropathy, episodic myoglobinuria, and respiratory failure in deficiency of the mitochondrial trifunctional protein. *Muscle Nerve* 2004; **29**: 66–72.
132. Tein I, Donner EJ, Hale DE, Murphy EG. Clinical and neurophysiologic response of myopathy and neuropathy in long-chain L-3-hydroxyacyl-CoA dehydrogenase deficiency to oral prednisone. *Pediatr Neurol* 1995; **12**: 68–76.
133. Thyagarajan D, Bressman S, Bruno C et al. A novel mitochondrial 12S rRNA point mutation in parkinsonism, deafness, and neuropathy. *Ann Neurol* 2000; **48**: 730–736.
134. Schoffer JM, Brown M, Huoponen K. A mitochondrial DNA (mtDNA) mutation associated with maternally inherited deafness and Parkinson's disease (PD). *Neurology* 1996; **46**: S31.002.A331.
135. Mendell JR, Kissel JT, Cornblath DR. *Diagnosis and Management of Peripheral Nerve Disorders*. New York: Oxford University Press, 2001.
136. Di Rocco M, Lamba LD, Minniti G et al. Outcome of thiamine treatment in a child with Leigh disease due to thiamine-responsive pyruvate dehydrogenase deficiency. *Eur J Paediatr Neurol* 2000; **4**: 115–117.
137. Naito E, Ito M, Yokota I et al. Thiamine-responsive pyruvate dehydrogenase deficiency in two patients caused by a point mutation (F205L and L216F) within the thiamine pyrophosphate binding region. *Biochim Biophys Acta* 2002; **1588**: 79–84.
138. Goto Y, Tojo M, Tohyama J et al. A novel point mutation in the mitochondrial $tRNA^{Leu(UUR)}$ gene in a family with mitochondrial myopathy. *Ann Neurol* 1992; **31**: 672–675.
139. Bindoff LA, Howell N, Poulton J et al. Abnormal RNA processing associated with a novel tRNA mutation in mitochondrial DNA. A potential disease mechanism. *J Biol Chem* 1993; **268**: 19559–19564.
140. Hadjigeorgiou GM, Kim SH, Fischbeck KH et al. A new mitochondrial DNA mutation (A3288G) in the $tRNA^{Leu(UUR)}$ gene associated with familial myopathy. *J Neurol Sci* 1999; **164**: 153–157.
141. Moraes CT, Ciacci F, Bonilla E et al. A mitochondrial tRNA anticodon swap associated with a muscle disease. *Nat Genet* 1993; **4**: 284–288.
142. Kleinle S, Schneider V, Moosmann P et al. A novel mitochondrial $tRNA^{Phe}$ mutation inhibiting anticodon stem formation associated with a muscle disease. *Biochem Biophys Res Commun* 1998; **247**: 112–115.
143. Silvestri G, Rana M, DiMuzio A et al. A late-onset mitochondrial myopathy is associated with a novel mitochondrial DNA (mtDNA) point mutation in the $tRNA^{Trp}$ gene. *Neuromuscul Disord* 1998; **8**: 291–295.
144. Vissing J, Salamon MB, Arlien-Soborg P et al. A new mitochondrial $tRNA^{Met}$ gene mutation in a patient with dystrophic muscle and exercise intolerance. *Neurology* 1998; **50**: 1875–1878.
145. Weber K, Wilson JN, Taylor L et al. A new mtDNA mutation showing accumulation with time and restriction to skeletal muscle. *Am J Hum Genet* 1997; **60**: 373–380.
146. Cardaioli E, Da Pozzo P, Radi E et al. A novel heteroplasmic $tRNA^{Leu(CUN)}$ mtDNA point mutation associated with chronic progressive external ophthalmoplegia. *Biochem Biophys Res Commun* 2005; **327**: 675–678.
147. Mancuso M, Ferraris S, Nishigaki Y et al. Congenital or late-onset myopathy in patients with the T14709C mtDNA mutation. *J Neurol Sci* 2005; **228**: 93–97.
148. Spinazzola A, Carrara F, Mora M, Zeviani M. Mitochondrial myopathy and ophthalmoplegia in a sporadic patient with the 5698G→A mitochondrial DNA mutation. *Neuromuscul Disord* 2004; **14**: 815–817.
149. Bidooki S, Jackson MJ, Johnson MA et al. Sporadic mitochondrial myopathy due to a new mutation in the mitochondrial $tRNA^{Ser(UCN)}$ gene. *Neuromuscul Disord* 2004; **14**: 417–420.
150. Moslemi AR, Lindberg C, Toft J et al.

A novel mutation in the mitochondrial tRNA^{Phe} gene associated with mitochondrial myopathy. *Neuromuscul Disord* 2004; **14**: 46–50.

151. Horvath R, Lochmuller H, Scharfe C et al. A tRNA^{Ala} mutation causing mitochondrial myopathy clinically resembling myotonic dystrophy. *J Med Genet* 2003; **40**: 752–757.

152. Campos Y, Garcia A, del Hoyo P et al. Two pathogenic mutations in the mitochondrial DNA tRNA$^{Leu(UUR)}$ gene (T3258C and A3280G) resulting in variable clinical phenotypes. *Neuromuscul Disord* 2003; **13**: 416–420.

153. Karadimas CL, Salviati L, Sacconi S et al. Mitochondrial myopathy and ophthalmoplegia in a sporadic patient with the G12315A mutation in mitochondrial DNA. *Neuromuscul Disord* 2002; **12**: 865–868.

154. Taylor RW, Schaefer AM, McFarland R et al. A novel mitochondrial DNA tRNA^{Ile} (A4267G) mutation in a sporadic patient with mitochondrial myopathy. *Neuromuscul Disord* 2002; **12**: 659–664.

155. Bruno C, Sacco O, Santorelli FM et al. Mitochondrial myopathy and respiratory failure associated with a new mutation in the mitochondrial transfer ribonucleic acid glutamic acid gene. *J Child Neurol* 2003; **18**: 300–303.

156. Vives-Bauza C, Gamez J, Roig M et al. Exercise intolerance resulting from a muscle-restricted mutation in the mitochondrial tRNA$^{Leu(CUN)}$ gene. *Ann Med* 2001; **33**: 493–496.

157. Karadimas C, Tanji K, Geremek M et al. A5814G mutation in mitochondrial DNA can cause mitochondrial myopathy and cardiomyopathy. *J Child Neurol* 2001; **16**: 531–533.

158. Campos Y, Gamez J, Garcia A et al. A new mtDNA mutation in the tRNA$^{Leu(UUR)}$ gene associated with ocular myopathy. *Neuromuscul Disord* 2001; **11**: 477–480.

159. Uziel G, Carrara F, Granata T et al. Neuromuscular syndrome associated with the 3291T→C mutation of mitochondrial DNA: a second case. *Neuromuscul Disord* 2000; **10**: 415–418.

160. Bruno C, Kirby DM, Koga Y et al. The mitochondrial DNA C3303T mutation can cause cardiomyopathy and/or skeletal myopathy. *J Pediatr* 1999; **135**: 197–202.

161. Dumoulin R, Sagnol I, Ferlin T et al. A novel gly290asp mitochondrial cytochrome *b* mutation linked to a complex III deficiency in progressive exercise intolerance. *Mol Cell Probes* 1996; **10**: 389–391.

162. Keightley JA, Anitori R, Burton MD et al. Mitochondrial encephalomyopathy and complex III deficiency associated with a stop-codon mutation in the cytochrome *b* gene. *Am J Hum Genet* 2000; **67**: 1400–1410.

163. Andreu AL, Bruno C, Shanske S et al. Missense mutation in the mtDNA cytochrome *b* gene in a patient with myopathy. *Neurology* 1998; **51**: 1444–1447.

164. Andreu AL, Bruno C, Dunne TC et al. A nonsense mutation (G15059A) in the cytochrome *b* gene in a patient with exercise intolerance and myoglobinuria. *Ann Neurol* 1999; **45**: 127–130.

165. Lamantea E, Carrara F, Mariotti C et al. A novel nonsense mutation (Q352X) in the mitochondrial cytochrome *b* gene associated with a combined deficiency of complexes I and III. *Neuromuscul Disord* 2002; **12**: 49–52.

166. Rahman S, Taanman JW, Cooper JM et al. A missense mutation of cytochrome oxidase subunit II causes defective assembly and myopathy. *Am J Hum Genet* 1999; **65**: 1030–1039.

167. Keightley JA, Hoffbuhr KC, Burton MD et al. A microdeletion in cytochrome *c* oxidase (COX) subunit III associated with COX deficiency and recurrent myoglobinuria. *Nat Genet* 1996; **12**: 410–416.

168. Kollberg G, Moslemi AR, Lindberg C et al. Mitochondrial myopathy and rhabdomyolysis associated with a novel nonsense mutation in the gene encoding cytochrome *c* oxidase subunit I. *J Neuropathol Exp Neurol* 2005; **64**: 123–128.

169. McFarland R, Taylor RW, Chinnery PF et al. A novel sporadic mutation in cytochrome *c* oxidase subunit II as a cause of rhabdomyolysis. *Neuromuscul Disord* 2004; **14**: 162–166.

170. Kaufmann P, Engelstad K, Wei Y et al. A randomized placebo-controlled trial of dichloroacetate in MELAS. Toxicity overshadows potential benefit.

4

Mitochondrial cardiology

Jeffrey A Towbin

Introduction

The heart requires high levels of energy, mostly in the form of adenosine triphosphate (ATP), which is predominantly generated by mitochondria. Therefore, it is easy to see how defects in mitochondrial function can lead to a variety of negative effects on the heart. In this chapter, we will describe the typical cardiac diseases caused by mitochondrial dysfunction.

Normal cardiac structure

Cardiac muscle fibers comprise separate cellular units (myocytes) connected in series.[1] In contrast to skeletal muscle fibers, cardiomyocytes do not assemble in parallel arrays but rather bifurcate and recombine to form a complex three-dimensional network. They are joined at each end to adjacent myocytes at the intercalated discs, specialized areas of interdigitating cell membrane (Figure 4.1). The intercalated disc has gap junctions (containing connexins) and mechanical junctions, consisting of adherens junctions (containing N-cadherin, catenins, and vinculin) and desmosomes (containing desmin, desmoplakin, plakophilin, desmocollin, and desmoglein). Cardiomyocytes are surrounded by a thin membrane (sarcolemma) and contain bundles of longitudinally arranged myofibrils. The myofibrils are formed by repeating sarcomeres, which are the basic contractile units of cardiac muscle and consist of interdigitating thin (actin) and thick (myosin) filaments (Figure 4.1), giving cardiac muscle its characteristic striated appearance.[2,3] The thick filaments are composed primarily of myosin but also contain myosin-binding proteins C, H, and X. The thin filaments are composed of cardiac actin, α-tropomyosin (α-TM), and troponins T, I, and C (cTnT, cTnI, cTnC). In addition, myofibrils contain a third filament formed by the giant protein titin, which extends from the Z-disc to the M-line and acts as a molecular template for the layout of the sarcomere. The Z-disc at each end of the sarcomere is formed by a lattice of interdigitating proteins that maintain myofilament organization by cross-linking antiparallel titin and thin filaments from adjacent sarcomeres (Figure 4.2). Other proteins in the Z-disc include α-actinin, nebulette, telethonin/T-cap, capZ, muscle LIM protein (MLP), myopalladin, myotilin, Cypher/ZASP, filamin, and FATZ.[2,3]

Finally, the extrasarcomeric cytoskeleton, a complex network of proteins linking the sarcomere with the sarcolemma and the extracellular matrix (ECM), provides structural support for subcellular structures and transmits mechanical and chemical signals within and between cells. The extrasarcomeric cytoskeleton has intermyofibrillar and subsarcolemmal components. The intermyofibrillar

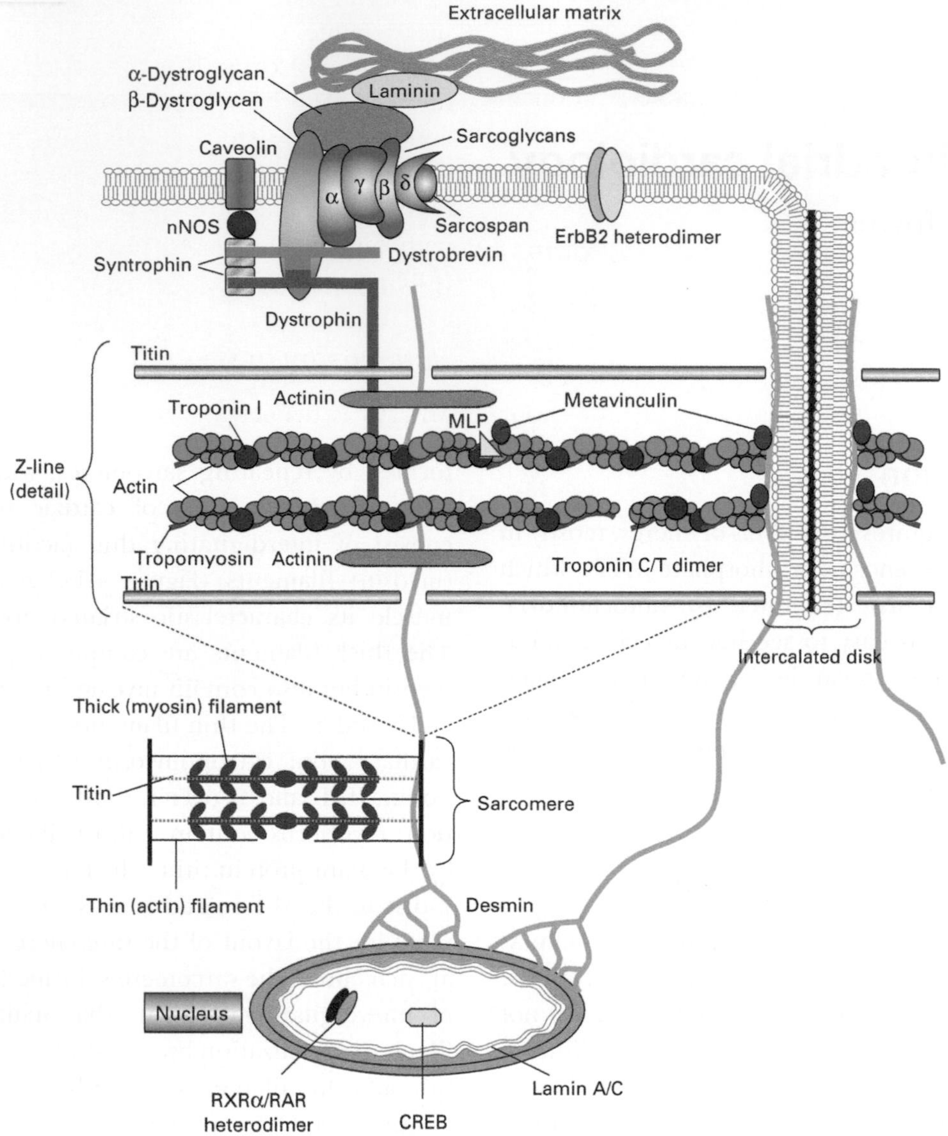

Figure 4.1 Cardiac myocyte structure. Note membrane proteins, intercalated disc, and sarcomeric structure

cytoskeleton is composed of intermediate filaments (IFs), microfilaments, and microtubules.[4–9] Desmin IFs form a three-dimensional scaffold throughout the extra-sarcomeric cytoskeleton, surrounding the Z-disc and allowing for longitudinal connections between adjacent Z-discs and lateral connections to subsarcolemmal costameres.[3–9] Microfilaments composed of non-sarcomeric actin (mainly γ-actin) also form complex networks linking the sarcomere (via α-actinin) to various components of the costameres. Costameres are subsarcolemmal domains located in a periodic, grid-like pattern,

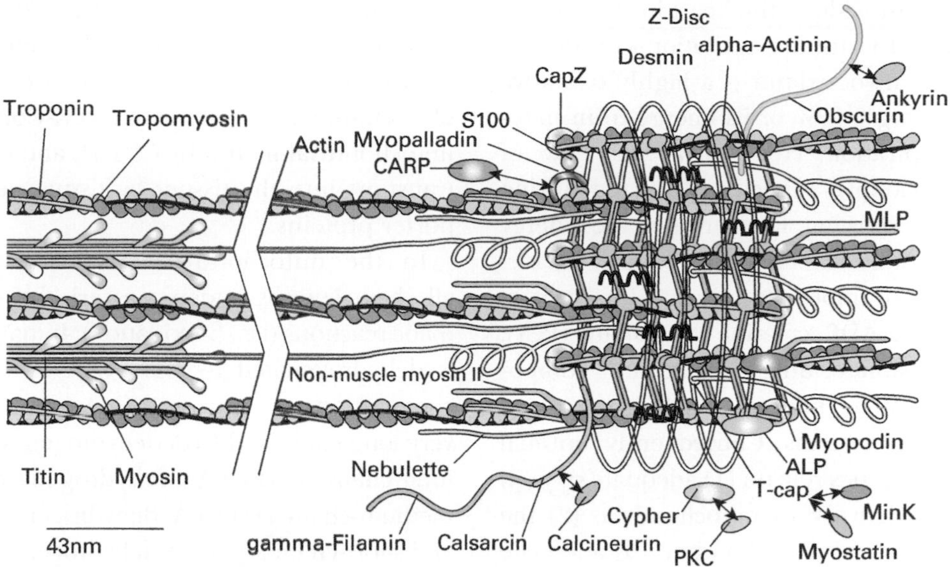

Figure 4.2 Z-disc architecture. The Z-disc of the sarcomere is comprised of multiple interacting proteins that anchor the sarcomere. The proteins involved in the Z-disc structure include alpha-actinin, MLP, Cypher (ZASP), and others, MLP = muscle LIM protein; ALP = actinin-associated LIM protein

flanking the Z-discs and overlying the I bands, on the cytoplasmic side of the sarcolemma. They are sites of interconnection between various cytoskeletal networks, linking sarcomere and sarcolemma and functioning as anchor sites for stabilization of the sarcolemma and for integration of pathways involved in mechanical force transduction. Costameres contain three principal components: focal adhesion-type complex, spectrin-based complex, and dystrophin/dystrophin-associated protein complex (DAPC).[10,11] The focal adhesion-type complex consists of cytoplasmic proteins (i.e., vinculin, talin, tensin, paxillin, zyxin) and connects with cytoskeletal actin filaments and with the transmembrane proteins α-, β-dystroglycan, α-, β-, γ-, δ-sarcoglycans, dystrobrevin, and syntrophin.[6,7] Several actin-associated proteins are located at sites of attachment of cytoskeletal actin filaments with costameric complexes, including α-actinin and the muscle LIM protein, MLP. The C-terminus of dystrophin binds β-dystroglycan (Figure 4.1), which in turn interacts with α-dystroglycan to link to the ECM (via α-2-laminin). The N-terminus of dystrophin interacts with actin. Notably, voltage-gated sodium channels co-localize with dystrophin, β-spectrin, ankyrin, and syntrophins, whereas potassium channels interact with the sarcomeric Z-disc and intercalated discs.[12–14] Since arrhythmias and conduction system diseases are common in children and adults with all forms of cardiomyopathy, this interaction could play an important role in pathogenesis. Hence, disruption of the links between the sarcolemma and the ECM at the dystrophin C-terminus and between the sarcomere and the nucleus via N-terminal dystrophin interactions could lead to a 'domino effect', disruption of systolic function, followed by diastolic dysfunction, and development of arrhythmias.

Normal cardiac metabolism

Cardiac function depends on a finely tuned balance between the work the heart must perform to meet the needs of the body and the energy that the body must provide to the heart in the form of ATP required to sustain excitation–contraction coupling. The myocardium is a highly oxidative tissue, producing >90% of its energy from mitochondrial respiration. However, at least 90% of the heart's oxidative capacity is utilized during exercise, thus allowing for considerable energy reserve.[15] Oxidative metabolism requires balancing a variety of molecules, including oxygen, substrates, ATP, ADP, creatine phosphate (PCr), inorganic phosphate, and calcium, and components necessary to maintain redox state and phosphotransfer systems. Consequently, optimal cellular bioenergetics rely on (1) adequate oxygen and substrate delivery to mitochondria, (2) the oxidative capacity of mitochondria, (3) adequate amounts of high-energy phosphate and the PCr/ATP ratio, (4) efficient energy transfer from mitochondria to sites of energy utilization, (5) adequate local regulation of ATP/ADP ratios near ATPases, and (6) efficient feedback signaling from utilization sites to maintain energy homeostasis. Defects at any step of the cardiac bioenergetics pathway can lead to cardiac disease.

Fatty acid oxidation

β-oxidation of free fatty acids is an important source of energy for multiple tissues, including the heart (see Figure 1.1 in Chapter 1). The heart, a highly aerobic organ, utilizes long-chain fatty acids as its primary source of energy. Therefore, it stands to reason that defects of β-oxidation would result in cardiovascular manifestations.[16] Free fatty acids of carbon length 20 or less are β-oxidized in the mitochondria. Short-chain and medium-chain fatty acids enter the mitochondrial matrix directly and upon entry are activated to their corresponding acyl-CoA thioesters by an acyl-CoA synthetase. In contrast, long-chain fatty acids are activated in the cytoplasm and require active transport into the mitochondria.[17] This complex process includes (1) conjugation to carnitine by carnitine palmitoyl transferase I (CPT I) at the outer mitochondrial membrane, (2) transfer to CPT II on the inner mitochondrial membrane via a carnitine-acylcarnitine translocase, (3) release of carnitine and long-chain acyl-CoAs into the mitochondrial matrix by CPT II, and (4) carnitine transport into the tissues by tissue-specific transporter proteins.[18]

In the mitochondrial matrix, acyl-CoAs of all chain lengths undergo a series of cyclic enzymatic reactions (i.e., β-oxidation). Initially, acyl-CoA is dehydrogenated to enoyl-CoA by the catalytic cooperation of four acyl-CoA dehydrogenases: very long-chain acyl-CoA dehydrogenase (VLCAD), long-chain acyl-CoA dehydrogenase (LCAD), medium-chain acyl-CoA dehydrogenase (MCAD), and short-chain acyl-CoA dehydrogenase (SCAD).[17] Electrons released during these reactions are channeled into the respiratory chain by electron transfer flavoprotein (ETF) and ETF dehydrogenase to produce adenosine triphosphate (ATP) (see Chapter 1, Figure 1.1). The enoyl-CoAs produced by the acyl-CoA dehydrogenases are further metabolized through three enzymatic reactions to release acetyl-CoA and a new acyl-CoA molecule that is two carbons shorter; these reactions, however, differ depending on the chain length of the substrate. In the case of long-chain acyl-CoA substrates, the reactions are carried out by a trifunctional protein, which has activities of acyl-CoA hydratase, hydroxyacyl-CoA dehydrogenase and acyl-CoA ketothiolase while for shorter-chain acyl-CoA substrates specific enzymes are needed.[18]

Oxidative phosphorylation

Oxidative phosphorylation disorders are a group of inherited metabolic diseases with variable clinical presentations (see Chapter 1).

The syndrome of heart failure

Traditionally, the syndrome of heart failure has been viewed as a constellation of clinical findings resulting from inadequate systolic function ('pump function'). Over the past decade, however, this view has been altered by clinical and research data, including the persistently poor outcome of patients despite therapies designed to improve systolic function.[19] In addition, new information on inflammatory mediators, apoptosis, structure–function studies, and genetics has suggested that heart failure results from a complex interaction of structural, functional, and biologic perturbations.

The current concept of heart failure integrates multiple diverse models, hemodynamic, neurohormonal, structural, and autocrine–paracrine.[20,21] The hemodynamic model focuses on alterations in load on the failing ventricle and attendant pump dysfunction. Based on this hypothesis, therapies employ inotropic agents and vasodilators to improve contractility. The neurohormonal model stresses the importance of the renin–angiotensin–aldosterone system (RAAS) and of the sympathetic nervous system in the pathogenesis of heart failure. Pharmacological therapy attempts to antagonize the effects of circulating norepinephrine and angiotensin II. The autocrine–paracrine model was based on the findings that norepinephrine, angiotensin II, and other vasoactive substances such as brain natriuretic peptide (BNP), are not only circulating but also synthesized within the myocardium, thus adding autocrine and paracrine modes of action to their systemic effects. Finally, the structural model focuses on the interactions between sarcomere and sarcolemma via cytoskeletal and other proteins. These, as well as models centered on inflammatory mediators and apoptosis, have all been invoked to account for features of heart failure. It is likely that all play roles in this clinical syndrome.

Yet another model of heart failure is the metabolic one, in which disparities between energy production, energy utilization, and energy requirements of the heart are key contributors. In this model, ATP production is required to drive the contractile apparatus because the thick filament protein myosin requires ATP at the β-myosin head for contraction to occur. Lack of energy causes disturbance in the contractile apparatus machinery, leading to pump dysfunction. To counter this problem, therapeutic strategies have included coenzyme Q10, carnitine, riboflavin, and thiamine, amongst other vitamins and cofactors.

Despite the complexity of interactions causing heart failure, a major abnormality at the center of the syndrome is the process of remodeling. Remodeling of the left ventricle is a process in which ventricular size, shape, and function are altered due to mechanical, genetic, and neurohormonal factors that lead to hypertrophy, myocyte loss, and interstitial fibrosis.[22] In dilated cardiomyopathy, progressive ventricular dilation and changes of the ventricle to a more spherical shape, together with changes in ventricular function and/or hypertrophy, occur without a known triggering event (except in patients with myocardial infarction). Due to these remodeling events, mitral regurgitation may develop as the geometric relationship between mitral valve apparatus, mitral ring, and papillary muscles is altered. Mitral regurgitation increases volume load on an already compromised ventricle, further contributing to remodeling, disease progression, and left atrial dilation. Improved outcomes may depend on the ability to reverse this remodeling process ('reverse remodeling').

Cardiopathies in children with mitochondrial disease

Mitochondrial disorders associated with abnormalities of oxidative phosphorylation are genetically, biochemically, and clinically heterogeneous (see Chapter 1). Organs such as brain, skeletal muscle, and heart are highly energy dependent and, therefore, especially vulnerable to defects in energy metabolism.[23]

The most common cardiopathies associated with mitochondrial dysfunction present in infants, who usually develop a hypertrophic dilated heart with systolic dysfunction.[24] Other presentations in young children include hypertrophic cardiomyopathy (HCM) with hypercontractile systolic function, left ventricular non-compaction (LVNC), or dilated cardiomyopathy (DCM). In addition, conduction system diseases, such as heart block, pre-excitation, or Wolff–Parkinson–White (WPW) syndrome, and even congenital heart disease have been described.[25] Older children, adolescents, and young adults typically present with DCM, DCM with conduction disease, or simply conduction disease, although LVNC has also been reported.[26]

The Baylor experience

Our group described the clinical spectrum, morbidity, and mortality associated with mitochondrial disease in 113 children seen at our institution.[27] We reviewed retrospectively the genetic, clinical, and laboratory records of 400 children referred to our hospital between 1997 and 2003 for evaluation of possible mitochondrial disease, based on neurologic, musculoskeletal, or cardiac features. Using the modified Walker criteria, the diagnosis of 'definite' mitochondrial disease was established in 113 children. This classification scheme utilizes objective clinical, histologic, biochemical, functional, molecular, and metabolic features to establish a diagnosis of mitochondrial disease. Patients with two major or one major and two minor criteria are assigned a definite diagnosis. Of the 113 children who met these criteria, 58% were boys and 42% were girls. Mean age of presentation was 40 months (range: 2 weeks to 18 years) and mean age at death was 5 years and 4 months. All ethnicities were represented. The inheritance pattern was unknown in the majority of cases, but 13/113 (11.5%) had maternal inheritance, 2/113 (1.8%) patients had autosomal recessive inheritance based on nuclear DNA mutations, and one child with Barth syndrome had X-linked inheritance.

In our cohort, 45 children had predominantly cardiac presentations and had earlier onset than those with encephalomyopathy (33 vs 44 months).[27] Of the patients with cardiac manifestations, 58% had HCM, 29% had DCM, and 13% had LVNC. Only 11% had arrhythmias, most commonly ventricular tachycardia (VT) while only two children had WPW. Survival by age 16 years differed between patients with cardiac disease and those with predominantly neurologic disease: only 18% of cardiac patients were alive at age 16 as opposed to 95% of neurologic patients.[27]

Diagnostic evaluation included urine and blood studies, genetic studies, and muscle biopsy for histology and biochemistry. Most patients, 102/113 (90%), underwent muscle biopsy. A significant respiratory chain defect was observed in 71% of patients, including complex I deficiency (32%), combined complex I, III, and IV deficiencies (26%), complex IV deficiency (19%), complex III deficiency (16%), and complex II deficiency (7%).

The most common mtDNA mutation was the A3243G, which was identified in eight patients. This mutation is usually associated with mitochondrial encephalomyopathy, lactic acidosis, and stroke-like episodes (MELAS) (see below). Cardiac manifestations of MELAS include hypertrophic, dilated, or hypertrophic-dilated cardiomyopathy, ventricular arrhythmias, pre-excitation and conduction block.[24,28] The A3243G mutation has been found in 80% of patients with MELAS (see Chapter 2).

The remaining mtDNA mutations identified in our patients included the A8344G mutation usually associated with myoclonic epilepsy and ragged-red fibers (MERRF) in two children, the G3460A mutation, usually associated with Leber hereditary optic neuropathy (LHON) in one child, the T8993C mutation in the ATPase 6 gene, associated with neuropathy, ataxia, and retinitis pigmentosa (NARP) in one child, and a 5-kilobase (kb) deletion, typically causing chronic progressive external ophthalmoplegia (CPEO) or Kearns–Sayre syndrome (KSS), in one child.[27]

MERRF, LHON and CPEO have all been associated with cardiovascular disease, although cardiomyopathy is not part of their typical presentations.[23,29,30] MERRF is characterized by progressive myoclonic epilepsy, mitochondrial myopathy with ragged red fibers, dementia, hearing loss, and ataxia (see Chapter 2).[31,32]

In LHON, three mtDNA point mutations, G3460A (as seen in our patient), G11778A, and T14484C account for more than 90% of all LHON cases (see Chapter 5). Sorajja and colleagues[29] studied 24 consecutive patients with LHON, eight of whom had the G3460A mutation; five of these had cardiac hypertrophy and one died suddenly. CPEO and KSS are typically caused by single or multiple deletions of mtDNA and frequently have cardiac manifestations, including conduction defects, dilated and hypertrophic cardiomyopathies, and pre-excitation (see below).[33–35]

Although our study offers a realistic view of the relative frequency of mitochondrial cardiomyopathies in a pediatric population and suggests that the most common mtDNA mutations (A3243G-MELAS, A8344G-MERRF, A3460G-LHON, T8993C-NARP, and single deletions-CPEO) are also the most common causes of childhood cardiomyopathy, there are many other, albeit rarer, mtDNA mutations, which have been associated with cardiomyopathy. In the following sections, we will consider sequentially the mitochondrial cardiomyopathies due to mutations in mtDNA and those due to mutations in nuclear DNA.

Cardiomyopathies due to mutations in mtDNA

Sporadic rearrangements

Large-scale rearrangements of mtDNA consisting of single deletions or duplications generally occur in sporadic patients. Frequently, both types of rearrangements are present in the same individual; in this situation, the deletion and duplication are structurally related. Specifically, the duplication corresponds to a full-length wild-type molecule plus the deleted mtDNA segment (see Box 3.2). Duplications are probably not directly pathogenic, but can produce deleted mtDNA molecules, which are pathogenic.[36,37] A key point is that each patient has a single type of rearranged molecule, which is clonally derived from a spontaneous rearrangement event that occurred in oogenesis or early in development.

Three major clinical entities are associated with sporadic mtDNA deletions and duplications: KSS, Pearson syndrome (PS), and sporadic CPEO with RRF (see Chapter 2). Of these disorders, cardiac involvement is most prominent in KSS, a multisystem disease defined by the obligate triad of onset before age 20 years, PEO, and pigmentary retinopathy, plus at least one of the following additional features: cardiac conduction block, cerebellar syndrome, and cerebrospinal fluid protein greater than 100 mg/dL.[38] A muscle biopsy is generally required to confirm the diagnosis by molecular analysis because the mtDNA rearrangements are much more abundant in post-mitotic tissues than in replicating cells, such as leukocytes. Muscle histology reveals marked mitochondrial proliferation with RRF in the modified Gomori trichrome stain. The RRF show increased histochemical stain for succinate dehydrogenase (SDH) and decreased or absent stain for cytochrome *c* oxidase (COX) (see Chapter 3).

Conduction block is the most common cardiac manifestation in KSS. In a review of 86 patients reported between 1982 and 1992, 61 of 73 (84%) had heart block (unpublished data from reference 39). The conduction defects include prolonged intraventricular conduction time, bundle-branch block, and atrioventricular block and are frequent causes of death. Placement of a pacemaker may be a lifesaving procedure, particularly in patients with second-degree or third-degree atrioventricular (AV) block or bifascicular block.[40] In comparison to cardiac conduction blocks, cardiomyopathy is much less frequent and seems to be a late-onset phenomenon; it was described in only two of 86 KSS patients,[39] who developed dilated cardiomyopathy at 21 and 33 years of age.[41,42] The cardiomyopathy can be fatal[43] and cardioembolic strokes have been reported as a complication.[44,45] Because of the dual risks of cardiac embolism and severe cardiomyopathy, cardiac transplantation should be considered for some KSS patients. For example, one 38-year-old man with incomplete KSS and a heteroplasmic 4.5-kilobase (kb) mtDNA deletion developed cardiac failure over several months and underwent a successful cardiac transplantation with a stable neurological status 18 months later.[46] We are following a similar KSS patient who developed an AV node conduction abnormality and underwent pacemaker placement at age 14 years. At age 29 years, he had pyramidal tract signs and moderate ataxia, but was intellectually intact and developed congestive heart failure. At age 29 years, he underwent cardiac transplantation and, 14 months later, was medically stable.

The increased vulnerability of the conduction system in KSS may be due to a selective concentration of the deletions in this specialized tissue. This hypothesis has been supported by postmortem data in a KSS patient, which revealed higher proportions of the mtDNA deletion in the sinus node, AV node, and bundle branches than in the contractile myocardium.[47] The uncommon occurrence and late onset of cardiomyopathy in KSS may be due to the relatively low abundance of rearranged mtDNA molecules in the myocardium. An alternative explanation was proposed by Fromenty and colleagues,[48] who employed a novel long polymerase chain reaction (PCR) method to quantitate deleted and duplicated mtDNAs. They demonstrated that duplications represented an unusually high proportion (41–91%) of all rearranged molecules in hearts from two KSS patients. By contrast, the percentage of mtDNA duplications in other tissues ranged from 0–39%. Because of the preferential accumulation of duplicated rather than deleted mtDNA molecules, the myocardium may be relatively spared in KSS.

Patients with isolated progressive external ophthalmoplegia and single mtDNA deletions generally do not develop cardiac conduction blocks. However, some patients have a disease of intermediate severity between myopathic PEO and multisystemic KSS. Such patients are at risk of developing cardiac conduction blocks, cardiomyopathy, or both.

Maternally inherited point mutations

At least 18 mtDNA mutations are associated with cardiomyopathies (Figure 4.3, Table 4.1 and Box 4.1). Fourteen point mutations are in tRNA genes, and two of these, $tRNA^{Leu(UUR)}$ and $tRNA^{Ile}$, seem to be hotspots for cardiomyopathies. It is not too surprising that mutations in $tRNA^{Leu(UUR)}$ are frequently encountered in patients with cardiomyopathies because 16 mutations in this gene have been associated with multisystemic human disorders. By contrast, it is striking that most mutations in $tRNA^{Ile}$ (five of nine) are associated with diseases that present primarily or exclusively with cardiomyopathy.

A prime example of a $tRNA^{Leu(UUR)}$ mutation associated with a multisystem disorder is A3243G-MELAS, as discussed above. In a review of 110 reported MELAS patients, cardiac manifestations included congestive heart failure in 18%, Wolff–Parkinson–White syndrome in 14%, and cardiac conduction block in 6%.[49] The cardiomyopathy is usually hypertrophic.[50,51] Isolated cardiomyopathy can also be the presenting manifestation of this mutation.[52–54]

Characteristic histological findings in patients with MELAS are 'strongly succinate-reactive vessels' (SSVs) in skeletal muscle and brain.[55,56] These abnormalities are due to mitochondrial proliferation in the walls of capillaries and small arterioles and have suggested that MELAS is due

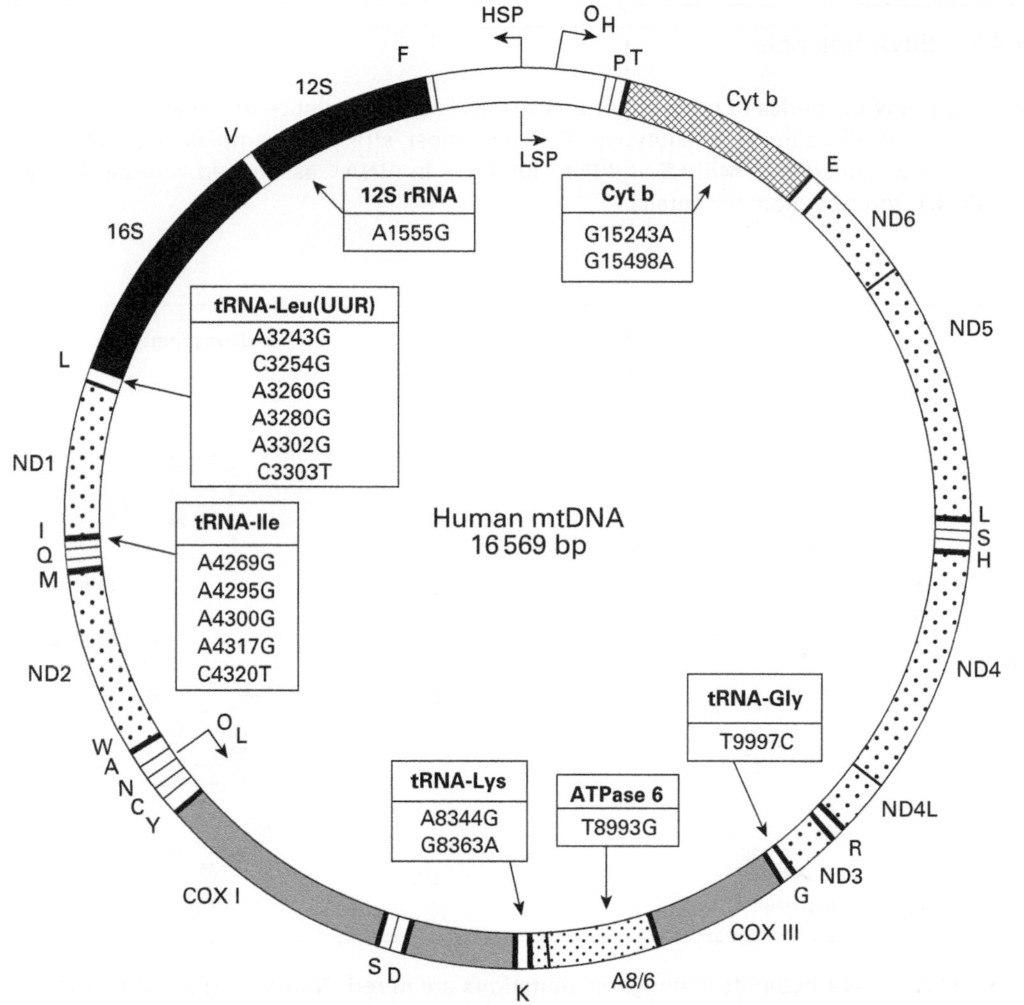

Figure 4.3 mtDNA mutations associated with cardiomyopathy. The differently shaded areas in the mtDNA circle represent the seven subunits of complex I (ND), the three subunits of cytochrome *c* oxidase (COX), cytochrome *b*, two subunits of ATP synthase (ATPase 6 and 8), the 12S and 16S ribosomal RNAs (rRNA), and the 22 transfer RNAs (tRNA) identified by one-letter codes for the corresponding amino acids

to a vasculopathy. Endomyocardial biopsies have revealed similar mitochondrial proliferation in the endothelium of cardiac blood vessels, suggesting that cardiac involvement may also be secondary to angiopathy.[57] Interestingly, in three patients studied with dipyridamole stress scintigraphy, there was cardiac hyperperfusion in early images and a 'filling-in' pattern in the late images.[57] These findings, along with the absence of narrowing of large vessels on coronary angiography, support the arteriolar vasculopathy hypothesis. In contrast, phosphorus magnetic resonance spectroscopy of cardiac muscle revealed evidence of bioenergetic defects in seven patients with cardiomyopathy and the A3243G mutation.[58]

Five other point mutations in the $tRNA^{Leu(UUR)}$ have been associated with cardiomyopathy alone (A3260G, C3303T), cardiopathy and myopathy

Box 4.1 tRNA hotspots

One of the many mysteries of mitochondrial diseases is the occurrence of mutational 'hotspots' associated with specific clinical phenotypes. The two most striking examples are the mutations in $tRNA^{Leu(UUR)}$ associated with MELAS and the mutations in $tRNA^{Ile}$ associated with cardiomyopathies. See Table 4.1 and Appendix for details.

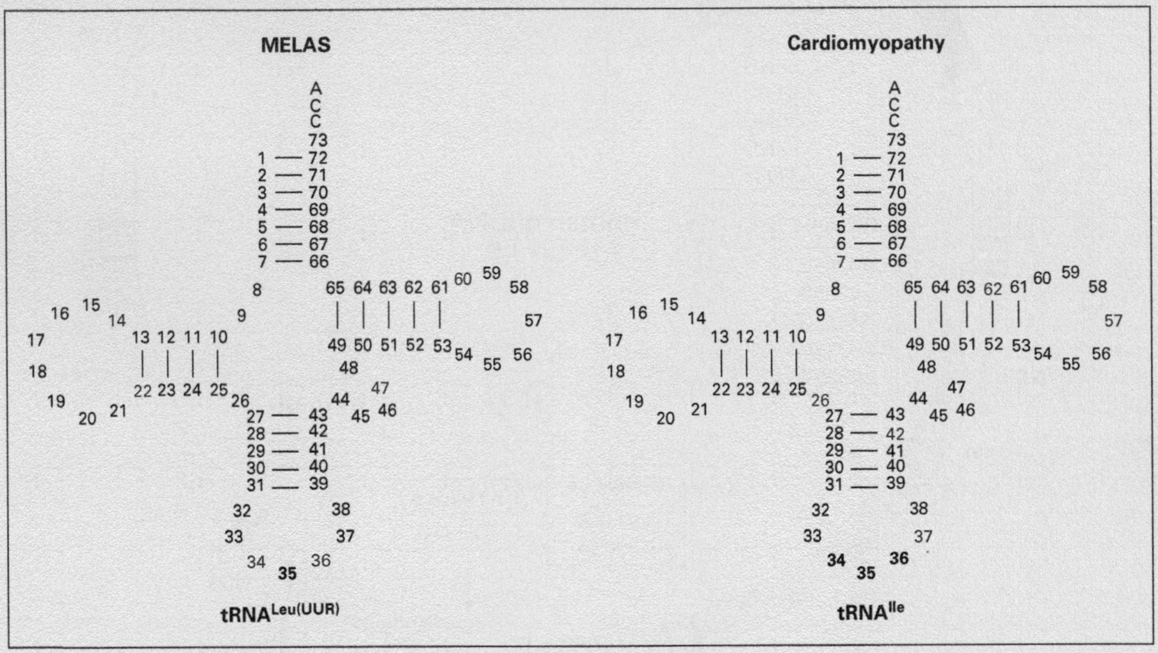

Figure B4.1.1 tRNA hotspots. Pathogenic mutations are in red. Numbering according to reference 1

References

1. Sprinzl M, Hartmann T, Weber J et al. Compilation of tRNA sequences and sequences of tRNA genes. *Nucleic Acids Res* 1989; **17**(suppl.): r1–r172.

(A3260G, C3303T), or cardiopathy as part of the MELAS syndrome (C3254G, A3260G).[52,59–64]

The A4269G mutation in the $tRNA^{Ile}$ gene was originally identified in a patient with a multisystem disorder characterized by growth failure, nephropathy, hearing loss, epilepsy, mild mental retardation, and dilated cardiomyopathy, which caused intractable cardiac failure and death at age 18 years.[65] The C4320T mutation was also associated with a multiorgan disorder in a child who died at age 7 months of cardiac failure and hypertrophic cardiomyopathy, but also had severe encephalopathy manifesting as seizures, nystagmus, and spastic tetraparesis.[66] Intriguingly, the

Table 4.1 Mitochondrial DNA point mutations associated with cardiomyopathy alone or as a major component of a multisystem disorder

Mutation	Gene	Clinical features	Reference
A3243G	$tRNA^{Leu(UUR)}$	MELAS; PEO; DM/De; cardiomyopathy(H)	(49–54)
C3254G	$tRNA^{Leu(UUR)}$	MELAS	(59)
A3260G	$tRNA^{Leu(UUR)}$	Myopathy/cardiomyopathy(H); MELAS	(60, 61)
A3280G	$tRNA^{Leu(UUR)}$	Myopathy/CCB/arrhythmia(H)	(64)
A3302G	$tRNA^{Leu(UUR)}$	Myopathy/cardiomyopathy(H)	(63)
C3303T	$tRNA^{Leu(UUR)}$	Cardiomyopathy(H)	(62)
A4269G	$tRNA^{Ile}$	Encephalomyopathy; cardiomyopathy	(65)
A4295G	$tRNA^{Ile}$	Cardiomyopathy(H)	(167)
A4300G	$tRNA^{Ile}$	Cardiomyopathy(H)	(168)
A4317G	$tRNA^{Ile}$	Cardiomyopathy(H+Di)	(171)
C4320T	$tRNA^{Ile}$	Cardiomyopathy(H)	(66)
A8344G	$tRNA^{Lys}$	MERRF/D/cardiomyopathy(H)	(170)
G8363A	$tRNA^{Lys}$	Encephalopathy/cardiomyopathy(H); MERRF	(68–70)
T8993G	ATPase 6	NARP/MILS; cardiomyopathy	(74)
T9997C	$tRNA^{Gly}$	Cardiomyopathy(H)/GI dysmotility	(171)
G15243A	Cyt *b*	Cardiomyopathy(H)	(75)
G15498G	Cyt *b*	Histiocytoid cardiomyopathy	(76)
A1555G	12S rRNA	De/AID; cardiomyopathy(R)	(79)

AID = aminoglycoside-induced deafness; CCB = cardiac conduction block; D = depression; De = deafness; Di = dilated (cardiomyopathy); DM = diabetes mellitus; GI = gastrointestinal; H = hypertrophic (cardiomyopathy); MELAS = mitochondrial encephalomyopathy, lactic acidosis, and strokelike episodes; MERRF = myoclonus epilepsy with ragged-red fibers; MILS = maternally inherited Leigh syndrome; NARP = neuropathy, ataxia, retinitis pigmentosa; PEO = progressive external ophthalmoplegia.

three other point mutations in the $tRNA^{Ile}$ gene, A4300G, A4317G, and C4320T, have been identified only in patients with isolated hypertrophic cardiomyopathies. It is not known why mutations in this particular tRNA are associated with heart disease. Even more intriguing is the finding of homoplasmic A4300G mutations in two unrelated families with isolated hypertrophic cardiomyopathy.[67] The pathogenic role for the mutation was confirmed by high-resolution Northern blot analysis of heart tissue from both families, showing profoundly decreased steady-state levels of the mature mitochondrial $tRNA^{Ile}$.

In addition to the MELAS A3243G mutation, mtDNA mutations pathogenically related to two other acronymic syndromes, MERRF and NARP, have been also linked to cardiomyopathies, as documented above by our retrospective study of children with mitochondrial diseases. In a review of 62 reported MERRF patients, about one-third had clinical cardiomyopathy while 22% had Wolff–Parkinson–White syndrome.[39] Cardiac evaluation of two MERRF patients revealed cardiomegaly, electrocardiographic abnormalities including ST depression, T-wave inversion, and premature ventricular contractions, and echocardiogram revealed asymmetric septal hypertrophy with diffuse hypokinesis of the left ventricle.[40] The G8363A mutation has been identified in two families with MERRF.[68,69] However, in two other families harboring this mutation, hypertrophic cardiomyopathy overshadowed the co-existing encephalopathy and hearing loss.[70] NARP is typically due to the T8993G mutation in the ATPase 6 gene.[71] When this mutation is present in high proportions, patients develop maternally inherited Leigh syndrome (MILS).[72,73] One infant with MILS also had a severe hypertrophic cardiomyopathy leading to death at age 6 months.[74] An endomyocardial biopsy revealed hypertrophic and vacuolated myocytes with abnormal mitochondria.

While most pathogenic mtDNA mutations affect tRNA genes, over the last few years, a growing number of mutations in polypeptide-encoding mtDNA genes have been identified. Two sporadic patients with cardiomyopathy were found to harbor mutations in the gene encoding cytochrome *b*, the only mtDNA-encoded subunit of complex III of the respiratory chain.[75,76] One patient, harboring a heteroplasmic G15243A mutation, had a severe hypertrophic cardiomyopathy with elevated sarcoplasmic enzymes in serum and lactic acidosis and died of cardiac failure at 9 years of age.[75] The other patient was a girl with histiocytoid cardiomyopathy, a rare disorder of infancy and childhood histologically characterized by pale granular foamy histiocyte-like cells within the myocardium.[77] This patient had clinical and pathological features of histiocytoid cardiomyopathy, but also had hepatic steatosis and acute tubular necrosis.[77] She was found to have a heteroplasmic G15498A mutation resulting in the substitution of a glycine by aspartic acid at amino acid 251 of cytochrome *b*.[76] Interestingly, a second case of histiocytoid cardiomyopathy was due to the A8344G-MERRF mutation.[78]

A point mutation, A1555G, in the 12S ribosomal RNA (rRNA) gene, typically associated with aminoglycoside-induced deafness or non-syndromic deafness, was identified in a family with maternally inherited restrictive cardiomyopathy.[79] Skeletal muscle biopsy of the proband revealed minicores and reduced COX activity.

In a patient with parkinsonism/MELAS overlap syndrome and a mildly hypertrophic cardiac left ventricle, a 4-base-pair deletion in the cytochrome *b* gene was associated with decreased complex III activity.[80] Using cybrid cell clones harboring high proportions of this mutation, Rana, Moraes and colleagues showed evidence of increased free-radical production.[81]

Fundamental questions regarding mtDNA point mutations remain to be resolved. Why is the heart selectively or predominantly affected by some mtDNA mutations? Why do certain individuals harboring a particular mtDNA mutation develop cardiomyopathy while others do not?

Cardiomyopathies due to mutations in nuclear DNA

Defects of respiratory chain subunits

To date, pathogenic mutations in genes encoding respiratory chain subunits have been found only for complex I and complex II.[82]

Patients with complex I deficiency were children who developed symptoms soon after birth and died before 3 years of age. Mutations were identified in ten genes that are highly conserved from bacteria to mammals. The clinical picture was dominated by encephalopathy with LS-like symmetrical brain lesions or with leukodystrophy. However, hypertrophic cardiomyopathy was the dominant clinical feature – and the cause of early death – in patients from two of three families with mutations in the *NDUFS2* gene[83] and in a family with three affected siblings of consanguineous parents with a *NDUFV2* mutation.[84] 'Moderate hypertrophic obstructive cardiomyopathy' was also reported in an infant with LS who died at 11 weeks of age and was compound heterozygous for two mutations in the *NDUFS8* gene. Complex I activity was reported as 'completely deficient' in postmortem cardiac tissue from this infant.[85] A third infant with LS and a homozygous mutation in the *NDUFS4* gene was described to also have 'severe hypertrophic cardiomyopathy', but no details were given on her cardiac condition.[86] Thus, cardiomyopathy may be underdiagnosed in children with complex I deficiency and devastating encephalopathies.

Complex II deficiency is a rare cause of mitochondrial disorders and the few reported patients had LS or late-onset encephalomyopathy without overt heart involvement.[82]

Other autosomal disorders causing mitochondrial dysfunction without directly affecting the mitochondrial respiratory chain include Friedreich ataxia (FA), an autosomal recessive disorder characterized by ataxia, dysarthria, loss of tendon reflexes, corticospinal tract dysfunction, and hypertrophic cardiomyopathy (see Chapter 13).[87] The cardiomyopathy is the most frequent cause of death. All patients with FA harbor pathological expansions of a GAA trinucleotide repeat within intron 1 of the frataxin gene, although a small number of patients also have point mutations.[88] The gene product is localized to mitochondria, where it plays a role in the metabolism of iron–sulfur (Fe–S) clusters.[89] A preliminary study of three FA patients treated for 4–9 months with the antioxidant idebenone revealed marked reduction of the cardiac left ventricular mass index.[90] The beneficial effect of idebenone or coenzyme Q10 on the cardiopathy of Friedreich's ataxia has been confirmed by other groups.[91,92]

Defects of ancillary proteins

Contrary to the experience with complexes I and II, there are no known mutations in nuclear genes encoding subunits of complex III, IV, or V. Defects in these complexes are due to 'indirect hits', that is, defects in proteins that are not components of the complexes but are needed for their proper assembly and functioning.[82]

Mutations in one ancillary protein of complex III, BCS1L, have been associated with a severe encephalomyopathy of infancy and childhood labeled GRACILE (growth retardation, aminoaciduria, cholestasis, iron overload, lactacidosis, and early death) by Finnish and British investigators. Despite its multisystemic nature and rapid downhill course, GRACILE seems to spare the heart.[93]

Cytochrome *c* oxidase (COX, complex IV) deficiency has been associated with mutations in at least six assembly proteins, all of which cause multisystem disorders, but with different 'targets', i.e. more severely affected, tissues. Thus, mutations in SURF1 affect predominantly the brain and are arguably the most common cause of LS. The only patient with mutations in the SCO1 assembly protein had predominant involvement of liver and brain, justifying the term 'hepatoencephalopathy' used to define this syndrome.[82] Although mutations in the COX10 assembly factor were associated with tubulopathy in the first reported case[94] and the condition was therefore labeled 'nephroencephalopathy', the clinical presentation is heterogeneous and includes, besides LS, hypertrophic cardiomyopathy.[95]

Rapidly fatal infantile hypertrophic cardiomyopathy dominates the clinical picture in patients with mutations in two genes, *SCO2* and *COX15*.[96,97] As these infants also have evidence of a LS-like encephalopathy, this syndrome is often dubbed 'cardioencephalopathy'. *SCO2* (like *SCO1*) encodes a copper-binding protein, whose presumed function is to transfer copper (an essential prosthetic group) to the COX holoprotein. Recent evidence from the crystal structure of human SCO1, however, suggests that both SCO proteins may act not only as copper chaperones but rather as mitochondrial redox signaling molecules.[98] *COX15* encodes a protein involved in the synthesis of heme A, another prosthetic group of COX.[97] Interestingly, for both *SCO2* and *COX15* mutations, compound heterozygosity for a common mutation and a rarer change is associated with the rapidly fatal phenotype, whereas homozygosity for the common mutation is compatible with delayed onset of cardiopathy, more prolonged course, and the appearance of typical LS lesions in the brain.[99,100] Although SCO2 may not be essential for the transport of copper to the COX holoenzyme, addition of copper to the culture medium of myoblasts corrected the biochemical defect in vitro[101,102] and copper supplementation to children with delayed-onset ameliorated their cardiac condition[103] (for more details, see Chapter 14).

Two infants with mutations in *ATP12*, an assembly gene for complex V, had severe encephalomyopathy: one died at 3 days of age, the other at 14 months. There was no mention of heart involvement in either child.[104] In contrast, a third infant with good evidence of a complex V deficiency of nuclear origin but no known molecular defect, had craniofacial anomalies, hypotonia, hepatomegaly, but also cardiomegaly with septal hypertrophy before dying on the second day of life.[105]

Defects of intergenomic signaling

A growing number of autosomal diseases have been associated with mtDNA depletion and multiple deletions.[106] These disorders are thought to disrupt the 'dialog' between the two genomes that regulates the integrity and quantity of mtDNA. Autosomal dominant progressive external ophthalmoplegia (AD-PEO) with multiple mtDNA deletions was the first of these disorders to be identified.[107] Cardiological evaluation of other family members revealed sinus bradycardia and electrocardiographic evidence of myocardial ischemia. Of the autosomal recessive PEO with multiple mtDNA deletions, one is particularly relevant to cardiology; autosomal recessive cardiomyopathy-ophthalmoplegia (ARCO) was identified in two unrelated families from the eastern seaboard of the Arabian peninsula.[108] In each family, three siblings presented with childhood-onset PEO, mild facial and proximal limb weakness, and severe cardiomyopathy, which was treated by cardiac transplantation in one individual.

Multiple mtDNA deletions have also been identified in patients without PEO. Severe dilated cardiomyopathy caused death of a mother and her son at ages 37 and 22; there were multiple deletions of mtDNA in the cardiac tissues of both patients.[109] Another sporadic patient with hypertrophic cardiomyopathy, mild proximal limb weakness, but not PEO, had multiple mtDNA deletions in skeletal muscle.[110]

MtDNA depletion syndrome was originally reported in infants with severe hepatopathy or myopathy[111] and mutations in two genes were later identified. Mutations in the deoxyguanosine kinase gene (*DGUOK*) are usually associated with the hepatocerebral presentation,[112] whereas mutations in the thymidine kinase 2 (*TK2*) gene usually cause predominantly myopathic phenotypes.[113] Involvement of the heart seems uncommon: of six children with mtDNA depletion in skeletal muscle reported by Macmillan and Shoubridge,[114] only one had congestive heart failure, but the amount of mtDNA in cardiac tissue was not determined. However, isolated hypertrophic non-obstructive cardiomyopathy was attributed convincingly to mtDNA depletion at least in one case, a girl whose older sister had died of acute heart failure at 9 months of age. The patient developed rapidly progressive and intractable cardiomyopathy at age 1 year: because there was no evidence that skeletal muscle or other tissues were involved, she was successfully treated with cardiac transplantation.[115] Thus, albeit probably rare, mtDNA depletion should be considered in the differential diagnosis of infantile isolated hypertrophic cardiomyopathy.

Mitochondrial neurogastrointestinal encephalomyopathy (MNGIE) was the first disease of intergenomic communication to be molecularly defined.[116,117] While the predominant clinical manifestation is gastrointestinal dysmotility, electrocardiograms have revealed left ventricular hypertrophy (11%) and cardiac conduction block (6%). This autosomal recessive disorder is associated with depletion and multiple deletions of mtDNA and is due to mutations in the gene encoding thymidine phosphorylase, a cytosolic enzyme that may be important in the regulation of nucleotide pools in the mitochondria. Kaukonen, Suomalainen and colleagues identified mutations in the gene encoding the heart/muscle adenine nucleotide translocator 1 (*ANT1*) in a subgroup of patients with AD-PEO.[118] Although symptoms of AD-PEO are predominantly confined to skeletal muscle, Kaukonen et al. documented multiple mtDNA deletions in the hearts of two members of a Finnish family with *ANT1* mutations.[119] ANT1 is localized to the inner mitochondrial membrane and exports ATP in exchange for ADP. Graham et al.[120] confirmed the importance of ANT for myocardial function. They developed a mouse model with deficient ANT1: affected mice developed neonatal HCM. These animals demonstrated hypertrophic myocytes with myofibrillas disarray and systolic hypercontractility. Early morbidity and mortality was notable in these animals. Ragged red fibers were seen on skeletal muscle histology.

A deficiency of the ANT1 translocator was documented by immunoblot analysis of muscle mitochondria and by functional studies in two unrelated children with Sengers syndrome (congenital cataracts, hypertrophic cardiomyopathy, mitochondrial myopathy, and lactic acidosis). As no mutations were detected in the *ANT1* gene, it was postulated that the ANT1 deficiency in these patients was due to transcriptional, translational, or post-translational anomalies.[121]

Mutations in two more genes, *PEO1* (formerly called *C10orf2* or *Twinkle*) and *POLG*, have been associated with PEO and multiple mtDNA deletions.[122] *PEO1* encodes a helicase and causes AD-PEO; *POLG* encodes the mitochondrial polymerase γ and causes either AD- or AR-PEO syndromes. In addition, *POLG* mutations have been associated with mtDNA depletion, especially in children with the hepatocerebral disorder known as Alpers syndrome.[123] Although these disorders are generalized, as a rule patients with mutations in *PEO1* and *POLG* do not have cardiomyopathy.

Defects of the lipid milieu

The components of the respiratory chain are embedded in the lipid bilayer of the inner mitochondrial membrane. This is not merely a scaffold, but participates in the respiratory chain function, largely due to the role of cardiolipin, an acidic phospholipid uniquely abundant in the inner mitochondrial membrane.[124] It stands to reason, therefore, that alterations of the lipid milieu of the membrane may cause disease. A case in point is Barth syndrome. Initially described as X-linked cardioskeletal myopathy with abnormal mitochondria and neutropenia by Neustein et al.[125] and Barth et al.[126] this disorder typically presents in male infants as CHF associated with neutropenia (cyclic) and 3-methylglutaconic aciduria.[127] Mitochondrial dysfunction is suggested by EM and electron transport chain biochemical analysis. Recently, abnormalities in cardiolipin have been noted.[128–130] Echocardiographically, these infants have left ventricular dysfunction with dilation, endocardial fibroelastosis, or a dilated hypertrophic left ventricle. In some cases, they succumb to CHF/sudden death VT/VF, or sepsis due to leukocyte dysfunction. Most children survive infancy and do well clinically, although DCM usually persists. In some cases, cardiac transplantation has been performed. Histopathologic evaluation

Table 4.2 Mitochondrial diseases with prominent cardiopathies

	Functional defect	Clinical features	Cardiac features	Molecular genetics
mtDNA mutations	Defects of mitochondrial protein synthesis	KSS MELAS; MERRF; myopathy	Conduction block; CM; HC; WPW; histiocytoid CM	mtDNA deletion $tRNA^{Leu(UUR)}$; $tRNA^{Lys}$; $tRNA^{Ile}$; 12SrRNA
	Mitochondrial protein coding gene mutations	LHON; NARP/MILS Myopathy	HC; WPW histiocytoid CM	ND genes ATPase 6 Cyt*b*; COX
Intergenomic signaling defects (nDNA)	Multiple mtDNA deletions	ARCO MNGIE	HC LVH; conduction block	*?* *TP*
	mtDNA depletion	Hepatocerebral; myopathic; Alpers	HC	*DGUOK, TK2* *POLG*
Other nDNA mutations	RC subunit gene mutations	LS	CHF	*NDUFS2; NDUFS4; NDUFS8; NDUFV2*
	Assembly protein defects	LS; cardioencephalopathy	CHF	*SCO2; COX15*
	Lipid milieu	Barth syndrome	CHF; LVNC	*G4.5 (TAZ)*

ARCO = autosomal recessive cardiomyopathy ophthalmoplegia; CHF = congestive heart failure; CM = cardiomyopathy; COX = cytochrome *c* oxidase; DGUOK = deoxyguanosine kinase; HC = hypertrophic cardiomyopathy; LHON = Leber hereditary optic neuropathy; LS = Leigh syndrome; LVNC = left ventricular non-compaction; MELAS = mitochondrial encephalomyopathy, lactic acidosis, and stroke-like episodes; MERRF = myoclonus epilepsy with ragged-red fibers; MILS = maternally inherited Leigh syndrome; MNGIE = mitochondrial neurogastrointestinal encephalomyopathy; mtDNA = mitochondrial DNA; NARP = neuropathy, ataxia, retinitis pigmentosa; ND = reduced nicotinamide adenine dinucleotide (NADH) dehydrogenase; nDNA = nuclear DNA; POLG = polymerase gamma; RC = respiratory chain; SCO2 = synthesis of cytochrome oxidase 2; TAZ = tafazzin gene; TK2 = thymidine kinase 2; TP = thymidine phosphorylase; WPW = Wolff–Parkinson–White

typically demonstrates the features of DCM, although endocardial fibroelastosis may be prominent and the mitochondria are abnormal in shape and abundance.

The genetic basis of Barth syndrome was first described by Bione et al.[131] who cloned the disease-causing gene, *G4.5 (TAZ)*. This gene encodes a novel protein called tafazzin, whose function is not currently known. It has been speculated, however, that the gene product is an acyltransferase based on the cardiolipin abnormalities.[132] Mutations in *G4.5* result in a wide clinical spectrum, which includes apparent classic DCM, hypertrophic DCM, endocardial fibroelastosis (EFE), or LVNC.[133–135] In the latter case, the left ventricle non-compaction is characterized by deep trabeculations giving the appearance of a 'spongiform' myocardium.[136,137] The mechanisms responsible for this clinical heterogeneity are not currently known. More detail will be provided regarding LVNC in the section on this disorder.

Table 4.2 summarizes all mitochondrial diseases with prominent cardiac involvement, dividing them into the three categories discussed above, defects of mtDNA, defects of intergenomic signaling, and defects of nuclear DNA (nDNA).

Cardiac phenotypes associated with mitochondrial disease

Congestive heart failure

Congestive heart failure (CHF) due to myocardial dysfunction is a serious malady and a major cause of morbidity and mortality in children and adults.[20] In this condition, ventricular arrhythmias are common and often result in sudden death. Disorders causing CHF are the most common reasons for cardiac transplantation, with an associated cost of billions of dollars annually in the United States.[138] In turn, DCM is the most common cause of CHF[20,139] and, although the overall incidence varies, DCM is thought to occur in at least 40/100 000 people.[139,140] Both prevalence and incidence of DCM appear to be increasing.[140] In the pediatric population, newborns and infants have the highest rates of disease, with an annual incidence of 1.13 per 100 000 children (range 5.98–10.72 per 100 000).[139,141] Symptomatic heart failure at all ages still has a poor prognosis, with one-year mortality rates of 45%.[20]

Dilated cardiomyopathy

Dilated cardiomyopathy is characterized by increased ventricular size (i.e., left ventricular or biventricular dilation) and reduced ventricular contractility (Figure 4.4), in the absence of coronary artery disease, valvular abnormalities or pericardial disease. Mitral regurgitation is common, as are ventricular arrhythmias, particularly ventricular tachycardia (VT), *torsade de pointes* (TdP), and ventricular fibrillation (VF). Clinical features include the signs and symptoms of CHF, i.e. breathlessness, fatigue, orthopnea, diaphoresis, chest pain, palpitations, exercise intolerance, and syncope.[21] In childhood, the male to female ratio is only 1.5.[139] Regardless of etiology, the clinical course of DCM is usually progressive and approximately 50% of patients die within 5 years of diagnosis if they do not undergo transplantation.[20] The cause of death is evenly divided between sudden death and pump

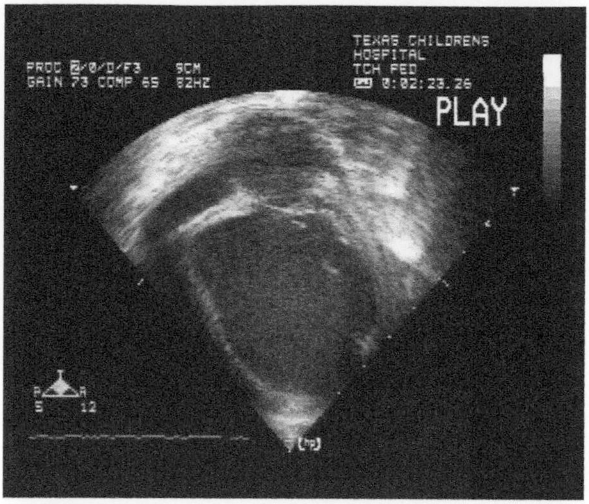

Figure 4.4 Echocardiographic features of dilated cardiomyopathy. Apical four-chamber view with atria superiorly and ventricles inferiorly. Note the extremely enlarged left ventricular chamber with the interventricular septum pushed rightward. The right ventricle is at the bottom left, somewhat compressed due to the large left ventricle

failure. Longer survival has been achieved with improved medical therapies (i.e. angiotensin converting enzyme [ACE] inhibitors, β-blockers) and interventions (i.e. implantable defibrillators, ventricular assist devices). However, neonates and infants with metabolic instability and bouts of lactic acidosis succumb early in life, commonly before their first birthday.[25,139]

In children, the underlying etiology of DCM may include mitochondrial (see above) or other metabolic derangement. Therefore, urine analysis for lactate, amino acids and organic acids may be useful and in some cases may help to narrow the differential diagnosis. For instance, elevated 3-methyl-glutaconic acid in a boy with neutropenia would be diagnostic of Barth syndrome. Blood studies, including complete blood count, acylcarnitine profile (for fatty acid oxidation defects), pyruvate dehydrogenase complex, electrolyte profile, creatine kinase (with isoform analysis if elevated), plasma amino acids, and blood for genetic testing should be obtained. Elevation of creatine kinase muscle isoform (CK-MM) suggests an associated skeletal myopathy and may help to identify the defective gene. Viral serologies may or may not be helpful. In some patients, particularly young children, skeletal muscle biopsy for light and electron microscopy, and electron transport chain biochemistry can be useful and, if abnormal, suggests blood studies to screen for mitochondrial DNA or nuclear DNA mutations or for disorders of fatty acid oxidation.

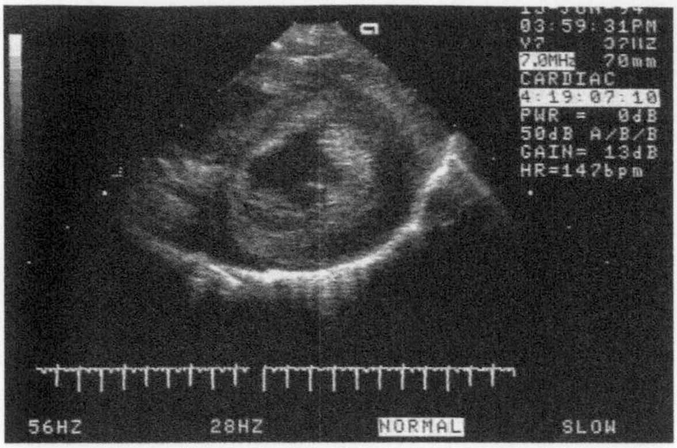

Figure 4.5 Echocardiography in hypertrophic cardiomyopathy. Concentric hypertrophy in a 1-month-old. Note the small left ventricular chamber and thickened interventricular septum and wall

Hypertrophic cardiomyopathy

Hypertrophic cardiomyopathy (HCM) is defined by wall thickening.[142] However, the major features of this disorder are its tendency to be inherited, its association with sudden death in young, healthy, athletic individuals,[143] and its frequent progression to heart failure.[144] Heart failure can be due to diastolic factors or to the development of systolic dysfunction, the so-called 'burned out' HCM.[144] Although generally less common than DCM, HCM is frequent in patients with mitochondrial diseases due to mutations in either mtDNA (Table 4.1) or nDNA (Table 4.2).

HCM is characterized by thickening of the interventricular septum and left ventricular free wall in an asymmetric (asymmetric septal hypertrophy, ASH) or concentric fashion (Figure 4.5). Left ventricular outflow tract obstruction (LVOTO) may also occur. Histological features include myocyte hypertrophy, myofibrillar disarray, and interstitial fibrosis[142] in the autosomal dominant form, whereas mitochondrial proliferation, vacuolization, and glycogen and lipid overabundance characterize mitochondrial or other metabolic forms of HCM.

In the pediatric age range, the underlying etiologies and the variable age-at-onset differentiate further the childhood form of disease from the adult counterpart.[25] In children less than one year of age, ventricular hypertrophy associated with systolic dysfunction is more the rule than the exception. In addition, overlap disorders in which HCM coexists with other features are also more common during childhood, further confounding the presentations, treatments, and outcomes compared to adult disease.

Individuals with HCM exhibit significant variability in their clinical presentation. They may be asymptomatic or present with symptoms ranging from frank heart failure to palpitations and dizziness, to syncope and sudden death. The age at onset of symptoms varies from birth or childhood to late life (fifth or sixth decade). Most children with mitochondrial disease present in the first days or weeks of life; those with autosomal dominant disease most commonly present in the first two decades of life but typically after age 10 years.[25] The physical examination in subjects with HCM may or may not be fruitful. Due to poor ventricular relaxation, ventricular stiffness may result in an S4 gallop. In patients with left ventricular outflow tract obstruction, an outflow murmur may be heard. Otherwise, the examination is normal unless there is a restrictive component or heart failure, in which case jugular venous distention, hepatomegaly, and other signs of heart failure may be in evidence.

The diagnosis of HCM relies on echocardiography, Holter monitoring, and exercise testing; histopathology may also be useful. In addition, in small children, metabolic studies may be useful in determining the etiology of the disease.[25]

The natural history of HCM is variable; some individuals remain asymptomatic throughout life, and others may develop progressive symptoms with or without heart failure or experience sudden death.[79–81] Longitudinal echocardiographic studies have documented left ventricular remodeling with age. Progressive increases of left ventricular wall thickness have been reported in individuals during adolescence and early adult life. In some individuals, left ventricular wall thickness may increase in later life.[93] Age-related reductions in left ventricular wall thickness, associated with myocyte loss and fibrosis, have also been described in individuals with long-standing disease ('burnt out' HCM).[86–88] Ten to 20% of individuals with HCM may develop dilated cardiomyopathy. Ten to 16% of adult individuals develop atrial fibrillation, a risk that is increased in patients with left atrial enlargement.[142]

In young children with mitochondrial disease, onset in the first days or weeks is common with symptoms of heart failure or murmur. In those with depressed systolic function and fragile metabolic status, death is common before the first year of life. In those who survive beyond the first year, there is commonly a clinical 'honeymoon period' when relative stability ensues and during which cardiac function is usually good. During puberty, significant symptoms (and death) commonly develop.

Left ventricular non-compaction (LVNC)

Left ventricular non-compaction (LVNC) is a form of primary myocardial disease that most commonly presents in infancy but may be diagnosed later in life, even in adulthood.[136] Typically, neonates with LVNC present with heart failure; clinical evaluation usually identifies cardiomegaly with pulmonary edema on chest X-ray and the electrocardiogram may show huge QRS voltages reminiscent of Pompe disease, evidence of pre-excitation, and ST-T wave abnormalities.[137] Echocardiography characteristically demonstrates a hypertrophic, dilated or combined dilated hypertrophic left ventricle with deep trabeculations and poor systolic function. The deep trabeculations in the endocardial surface of the left ventricle had led to terms such as 'fetal myocardium' and spongiform myocardium. The phenotype can change over time, with increasing levels of hypertrophy and improved contractile function before redevelopment of cardiac thinning and dysfunction.[137] The right ventricle may also be affected.

The non-compacted ventricular myocardium, with its excessively prominent trabecular meshwork and deep intertrabecular recesses, is seen in the early period of embryogenesis and the postnatal disorder is attributed to developmental arrest.[136,137] The recesses are lined with endothelium continuous with that of the ventricular endocardium. Two forms of LVNC occur in neonates, an isolated form (isolated LVNC, ILVNC) without other structural abnormalities, and a non-isolated form (non-isolated LVNC, NLVNC) with associated congenital cardiac defects, including ventricular or atrial septal defects (VSD, ASD), pulmonic stenosis (PS) or other right heart obstruction, hypoplastic left heart syndrome (HLHS), or other left heart obstructive disorders.[145] Dysmorphic features and neurologic/neuromuscular disorders have also been associated, and ventricular arrhythmias and embolic phenomena have been routinely reported.

The inheritance of LVNC is heterogeneous. In some cases of ILVNC, X-linked inheritance has been identified.[25,145] The gene locus has been mapped to Xq28, and mutations in the gene *G4.5*

(TAZ), which encodes tafazzin protein, have been reported.[131,145] This gene has also been shown to cause Barth syndrome, suggesting that these may be allelic disorders.[146]

Other cases of ILVNC and most NLVNC are inherited as autosomal dominant traits. We have identified mutations in α-dystrobrevin in some of these patients.[145] Although abnormalities of skeletal muscle with abnormal-appearing mitochondria have been noted,[137,147] the gene encodes a structural protein with signaling properties.[145] In some cases, the disease also appears to have a mitochondrial basis.[148]

Fatty acid oxidation defects

Although throughout this book we have stuck to the restrictive definition of mitochondrial diseases as being due to defects of the respiratory chain, in the chapter on cardiology (and in Chapter 3, when discussing peripheral neuropathies) we extend the term to include defects of fatty acid oxidation. We do so because inborn errors of lipid metabolism are important causes of cardiomyopathy (and peripheral neuropathy).

Most myocardial energy is derived from long-chain fatty acids via mitochondrial β-oxidation after transport of long-chain fatty acids and carnitine across the cardiomyocyte plasma membrane.[18] A variety of proteins are required for efficient functioning of this system and all genetic defects in this metabolic pathway are inherited as autosomal recessive traits. We will briefly describe defects of the carnitine transporter, the carnitine palmitoyl-transferase (CPT) step, and of the enzymes of the β-oxidation spiral.

Carnitine deficiency

L-carnitine, a small, water-soluble molecule containing seven carbon atoms, is important in the shuttling of long-chain fatty acids and activated acetate across the intermitochondrial membrane. A specific translocase facilitates this exchange. Carnitine also serves as the shuttle for the end-products of peroxisomal fatty acid oxidation and for α-keto-acids derived from branched chain amino acids. These metabolites are transferred into the mitochondrial matrix for terminal oxidation.[149]

Primary carnitine deficiency is characterized by severe decrease of carnitine in affected tissues; serum carnitine concentration is also markedly decreased in the systemic form of primary carnitine deficiency. The mechanism underlying primary carnitine deficiency is defective transport of carnitine from blood into affected tissues.[150] Secondary carnitine deficiencies are characterized by less-striking decreases in total or free serum carnitine and by an increase in esterified:free ratio. The secondary forms are heterogeneous and include underlying inherited metabolic errors, diverse acquired diseases, and iatrogenic factors, such as drug administration. Carnitine deficiency is usually divided into two forms – a myopathic form and a systemic form – based on carnitine levels in blood and affected tissues. In the myopathic form, carnitine levels are only decreased in muscle, while in the systemic form carnitine is low in multiple tissues, including muscle, liver, and plasma.[18,149] The systemic form presents in infancy or early childhood with episodes of hypoglycemia, ammonemia, acidemia, hepatomegaly, and endocardial fibroelastosis (EFE).[151,152] However, the most common clinical presentation is progressive cardiomyopathy: echocardiography and ECG show dilated cardiomyopathy, peaked T waves, and signs of ventricular hypertrophy. Myopathy is usually associated with cardiomyopathy and is manifested by mild motor delay, hypotonia, or slowly progressive proximal weakness. Muscle biopsy shows severe lipid storage. Endomyocardial biopsies or postmortem studies also show massive lipid storage in the heart.

Both total and free carnitine concentrations are extremely low (usually below 10% of normal) in skeletal muscle and in the myocardium.

Linkage analysis has localized the gene responsible for primary carnitine deficiency to chromosome 5q. The gene, (*OCTN2*) which encodes one member of a family of organic cation transporters, has been isolated and several pathogenic mutations have been identified in patients and their asymptomatic parents.[153,150,154] Both cardiac dysfunction and muscle weakness respond dramatically to oral carnitine supplementation, and these patients can live normal lives with continuous replacement therapy.[151,152]

Carnitine palmitoyl-transferase (CPT) deficiency

Two CPTs exist in mitochondria.[18,155] CPT I is located within the inner mitochondrial membrane and it exists as two different tissue-specific isoforms, a liver isozyme (IA) and a muscle isozyme (IB).[18,149] CPT IA deficiency manifests with metabolic crises without cardiac involvement and occurs in the first 2 years of life. The human CPT I genes have been cloned and mutations in isozyme IA have been identified in patients.[156]

CPT II is present on the inner mitochondrial membrane and exists as a single isoform.[18] Mutations in this gene result in three differing clinical presentations, the most severe of which occurs in the neonate and manifests with metabolic decompensation (hypoketotic hypoglycemia, metabolic acidosis), respiratory distress, hepatomegaly and congestive heart failure, with or without arrhythmias.[157] Death usually occurs in the first month of life. Null mutations associated with complete lack of protein expression have been identified in these patients. An intermediate form, which presents between 3 and 24 months of life and may manifest as sudden death, has also been described. This hepato-cardio-muscular form is similar to the severe form except that ventricular tachycardia and heart block are common and probably due to accumulation of toxic long-chain acylcarnitines.[158] A homozygous arginine to cysteine missense mutation (R613C) has been found to cause this form.[159] Finally, the least severe (but most common) form, recurrent and paroxysmal myoglobinuria, occurs in young adults and is not associated with cardiac disease.[160]

β-oxidation spiral defects

This cascade of events consists of four enzymatic steps which utilize fatty acyl-CoA as substrates and shorten them by two carbons during each round of the spiral (see Chapter 1, Figure 1.1).[18,161] The first step is a straight chain acyl-CoA dehydrogenase reaction which utilizes four related enzymes with differing substrate specificities (short-chain acyl-CoA dehydrogenase, medium-chain acyl-CoA dehydrogenase, long-chain acyl-CoA dehydrogenase, and very-long-chain acyl-CoA dehydrogenase).[18] The second step involves an enoyl-CoA hydratase reaction, which is followed by a 3-hydroxyacyl-CoA dehydrogenase reaction catalyzed by the short-chain 3-hydroxycyl-CoA dehydrogenase and the long-chain 3-hydroxyacyl CoA dehydrogenase. The final reaction catalyzes a 3-keto-thiolase cleavage.

Medium chain acyl-CoA dehydrogenase (MCAD) deficiency

This disorder appears to be the most common inborn error of fatty acid oxidation, affecting one in 6 000–10 000 live Caucasians.[18,162] It is characterized by recurrent illnesses, provoked by fasting for more than12 hours, with the first episode generally occurring between 6 and 24 months of life. The most common symptoms include vomiting and severe lethargy often progressing to coma. Less dramatic symptoms include muscle weakness and exercise intolerance. Hypoglycemia is often present between episodes, when patients appear normal. Hepatomegaly and sudden death related to DCM occur, but cardiomyopathy is rare. The gene responsible for this autosomal recessive disorder has been localized to chromosome 1p31; the entire human *MCAD* gene has been cloned and sequenced.[162]

Very long chain acyl-CoA dehydrogenase (VLCAD) deficiency

This disorder manifests with recurrent episodes of coma, vomiting, and hypoglycemia triggered by fasting.[163] Some patients have much more severe illness with notable involvement of cardiac and skeletal muscle. Both HCM and DCM have been seen and are often fatal. Like MCAD, VLCAD patients have secondary carnitine deficiency and their fasting urine organic acid profile is abnormal, with low ketones and increased levels of dicarboxylic acids. More than 15 mutations in the VLCAD gene have been identified,[164] including missense mutations, premature termination codon mutations, and splice site mutations. Many result in undetectable protein levels.

Therapy for these patients includes aggressive treatment with glucose and hemodynamic support that may reverse the cardiac phenotype. When cardiac disease persists, chronic therapy for the dilated or hypertrophic heart disease should be instituted.

Long-chain 3-hydroxyacyl-CoA dehydrogenase (LCHAD) deficiency

This abnormality typically manifests as infantile cardiomyopathy with a Reye syndrome-like metabolic crisis, and may present initially with sudden death.[165] The crisis is commonly precipitated by reduced caloric intake, especially in the setting of a viral syndrome. Approximately 50% of these infants die but those that survive commonly recover substantial myocardial function. Later-onset morbidity and mortality occurs in a substantial percentage of these infantile survivors. The gene has been identified and mutations are known. A mutation 'hotspot', G1528C, accounts for approximately 90% of all mutations.[166]

References

1. Schwartz SM, Duffy JY, Pearl JM, Nelson DP. Cellular and molecular aspects of myocardial dysfunction. *Crit Care Med* 2001; **29**: S214–S219.
2. Gregorio CC, Antin PB. The heart of myofibril assembly. *Trends Cell Biol* 2000; **10**: 355–362.
3. Squire JM. Architecture and function in the muscle sarcomere. *Curr Opin Struct Biol* 2000; **7**: 247–257.
4. Clark KA, McElhinny AS, Beckerle MC, Gregorio CC. Striated muscle cytoarchitecture: An intricate web of form and function. *Annu Rev Cell Dev Biol* 2002; **18**: 637–706.
5. Vigoreaux JO. The muscle Z band: Lessons in stress management. *J Muscle Res Cell Motil* 1994; **15**: 237–255.
6. Barth AL, Nathke IS, Nelson WJ. Cadherins, catenins and APC protein: interplay between cytoskeletal complexes and signaling pathways. *Curr Opin Cell Biol* 1997; **9**: 683–690.
7. Burridge K, Chrzanowska-Wodnicka M. Focal adhesions, contractility, and signaling. *Annu Rev Cell Dev Biol* 1996; **12**: 463–518.
8. Capetanaki Y. Desmin cytoskeleton: A potential regulator of muscle mitochondrial behaviour and function. *Trends Cardiovasc Med* 2002; **12**: 339–348.
9. Stewart M. Intermediate filament structure and assembly. *Curr Opin Cell Biol* 1993; **5**: 3–11.
10. Sharp WW, Simpson DG, Borg DG et al. Mechanical forces regulate focal adhesions and costamere assembly in cardiac myocytes. *Am J Physiol* 1997; **273**: H546–556.
11. Straub V, Campbell KP. Muscular dystrophies and the dystrophin-glycoprotein complex. *Curr Opin Neurol* 1997; **10**: 168–175.
12. Furukawa T, Ono Y, Tsuchiya H et al. Specific interactions of the potassium channel β-subunit minK with the sarcomeric protein T-cap suggests a T-tubule-myofibril linking system. *J Mol Biol* 2001; **313**: 775–784.
13. Kucera JP, Rohr S, Rudy Y. Localization of sodium channels in intercalated disks modulate cardiac conduction. *Circ Res* 2002; **91**: 1176–1182.

14. Ribaux P, Bleicher F, Couble ML et al. Voltage-gated sodium channel (SkM1) content in dystrophin-deficient muscle. *Pflugers Arch* 2001; **441**: 746–755.
15. Mootha VK, Arai AE, Balaban RS. Maximum oxidative phosphorylation capacity of the mammalian heart. *Am J Physiol* 1997; **441**: 746–755.
16. Hale D, Bennett MJ. Fatty acid oxidation disorders: A new class of metabolic diseases. *Pediatrics* 1992; **121**: 1–11.
17. Vockley J. The changing face of disorders of fatty acid oxidation. *Mayo Clin Proc* 1994; **69**: 249–257.
18. DiDonato S, Taroni F. Disorders of lipid metabolism. In: Engel AG, Franzini-Armstrong C, eds. *Myology*. Vol. 2. New York: McGraw-Hill, 2004: 1587–1621.
19. Hunt SA, Baker DW, Chin MH. ACC/AHA guidelines for the evaluation and management of chronic heart failure in the adult: Executive Summary. *J Am Coll Cardiol* 2001; **38**: 2101–2113.
20. Jessup M, Brozena S. Heart failure. *New Engl J Med* 2003; **348**: 2007–2018.
21. Francis GS, Wilson-Tang WH. Pathophysiology of congestive heart failure. *Rev Cardiovasc Med* 2003; **4** (Suppl 2): S14–S20.
22. Sutton MGSJ, Sharpe N. Left ventricular remodeling after myocardial infarction: pathophysiology and therapy. *Circulation* 2000; **101**: 2981–2988.
23. Wallace DC. Mitochondrial defects in cardiomyopathy and neuromuscular disease. *Am Heart J* 2000; **139**: S70–S85.
24. Shoffner JM, Wallace DC. Oxidative phosphorylation diseases. In: Scriver CR, Beaudet AL, Sly WS, Valle D, eds. *The Metabolic and Molecular Bases of Inherited Disease*. Vol. 1. New York: McGraw-Hill, 1995: 1535–1609.
25. Towbin JA, Lipshultz SE. Genetics of neonatal cardiomyopathy. *Curr Opin Cardiol* 1999; **14**: 250–262.
26. Towbin JA, Bowles NE. The failing heart. *Nature* 2002; **415**: 227–233.
27. Scaglia F, Towbin JA, Craigen WJ et al. Clinical spectrum, morbidity, and mortality in 113 pediatric patients with mitochondrial disease. *Pediatrics* 2004; **114**: 925–931.
28. Goto Y, Horai S, Matsuoka T et al. Mitochondrial myopathy, encephalopathy, lactic acidosis, and stroke-like episodes (MELAS): A correlative study of the clinical features and mitochondrial DNA mutation. *Neurology* 1992; **42**: 545–550.
29. Sorajja P, Sweeney MG, Chalmers RA et al. Cardiac abnormalities in patients with Leber's hereditary optic neuropathy. *Heart* 2003; **89**: 791–792.
30. Holmgren D, Wahlander H, Eriksson BO et al. Cardiomyopathy in children with mitochondrial disease. *Eur Heart J* 2003; **24**: 280–288.
31. Shoffner JM, Lott MT, Lezza A et al. Myoclonic epilepsy and ragged-red fiber disease (MERRF) is associated with a mitochondrial DNA $tRNA^{Lys}$ mutation. *Cell* 1990; **61**: 931–937.
32. DiMauro S, Hirano M, Kaufmann P et al. Clinical features and genetics of myoclonic epilepsy with ragged red fibers. In: Fahn S, Frucht SJ, eds. *Myoclonus and Paroxysmal Dyskinesia*. Philadelphia: Lippincott Williams & Wilkins, 2002: 217–229.
33. Berenberg RA, Pellock JM, DiMauro S, Rowland LP. Lumping or splitting? 'Ophthalmoplegia plus' or Kearns-Sayre syndrome? *Ann Neurol* 1977; **1**: 37–43.
34. Moraes CT, DiMauro S, Zeviani M et al. Mitochondrial DNA deletions in progressive external ophthalmoplegia and Kearns-Sayre syndrome. *N Engl J Med* 1989; **320**: 1293–1299.
35. Zeviani M, Moraes CT, DiMauro S. Deletions of mitochondrial DNA in Kearns-Sayre syndrome. *Neurology* 1988; **38**: 1339–1346.
36. Manfredi G, Vu T, Bonilla E et al. Association of myopathy with large-scale mitochondrial DNA duplications and deletions: Which is pathogenic? *Ann Neurol* 1997; **42**: 180–188.
37. Tang Y, Manfredi G, Hirano M, Schon EA. Maintenance of human rearranged mitochondrial DNAs in long-term cultured transmitochondrial cell lines. *Mol Biol Cell* 2000; **11**: 2349–2358.
38. Rowland LP, Hays AP, DiMauro S et al. Diverse clinical disorders associated with morphological abnormalities in mitochondria. In: Scarlato G, Cerri C, eds. *Mitochondrial Pathology in Muscle Diseases*. Padua: Piccin, 1983: 141–158.
39. Hirano M, DiMauro S. Clinical features of mitochondrial myopathies and encephalomyopathies. In: Lane RJM, ed. *Handbook of Muscle Disease* vol. 1st ed. New York: Marcel Dekker, Inc., 1996: 479–504.
40. Anan R, Nakagawa M, Miyata M et al. Cardiac involvement in mitochondrial diseases. A study of 17 patients with mitochondrial DNA defects. *Circulation* 1995; **91**: 955–961.

41. Channer K, Channer J, Campbell M, Russel Rees J. Cardiomyopathy in the Kearns-Sayre syndrome. *Br Heart J* 1988; **59**: 486–490.
42. Tveskov C, Angelo-Nielsen K. Kearns-Sayre syndrome and dilated cardiomyopathy. *Neurology* 1990; **40**: 553–554.
43. Hubner G, Gokel JM, Pongratz D et al. Fatal mitochondrial cardiomyopathy in Kearns-Sayre syndrome. *Virchows Arch* [a]. 1986; **408**: 611–621.
44. Koksinski C, Mull M, Lethen H, Topper R. Evidence for cardioembolic stroke in a case of Kearns-Sayre syndrome. *Stroke* 1995; **26**: 1950–1952.
45. Provenzale JM, VanLandingham K. Cerebral infarction associated with Kearns-Sayre syndrome-related cardiomyopathy. *Neurology* 1996; **46**: 826–828.
46. Tranchant C, Mousson B, Mohr M et al. Cardiac transplantation in an incomplete Kearns-Sayre syndrome with mitochondrial DNA deletion. *Neuromusc Disord* 1993; **3**: 561–566.
47. Muller-Hocker J, Jacob U, Seibel P. The common 4977 base pair deletion of mitochondrial DNA preferentially accumulates in the cardiac conduction system of patients with Kearns-Sayre syndrome. *Mod Pathol* 1998; **11**: 295–301.
48. Fromenty B, Carrozzo R, Shanske S, Schon EA. High proportions of mtDNA duplications in patients with Kearns-Sayre syndrome occur in the heart. *Am J Med Genet* 1997; **71**: 443–452.
49. Hirano M, Pavlakis S. Mitochondrial myopathy, encephalopathy, lactic acidosis, and stroke-like episodes (MELAS): current concepts. *J Child Neurol* 1994; **9**: 4–13.
50. Suzuki Y, Harada K, Miura Y et al. Mitochondrial myopathy, encephalopathy, lactic acidosis, and stroke-like episodes (MELAS): decrease in diastolic left ventricular function assessed by echocardiography. *Pediatr Cardiol* 1993; **14**: 162–166.
51. Okajima Y, Tanabe Y, Takayanagi M, Aotsuka H. A follow-up study of myocardial involvement in patients with mitochondrial encephalomyopathy, lactic acidosis, and stroke-like episodes (MELAS). *Heart* 1998; **80**: 292–295.
52. Silvestri G, Bertini E, Servidei S et al. Maternally inherited cardiomyopathy: A new phenotype associated with the A to G at nt. 3243 of mitochondrial DNA (MELAS mutation). *Muscle Nerve* 1997; **20**: 221–225.
53. Vilarinho L, Santorelli FM, Rosas MJ et al. The mitochondrial A3243G mutation presenting as severe cardiomyopathy. *J Med Genet* 1997; **34**: 607–609.
54. Hiruta Y, Chin K, Shitomi K et al. Mitochondrial encephalomyopathy with A to G transition of mitochondrial transfer $RNA^{Leu(UUR)}$3,243 presenting hypertrophic cardiomyopathy. *Inter Med* 1995; **34**: 670–673.
55. Hasegawa H, Matsuoka T, Goto I, Nonaka I. Strongly succinate dehydrogenase-reactive blood vessels in muscles from patients with mitochondrial myopathy, encephalopathy, lactic acidosis, and stroke-like episodes. *Ann Neurol* 1991; **29**: 601–605.
56. Sakuta R, Nonaka I. Vascular involvement in mitochondrial myopathy. *Ann Neurol* 1989; **25**: 594–601.
57. Sato W, Tanaka M, Sugiyama S et al. Cardiomyopathy and angiopathy in patients with mitochondrial myopathy, encephalopathy, lactic acidosis, and stroke-like episodes. *Am Heart J* 1994; **128**: 733–741.
58. Lodi R, Rajagopalan B, Blamire AM et al. Abnormal cardiac energetics in patients carrying the A3243G mtDNA mutation measured in vivo using phosphorus MR spectroscopy. *Biochim Biophys Acta* 2004; **1657**: 146–150.
59. Kawarai T, Kawakami H, Kozuka K et al. A new mitochondrial DNA mutation associated with mitochondrial myopathy: $tRNA^{Leu(UUR)}$ 3254 C-to-G. *Neurology* 1997; **49**: 598–600.
60. Zeviani M, Gellera C, Antozzi C et al. Maternally inherited myopathy and cardiomyopathy: association with mutation in mitochondrial DNA $tRNA^{Leu(UUR)}$. *Lancet* 1991; **338**: 143–147.
61. Nishino I, Komatsu M, Kodama S et al. The 3260 mutation in mitochondrial DNA can cause mitochondrial myopathy, encephalopathy, lactic acidosis, and stroke-like episodes (MELAS). *Muscle Nerve* 1996; **19**: 1603–1604.
62. Bruno C, Kirby DM, Koga Y et al. The mitochondrial DNA C3303T mutation can cause cardiomyopathy and/or skeletal myopathy. *J Pediatr* 1999; **135**: 197–202.
63. Campos Y, Garcia A, del Hoyo P et al. Two pathogenic mutations in the mitochondrial DNA $tRNA^{Leu(UUR)}$ gene (T3258C and A3280G) resulting in variable clinical phenotypes. *Neuromusc Disord* 2003; **13**: 416–420.

64. van den Bosch BJC, de Coo IFM, Hendrickx ATM et al. Increased risk for cardiorespiratory failure associated with the A3302G mutation in the mitochondrial DNA encoded $tRNA^{Leu(UUR)}$ gene. *Neuromusc Disord* 2004; **14**: 683–688.
65. Taniike M, Fukushima H, Yanagihara I et al. Mitochondrial $tRNA^{Ile}$ mutation in fatal cardiomyopathy. *Biochem Biophys Res Commun* 1992; **186**: 47–53.
66. Santorelli F, El-Schahawi M, Shanske S et al. A novel mtDNA mutation associated with human cardiomyopathy. *Circulation* 1995; **92**(Suppl 1): 232–233.
67. Taylor RW, Giordano C, Davidson MM et al. A homoplasmic mitochondrial transfer ribonucleic acid mutation as a cause of maternally inherited cardiomyopathy. *J Am Coll Cardiol* 2003; **41**: 1786–1796.
68. Ozawa M, Nishino I, Horai S et al. Myoclonus epilepsy associated with ragged-red fibers: A G-to-A mutation at nucleotide pair 8363 in mitochondrial $tRNA^{Lys}$ in two families. *Muscle Nerve* 1997; **20**: 271–278.
69. Shtilbans A, Shanske S, Goodman S et al. G8363A mutation in the mitochondrial DNA transfer ribonucleic acid Lys gene: another cause of Leigh syndrome. *J Child Neurol* 2000; **15**: 759–761.
70. Santorelli FM, Mak S-C, El-Schahawi M et al. Maternally inherited cardiomyopathy and hearing loss associated with a novel mutation in the mitochondrial DNA $tRNA^{Lys}$ gene (G8363A). *Am J Hum Genet* 1996; **58**: 933–939.
71. Holt IJ, Harding AE, Petty RK, Morgan Hughes JA. A new mitochondrial disease associated with mitochondrial DNA heteroplasmy. *Am J Hum Genet* 1990; **46**: 428–433.
72. Tatuch Y, Christodoulou J, Feigenbaum A et al. Heteroplasmic mtDNA mutation (T→G) at 8993 can cause Leigh disease when the percentage of abnormal mtDNA is high. *Am J Hum Genet* 1992; **50**: 852–858.
73. Santorelli FM, Shanske S, Macaya A et al. The mutation at nt 8993 of mitochondrial DNA is a common cause of Leigh syndrome. *Ann Neurol* 1993; **34**: 827–834.
74. Pastores GM, Santorelli FM, Shanske S et al. Leigh syndrome and hypertrophic cardiomyopathy in an infant with a mitochondrial DNA point mutation (T8993G). *Am J Med Genet* 1994; **50**: 265–271.
75. Valnot I, Kassis J, Chretien D et al. A mitochondrial cytochrome *b* mutation but no mutations of nuclearly encoded subunits in ubiquinol cytochrome *c* reductase (complex III) deficiency. *Hum Genet* 1999; **104**: 460–466.
76. Andreu AL, Checcarelli N, Iwata S et al. A missense mutation in the mitochondrial cytochrome *b* gene in a revisited case with histiocytoid cardiomyopathy. *Pediatr Res* 2000; **48**: 311–314.
77. Papadimitriou A, Neustein HB, DiMauro S et al. Histiocytoid cardiomyopathy of infancy: deficiency of reducible cytochrome *b* in heart mitochondria. *Pediatr Res* 1984; **18**: 1023–1028.
78. Vallance HD, Jeven G, Wallace DC, Brown MD. A case of sporadic infantile histiocytoid cardiomyopathy caused by the A8344G (MERRF) mitochondrial DNA mutation. *Pediatr Cardiol* 2004; **25**: 538–540.
79. Santorelli FM, Tanji K, Manta P et al. Maternally inherited cardiomyopathy: An atypical presentation of the 12S rRNA A1555G mutation. *Am J Hum Genet* 1999; **64**: 295–300.
80. De Coo IFM, Renier WO, Ruitenbeek W et al. A 4-base pair deletion in the mitochondrial cytochrome *b* gene associated with Parkinsonism/MELAS overlap syndrome. *Ann Neurol* 1999; **45**: 130–133.
81. Rana M, de Coo I, Diaz F et al. An out-of-frame cytochrome *b* gene deletion from a patient with Parkinsonism is associated with impaired complex III assembly and an increase in free radical production. *Ann Neurol* 2000; **48**: 774–781.
82. DiMauro S, Hirano M. Mitochondrial encephalomyopathies: an update. *Neuromusc Disord* 2005; **15**: 276–286.
83. Loeffen J, Elpeleg O, Smeitink J et al. Mutations in the complex I *NDUFS2* gene of patients with cardiomyopathy and encephalomyopathy. *Ann Neurol* 2001; **49**: 195–201.
84. Benit P, Beugnot R, Chretien D et al. Mutant NDUFV2 subunit of mitochondrial complex I causes early onset hypertrophic cardiomyopathy and encephalopathy. *Hum Mut* 2003; **21**: 582–586.
85. Loeffen J, Smeitink J, Triepels R et al. The first nuclear-encoded complex I mutation in a patient with Leigh syndrome. *Am J Hum Genet* 1998; **63**: 1598–1608.
86. Petruzzella V, Vergari R, Puzziferri I et al. A nonsense mutation in the *NDUFS4* gene encoding the 18 kDa (AQDQ) subunit of complex I abolishes assembly and activity of the complex in a patient with Leigh-like syndrome. *Hum Mol Genet* 2001; **10**: 529–535.

87. Delatycki MB, Williamson R, Forrest SM. Friedreich's ataxia: an overview. *J Med Genet* 2000; **37**: 1–8.
88. Campuzano V, Montermini L, Molto MD et al. Friedreich's ataxia: autosomal recessive disease caused by an intronic GAA triplet repeat expansion. *Science* 1996; **271**: 1374–1375.
89. Babcock M, de Silva D, Oaks R et al. Regulation of mitochondrial iron accumulation by Yfh1p, a putative homolog of frataxin. *Science* 1997; **276**: 1709–1712.
90. Rustin P, von Kleist-Retzow J-C, Chantrel-Groussard K et al. Effect of idebenone on cardiomyopathy in Friedreich's ataxia: a preliminary study. *Lancet* 1999; **354**: 477–479.
91. Mariotti C, Solari A, Torta D et al. Idebenone treatment in Friedreich patients: one-year-long randomized placebo-controlled trial. *Neurology* 2003; **60**: 1676–1679.
92. Lodi R, Hart PE, Rajagopalan B et al. Antioxidant treatment improves in vivo cardiac and skeletal muscle bioenergetics in patients with Friedreich's ataxia. *Ann Neurol* 2001; **49**: 590–596.
93. Fellman V. The GRACILE syndrome, a neonatal lethal metabolic disorder with iron overload. *Blood Cells Mol Dis* 2002; **29**: 444–450.
94. Valnot I, von Kleist-Retzow J-C, Barrientos A et al. A mutation in the human heme-A:farnesyltransferase gene (*COX 10*) causes cytochrome c oxidase deficiency. *Hum Mol Genet* 2000; **9**: 1245–1249.
95. Antonicka H, Leary SC, Guercin G-H et al. Mutations in *COX10* result in a defect in mitochondrial heme A biosynthesis and acount for multiple, early-onset clinical phenotypes associated with isolated COX deficiency. *Hum Mol Genet* 2003; **12**: 2693–2702.
96. Papadopoulou LC, Sue CM, Davidson MM et al. Fatal infantile cardioencephalomyopathy with COX deficiency and mutations in *SCO2*, a COX assembly gene. *Nature Genet* 1999; **23**: 333–337.
97. Antonicka H, Mattman A, Carlson CG et al. Mutations in *COX15* produce a defect in the mitochondrial heme biosynthetic pathway, causing early-onset fatal hypertrophic cardiomyopathy. *Am J Hum Genet* 2003; **72**: 101–114.
98. Williams JC, Sue CM, Banting GS et al. Crystal structure of human SCO1. *J Biol Chem* 2005; **280**: 15202–15211.
99. Jaksch M, Horvath R, Horn N et al. Homozygosity (E140K) in *SCO2* causes delayed infantile onset of cardiomyopathy and neuropathy. *Neurology* 2001; **57**: 1440–1446.
100. Oquendo CE, Antonicka H, Shoubridge EA et al. Functional and genetic studies demonstrate that mutation in the COX15 gene can cause Leigh syndrome. *J Med Genet* 2004; **41**: 540–544.
101. Jaksch M, Paret C, Stucka R et al. Cytochrome *c* oxidase deficiency due to mutations in *SCO2*, encoding a mitochondrial copper-binding protein, is rescued by copper in human myoblasts. *Hum Mol Genet* 2001; **10**: 3025–3035.
102. Salviati L, Hernandez-Rosa E, Walker WF et al. Copper supplementation restores cytochrome *c* oxidase activity in cultured cells from patients with *SCO2* mutations. *Biochem J* 2002; **363**: 321–327.
103. Freisinger P, Horvath R, Macmillan C et al. Reversion of hypertrophic cardiomyopathy in a patient with deficiency of the mitochondrial copper binding protein Sco2: Is there a potential effect of copper? *J Inher Metab Dis* 2004; **27**: 67–79.
104. De Meirleir L, Seneca S, Lissens W et al. Respiratory chain complex V deficiency due to a mutation in the assembly gene *ATP12*. *J Med Genet* 2004; **41**: 120–124.
105. Houstek J, Mracek T, Vojtiskova A, Zeman J. Mitochondrial diseases and ATPase defects of nuclear origin. *Biochim Biophys Acta* 2004; **1658**: 115–121.
106. Hirano M, Marti R, Ferreira-Barros C et al. Defects of intergenomic communication: autosomal disorders that cause multiple deletions and depletion of mitochondrial DNA. *Semin Cell Develop Biol* 2001; **12**: 417–427.
107. Zeviani M, Servidei S, Gellera C et al. An autosomal dominant disorder with multiple deletions of mitochondrial DNA starting at the D-loop region. *Nature* 1989; **339**: 309–311.
108. Bohlega S, Tanji K, Santorelli FM et al. Multiple mitochondrial DNA deletions associated with autosomal recessive ophthalmoplegia and severe cardiomyopathy. *Neurology* 1996; **46**: 1329–1334.
109. Takei Y-I, Ikeda S-I, Yanagisawa N et al. Multiple mitochondrial DNA deletions in a patient with mitochondrial myopathy and cardiomyopathy but no ophthalmoplegia. *Muscle Nerve* 1995; **18**: 1321–1325.

110. Suomalainen A, Paetau A, Leinonen H et al. Inherited idiopathic dilated cardiomyopathy with multiple deletions of mitochondrial DNA. *Lancet* 1992; **340**: 1319–1320.
111. Moraes CT, Shanske S, Tritschler HJ et al. MtDNA depletion with variable tissue expression: A novel genetic abnormality in mitochondrial diseases. *Am J Hum Genet* 1991; **48**: 492–501.
112. Mandel H, Szargel R, Labay V et al. The deoxyguanosine kinase gene is mutated in individuals with depleted hepatocerebral mitochondrial DNA. *Nature Genet* 2001; **29**: 337–341.
113. Saada A, Shaag A, Mandel H et al. Mutant mitochondrial thymidine kinase in mitochondrial DNA depletion myopathy. *Nature Genet* 2001; **29**: 342–344.
114. Macmillan CJ, Shoubridge EA. Mitochondrial DNA depletion: Prevalence in a pediatric population referred for neurologic evaluation. *Pediatr Neurol* 1996; **14**: 203–210.
115. Santorelli FM, Gagliardi MG, Dionisi-Vici C et al. Hypertrophic cardiomyopathy and mtDNA depletion. Successful treatment with heart transplantation. *Neuromusc Disord* 2002; **12**: 56–59.
116. Hirano M, Silvestri G, Blake D et al. Mitochondrial neurogastrointestinal encephalomyopathy (MNGIE): Clinical, biochemical and genetic features of an autosomal recessive mitochondrial disorder. *Neurology* 1994; **44**: 721–727.
117. Nishino I, Spinazzola A, Hirano M. Thymidine phosphorylase gene mutations in MNGIE, a human mitochondrial disorder. *Science* 1999; **283**: 689–692.
118. Kaukonen J, Juselius JK, Tiranti V et al. Role of adenine nucleotide translocator 1 in mtDNA maintenance. *Science* 2000; **289**: 782–785.
119. Suomalainen A, Majander A, Wallin M et al. Autosomal dominant progressive external ophthalmoplegia with multiple deletions of mtDNA: Clinical, biochemical, and molecular genetic features of the 10q-linked disease. *Neurology* 1997; **48**: 1244–1253.
120. Graham BH, Waymire KG, Cottrell B et al. A mouse model for mitochondrial myopathy and cardiomyopathy resulting from a deficiency in the heart/muscle isoform of the adenine nucleotide translocator. *Nature Genet* 1997; **16**: 226–234.
121. Jordens EZ, Palmieri L, Huizing M et al. Adenine nucleotide translocator 1 deficiency associated with Sengers syndrome. *Ann Neurol* 2002; **52**: 95–99.
122. Hirano M, DiMauro S. *ANT1, Twinkle, POLG*, and *TP*: New genes open our eyes to ophthalmoplegia. *Neurology* 2001; **57**: 2163–2165.
123. Naviaux RK, Nguyen KV. *POLG* mutations associated with Alpers' syndrome and mitochondrial DNA depletion. *Ann Neurol* 2004; **55**: 706–712.
124. Schlame M, Rua D, Greenberg ML. The biosynthesis and functional role of cardiolipin. *Progr Lipid Res* 2000; **39**: 257–288.
125. Neustein HD, Lurie PR, Dahms B, Takahashi M. An X-linked recessive cardiomyopathy with abnormal mitochondria. *Pediatrics* 1979; **64**: 24–29.
126. Barth PG, Scholte HR, Berden JA et al. An X-linked mitochondrial disease affecting cardiac muscle, skeletal muscle and neutrophil leucocytes. *J Neurol Sci* 1983; **62**: 327–355.
127. Kelley RI, Cheatham JP, Clark BJ et al. X-linked dilated cardiomyopathy with neutropenia, growth retardation, and 3-methylglutaconic aciduria. *J Pediatr* 1991; **119**: 738–747.
128. Schlame M, Towbin JA, Heerdt PM et al. Deficiency of tetralinoleoyl-cardiolipin in Barth syndrome. *Ann Neurol* 2002; **51**: 634–637.
129. Vreken P, Valianpour F, Nijtmans LG et al. Defective remodeling of cardiolipin and phosphatidylglycerol in Barth syndrome. *Biochem Biophys Res Commun* 2000; **279**: 378–382.
130. Schlame M, Kelley RI, Feigenbaum A et al. Phospholipid abnormalities in children with Barth syndrome. *J Am Coll Cardiol* 2003; **42**: 1994–1999.
131. Bione S, D'Adamo P, Maestrini E et al. A novel X-linked gene, *G4.5*, is responsible for Barth syndrome. *Nature Genet* 1996; **12**: 385–389.
132. Neuwald AF. Barth syndrome may be due to an acyltransferase deficiency. *Curr Biol* 1997; **7**: R465–R466.
133. D'Adamo P, Fassone L, Gedeon A et al. The X-linked gene *G4.5* is responsible for different infantile dilated cardiomyopathies. *Am J Hum Genet* 1997; **61**: 862–867.
134. Johnston J, Kelley RI, Feigenbaum A et al. Mutation characterization and genotype-phenotype

correlation in Barth syndrome. *Am J Hum Genet* 1997; **61**: 1053–1058.
135. Chen R, Tsuji T, Ichida F et al. Mutation analysis of the G4.5 gene in patients with isolated left ventricular noncompaction. *Mol Genet Metab* 2002; **77**: 319–325.
136. Chin TK, Perloff JK, Williams RG et al. Isolated noncompaction of left ventricular myocardium. A study of eight cases. *Circulation* 1990; **82**: 507–513.
137. Pignatelli RH, McMahon CJ, Dreyer WJ et al. Clinical characterization of left ventricular noncompaction in children. A relatively common form of cardiomyopathy. *Circulation* 2003; **108**: 2672–2678.
138. O'Connell JB, Bristow MR. Economic impact of heart failure in the United States: Time for a different approach. *J Heart Lung Transplant* 1994; **13**: S107–S112.
139. Lipshultz SE, Sleeper LA, Towbin JA et al. The incidence of pediatric cardiomyopathy in two regions of the United States. *New Engl J Med* 2003; **348**: 1703–1705.
140. Towbin JA. Familial dilated cardiomyopathy. In: Berul CI, Towbin JA, eds. *The Molecular and Clinical Genetics of Cardiac Electrophysiological Disease*. Boston: Kluwer Academic Publishers, 2000: 195–218.
141. Nugent AW, Daubeney PEF, Chondros P et al. The epidemiology of childhood cardiomyopathy in Australia. *New Engl J Med* 2003; **348**: 1703–1705.
142. Ommen SR. Hypertrophic cardiomyopathy. *Curr Probl Cardiol* 2004; **29**: 239–291.
143. Frenneaux MP. Assessing the risk of sudden cardiac death in a patient with hypertrophic cardiomyopathy. *Heart* 2004; **90**: 570–575.
144. Gaasch WH, Zile MR. Left ventricular diastolic dysfunction and diastolic heart failure. *Annu Rev Med* 2004; **55**: 373–394.
145. Ichida F, Tsubata S, Bowles KR et al. Novel gene mutation in patients with left ventricular noncompaction or Barth syndrome. *Circulation* 2001; **103**: 1256–1263.
146. Bleyl SB, Mumford BR, Thompson V et al. Neonatal, lethal noncompaction of the left ventricular myocardium is allelic with Barth syndrome. *Am J Hum Genet* 1997; **61**: 868–872.
147. Stromberg D, Gajarski RJ, Exil V et al. Left ventricular noncompaction: Evidence for a mitochondrial etiology. *J Am Coll Cardiol* 1998; 31: 30A.
148. Stollberger C, Finsterer J. Left ventricular hypertrabeculation/noncompaction. *J Am Soc Echocardiogr* 2004; **17**: 91–100.
149. Tein I. Lipid storage muscular disorders. In: Jones HR, De Vivo DC, Darras BT, eds. *Neuromuscular Disorders of Infancy, Childhood, and Adolescence*. Boston: Butterworth-Heinemann, 2003: 833–860.
150. Tein I. Carnitine transport: Pathophysiology and metabolism of known molecular defects. *J Inher Metab Dis* 2003; **26**: 147–169.
151. Waber LJ, Valle D, Neill C et al. Carnitine deficiency presenting as familial cardiomyopathy: a treatable defect in carnitine transport. *J Pediatr* 1982; **101**: 700–705.
152. Bennett MJ, Hale DE, Pollitt RJ et al. Endocardial fibroelastosis and primary carnitine deficiency due to a defect in the plasma membrane carnitine transporter. *Clin Cardiol* 1996; **19**: 243–246.
153. Lamhonwah A-M, Tein I. Carnitine uptake defect: Frameshift mutations in the human plasmalemmal carnitine transporter gene. *Biochem Biophys Res Commun* 1998; **252**: 396–401.
154. Tang NLS, Ganapathy V, Wu X et al. Mutations of *OCTN2*, an organic cation/carnitine transporter, lead to deficient cellular carnitine uptake in primary carnitine deficiency. *Hum Mol Genet* 1999; **8**: 655–660.
155. McGarry JD, Brown NF. The mitochondrial carnitine palmitoyltrasferase system. From concept to molecular analysis. *Eur J Biochem* 1997; **15**: 1–14.
156. Britton CH, Schultz RA, Zhang B et al. Human liver mitochondrial carnitine palmitoyltransferase I: characterization of its cDNA and chromosomal localization and partial analysis of the gene. *Proc Natl Acad Sci USA* 1995; **92**: 1984–1988.
157. Hiug G, Bove KE, Soukup S. Lethal neonatal multiorgan deficiency of CPT-II. *New Engl J Med* 1991; **325**: 1862–1865.
158. Demaugre F, Bonnefont J-P, Colonna M et al. Infantile form of carnitine palmitoyltransferase II deficiency with hepatomuscular symptoms and sudden death. Physiopathological approach to carnitine palmitoyltransferase II deficiencies. *J Clin Invest* 1991; **87**: 859–864.

159. Strauss A. Defects of mitochondrial proteins and pediatric heart disease. *Progr Pediatr Cardiol* 1996; **6**: 83–90.
160. DiMauro S, DiMauro-Melis PM. Muscle carnitine palmityltransferase deficiency and myoglobinuria. *Science* 1973; **182**: 929–931.
161. Kelly DP, Strauss AW. Inherited cardiomyopathies. *New Engl J Med* 1994; **330**: 930–932.
162. Kelly DP, Kim JB, Billadello JJ et al. Nucleotide sequence of medium-chain acyl-CoA dehydrogenase mRNA and its expression in enzyme-deficient human tissue. *Proc Natl Acad Sci USA* 1987; **84**: 4068–4072.
163. Strauss AW, Powell CK, Hale DF et al. Molecular basis of human mitochondrial very-long-chain acyl-CoA dehydrogenase deficiency causing cardiomyopathy and sudden death in childhood. *Proc Natl Acad Sci USA* 1995; **92**: 10496–10500.
164. Andresen BS, Bross P, Vianey-Saban C et al. Cloning and characterization of human very-long-chain acyl-CoA dehydrogenase cDNA, chromosomal assignment of the gene and identification in four patients of nine different mutations within the *VLCAD* gene. *Hum Mol Genet* 1996; **5**: 461–472.
165. Wanders RJA, Duran M, Ijlst L et al. Sudden infant death and long-chain 3-hydroxyacyl-CoA dehydrogenase. *Lancet* 1989; **2**: 52–53.
166. Ijlst L, Wanders RJA, Ushikubo S et al. Molecular basis of long-chain 3-hydroxyacyl-CoA dehydrogenase deficiency: identification of the major disease-causing mutation in the alpha-subunit of the mitochondrial trifunctional protein. *Biochim Biophys Acta* 1994; **1215**: 347–350.
167. Merante F, Myint T, Tein I et al. An additional mitochondrial $tRNA^{Ile}$ point mutation (A-to-G at nucleotide 4295) causing hypertrophic cardiomyopathy. *Hum Mut* 1996; **8**: 216–222.
168. Casali C, Santorelli FM, D'Amato G et al. A novel mtDNA point mutation in maternally inherited cardiomyopathy. *Biochem Biophys Res Commun* 1995; **213**: 588–593.
169. Tanaka M, Ino H, Ohno K et al. Mitochondrial mutation in fatal infantile cardiomyopathy. *Lancet* 1990; **2**: 1452.
170. Silvestri G, Ciafaloni E, Santorelli FM et al. Clinical features associated with the A→G transition at nucleotide 8344 of mtDNA ("MERRF mutation"). *Neurology* 1993; **43**: 1200–1206.
171. Merante F, Tein I, Benson L et al. Maternally inherited hypertrophic cardiomyopathy due to a novel T-to-C transition at nucleotide 9997 in the mitochondrial tRNAglycine gene. *Am J Hum Genet* 1994; **55**: 437–446.

5

Mitochondrial ophthalmology

Valerio Carelli, Piero Barboni and Alfredo A Sadun

Mitochondrial ophthalmology

In 1988, the birthdate of molecular mitochondrial medicine, two disorders were associated with pathogenic defects of mitochondrial DNA (mtDNA), both with predominant neuro-ophthalmologic involvement.

The first disorder was characterized by progressive external ophthalmoplegia (PEO), mitochondrial myopathy with ragged-red fibers (RRF), and large-scale deletions of mtDNA.[1] This molecular defect was shortly thereafter associated with Kearns–Sayre syndrome (KSS),[2] a multisystemic disorder,[3] which includes PEO, pigmentary retinopathy, onset before 20 years of age, and one or more of the following: complete heart block, ataxia, cerebrospinal fluid (CSF) protein higher than 1 g/liter.

The second disorder associated with a mtDNA point mutation in the *ND4* gene of complex I, was Leber's hereditary optic neuropathy (LHON),[4] a form of optic nerve degeneration inherited through the maternal lineage but affecting predominantly young men.[5]

Since 1988, mitochondrial medicine has progressed so fast that it has become mandatory for both specialists and general practitioners to familiarize themselves with the general concepts of this new exciting chapter of medicine and biology.[6] While new mtDNA mutations are still being identified,[7] recent years have been characterized by the initially slow,[8] but rapidly accelerating, identification of nuclear genes responsible for mitochondrial disorders.[9] Frequently, well-known diseases, which were not suspected to be mitochondrial, have revealed a mitochondrial etiology.[10,11] Within the larger picture of mitochondrial medicine, the importance of the visual system as an especially vulnerable target of mitochondrial dysfunction was clear from the beginning. Thus, mitochondrial ophthalmology itself is a dynamic and fast-evolving subspecialty of mitochondrial medicine.

The mitochondrial dependence of the visual system: retina and optic nerve

The visual sensory system begins at the retina. This thin and transparent neural membrane covers the inner surface of the posterior part of the eyeball. Much information processing occurs within the three layers of neurons, the two layers of neuropil, and the ultimate component, the retinal nerve fiber layer. The latter coalesces to form the optic nerve, which then carries these fibers to the primary visual nuclei in the brain.[12] The precise geometry and anatomy of the retina can be appreciated at two levels.[13] First, there is a radial symmetry centered on the fovea, the area with the highest visual sensitivity and acuity. The concentration of retinal elements, and the retinal sensitivity, decreases with increasing distance from the fovea.

Orthogonal to the retinal plane is a precise layered cytoarchitecture (Figure 5.1).[14] The retina can be divided into ten layers that we will describe from the outside to the inside in relation to the center of the eye (this is also the direction of information transfer).[15]

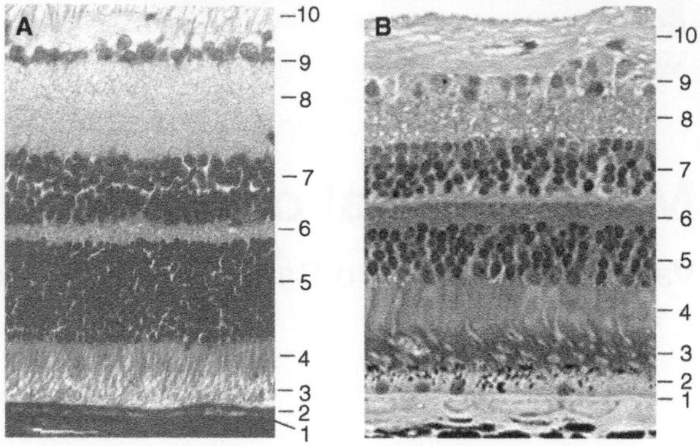

Figure 5.1 Normal retina (courtesy of Prof Alfredo A Sadun and Fred N Ross-Cisneros). Sections of human (**A**) and monkey (**B**) retina embedded in glycol methacrylate (plastic), 1-μm thick, stained with 1% toluidine blue: (1) Bruch's membrane; (2) retinal pigmented epithelium (RPE); (3) outer segments of rods and cones; (4) inner segments of rods and cones; (5) outer nuclear layer; (6) outer plexiform layer; (7) inner nuclear layer; (8) inner plexiform layer; (9) retinal ganglion cell (RGC) layer; (10) nerve fiber layer (NFL)

- A basement membrane of collagen termed *Bruch's membrane* separates the neuro-retina from the outer vascular choroid.
- A single layer of *retinal pigmented epithelium* (RPE) lines the basement membrane, provides a tight junction-based blood–retina barrier, and supports both physically (through processes that interdigitate with the outer segments of rods and cones) and biochemically the outer segment of the percipient cells.
- The *outer segment of the rods and cones* contains tightly packed cylinders of rhodopsin-containing membrane folded into discs; it is this system that transduces light signals into changes in membrane electrical potential.
- The *inner segment of the rods and cones* contains the enormous concentrations of mitochondria that are needed to provide the ATP to replace the light-bleached ('spent') all-*trans*-rhodopsin with 'fresh' 11-*cis*-rhodopsin.
- The nuclei of the rods and cones form the *outer nuclear layer* of the retina.
- The spherules and pedicles of the rods and cones form the complex neuropil of the *outer plexiform layer*.
- The nuclei of bipolar cells, Müller cells, many amacrine cells, and horizontal cells constitute the *inner nuclear layer*.
- The synaptic neuropil between bipolar cells, amacrine cells, and ganglion cells create the *inner plexiform layer*.
- The *retinal ganglion cell layer* (RGC) lies innermost to the other cells of the retina.
- Axons of the RGCs line the inner aspects of the retina to form the *nerve fiber layer* (NFL): these axons converge, like spokes to the hub of a wheel, to produce the optic nerve head.

This is not to be confused with the scheme of ten retinal layers originally drawn up by Ramón y Cajal, whose pioneering work established the basic circuitry of the retina.[16] Cajal described external and internal limiting membranes, which are not, in fact, true membranes. The 'external limiting membrane' of Cajal is a line of gap and occlusion junctions formed by the inner elements of RPE cells.[17,18] His 'internal limiting membrane' is a collagen condensation formed by the interweaving innermost processes of the Müller cells and their attachments to the collagen elements of the vitreous face.[18] Müller cells form the glial skeleton of the retina as they bridge the outer to inner aspects of the retina.[15]

For our purposes, the ten retinal layers schematize the functional and metabolic organization of the retina. It is particularly useful to consider the three layers formed by rods and cones.[19] The outer segments of these cells are the sites of the rhodopsin-based transduction of light. The inner segments are bulging cylinders packed with mitochondria, while the nuclei lie innermost and near the spherules and pedicles that form the inner plexiform layer. The inner segments of rods and cones have the highest concentration of mitochondria of any tissue in the body.[20] The oxygen tension provided by the rich arterial plexus of the nearby choroid is also the highest in the body.[21]

There are approximately 110 million rods, 6 million cones and 1.2 million RGCs, whose axons form the optic nerve.[22] Humans have a cone-based visual system, as reflected by our excellent color vision and central visual acuity in the light. Even so, 6 million cones connect, through bipolars, to only 1.2 million RGCs, resulting in convergence of information downstream.

Three cellular components of the retina are particularly dependent on mitochondrial function, and each cell type has special energy requirements. The RPE cells are constantly pumping ions to preserve the blood–retinal barrier and to keep out water and electrolytes from the potential space between the RPE and the basement membrane.[23] Through this process, the retina remains attached by 'a vacuum seal' and failure of this system produces retinal detachment. The photoreceptors are constantly replenishing their 11-*cis*-rhodopsin through ATP. Light causes bleaching of 11-*cis*-rhodopsin into its lower energy all-*trans* form. The RGCs not only have to transmit under all optical conditions (on-cells fire in the light and off-cells in the dark), but they also have to ensure axoplasmic transport all the way to distant primary visual nuclei.[24] However, the greatest energetic disadvantage for RGCs and their axons might be that retinal nerve fibers run a long course without the saltatory conduction provided by myelin. In order to maintain the optical transparency that permits good visual resolution, these axons become myelinated only after they have exited the eye and formed the optic nerve. The high dependence of these cells on mitochondrial oxidative phosphorylation may well explain why visual loss due to mitochondrial dysfunction affects mostly either the outer retina (e.g. retinal dystrophy in KSS) or RGCs (e.g. optic atrophy in LHON). Correspondingly, experimental disruption of mitochondrial oxidative phosphorylation produces both outer retinal and inner retinal damage.[25]

The blood supply to the outer retina, including the mitochondria-rich inner segments of the 120 million rods and cones, comes from the choroidal circulation.[15] The retinal vessels emanate from the central retinal artery at the optic nerve head and supply the inner retina, specifically the RGCs.[26] Each RGC contributes one axon, which exits inwardly and travels in the retinal NFL, where it coalesces with other axons to form the optic nerve head.[27] Studies of the intraretinal ganglion cell axons have shown that single axons may form varicosities, which are rich in mitochondria and in desmosome- and hemidesmosome-like junctions with other axons or glial cells.[28] These were interpreted as functional sites with local high-energy demand, probably important for signal transmission.

The 1.2 million axons of the retinal nerve fiber layer course along the inner retina towards the optic disc, then make an orthogonal turn and proceed posteriorly as they penetrate the openings in collagen plates of the lamina cribrosa.[29] Further behind the lamina cribrosa, the axons take on oligodendroglia and become rather heavily myelinated (Figure 5.2).[30] At this point, the energy demand of these fibers closely resembles that of other axons in the central nervous system.[31]

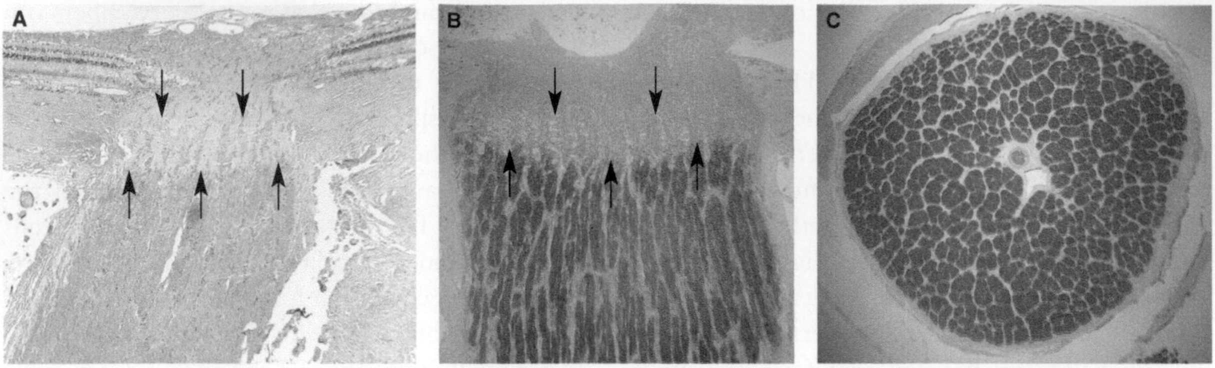

Figure 5.2 Sagittal and cross-section of normal optic nerve (courtesy of Prof Alfredo A Sadun and Fred N Ross-Cisneros). Sagittal section of the optic nerve head and retina stained with immunoperoxidase for myelin basic protein (**A**); sagittal section of the optic nerve head embedded in plastic (epon) and stained with *p*-phylenedyamine to show myelinated fibers (**B**); cross-section of the optic nerve embedded in plastic (epon) and stained with *p*-phylenedyamine to show myelinated fibers (**C**). The sagittal sections show a parallel transition from the retina to the optic nerve head, with well-organized bundles of myelinated axons (in brown) exiting behind the lamina cribrosa (between arrows). The lamina cribrosa shows a regular pattern of collagen fibers forming the laminar connective tissue running orthogonal to both vertical glial columns and unmyelinated nerve fibers. The cross-section shows the normal bundle organization of myelinated axons with densely packed axonal profiles within each bundle

Extraocular muscles, a specific target for mitochondrial dysfunction

In humans, each eye has six muscles. Depending on their points of insertion, their origins, and their fulcrum fixations, each of these muscles produces different torque and hence different movements of the eyeball. The four recti muscles and the superior oblique arise from the apex of the orbit at the annulus of Zinn, whereas the inferior oblique arises from the inferior nasal orbit.[32] The recti muscles insert into the sclera anteriorly to the equator and hence rotate the eye in the direction of their insertion in the horizontal or vertical plane. The oblique muscles attach behind the equator and at odd angles, such that the superior oblique produces incyclotortion and some depression whereas the inferior oblique produces excyclotortion and some elevation. The sixth cranial nerve innervates the lateral rectus; the fourth cranial nerve innervates the superior oblique, and the third cranial nerve innervates the other four muscles and is also responsible for other ocular functions. Neural computation allows the eyes to work in concert both for ductions (paired movements up, down, left, or right) and for vergences (movements that permit the object of regard to remain on corresponding areas of the two retinas despite positional variances of the object from the eyes).

The extraocular muscles (EOMs) differ from ordinary skeletal muscle in both anatomy and physiology.[33] The fibers of EOMs are smaller and more richly innervated than ordinary skeletal muscle fibers. EOMs are among the fastest and yet most fatigue-resistant muscles in the body.[34] The complex actions performed by the EOMs are reflected in their cytoarchitecture, fiber-type composition, and motor unit properties, which differ from those of ordinary skeletal muscles.[35,36] Classification of EOM fiber types includes the four types of 'ordinary' skeletal muscle (types I, IIA, IIB, and IIX) but also distinguishes types based on color, location, and innervation pattern, as recently reviewed.[36] Some EOM fibers are innervated by multiple axons and have multiple neuromuscular junctions along their lengths: stimulation results in tonic contractions without propagation of action potentials. In contrast, other EOM fibers are innervated by single axons, whose action potentials induce twitch contractions.[37] Another peculiarity of EOMs is that they express almost all myosin heavy chain (MyHC) isoforms and that the same muscle fiber can express more than one, including embryonic and neonatal isoforms, which persist in adult EOMs.[38]

Humans, as foveate animals with high levels of visual acuity, use quick saccadic eye movements to fixate on a target. In approximately 200 milliseconds, an object is targeted and saccadic eye movements are initiated. The reflex involves neural elements in the visual cortex, the superior colliculus, the cerebellum, and the paramedian reticular formation, such that the three ocular cranial nerves stimulate the EOMs to quickly move each eye. The maximum velocity for a saccade is 500 degrees/second.[39] Once an image is placed on the fovea, it is often desirable to keep it there. If the image is stationary, this is done by fixation. However, if the object of regard is moving, then the pursuit system generates smooth tracking movements of the eyes to match the pace of the target. Predictive mechanisms compensate for the latency (about 100 milliseconds) of the neural reflex.[32]

The EOM activity (of both saccades and pursuit movements) is both continuous and highly energy-dependent.[34] Two main factors may explain the remarkable resistance to fatigue of EOMs: (i) their high mitochondrial content[40] and metabolic rate;[41] and (ii) their extensive capillary network and high blood flow.[42] However, these metabolic features also render the EOMs more vulnerable to mitochondrial dysfunction, explaining why PEO is one of the commonest clinical manifestations of mitochondrial diseases.[6] Mitochondrial dysfunction may trigger a compensatory increase of mitochondrial numbers in EOMs, as described in patients with LHON or PEO.[43,44] Furthermore, age-related decline in respiratory efficiency may occur faster in EOMs than in other skeletal muscles, thus explaining the higher accumulation of cytochrome *c* oxidase-deficient fibers seen in the EOM of aged individuals.[45]

Mitochondrial optic neuropathies: non-syndromic inherited optic neuropathies

This category of mitochondrial disorders is characterized by extreme selectivity of tissue expression, as the RGCs and the optic nerve are the only affected sites. Another common feature, and a hallmark of mitochondrial optic neuropathies, is the early and preferential involvement of the small fibers in the papillomacular bundle that serves central vision.[46]

Two diseases with both overlapping features and important differences belong to this category, LHON and DOA.[31] LHON is due to mtDNA point mutations and obeys the rules of mitochondrial genetics, whereas DOA is due to nuclear gene mutations and is transmitted as an autosomal dominant trait. Although the two disorders have different genetic etiologies and different progressions (one is subacute, the other slowly progressive), both show variable penetrance, which is not easily explained.

Leber's hereditary optic neuropathy (LHON): an mtDNA disease with tissue-specific expression

LHON is a maternally inherited subacute loss of central vision affecting predominantly young men. Initially described by Von Graefe,[47] it was formally defined as a clinical entity by Leber[5] and is now recognized as the most frequent mitochondrial

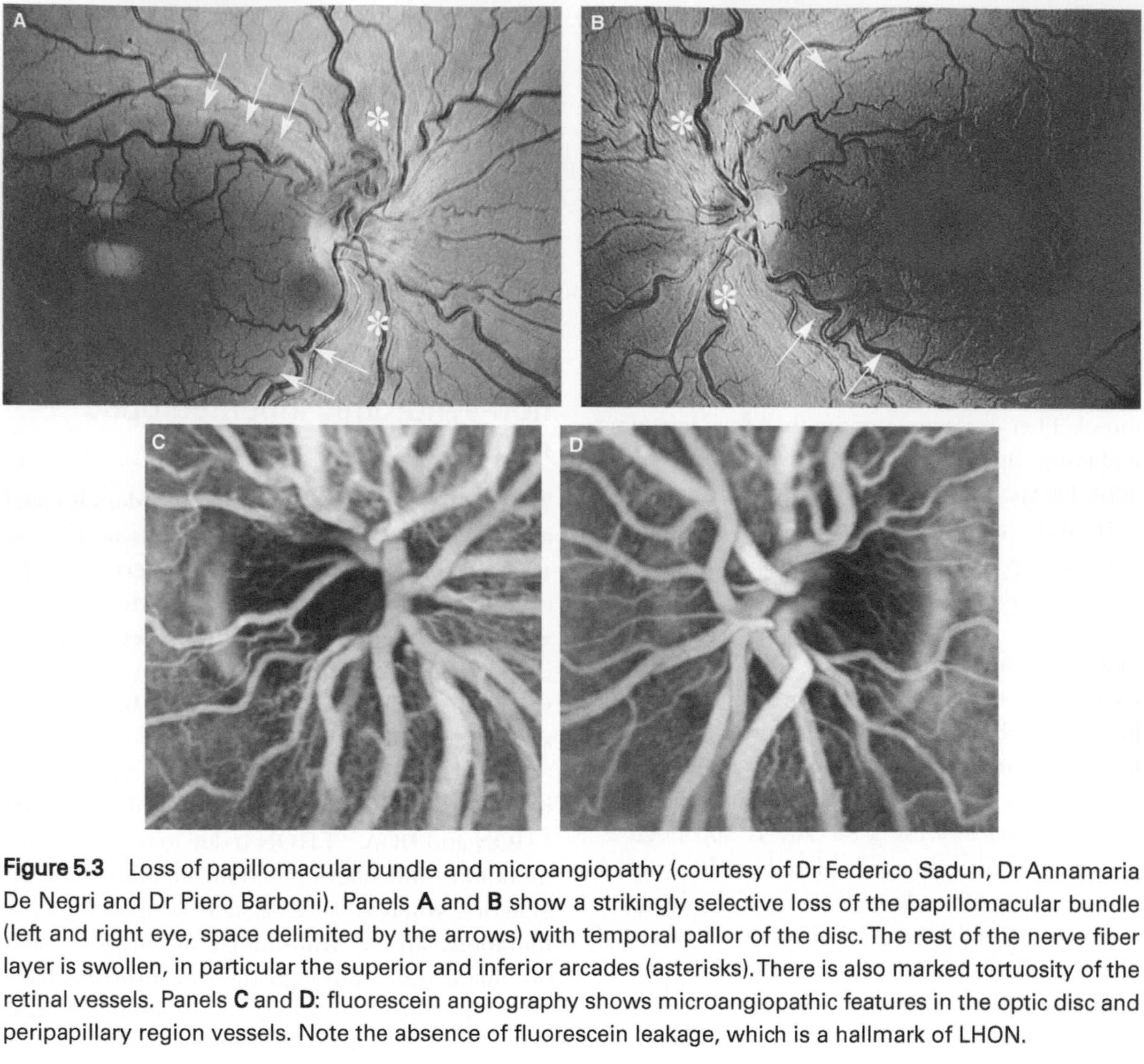

Figure 5.3 Loss of papillomacular bundle and microangiopathy (courtesy of Dr Federico Sadun, Dr Annamaria De Negri and Dr Piero Barboni). Panels **A** and **B** show a strikingly selective loss of the papillomacular bundle (left and right eye, space delimited by the arrows) with temporal pallor of the disc. The rest of the nerve fiber layer is swollen, in particular the superior and inferior arcades (asterisks). There is also marked tortuosity of the retinal vessels. Panels **C** and **D**: fluorescein angiography shows microangiopathic features in the optic disc and peripapillary region vessels. Note the absence of fluorescein leakage, which is a hallmark of LHON.

disease,[48] with a minimum point prevalence of 3.22:100 000 in northeastern England.[49]

Clinically, LHON is characterized by rapid and painless loss of central vision in one or both eyes accompanied by fading of colors (dyschromatopsia). The second eye may become involved within days, months, or more rarely, years.[50,51] Visual acuity reaches stable residual values at or below 20/200 within a few months and the visual field defect shows a large centro-cecal absolute scotoma.

Fundus examination during the subacute stage frequently reveals a characteristic triad of signs,[52–54] including circumpapillary telangiectatic microangiopathy; swelling of the nerve fiber layer around the disc (pseudoedema); and lack of leakage on fluorescein angiography (in contrast to true edema) (Figure 5.3). The optic disc appears hyperemic, with occasional peripapillar hemorrhages, and axonal loss in the papillomacular bundle rapidly leads to temporal pallor of the disc (Figure 5.4). In time, the

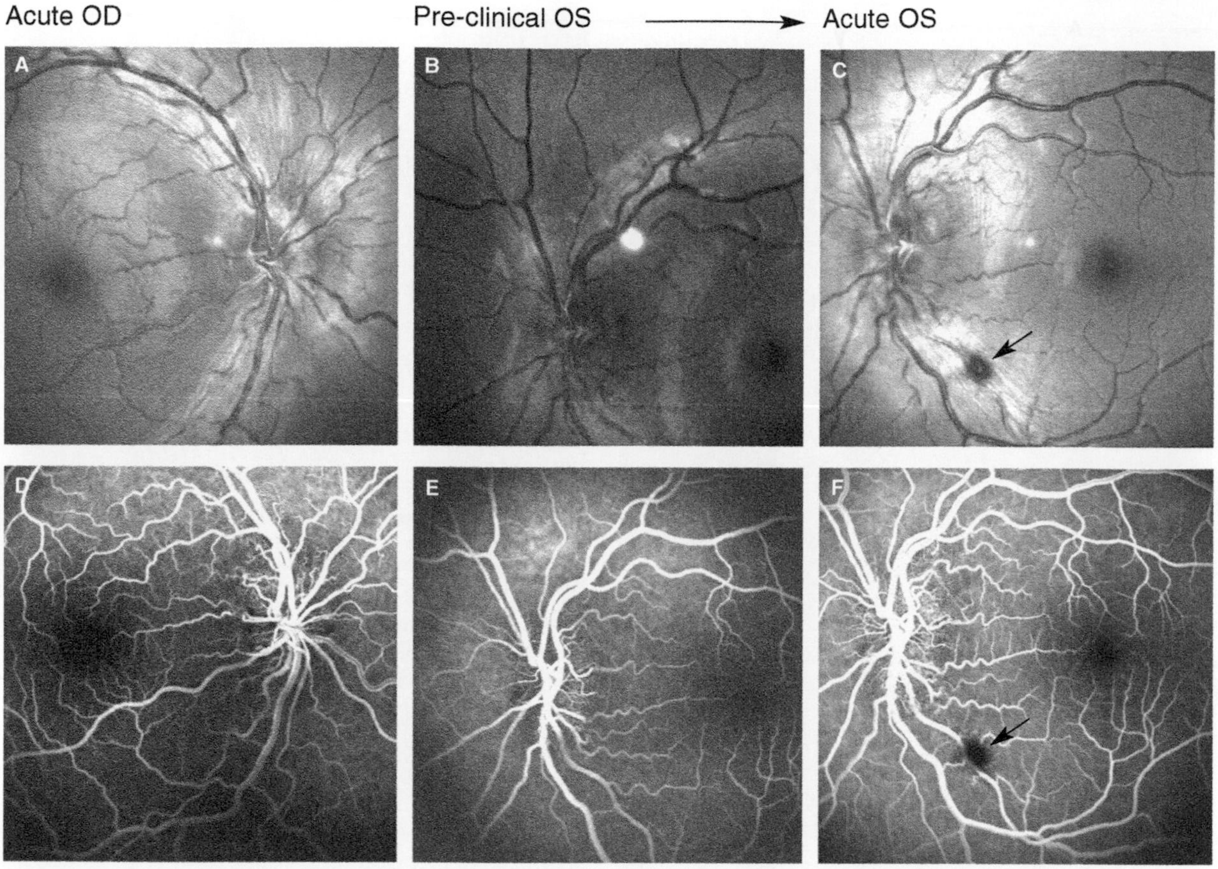

Figure 5.4 Progressive changes of the fundus in a LHON case (courtesy of Dr Arturo Carta). Panels **A** (red free fundus picture) and **D** (fluorescein angiography) show the right affected eye in a LHON/11778 case shortly after disease onset, with loss of the papillomacular bundle and swelling of the superior and inferior nerve fiber layer arcades, as well as microangiopathy. Panels **B** and **E** show the left eye, still in a pre-clinical stage. Panels **C** and **F** show the left eye 3 months later, now in the acute phase, showing microangiopathy, initial loss of temporal fibers belonging to the papillomacular bundle, and swollen nerve fiber layer, with a superficial hemorrhage (arrow)

optic disc turns completely pale. These fundus changes may be absent or minimal in affected individuals, while the microangiopathy may be present in asymptomatic maternal family members.[55]

The endpoint of LHON is usually optic atrophy with permanent loss of central vision and relative sparing of pupillary light responses.[50,51,56] Spontaneous recovery of visual acuity has occasionally been reported even years after onset.[57–59] Vision may improve progressively, sometimes suddenly, with contraction of the scotoma or reappearance of small islands of vision within it (fenestrations). The most favorable prognostic factors are young age of onset and type of pathogenic mutation, the 14484/ND6 mutation being most commonly associated with spontaneous recovery.[60,61] Cupping of the optic disc has frequently been reported in long-lasting LHON as a sign of chronicity.[62]

Only a few LHON patients have been studied histopathologically and none during the acute

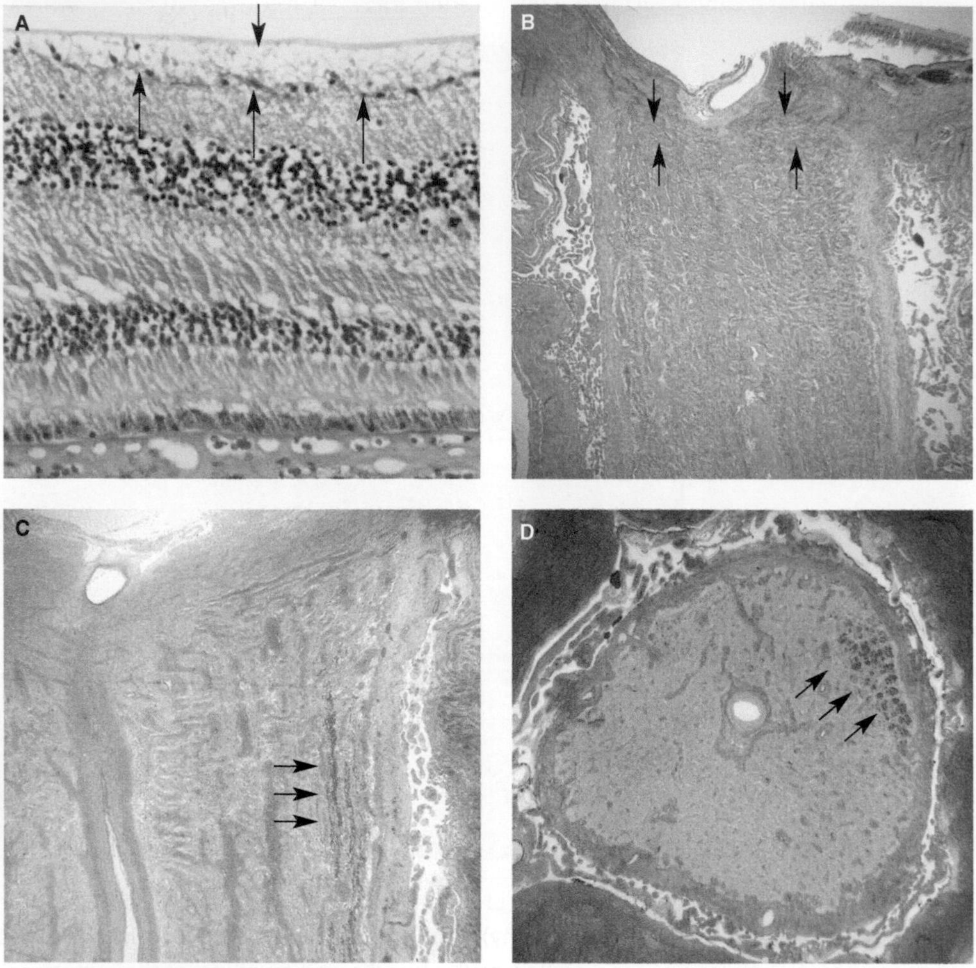

Figure 5.5 LHON histopathology (courtesy of Prof Alfredo A Sadun and Fred N Ross-Cisneros). In panel **A**, the retina of a patient with LHON/3460, stained by hematoxylin and eosin, is characterized by massive loss of retinal ganglion cells (arrows, most of the remaining cells are displaced amacrine cells) and of the nerve fiber layer (between arrows) whereas the remaining layers are fairly normal. In panel **B**, a sagittal section of the optic nerve head from the same LHON case stained with trichrome, shows marked loss of axons and gliotic substitution of the nerve. The collapse of the lamina cribrosa can be also noted (between arrows). In panel **C**, a sagittal section of the same optic nerve head stained with *p*-phylenedyamine highlights the dramatic loss of myelinated axons, of which only a few peripheral bundles (arrows) are recognizable as darker columns in the midst of extensive gliosis. In panel **D**, a cross-section of the same optic nerve shows that only a few bundles are spared in the far periphery (arrows) of a very atrophic nerve

stage of the disease (reviewed in reference 31): in all cases the major retinal finding was a drastic loss of RGC and NFL. The two cases investigated in our laboratories by serial sagittal- and cross-sectioning through the optic nerve head and the postlaminar optic nerve showed a complete loss of central fibers with various degrees of axonal sparing in the periphery and absence of inflammatory signs (Figure 5.5).[31,43,46,51,63,64] Larger axon profiles were selectively spared and found within the reactive gliotic tissue replacing the fiber loss.

Ultrastructural studies revealed axoplasmic abnormalities, such as patchy accumulations of mitochondria, cytoplasmic debris, and cytoskeleton changes.[31,43,46,51] Wide variability in myelin thickness was also evident, with some axons being almost denuded of the myelin sheath. Most demyelinated fibers showed accumulation of mitochondria, which sometimes filled the entire axonal profile.[31,46,51] There was also some evidence of remyelination, indicating that the physiopathological process may be much more dynamic than originally thought. Overall, these findings in both axons and myelin suggest a surprisingly persistent low-grade degenerative process long after the clinical onset of LHON.[31,46,51]

The maternal inheritance of LHON, clearly recognized only a few decades ago,[65] led to the identification of frequent point mutations at positions 11778/ND4, 3460/ND1, and 14484/ND6.[31,50,51] An array of rarer but truly pathogenic mtDNA point mutations affects different subunits of complex I, more commonly ND6 and ND1.[66,67] Common polymorphic variants often occur together with one of the pathogenic mutations and are considered weak genetic determinants, but their real role remains unclear.[68–70] mtDNA mutations do not explain at least two features of LHON: the male prevalence and the incomplete and variable penetrance.[31,50,51] Although most LHON families carry the mtDNA pathogenic mutation in the homoplasmic condition (100% of the mtDNA molecules are mutated), not all maternally related individuals develop LHON. Thus, the mtDNA mutation is a necessary but not a sufficient condition to determine the pathology, and additional genetic determinants, such as nuclear modifying genes, have been postulated and debated.[71,72] The X chromosome is a good candidate for modifying genes because this would explain the male prevalence. Formal compatibility with a two-locus model (mitochondrial pathogenic plus nuclear modifying) has been confirmed by segregation studies in LHON pedigrees.[71,73,74] However, to date no modifying gene on the X chromosome has been identified by numerous studies based on linkage analysis,[75–77] X-inactivation pattern,[78–80] or direct screening of candidate genes.[81] The gender difference could also be due to a gender-specific metabolic factor, which influences the pathogenicity of the mtDNA mutation. Indeed, a protective role of estrogens against oxidative stress has been shown in animal models,[82] and used to explain the gender bias in LHON.[80]

Another controversial topic regards the influence that certain environmental factors may exert on LHON penetrance, triggering the pathologic process in previously unaffected mutation carriers. Tobacco smoking and alcohol consumption are the most likely risk factors,[50,51] but exposures to a variety of less common factors have also been described,[83] including head trauma,[84,85] uncontrolled diabetes,[86] or pharmaceutical agents that interfere with mitochondrial metabolism, such as ethambutol,[87,88] and antiretroviral drugs in HIV patients.[89,90] Two recent studies of large LHON pedigrees with the 11778/ND4 mutation provided convincing evidence of a strong association between tobacco use and disease expression.[83,91] It is not surprising that environmental factors such as tobacco and alcohol may increase LHON penetrance, given that the clinical presentation of toxic and nutritional optic neuropathies is remarkably similar to LHON.[46]

The biochemical effects of LHON mutations proved to be complex, but at least two main consequences of complex I dysfunction have been documented, i.e. reduction of ATP synthesis and increase of ROS production.[92] Reduced availability of ATP may slow the axoplasmic transport of mitochondria, particularly if additional stressful conditions, such as exposure to toxic environmental factors, coexist. Oxidative stress may damage vulnerable cells, such as oligodendrocytes, and the turnover of axonal myelination may suffer.[93] Respiratory impairment may induce compensatory proliferation of mitochondria in

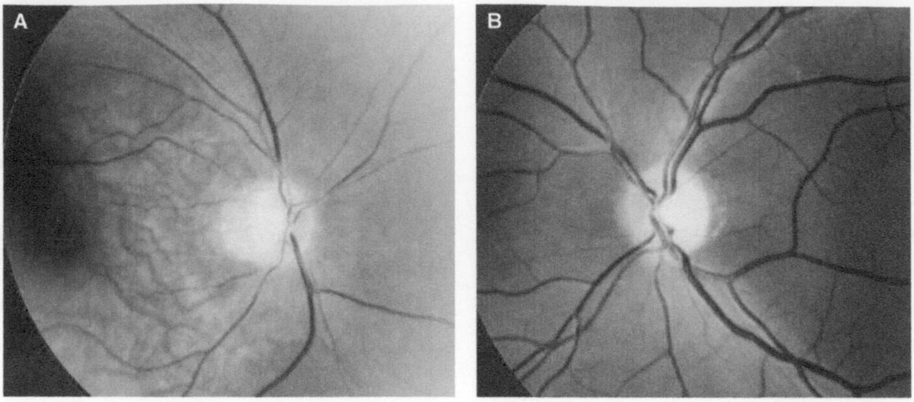

Figure 5.6 Fundus in DOA (courtesy of Dr Piero Barboni). Panel **A** shows a color fundus picture of the right eye from a DOA patient with severe and diffuse optic atrophy. Panel **B** shows the left eye from a DOA patient of comparable age with a mild form of optic neuropathy, illustrating the wide variability in the clinical expression of DOA.

some tissues, which was actually documented in skeletal muscle[43,51,94] and in the endothelial and smooth muscle cells of blood vessels.[95] The interplay of bioenergetic impairment and oxidative stress with anatomo-physiological tissue-specific features can influence the pathways of neuronal cell death. For example, RGCs, the target tissue in LHON, are functionally skewed because the initial unmyelinated portions of the axons have high-energy demand whereas the retrobulbar portion of the nerve, which is myelinated and has saltatory action potentials, has lower energy requirement. Therefore, abundant mitochondria characterize the first portion, whereas the retrobulbar part of the nerve only has a few docked mitochondria at the regions that require the most energy, the nodes of Ranvier. Differential mitochondrial distribution seems to be a crucial feature for the correct functioning of the axons.[31]

Dominant optic neuropathy (DOA): the Mendelian version of a mitochondrial optic neuropathy

DOA, also known as Kjer's optic neuropathy,[96] is characterized by slowly progressive, roughly bilaterally symmetrical visual loss in childhood, accompanied by temporal pallor of the optic discs (Figure 5.6).[31] Examination also demonstrates centrocecal scotomas and impairments of color vision (tritanopia). The disease is frequently recognized during routine vision testing (school or driving license eye screenings). Disease progression may be quite variable within the same family, ranging from mild cases with visual acuity that stabilizes in adolescence, to slowly but relentlessly progressing cases, to cases with sudden, step-like decreases of visual acuity. This variability of clinical expression is reflected by the different extent of optic atrophy shown by different patients (Figure 5.6).

Despite the remarkably different clinical course, the endpoint of the pathological process in DOA is often clinically indistinguishable from that in LHON.[97] A frequent feature of DOA's end-stage fundus is optic disc excavation,[98] which is also reported in LHON.[62] A recent detailed study of optic disc morphology in DOA patients with *OPA1* mutations showed optic disc excavation with enlarged cup-to-disc ratio, frequent peripapillary atrophy, and temporal gray crescent features, also seen in glaucomatous optic neuropathy.[98] Overall, despite a remarkably different natural history,

LHON and DOA share a similar endpoint with predominant involvement of the papillomacular bundle. Both diseases also share a remarkable variability in penetrance.

DOA histopathology is limited to a few cases, which showed selective loss of RGCs, particularly in the macular area, with a substantially normal appearance of the rest of the retina.[99,100] The optic nerve showed axonal loss and swelling, demyelination, and increased content of collagen especially in the temporal aspect (suggesting vulnerability of the small papillo-macular bundle (PMB) fibers), and no sign of inflammation.[31]

DOA has been linked to three different loci. Most cases have been mapped to chromosome 3q28-qter (*OPA1* gene),[101] but a single family of German descent has been mapped to chromosome 18q12.2–12.3 (*OPA4* gene)[102] and a further locus has been recently reported in chromosome 22q (*OPA5* gene).[103] Further genetic heterogeneity probably exists; for example, some families with a DOA variant associated with sensorineural deafness do not link to the above loci.[104] In 2000, two different groups simultaneously identified mutations in the *OPA1* gene, and described the encoded protein as a dynamin-related GTPase targeted to mitochondria.[105,106] Large series of DOA patients have since been investigated and over 60 mutations have been reported, including missense, nonsense, deletion/insertion, and splicing changes.[107–110] Mutations are found throughout the gene and most of them produce a truncated protein, suggesting that haploinsufficiency is the mechanism underlying DOA. However, a few truncation mutations affect the C-terminus, a putative dimerization domain, and a dominant negative effect has been hypothesized in these cases.[111] Finally, semi-dominant alleles have also been reported, with compound heterozygous patients being much more severely affected than their heterozygous parents or siblings.[107] A number of asymptomatic carriers of OPA1 mutations have been identified within families, suggesting lower penetrance.[108] One frameshift mutation, 2708del(TTAG), seems to be the most frequent in white patients and may be a hotspot.[109,110] Another mutation has been associated, by different authors, with the more severe phenotype of DOA and sensorineural deafness, which in two families also included ptosis and ophthalmoplegia.[112,113] However, in general the genotype–phenotype correlation is weak, with great variability in both penetrance and clinical severity. As is the case for LHON, other as yet unknown genetic or epigenetic/environmental factors may play a role in the phenotypic expression of DOA.

The *OPA1* gene encodes a protein that is targeted to mitochondria by a leader sequence. This protein is closely related to a family of proteins involved in mitochondrial fusion and is anchored to the mitochondrial inner membrane, facing the inter-membrane space.[114] OPA1 has eight mRNA isoforms resulting from alternative splicing. These are expressed in a variety of tissues, with the highest levels in retina, brain, testis, heart, and muscle.[109,111]

Down-regulation of *OPA1* gene expression in HeLa cells by RNA interference (RNAi) led to fragmentation of the mitochondrial network, loss of mitochondrial membrane potential, and drastic disorganization of the cristae.[115] Moreover, these events were followed by release of cytochrome *c* and caspase-dependent activation of the apoptotic cascade.[115] These experiments suggest that *OPA1* is a major organizer of the mitochondrial inner membrane, contributing to cristae maintenance and mitochondrial morphology.

Mitochondrial optic neuropathies: syndromic inherited optic neuropathies due to mtDNA or nuclear DNA defects

An optic neuropathy similar to that seen in LHON or DOA is frequently part of mitochondrial syndromes due to mtDNA mutations, such as myoclonic epilepsy, ragged red fibers (MERRF),[116] mitochondrial encephalomyopathy, lactic acidosis, stroke-like episodes (MELAS),[116–119] or Leigh syndrome,[120,121] to mention only the most common. Optic neuropathy is also common in mitochondrial disorders due to nuclear gene mutations, such as Friedreich ataxia (FRDA),[122] Costeff syndrome (OPA3),[123] X-linked deafness-dystonia-optic atrophy syndrome (Mohr–Tranebjaerg syndrome),[124] hereditary spastic paraplegia,[11] or a syndrome of late-onset optic atrophy and ataxia linked to a mutation in complex II.[125,126]

A large study of the genotype–phenotype correlation in mitochondrial encephalomyopathies due to mtDNA mutations reported that optic atrophy is more frequent in MERRF than in MELAS, whereas retinal pigmentary abnormalities are more frequent in MELAS.[116] However, optic neuropathy has also been reported in a few patients carrying the typical A3243G/tRNA$^{Leu(UUR)}$ MELAS mutation.[119,127] Recently, much interest has been generated by the observation that point mutations in the mitochondrially encoded ND genes, mainly ND5, ND6, and ND1, are frequently associated with a syndromic form of LHON, with LHON/MELAS/Leigh syndrome,[128–132] with LHON/dystonia/Leigh syndrome,[133–135] or with LHON/MELAS overlaps.[136] A few 'LHON-plus' cases of slowly evolving or adult-onset Leigh syndrome have also been reported in association with the 'classical' 11778/ND4, 3460/ND1, or 14484/ND6 LHON mutations.[137] These observations point to a possible common pathogenic mechanism with different degrees of central nervous system involvement, where the LHON-like optic neuropathy represents only the tip of the iceberg. Remarkably, the few histopathological studies of the eye in Leigh cases present features indistinguishable from LHON.[120,121,138] The link between LHON, MELAS, and Leigh syndromes may relate to mitochondrial angiopathy as a shared common feature and to a possible vascular involvement in the pathophysiology of these phenotypes.[31,95,139] Mitochondrial encephalomyopathies with prominent optic atrophy have also been associated with cytochrome *c* oxidase subunit I (COX I) mutation[140] or to mtDNA deletion.[141]

Optic atrophy is an underestimated feature of Friedreich ataxia (FDRA), the most common inherited ataxia[142] due to recessive GAA triplet expansion or point mutations in the frataxin gene on chromosome 9q13.[143] Old studies had showed VEP abnormalities, temporal paleness of the optic disc, and moderate reduction of visual acuity reminiscent of DOA.[122] A single report described visual loss followed by recovery, closely resembling LHON, in a FRDA patient.[144] A recent study of the optic neuropathy in 25 FRDA Italian patients provided the first thorough description.[145] All patients showed predominantly peripheral loss of vision by computerized visual fields and optical coherence tomography (OCT), but visual acuity was impaired only in the most severe or advanced cases. Both fiber loss (evaluated by OCT) and age at onset were related to the size of the triplet expansion. An LHON-like subacute loss of central vision occurred in two patients of this cohort, validating the single case previously reported.[144] Studies of a different cohort of 99 FRDA Italian patients showed that mtDNA haplogroup U has a protective effect on the development of cardiomyopathy.[146] The pattern of optic atrophy in FRDA patients is similar to that seen in a neurological syndrome characterized by late-onset optic atrophy and cerebellar ataxia, which has been associated with mutations in a complex II gene.[125,126] It is worth noting that defective complex II is also found in patients with FRDA, in whom biochemical analyses have shown increased mitochondrial iron and impaired activities of iron–sulfur (Fe–S) cluster-containing mitochondrial enzymes, including respiratory complexes I, II, and III, and the matrix enzyme aconitase.[147] Another related disorder is vitamin-E-deficient ataxia, which can be due to mutations in the α-tocopherol transfer protein,[148] or to abetalipoproteinemia.[149] We observed recurrent optic atrophy in a family with abetalipoproteinemia, in which ^{31}P-MRS studies showed defective mitochondrial bioenergetics.[149]

Optic atrophy and increased urinary excretion of 3-methylglutaconic acid and of 3-methylglutaric acid are the main features of Costeff syndrome,[150] which has been associated with mutations in *OPA3*, a gene encoding a poorly characterized mitochondrial protein.[123] Besides optic atrophy, these patients also have extrapyramidal signs, spasticity, ataxia, dysarthria, and cognitive deficit. After the initial definition of the syndrome in an Iraqi Jew genetic isolate, mutations in *OPA3* have been reported in other populations.[151] Furthermore, at variance with the autosomal recessive Costeff syndrome, allelic mutations in *OPA3* have also been reported in families with autosomal dominant optic atrophy and cataract.[152]

Finally, optic atrophy has also been associated with other Mendelian mitochondrial diseases, such as the deafness-dystonia-optic atrophy syndrome (Mohr–Tranebjaerg syndrome) due to mutations in the X-linked DDP1/TIMM8a gene,[124,153–156] or hereditary spastic paraplegia due to mutations in the paraplegin gene.[11] Although visual loss is mainly due to neurodegeneration of the visual cortex, degeneration of the retina and the optic nerve contributes to the visual impairment.[155,156] DDP1/TIMM8a is similar to a family of yeast proteins located in the mitochondrial intermembrane space, which mediate the import and insertion of inner membrane proteins.[153] A lymphoblast cell line derived from a Mohr–Tranebjaerg syndrome patient had decreased NADH levels and defects in mitochondrial protein import.[157]

Optic atrophy frequently complicates the clinical picture of families with autosomal recessive spastic paraplegia due to mutations in the paraplegin gene. It is interesting to note that paraplegin, a putative mitochondrial metallopeptidase of the AAA family, has been reported to co-assemble with a homologous protein, AFG3L2, to form a complex in the mitochondrial inner membrane.[158] The lack of this complex impairs complex I activity in mitochondria and increases sensitivity to oxidative stress, a general paradigm of mitochondrial optic neuropathies.[31] This paradigm is bolstered by studies of paraplegin-deficient mice, which show axonal swellings due to massive accumulation of organelles and neurofilaments, suggestive of impaired axonal transport.[159] These changes are also seen in the optic nerve axons of this animal model and closely resemble the ultrastructural abnormalities described in LHON.[31,43,46,51]

Mitochondrial optic neuropathies: environmentally acquired forms

Tobacco-alcohol amblyopia (TAA),[160] the Cuban epidemic of optic neuropathy (CEON),[161] and other dietary (vitamin B, folate deficiencies) optic neuropathies,[162] as well as toxic optic neuropathies such as those due to chloramphenicol,[163] ethambutol,[164] or – more rarely – to carbon monoxide, methanol, and cyanide[165] are probably all related and due to acquired mitochondrial dysfunction.

Tobacco-alcohol amblyopia

Tobacco-alcohol amblyopia (TAA) characteristically affects men with a history of heavy tobacco and/or alcohol use.[160,166] Subacute loss of central vision with cecocentral scotomas, dyschromatopsia, and decreased visual acuity characterize this syndrome, together with tortuosity of small retinal vessels at fundoscopy. Temporal optic atrophy characterizes later stages of the disease, and histopathology shows pronounced loss of RGCs in the macula, with marked loss of papillomacular bundle fibers.[167] Cessation of drinking and smoking and timely administration of hydroxycobalamin may lead to visual recovery.[168]

Combined toxic insults from tobacco compounds and ethyl alcohol and concurrent nutritional deficiencies have been proposed as causes of the optic neuropathy.[160,168] The sharp decrease of new TAA cases in Western countries points to an important role of nutritional deficiencies. However, a wide body of evidence indicates that tobacco-derived compounds, including reactive oxygen species (ROS) and cyanide, impair mitochondrial respiration,[169] damage mtDNA,[170] and induce alterations of mitochondrial morphology.[171] Given the remarkable similarities between LHON and TAA, it was not surprising to find LHON-related mutations in TAA patients, indicating that some presumed TAA patients were, in fact, cases of LHON.[172]

Cuban epidemic of optic neuropathy (CEON) and other dietary optic neuropathies

Between 1992 and 1993, an epidemic of nutritional deficiency optic neuropathy affected tens of thousands of severely malnourished individuals in Cuba.[161] These patients all reported marked weight loss associated with deficient protein and vitamin intake, involving especially vitamin B12 and folate. The most striking fundoscopic finding was marked thinning of the nerve fiber layer of the papillomacular bundle, which formed a wedge defect bordered by swollen nerve fibers above and below.[173] The clinical presentation of CEON required at least three of the following five signs: bilateral progressive loss of visual acuity, bilateral cecocentral scotomas, bilateral dyschromatopsia, bilateral loss of high spatial frequency contrast sensitivity, or saccadic eye movements.[173] Besides the visual symptoms, over one third of the patients also had neurological symptoms, including peripheral neuropathy, ataxia, and hearing loss. Prompt administration of cyanocobalamin (3 mg daily) and folate (250 mg daily) led to recovery of visual acuity in a significant number of cases and dietary supplementation brought the epidemic to an end.

In general, loss of central vision together with dyschromatopsia, cecocentral scotomas, and selective loss of the papillomacular bundle characterizes the following vitamin deficiencies: vitamin B12 (cobalamin), vitamin B1 (thiamine; this is often associated with photophobia and eye pain), vitamin B2 (riboflavin), and folic acid. CEON, a recent similar epidemic in Tanzania,[174] and TAA may all involve a combination of dietary deficiencies and toxic exposures.

Chloramphenicol and ethambutol optic neuropathies

An optic neuropathy characterized by sudden onset, bilateral loss of central vision with cecocentral scotoma, selective involvement of the papillomacular bundle, and tortuosity of the retinal vessels may be induced in a dose-dependent fashion by the administration of at least two antibiotics, chloramphenicol[163] and ethambutol.[164]

Until 1970, chloramphenicol was used frequently to treat children with cystic fibrosis,[163] until toxicity was revealed by the many patients developing optic and peripheral neuropathy during treatment. Prompt cessation of the drug and supplementation of vitamin B complex usually restored visual function. Histopathological studies showed loss of RGCs and nerve fibers, and demyelination of the optic nerve involving predominantly the papillomacular bundle.[164] Chloramphenicol is a well-known inhibitor of mitochondrial protein synthesis. A similar toxic optic neuropathy has been recently ascribed to an antibiotic belonging to the oxazolidinone class (linezolid),[175,176] which shares with chloramphenicol the binding site on mitochondrial ribosomal RNA (rRNA), though not the mechanism of action.[177]

Ocular toxicity is also well established for ethambutol, an antimycobacterial agent used in the treatment of tuberculosis.[164] Symptoms are generally reversed by early withdrawal of the drug, but some visual loss may persist in conjunction with mild temporal pallor of the optic disc. The only histopathological study showed demyelination in the optic chiasm.[178] Ethambutol is a metal chelator and might interact with Cu-containing cytochrome oxidase (complex IV) and Fe-containing NADH:Q oxidoreductase (complex I), thus potentially damaging the mitochondrial respiratory chain.[46]

Toxic optic neuropathies

Toxins that are known to induce optic neuropathy include arsacetin, carbon monoxide, clioquinol, cyanide, hexachlorophene, isoniazid, lead, methanol, plasmocid, and triethyl tin.[165] Most of these interfere with oxidative phosphorylation. Other agents whose toxicity to the optic nerve is less well established include carbon disulfide, pheniprazine, quinine, and thallium.[165] Toxins suspected to cause optic neuropathy are carbon tetrachloride, cassava, daspasone, and suramin.[165]

Retinal dystrophies in mitochondrial syndromes

Besides the RGCs and the optic nerve, the RPE and photoreceptors are two other cell types within the retina that depend strictly on energy metabolism to carry out their functions. Given the atypical retinal pathology in mitochondrial disorders, it is preferable to refer to these disorders as 'retinal dystrophies' or simply retinopathies. The most prominent involvement of the retina is seen in three well-characterized syndromes: KSS,[3] MELAS,[179] and neuropathy, ataxia, retinitis pigmentosa (NARP).[180] We will focus on the retinopathy seen in these syndromes as a paradigm of what can be frequently found in other mitochondrial encephalomyopathies due to rarer mtDNA mutations. We will also limit our description to the ocular manifestations because these disorders are described in Chapters 2 and 3.

Retinopathy in Kearns–Sayre syndrome

The invariant triad of PEO, pigmentary retinopathy, and onset before 20 years of age characterizes this usually sporadic multisystem disorder.[3,181] Frequent additional symptoms include poor growth, progressive cerebellar syndrome, heart block, and increased protein content (above 100 mg/dl) in the cerebrospinal fluid (CSF). RRF and COX-negative fibers are the morphological hallmarks of the muscle biopsy (see Chapter 3). KSS is usually associated with a single mtDNA deletion,[2] which in most cases is not transmitted and is probably a somatic mutational event occurring very early during embryogenesis. After the original descriptions,[3,181] a few KSS cases have come to autopsy and the histopathology of the retina has been described.[182,183]

The pigmentary changes seen at fundoscopy are different from those of retinitis pigmentosa and are frequently described as 'salt and pepper' pigment clumping with a 'moth-eaten appearance'. They consist of mottled hypopigmented and hyperpigmented areas, which histologically show primary degeneration of RPE and alterations of photoreceptors and choriocapillaries.[3,181–183] There are alternating areas with complete absence of RPE and rod and cones and areas with fairly preserved outer retina. The inner retina seems to be always preserved, with normal appearance of RGCs and RNFL. Optic atrophy may develop only in advanced cases. The retinal degeneration in KSS often occurs in the peripapillary zone, sparing the peripheral retina (Figure 5.7). In the most advanced cases, the choroid vessels surrounding the disc may have a sclerotic appearance. Ultrastructural features include disappearance of the apical villi and basal infoldings of RPE, and loss of melanosomes without evidence of phagocytosis of photoreceptor debris.[182,183] The RPE contains proliferated mitochondria, which are often enlarged and irregularly shaped. Clinically, KSS patients complain of increasing difficulty seeing in the dark, culminating in night blindness. The retinal pathology is reflected by the electroretinographic (ERG) abnormalities.[184]

Retinopathy in MELAS

MELAS is defined by the presence of stroke-like episodes due to focal brain lesions, often localized

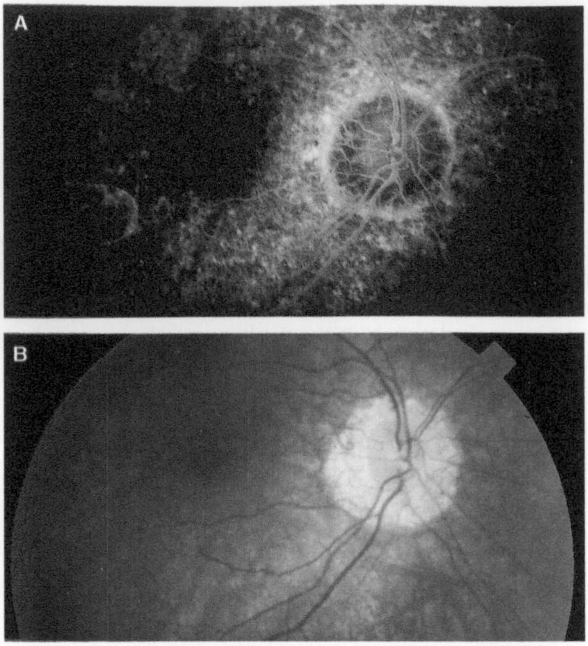

Figure 5.7 KSS fundus (courtesy of Dr Piero Barboni). 'Salt and pepper' retinopathy in Kearns–Sayre syndrome. In panel **A**, a fluorescein angiography of the right eye shows diffuse retinal pigment, epithelial atrophy, and peripapillary chorioretinal atrophy. In panel **B**, a color picture shows the mottled hypopigmented and hyperpigmented appearance of central and peripheral retina

to the parieto-occipital lobes, lactic acidosis, and RRF.[179,185] Other signs of central nervous system involvement include dementia, recurrent headache and vomiting, focal or generalized seizures, pigmentary retinopathy, and sensorineural deafness, and ataxia.[179,185] Non-neurological signs include diabetes, intestinal pseudo-obstruction, and cardiomyopathy (see Chapter 2). MELAS was first associated with a heteroplasmic point mutation (A3243G) in the $tRNA^{Leu(UUR)}$ gene.[186] Many other MELAS-associated point mutations were later reported,[187] although the A3243G is by far the most frequent.

We have already mentioned the relatively rare occurrence of optic neuropathy in MELAS.[117–119] Retinal changes have been reported more frequently,[116,184] although they are far less prominent than in KSS and often asymptomatic. However, they are clearly recognizable by fundoscopy, fluorescein angiography, visual evoked potentials, or ERG.[188–190] In one study, the retinal pigmentary abnormalities were described as symmetric areas of depigmentation involving predominantly the posterior pole and midperipheral retina.[188] However, as for KSS, patchy hyperpigmentation at the posterior pole of the fundus was also reported in MELAS, particularly in the macular area, alternating with focal areas of depigmentation.[189] Histopathologic and ultrastructural examinations showed degeneration of the photoreceptor outer segment in the macula, hyperpigmentation and atrophy of the RPE of the macula, and many, often enlarged, structurally abnormal mitochondria containing paracrystalline inclusions and circular cristae.[117,118]

Retinopathy in NARP

As the acronym implies, the cardinal manifestations of NARP, a maternally inherited syndrome, include ataxia, pigmentary retinopathy, and peripheral neuropathy.[180] MRI of the brain in NARP patients shows moderate, diffuse cerebral and cerebellar atrophy, and, in severely affected infants and children, Leigh-like symmetric lesions of the basal ganglia.[191] NARP is associated with a heteroplasmic T→G transversion[180] or T→C transition[192] at position 8993 in the ATPase 6 subunit gene. RRF fibers are consistently absent from the muscle biopsy. When the load of mutant mtDNA is very high (usually above 95%), patients have maternally inherited Leigh syndrome (MILS).[193] NARP and MILS may coexist in the same family. Impairment of ATP synthesis has been reported in cell cultures harboring the T8993G mutation, as well as in tissue-derived mitochondria, showing a strict orrelation with the mutation load.[194]

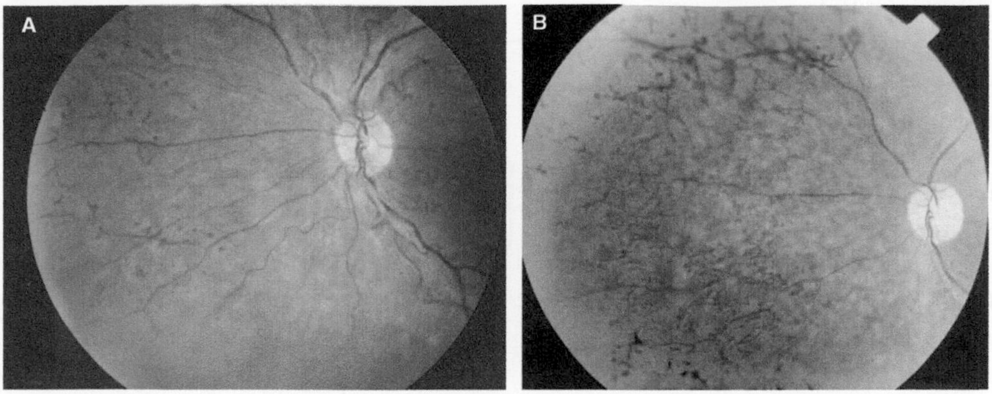

Figure 5.8 Progression of retinal dystrophy in NARP (courtesy of Dr Piero Barboni). In panel **A**, a color picture of the left eye shows bone spicule-like pigmentation of peripheral retina (originally published in Puddu et al. *Br J Ophthalmol* 1993; **77**: 84–88). In panel **B**, a color picture taken 12 years later illustrates the progression of the pigmentary retinopathy. Optic atrophy and attenuated retinal vessels are also evident at this time

Retinal dystrophy, a hallmark of the NARP syndrome, leads to severe night blindness and – in later stages – when it is complicated by optic neuropathy, may result in loss of visual acuity and blindness.[195–199] Retinal dystrophy has been described as 'salt-and-pepper retinopathy' or as 'diffuse pigmentary retinopathy'.[195] Variable degrees of cone and rod dysfunction have been described in different members of the same family carrying the T8993G mutation.[196] The variable severity of retinal dystrophy is not only related to different loads of mutant mtDNA but also to progression over time: this is exemplified by an American patient, whose retinopathy was first labeled 'salt-and-pepper' and later 'bone spicule pigment formation' (Figure 5.8).[197] The single case of a MILS patient with the T8993G mutation studied at autopsy showed both features of mitochondrial optic neuropathy similar to LHON and ultrastructural changes of mitochondria in the RPE.[121] These results do not differ from ocular findings in patients with other forms of Leigh syndrome,[120] and show that severe mtDNA point mutations, such as those causing NARP/MILS, MELAS, and KSS have overlapping features.[138]

Progressive external ophthalmoplegia (PEO): a common hallmark of mitochondrial myopathy

PEO is one of the commonest clinical manifestations of mitochondrial myopathy.[6,7] It can present as an isolated feature, or as one of many clinical features in mitochondrial syndromes due to mtDNA or nuclear DNA defects (see Chapter 2). Thus, inheritance of PEO can be sporadic, maternal or Mendelian. Onset can be early in life or in adulthood. Usually, patients or their relatives recall ptosis as the first sign, and old pictures are frequently helpful to establish age of onset and, in familial forms, which family members have been affected. The ophthalmoplegia develops over years in a slowly progressive fashion, but may lead to complete ocular paralysis and the ptosis may be severe enough to require surgical intervention.

At EOMs histopathology, the main finding is mitochondrial proliferation, documented by strong SDH stain contrasting with defective or absent COX activity in RRF.[200–203] At ultrastructure, the overabundant mitochondria show a wide range of morphological abnormalities, including swelling, irregular shapes, paracrystalline 'parking lot' inclusions, 'onion-ring like' cristae, tubular cristae, or light matrix conferring a 'ghost' appearance.[200–203] Myofibers with these pathological features may be present in one fiber or fiber segment and not in adjacent fibers or next fiber segments, probably due to differences in mutant load between fibers and fiber segments (Figure 5.9). The endstage pathology of PEO is fibrotic substitution of the EOMs, the anatomical substrate for complete ophthalmoplegia.

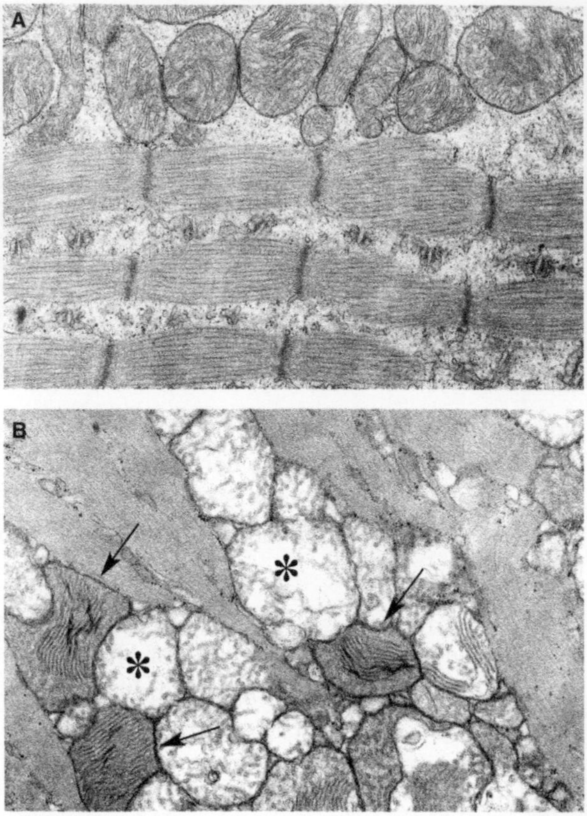

Figure 5.9 Ultrastructural features of PEO with single deletion (courtesy of Dr Arturo Carta). Panel **A** shows the ultrastructural organization of a normal extraocular muscle (medial rectus). Panel **B** is a high-magnification micrograph of an ultrastructurally altered muscle fiber (medial rectus) from a patient with PEO and a single mtDNA deletion. Many abnormal mitochondria have lost the cristae and look like 'ghosts' with light matrix (asterisks). In some mitochondria, aberrant parallel cristae are densely packed in an 'onion-like' pattern (arrows). The accumulation of proliferated mitochondria distorts and displaces the myofibrils

PEO in mtDNA disorders

Sporadic PEO is a muscle-specific milder variant of KSS.[204] It usually presents in young adults and is characterized by bilateral ptosis and ophthalmoplegia, exercise intolerance, and variable degrees of proximal muscle weakness and wasting. As in KSS, there are numerous RRF and COX-deficient fibers in the muscle biopsy.[205] Sporadic PEO, like KSS, is associated with single large-scale heteroplasmic rearrangements of mtDNA,[1,2,204] which are easily detected by Southern-blot (or quantitative PCR) analysis of muscle DNA. The mtDNA deletions are usually absent in lymphocytes or fibroblasts.

However, PEO is frequently associated with maternally inherited point mutation of mtDNA, like those typically causing MELAS and MERRF.[116] PEO, alone or within a complex syndrome, can be associated with any mtDNA mutation affecting tRNA genes (see Chapter 2).[206,207]

PEO in mitochondrial disorders due to nDNA mutations

These syndromes are characterized by multiple rearrangements and/or decreased copy number (depletion) of mtDNA in affected tissues, such as skeletal muscle and brain. The Mendelian transmission of these traits indicates that the primary causes reside in nuclear genes, whose defects impair the structural integrity and/or replication of mtDNA.[208–210] However, it is the progressive damage of mtDNA that ultimately leads to organ failure and disease. Mendelian PEO disorders are genetically heterogeneous, and linkage analysis has identified loci responsible for autosomal dominant PEO (adPEO) on chromosomes 10q,[211] 4q,[212] and 15q.[213] Additional loci must exist because several adPEO families fail to map to these loci. Autosomal-recessive PEO (arPEO), also characterized by the accumulation of multiple mtDNA deletions, has also been reported in several families.

The gene responsible for the adPEO form linked to the 4p locus encodes the muscle-specific isoform of the mitochondrial adenine nucleotide translocator (ANT1).[214] ANT1 predominates in skeletal muscle, but is also abundant in heart and brain. The gene responsible for the adPEO form linked to the 10q locus (*PEO1*) encodes a mitochondrially targeted protein named Twinkle, a helicase involved in the replication of the mitochondrial genome.[215] Finally, *POLG*, the gene responsible for the adPEO form linked to the 15q locus, encodes the main (catalytic) subunit of polymerase gamma, the only mitochondrial DNA polymerase.[213] This gene is probably the most frequent cause of adPEO,[216] but is also responsible for most arPEO cases and for approximately one-third of apparently sporadic PEO cases associated with multiple mtDNA deletions.[213,216,217] The severity of these syndromes depends on the type of mutant gene and on the type of mutation. For instance, mutations in *ANT1* seem to cause a relatively mild, slowly progressive myopathy, with little or no extramuscular symptoms. Mutations in Twinkle have variable severity, while the most severe syndromes have been associated with *POLG* mutations. In adPEO or arPEO due to *POLG* mutations, prominent features include dysphagia and dysphonia, sensory ataxia and, occasionally, parkinsonism, cerebellar ataxia, and chorea.[218–220] Unipolar or bipolar affective disorder, hypogonadism, and gastrointestinal dysmotility may be additional findings.[221,222]

A distinctive autosomal recessive syndrome is mitochondrial neurogastrointestinal encephalomyopathy (MNGIE), which is clinically defined by PEO, severe gastrointestinal dysmotility, cachexia, peripheral neuropathy, white matter changes in brain MRI, and mitochondrial abnormalities.[223,224] Loss-of-function mutations in the thymidine phosphorylase (*TP*) gene[225] lead to pathologic accumulations of thymidine and deoxyuridine, which somehow generate mtDNA defects (depletion, multiple deletions, and point mutations).[226] In the case of MNGIE, the prominent gastrointestinal problems result in a very characteristic cachectic appearance, which facilitates the diagnosis.

Clinical, laboratory and ancillary testing for neuro-ophthalmological mitochondrial disorders

The correct diagnosis of a mitochondrial neuro-ophthalmological disorder requires the close collaboration of neurologists, ophthalmologists and molecular biologists. Careful family history is extremely important in elucidating the hereditary pattern, sporadic, maternal or Mendelian, and in directing the molecular investigation towards studies of mtDNA or nDNA.

The neuro-ophthalmologist's task includes assessment of visual acuity, color vision and other measures of vision, slit-lamp examination of the anterior segment of the eye (cornea and lens), evaluation of intraocular pressure, fundus, extraocular motility, and pupillary reaction and accomodation. Instrumental examinations include visual field test (computerized perimetry), fluorescein angiography, contrast sensitivity, coordimetry, and electrophysiological examinations such as visual evoked potentials (VEP) and electroretinogram (ERG), and, more recently, multifocal VEP and ERG. A promising new tool is optical coherence tomography (OCT), which is described separately in the next section. Additional instruments for evaluation of NFL, optic nerve head, and macula include GDx Nerve Fiber Analyzer (scanning laser polarimetry), Heidelberg Retina Tomograph (HRT), and Retinal Thickness Analyzer (RTA).

The neurologist's task is particularly important when the ophthalmological features are part of more complex syndromes, like mitochondrial encephalomyopathies. Accurate family history is again the starting point. In maternally inherited mitochondrial encephalomyopathies, such as MELAS, MERRF and NARP, it is particularly important to identify oligosymptomatic individuals along the maternal line. For example, diabetes and sensorineural deafness, isolated cardiomyopathy, migraine, or epilepsy may all be expressions of the extreme intrafamilial variability of mtDNA mutations. Thus, a comprehensive neurological examination is essential for the clinical definition of a multisystem syndrome. Laboratory investigations of the central nervous system (CNS) include cerebrospinal fluid (CSF) analysis, computerized tomography (CT) scans, and magnetic resonance imaging (MRI). The response of venous lactate to standardized exercise on a cycloergometer is a valuable tool to reveal respiratory chain defects, even in 'mild' disorders, such as LHON.[67,227] CNS and muscle mitochondrial functions can also be investigated by phosphorus or proton MR spectroscopy (MRS),[228,229] which has proven very sensitive in documenting abnormalities of oxidative metabolism and may be of value both in longitudinal studies and in assessing the effectiveness of treatments.[230]

Genetic analysis is now available for a wide range of mtDNA-related ophthalmological disorders such as LHON, MELAS, MERRF, KSS, and PEO, as well as for several nuclear genes, including *ANT1*, *PEO1*, *POLG1*, *TP*, *OPA1*, *OPA3*, *DDT1/TIMM8a*, *FRDA*, and *SPG7*. Genetic screening based on polymerase chain reaction (PCR)/restriction fragment length polymorphisms (RFLP) of blood DNA for the 11778/ND4, the 3460/ND1, and the 14484/ND6 LHON mutations has widened the diagnosis of LHON to cases with many atypical features and is now suggested in anyone with unexplained bilateral optic neuropathy.[50,51] Conversely, systematic sequence analysis of ND subunit genes in patients with clinically typical LHON, but without any of the three frequent mtDNA mutations, revealed novel mtDNA mutations, which have been confirmed as pathogenic in multiple cases worldwide.[31,66,67] This may be considered the second line of molecular investigation in LHON. A third line of molecular investigations has to include mtDNA mutations in the ND5 subunit gene of complex I, which have been associated with overlapping phenotypes of LHON, MELAS, and Leigh syndrome in the same maternal lineage.[128–132] The clinical presentation of a mitochondrial encephalomyopathy, with a syndromic occurrence of LHON-like optic neuropathy, retinal dystrophy, and/or PEO must direct molecular screening towards specific pathogenic mutations in structural or tRNA genes or towards mtDNA single/multiple deletions.

Optical coherence tomography (OCT), a new tool in the study of mitochondrial optic neuropathies and retinopathies

OCT is a non-contact, non-invasive imaging technique developed to enable real-time, in vivo quantitative examination of the retina and the optic disc. The latest version of the machine, Stratus OCT, employs low-coherence interferometry to generate cross-sectional images of the retina, the optic disc, and the NFL with an axial resolution of ≤ 10 microns and a transverse resolution of 20 μm. The OCT contains an interferometer that resolves posterior pole structures by measuring the echo delay time of light reflected and backscattered from different layers in the retina and optic disc. With each scan pass, the OCT captures from 128 to 768 axial A-scans, and each A-scan consists of 1024 data points over 2 mm of depth. Therefore, the OCT integrates from 131 072 to 786 432 data points to construct a cross-sectional image of retinal and optic nerve anatomy.

The NFL thickness algorithm works in a two-pass process: it looks first for the highest rates of changes in reflectivity at the vitreoretinal interface, then for reflectivity above a threshold value

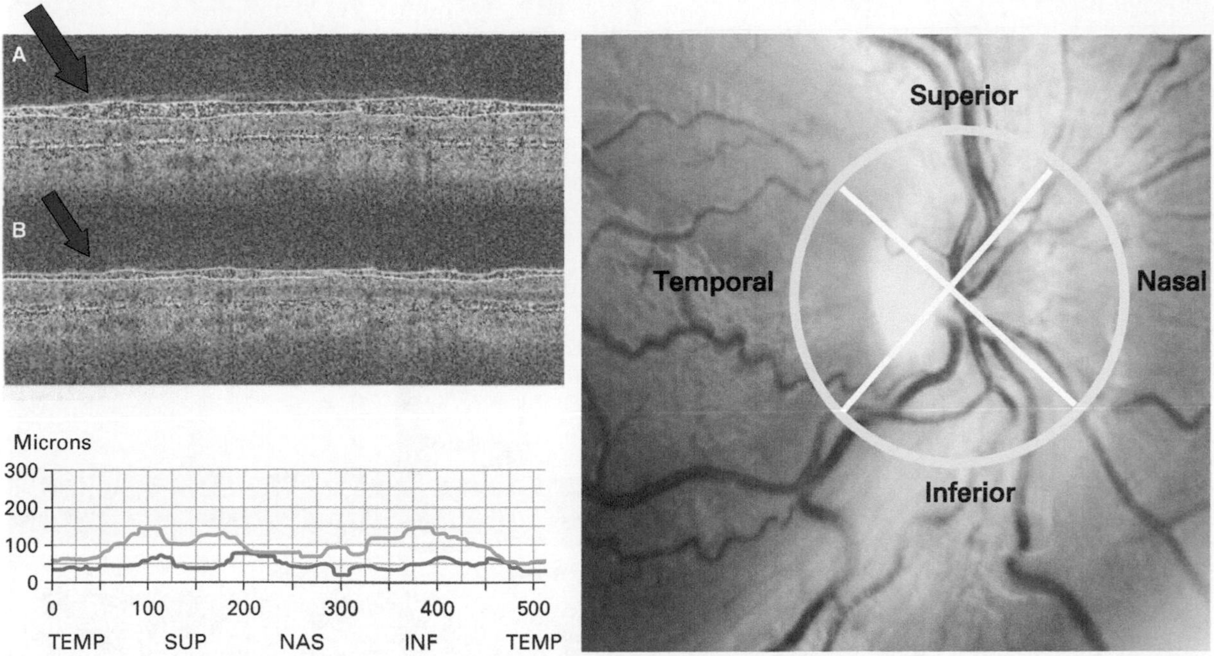

Figure 5.10 OCT RNFL analysis. The right panel shows the circular scan around the optic disc performed by OCT. In the left panel, the corresponding linear image of the retinal scan is shown with the nerve fiber layer in evidence as a more reflective layer in red (arrows). The picture on the left shows the clear difference between a thicker (**A**) and a thinner (**B**) nerve fiber layer. At the bottom of the left panel, the corresponding diagram of the two different cases is represented in the different quadrants (the green line indicates the thicker layer case and the blue line the thinner layer case)

in its adjacent highly reflective layer.[231] The threshold is individually determined for each scan as a multiple of the local maximum reflectance to correct for variations in optical alignment, drying of the corneal surface, or changes in pupil size. The NFL thickness is defined as a multiple of the number of pixels between the anterior and posterior edges of the NFL (Figure 5.10).

Two scan acquisition protocols can be used for NFL analysis: NFL thickness (3.4) and fast NFL thickness (3.4). In the first protocol, measurement is made along a circle concentric to the optic disc at a radius of 1.73 mm (the 3.4 mm diameter was found to be optimal for NFL analysis in a prototype instrument),[232] using a scanning mode that samples 512 data points (NFL Thickness 3.4 acquisition protocol). The second protocol acquires and compresses three 3.4 mm NFL thickness circle scans into one scan. Each scan consists of 256 linear A-scans. Scanning time is 1.92 seconds. The OCT software automatically calculates mean NFL thickness (360° measure), temporal quadrant thickness (316°–45° unit circle), superior quadrant thickness (46°–135°), nasal quadrant thickness (136°–225°) and inferior quadrant thickness (226°–315°) (Figure 5.10).

OCT is a reproducible tool to measure NFL thickness and is increasingly used to evaluate optic neuropathies, for example differentiating between normal and glaucomatous eyes.[233–237] We recently applied the OCT to study NFL thickness in LHON patients[238] and in unaffected carriers of LHON mtDNA mutations (Figure 5.11).[239] We characterized the NFL features during the acute

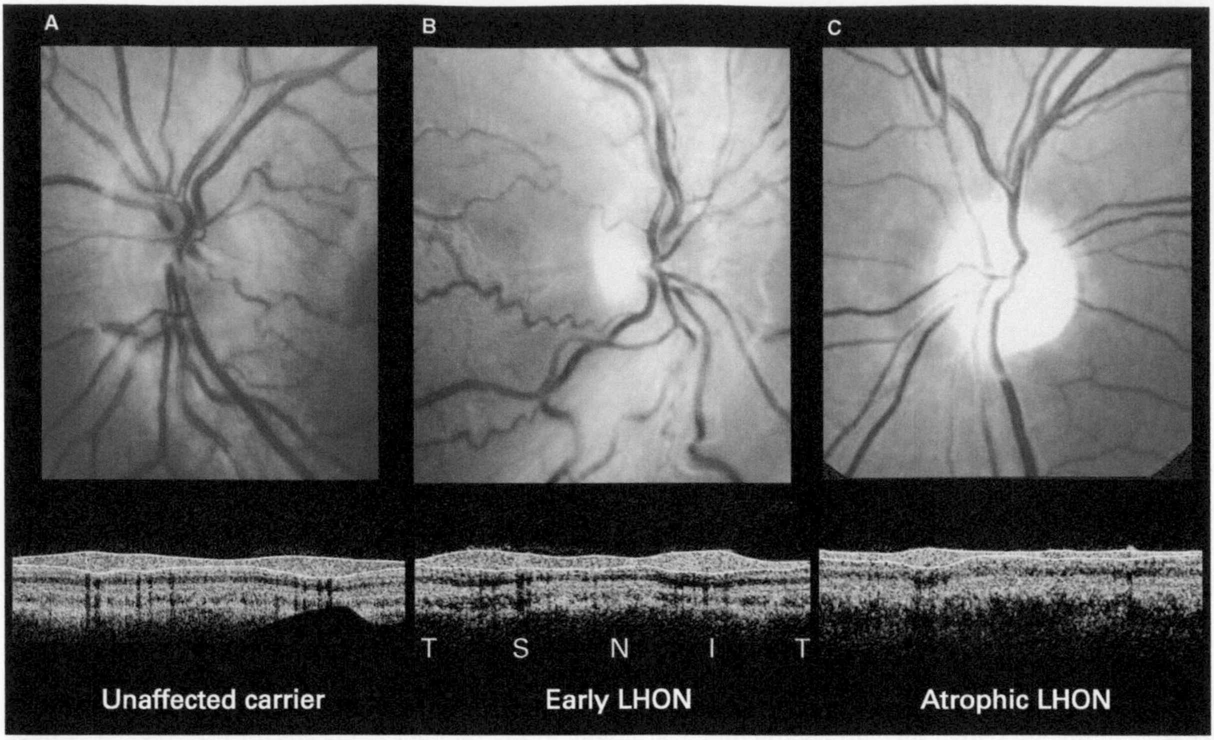

Figure 5.11 OCT in LHON. The three pictures show the fundus appearance (top) and the corresponding pattern of nerve fiber layer thickness detected by OCT (bottom; T=temporal, S=superior, N=nasal, I= inferior) in an unaffected carrier (**A**) and in patients with early (**B**) and late (**C**) stages of LHON. The OCT recognizes the thickening of the temporal quadrant in the unaffected carrier (**A**), the thinning of the temporal quadrant and the thickening of the other quadrants in the acute phase of LHON (**B**), and the diffuse thinning in the late (atrophic) stage of LHON (**C**)

phase of LHON (6 months from the disease onset) and during the chronic phase (more than 6 months from disease onset). OCT evaluation of NFL thickness also clearly distinguished patients that experienced some degrees of visual recovery from those who did not.[238] Furthermore, OCT evaluation of unaffected carriers has documented very early changes in NFL thickness,[239] raising the hope that OCT will be helpful in the longitudinal follow-up of both LHON carriers and patients as well as of some prognostic value. OCT evaluation could help us to understand which probability LHON patients have of experiencing a visual recovery and to predict the onset of the acute phase in unaffected mutation carriers. This information could then be used to establish a potential therapy in a timely manner.[240]

A rational diagnostic workup

A mitochondrial disorder is diagnosed on the basis of family history, clinical examination, and laboratory data pointing to mitochondrial dysfunction.[241,242] These tests include histology

Box 5.1 Cybrid technology

There is no known way to transfect human mitochondria with exogenous DNA in a stable and heritable manner. However, one can transfer patient mitochondria containing mutated mtDNAs from one cell to another, and then study these mutated mtDNAs in a neutral nuclear background. This is accomplished by making cytoplasmic hybrids, or 'cybrids' in which patient cells devoid of their nuclei (cytoplasts) but still containing mitochondria (cytoplasts) are fused with cells containing mitochondria that are devoid of their endogenous mtDNA (called ρ^0 cells, based on the yeast nomenclature).[1]

How are ρ^0 cells made? Typically, a transformed cell line – most commonly a human osteosarcoma line called 143B – that is deficient in thymidine kinase activity (TK^-) becomes ρ^0 following long-term exposure to ethidium bromide, an inhibitor of mtDNA replication that is preferentially taken up by mitochondria, owing to its high membrane potential (EtBr is a charged molecule). The ρ^0 line is auxotrophic for pyrimidines (such as uridine), due to the loss of a functional respiratory chain (because without a respiratory chain, the mitochondrial protein dihydroorotate dehydrogenase, a key enzyme in uridine biosynthesis, cannot function). For reasons that are less well understood, the cells are also auxotrophic for pyruvate.

This auxotrophy provides two selection schemes for the repopulation of these cells by exogenous mtDNA, based on complementation of the metabolic defects with exogenous mitochondria (and mtDNAs). The ρ^0 cells are repopulated by forming 'cytoplasmic hybrids' (cybrids) between the ρ^0 cells and cytoplasts (enucleated cells) from an mtDNA donor cell line. After cell fusion, cells are plated in medium containing bromodeoxyuridine (BrdU) and lacking either pyruvate or uridine. These selective media permit only the growth of ρ^0 cells which had fused with cytoplasts containing functional mitochondria, because the ρ^0 cells (which have defective thymidine kinase (TK) activity, another enzyme required for pyrimidine biosynthesis) are not able to grow in the absence of uridine or pyruvate, and TK^+ donor cells are not able to grow in the presence of BrdU (Figure B5.1.1).

Once the cybrids are made, they can be grown as cellular clones. Because the pool of cybrid cells reflects the distribution of heteroplasmy represented in the original population of patient cells, one can isolate cybrid clones harboring varying proportions of mutated mtDNAs, ranging from 0% mutant (100% wild-type (homoplasmic)) to 100% mutant (i.e. 0% wild-type (also homoplasmic)), plus anything in between (i.e. heteroplasmic). If one cannot find homoplasmic mutant clones, a clone with a high % heteroplasmy can be subjected to a second round of EtBr treatment, in which the mtDNA copy number is reduced from about 10 000 copies/cell to less than 50 copies/cell.[2] At that point, the EtBr is removed and the cells are allowed to repopulate their mtDNAs, resulting in a new population of cells with a skewed proportion of mtDNAs, including cells that are both homoplasmic wild-type and homoplasmic mutant (Figure B5.1.1).

Cybrid technology has been used successfully to study many pathogenic mtDNA mutations, including those causing MELAS, MERRF, NARP/MILS, and KSS.

(Continued)

Box 5.1 (Continued)

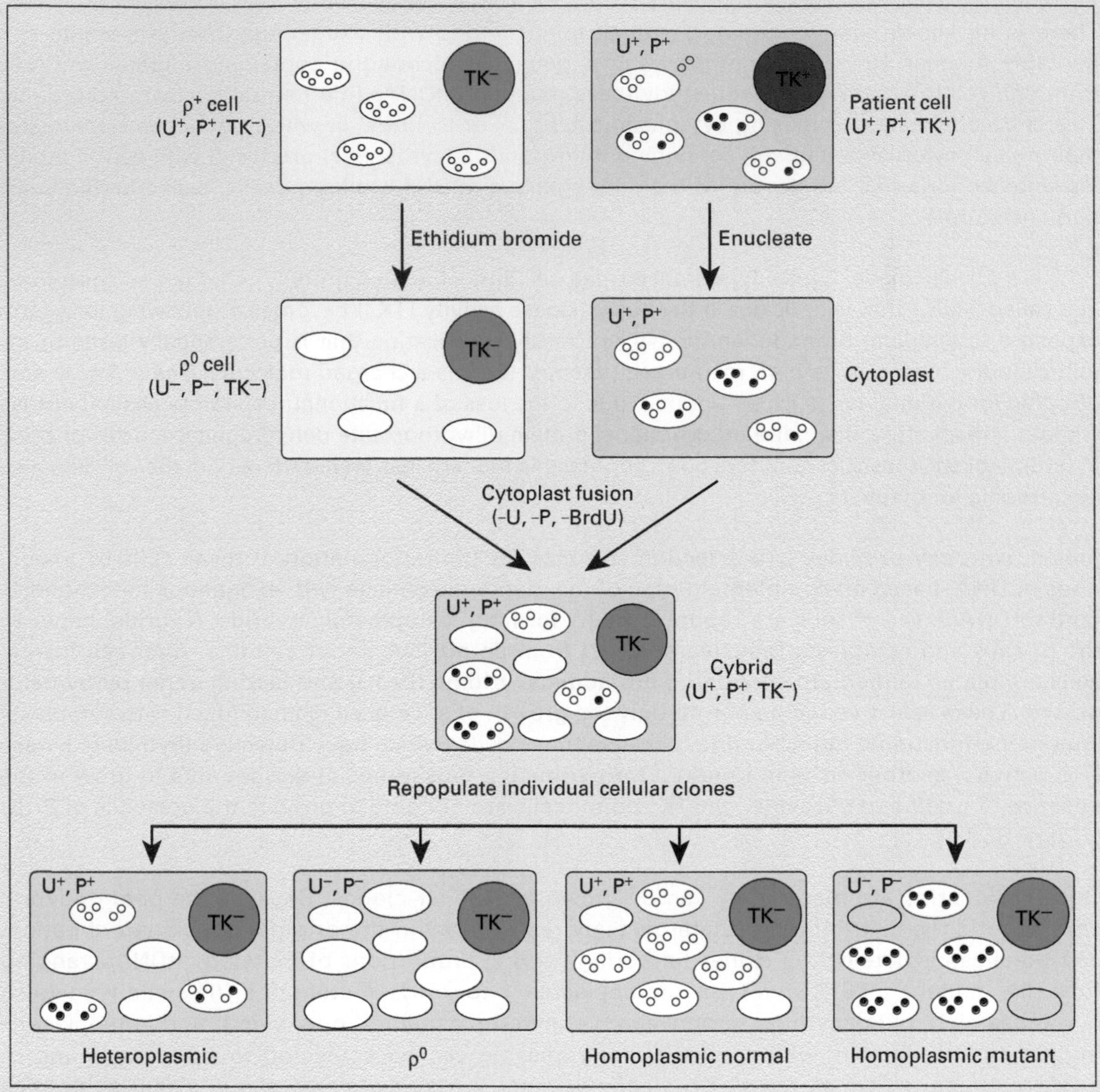

Figure B5.2.1 Making ρ^0 cells and cybrids. U, uridine; P, pyruvate; TK, thymidine kinase.

References

1. King MP, Attardi G. Human cells lacking mtDNA: repopulation with exogenous mitochondria by complementation. *Science* 1989; **246**: 500–503.
2. King MP. Use of ethidium bromide to manipulate ratio of mutated and wild-type mitochondrial DNA in cultured cells. *Methods Enzymol* 1996; **264**: 339–344.

and histoenzymology of muscle, serum lactate at rest or after standardized exercise, CSF analysis (protein and lactate), MR spectroscopy of muscle and/or brain, and biochemical evaluation of respiratory chain enzymes in tissues or cell lines. The family history can suggest maternal or Mendelian inheritance, or sporadic occurrence of the disorder.[243,244] Clinical features may suggest one of the well-defined mitochondrial encephalomyopathies (MELAS, MERRF, KSS, NARP, Leigh syndrome, etc.).[243,244] The diagnosis of neuro-ophthalmological non-syndromic disorders is based on the identification of typical mitochondrial patterns of degeneration, such as the early and prevalent involvement of the PMB in mitochondrial optic neuropathies,[31,46] or the atypical retinitis pigmentosa-like features of mitochondrial retinal dystrophies.[3,181–184]

If a molecular diagnosis is not rapidly reached, a frequent dilemma is whether to orient the molecular search towards mtDNA or towards nDNA. A helpful strategy, which is well established in many diagnostic and research centers wordwide, is the use of transmitochondrial cytoplasmic hybrid (cybrid) cell lines (Box 5.1).[245,246] Essentially, if the biochemical/metabolical phenotype is co-transferred with the mtDNA into the fusion cybrids, this is solid proof that the genetic defect is in the mitochondrial genome.[247] Conversely, given the variability of mtDNA, validation of new nucleotide change in a patient may require transfer of mutant mtDNA into the cybrid cell system to prove the pathogenicity of the mutation.[241–244]

If the biochemical/metabolical phenotype is complemented in the cybrid cell system, it is very likely that the mutation is in nDNA, and different approaches will then be needed to identify the responsible gene. These approaches include functional complementation of OXPHOS phenotypes expressed in cell culture, for example by growing the patient's defective fibroblasts in a highly selective medium, and testing the effect of human chromosome fragments after microcell-mediated transfer.[248] In the absence of carbohydrates in the culture medium, respiratory-deficient cells rapidly die unless a chromosome fragment carrying the disease gene rescues them. This is how the *SURF1* gene was implicated in a recessive form of Leigh syndrome.[249,250] Another strategy exploited the availability of whole-genome data sets of RNA and protein expression to identify culprit genes in two recessive mitochondrial disorders, the *LRPPRC* gene in the French-Canadian type (LSFC) variant of Leigh syndrome, and the *ETHE1* gene in ethylmalonic encephalopathy.[251,252] Detailed description of these techniques, which require collaboration with highly specialized research laboratories, is beyond the scope of this chapter.

Therapy and experimental treatments

Despite the rapid progress in our understanding of the genetic and biochemical basis of mitochondrial disorders, there are no effective therapeutic options for patients with mitochondrial diseases.[253] The only exceptions seem to be some Coenzyme Q (CoQ)-deficient syndromes, where CoQ administration may dramatically improve the clinical conditions of the patients.[254]

Therapeutic approaches to mitochondrial diseases are discussed in Chapter 14; here, we will limit our considerations to neuro-ophthalmological conditions. LHON is the most common disease due to an mtDNA defect, and DOA is considered the most common inherited optic neuropathy. Recurrence risks have been calculated for both the 11778/ND4 and the 14484/ND6 LHON pathogenic mutations, making it possible to provide some genetic counseling to patients and to unaffected relatives at risk.[255,256] In heteroplasmic cases, mtDNA analysis of peripheral tissues cannot be used to predict the mutation load in the optic nerve because skewed segregation may occur in different tissues.[257] Hence, no risk evaluation can be performed on this basis. None of the treatments used so far, including vitamins, co-factors, steroids, and surgery have proved effective.[31,46] Partial improvement of visual and neurological symptoms has been reported in a few patients treated with the quinone analog idebenone,[258–261] but more extensive experience is needed.[262] The results of a recent US trial with the putative neuroprotective agent brimonidine[263] were also disappointing.[264] Included in this trial were LHON patients in the acute phase, who had lost central vision in one eye, while the other eye was still unaffected. The unaffected eye was then chosen for brimonidine administration in the hope of rescuing or delaying the onset of visual loss, which, based on the natural history of LHON, is usually unavoidable days, weeks, or months after onset of the disease in the first eye. None of the patients enrolled in the study were protected from visual loss in the treated eye, although preliminary data from follow-up suggest a better preservation of the peripheral visual field. This trial with brimonidine raises concern about a realistic 'window of opportunity' for treating LHON. As suggested in the previous section, OCT could predict the onset of the acute phase in unaffected mutation carriers, thus widening this 'window of opportunity'. At present, avoidance of identified risk factors is the only consensus recommendation for LHON patients.

One experimental strategy proposed recently is allotopic expression, based on the expression of re-coded mtDNA genes as nuclear genes, whose wild-type protein products are targeted to defective mitochondria, where they rescue a specific mtDNA defect. The feasibility of this approach has been demonstrated in cell culture for the 8993T→G NARP/MILS mutation in the ATPase 6 gene[265] and for the 11778/ND4 mutation associated with LHON.[266] However, doubts have been raised about the efficiency and general applicability of this technique.[267]

Another novel strategy is aimed at reducing or eliminating heteroplasmic mutations by delivery of restriction enzymes into mitochondria. This approach, whose feasibility was first demonstrated in mouse cells, was applied later to human cybrid cell lines carrying the 8993T→G NARP/MILS mutation. This mutation creates a new, unique SmaI restriction site (GGGCCC). After adding a 5′ extension encoding a mitochondrial leader peptide to a recombinant SmaI cDNA, this was inserted into a mammalian expression vector. Expression of this recombinant SmaI endonuclease in 8993T→G heteroplasmic cybrids led to specific elimination of the mutant mtDNA, followed by repopulation of the cells with wild-type mtDNA.[268,269]

Conclusions and future directions

We have witnessed, since 1988, a very rapid development of mitochondrial medicine, which now integrates 'easier' investigations of mtDNA with the 'slower and harder' identification of the nuclear genetic counterpart needed to make the oxidative phosphorylation functioning.[6–9] For some mitochondrial disorders such as LHON, we now begin to explore the possibility of 'digenic' determination, that is an mtDNA pathogenic mutation acting in conjunction with nuclear-modifying genes.[72] However, the mitochondrial proteome has proven to be larger than initially thought and very complex.[270] Thus, besides the protein components of the respiratory chain, a complex array of genes and proteins is emerging as crucial determinants of mitochondrial function and pathology. Reactive oxygen species, their signaling roles and their control systems are major players in mitochondrial medicine and ophthalmology. Proteins involved in signaling and regulating the apoptotic process have the mitochondria as central players in the life and death of cells.[271] A number of these proteins show a Dr Jeckyll and Mr Hyde character, including cytochrome *c*, endonuclease G, apoptosis induction factor, just to mention a few, suggesting that these proteins may have multiple and sometimes opposite functional roles in different scenarios of cell life.[271] New categories of proteins are emerging, such as those involved in fission/fusion of mitochondria, the morphology of the cristae, the control of mtDNA copy number, as well as its replication and transcription. Since its beginning, in 1988, mitochondrial medicine has involved ophthalmology and has contributed to our understanding of the pathophysiology of optic nerve degeneration, retinal dystrophy, and EOM myopathy, just to mention the main topics of mitochondrial ophthalmology. Mitochondrial ophthalmology now needs good animal models that can help to understand pathogenic mechanisms and to experiment with therapeutic strategies.

There have been some attempts to develop 'mitomice', but this is still a formidable challenge, particularly when the purpose is to generate true models of human mtDNA diseases in mice.[272] It is much easier to knock out nuclear genes encoding mitochondrial proteins, and a few such mice models have been generated (Box 14.1).[273]

The ophthalmologic features in some of these nDNA and mtDNA mitomice are being reported.[274–276] Other animal models were created with the specific purpose of reproducing a mitochondrial optic neuropathy by biochemical manipulations,[277,278] or by ingenious engineering of gene expression.[279,280] The first attempts to prevent in vivo the development of optic neuropathy[281] and to foster regeneration of the optic nerve[282] are being reported in mouse models, and these findings bode well for the future.

References

1. Holt IJ, Harding AE, Morgan-Hughes JA. Deletions of muscle mitochondrial DNA in patients with mitochondrial myopathies. *Nature* 1988; **331**: 717–719.
2. Zeviani M, Moraes CT, DiMauro S et al. Deletions of mitochondrial DNA in Kearns-Sayre syndrome. *Neurology* 1988; **38**: 1339–1346.
3. Kearns TP, Sayre GP. Retinitis pigmentosa, external ophthalmoplegia and complete heart block. Unusual syndrome with histologic study in one of two cases. *Arch Ophthalmol* 1958; **60**: 280–289.
4. Wallace DC, Singh G, Lott MT et al. Mitochondrial DNA mutation associated with Leber's hereditary optic neuropathy. *Science* 1988; **242**: 1427–1430.
5. Leber T. Uber hereditare und congenital-angelegte Sehnervenleiden. *Archiv Ophthalmol* 1871; **17**: 249–291.
6. DiMauro S. Mitochondrial medicine. *Biochim Biophys Acta* 2004; **1659**: 107–114.
7. DiMauro S, Andreu AL. Mutations in mtDNA: are we scraping the bottom of the barrel? *Brain Pathol* 2000; **10**: 431–441.
8. DiMauro S, Schon EA. Nuclear power and mitochondrial disease. *Nat Genet* 1998; **19**: 214–215.
9. Zeviani M, Spinazzola A, Carelli V. Nuclear genes in mitochondrial disorders. *Curr Opin Genet Dev* 2003; **13**: 262–270.
10. Koutnikova H, Campuzano V, Foury F et al. Studies of human, mouse and yeast homologues indicate a mitochondrial function for frataxin. *Nat Genet* 1997; **16**: 345–351.
11. Casari G, De Fusco M, Ciarmatori S et al. Spastic paraplegia and OXPHOS impairment caused by mutations in paraplegin, a nuclear-encoded mitochondrial metalloprotease. *Cell* 1998; **93**: 973–983.
12. Dowling J. *The Retina: An Approachable Part of the Brain*. Cambridge, MA, The Belknap Press of Harvard University Press: 1987.
13. Rodieck RW. *The Vertebrate Retina: Principles of Structure and Function*. San Francisco, Freeman WH: 1973.
14. Rodieck RW. The primate retina. In: Steklis HD and Erwin J (eds.). *From Pigments to Perception: Advances in Understanding Visual Processes*. New York, Plenum Press. 1988; 83–89.
15. Duke-Elder S. *System of Ophthalmology: The Anatomy of the Visual System*. London, Kimpton: 1961.
16. Ramón y Cajal S. La rétine des vertébrés. *La Cellule* 1893; **9**: 17–257.
17. Cohen AI. The Retina. In: Hart WM eds. *Adler's Physiology of the Eye*. Mosby-Year Book. St. Louis. 9th Ed. 1992; **19**: 579–615.
18. Hogan MJ, Alvarado JA, Weddell JE. *Histology of the Human Eye: An Atlas and Textbook*. Philadelphia, Saunders WB: 1971.

19. Sterling P. Retina. In: Shepard GM (ed.), *The Synaptic Organization of the Brain*. New York, Oxford University Press. 1990; 170–213.
20. Hoang QV, Linsenmeier RA, Chung CK, Curcio CA. Photoreceptor inner segments in monkey and human retina: mitochondrial density, optics, and regional variation. *Vis Neurosci* 2002; **19**: 395–407.
21. Yu DY, Cringle SJ. Outer retinal anoxia during dark adaptation is not a general property of mammalian retinas. *Comp Biochem Physiol A Mol Integr Physiol* 2002; (**1**): 47–52.
22. Polyak S. *The Retina*. Chicago, University of Chicago Press: 1941.
23. Steuer H, Jaworski A, Elger B et al. Functional characterization and comparison of the outer blood–retina barrier and the blood–brain barrier. *Invest Ophthalmol Vis Sci* 2005; **46**: 1047–1053.
24. Minckler DS. Correlations between anatomic features and axonal transport in primate optic nerve head. *Trans Am Ophthalmol Soc* 1986; **84**: 429–452.
25. Seme MT, Summerfelt P, Henry MM et al. Formate-induced inhibition of photoreceptor function in methanol intoxication. *J Pharmacol Exp Ther* 1999; **289**: 361–370.
26. Onda E, Cioffi GA, Bacon DR, van Buskirk EM. Microvasculature of the human optic nerve. *Am J Ophthalmol* 1995; **120**: 92–101.
27. Ogden TE. Nerve fiber layer of the owl monkey retina: retinotopic organization. *Invest Ophthalmol Vis Sci* 1983; **24**: 265–269.
28. Wang L, Dong J, Cull G et al. Varicosities of intraretinal ganglion cell axons in human and non-human primates. *Invest Ophthalmol Vis Sci* 2003; **44**: 2–9.
29. Glaser J, Sadun AA. *Anatomy of the Visual Sensory System in Neuro-Ophthalmology*. Philadelphia, JB Lippincott Co: 1999; **3**: 75–94.
30. Sadun AA. *Anatomy of the Optic Nerve in Walsh and Hoyt's Clinical Neuro-ophthalmology*. Baltimore, Williams & Wilkins: 1997: 57–83.
31. Carelli V, Ross-Cisneros F, Sadun A. Mitochondrial dysfunction as a cause of optic neuropathies. *Prog Retinal Eye Res* 2004; **23**: 53–89.
32. Leigh RJ, Zee DS. Diagnosis of diplopia and strabismus. Chapter 9 in *The Neurology of Eye Movements*, 3rd Ed. Oxford, Oxford University Press: 1999; 321–404.
33. Porter JD, Baker RS. Muscles of a different 'color': the unusual properties of the extraocular muscles may predispose or protect them in neurogenic and myogenic disease. *Neurology* 1996; **46**: 30–37.
34. Fuchs AF, Binder MD. Fatigue resistance of human extraocular muscles. *J Neurophysiol* 1983; **49**: 28–34.
35. Porter JD, Baker RS, Ragusa RJ et al. Extraocular muscles: basic and clinical aspects of structure and function. *Surv Ophthalmol* 1995; **39**: 451–484.
36. Yu Wai Man CY, Chinnery PF, Griffiths PG. Extraocular muscles have fundamentally distinct properties that make them selectively vulnerable to certain disorders. *Neuromusc Disord* 2005; **15**: 17–23.
37. Khanna S, Richmonds CR, Kaminski HJ, Porter JD. Molecular organization of the extraocular muscle neuromuscular junction: partial conservation of and divergence from the skeletal muscle prototype. *Invest Ophthalmol Vis Sci* 2003; **44**: 1918–1926.
38. McLoon LK, Rios L, Wirtschafter JD. Complex three-dimensional patterns of myosin isoform expression: differences between and within specific extraocular muscles. *J Muscle Res Cell Motil* 1999; **20**: 771–783.
39. Yee RD. Nystagmus and saccadic intrusions and oscillations. Chapter 202 in Neuro-Ophthalmology (Sadun, Ed.) of *Yanoff and Dukar Ophthalmology*, 2nd Ed. St. Louis, Mosby: 2004: 1350–1359.
40. Carry MR, Ringel SP, Starcevich JM. Mitochondrial morphometrics of histochemically identified human extraocular muscle fibers. *Anat Rec* 1986; **214**: 8–16.
41. Chang TS, Johns DR, Walker D et al. Ocular clinicopathologic study of the mitochondrial encephalomyopathy overlap syndromes. *Arch Ophthalmol* 1993; **111**: 1254–1262.
42. Spencer RF, Porter JD. Structural organization of the extraocular muscles. In: Buttner-Enever JA, (ed.) *Reviews in Oculomotor Research*. New York; Elsevier: 1988.
43. Sadun AA, Kashima Y, Wurdeman AE et al. Morphological findings in the visual system in a case of Leber's hereditary optic neuropathy. *Clin Neurosci* 1994; 2: 165–172.
44. Carta A, Carelli V, D'Adda T et al. Human extraocular muscles in mitochondrial disease: comparing chronic progressive external ophthalmoplegia with Leber's hereditary optic neuropathy. *Br J Ophthalmol* 2005; **89**: 825–827.
45. Muller-Hocker J, Schneiderbanger K, Stefani FH, Kadenbach B. Progressive loss of cytochrome c oxi-

dase in the human extraocular muscles in ageing – a cytochemical-immunohistochemical study. *Mutat Res* 1992; **275**: 115–124.
46. Carelli V, Ross-Cisneros FN, Sadun AA. Optic nerve degeneration and mitochondrial dysfunction: genetic and acquired optic neuropathies. *Neurochem Int* 2002; **40**: 573–584.
47. Von Graefe A. Ein ungewohnlicher Fall von hereditarer Amaurose. *Archiv Ophthalmol* 1858; **4**: 266–268.
48. Chinnery PF, Johnson MA, Wardell TM et al. The epidemiology of pathogenic mitochondrial DNA mutations. *Ann Neurol* 2000; **48**: 188–193.
49. Man PY, Griffiths PG, Brown DT et al. The epidemiology of Leber hereditary optic neuropathy in the North East of England. *Am J Hum Genet* 2003; **72**: 333–339.
50. Newman NJ. Leber's optic neuropathy. In: Miller NR, Newman NJ eds. *Walsh and Hoyt's Clinical Neuro-Ophthalmology*. Baltimore: Williams & Wilkins, 1998; 742–753.
51. Carelli V. Leber's hereditary optic neuropathy. In: Schapira AHV, DiMauro S, ed. *Mitochondrial Disorders in Neurology*, 2nd Ed. Boston: Butterworth-Heinemann, 2002; 115–142.
52. Smith JL, Hoyt WF, Susac JO. Ocular fundus in acute Leber optic neuropathy. *Arch Ophthalmol* 1973; **90**: 349–354.
53. Nikoskelainen E, Hoyt WF, Nummelin K. Ophthalmoscopic findings in Leber's hereditary optic neuropathy. II. The fundus findings in affected family members. *Arch Ophthalmol* 1983; **101**: 1059–1068.
54. Nikoskelainen E, Hoyt WF, Nummelin K, Schatz H. Fundus findings in Leber's hereditary optic neuropathy. III. Fluorescein angiographic studies. *Arch Ophthalmol* 1984; **102**: 981–989.
55. Nikoskelainen E, Hoyt WF, Nummelin K. Ophthalmoscopic findings in Leber's hereditary optic neuropathy. I. Fundus findings in asymptomatic family members. *Arch Ophthalmol* 1982; **100**: 1597–1602.
56. Bose S, Bose S, Dhillon N et al. Relative sparing of afferent pupil fibers in a patient with 3460 Leber's hereditary optic neuropathy study using Di-I. *Graefes Arch Clin Exp Ophthalmol* 2005; **243**: 1175–1179.
57. Stone EM, Newman NJ, Miller NR et al. Visual recovery in patients with Leber's hereditary optic neuropathy and the 11778 mutation. *J Clin Neuro-ophthalmol* 1992; **12**: 10–14.
58. Mackey D, Howell N. A variant of Leber hereditary optic neuropathy characterized by recovery of vision and by an unusual mitochondrial genetic etiology. *Am J Hum Genet* 1992; **51**: 1218–1228.
59. Pezzi PP, De Negri AM, Sadun F et al. Childhood Leber's hereditary optic neuropathy (ND1/3460) with visual recovery. *Pediatr Neurol* 1998; **19**: 308–312.
60. Oostra RJ, Bolhuis PA, Wijburg FA et al. Leber's hereditary optic neuropathy: correlations between mitochondrial genotype and visual outcome. *J Med Genet* 1994; **31**: 280–286.
61. Riordan-Eva P, Sanders MD, Govan GG et al. The clinical features of Leber's hereditary optic neuropathy defined by the presence of a pathogenic mitochondrial DNA mutation. *Brain* 1995; **118**: 319–337.
62. Mashima Y, Kimura I, Yamamoto Y et al. Optic disc excavation in the atrophic stage of Leber's hereditary optic neuropathy: comparison with normal tension glaucoma. *Graefe's Arch Clin Exp Ophthalmol* 2003; **241**: 75–80.
63. Sadun AA, Win PH, Ross-Cisneros FN et al. Leber's hereditary optic neuropathy differentially affects smaller axons in the optic nerve. *Trans Am Ophthalmol Soc* 2000; **98**: 223–232.
64. Sadun AA, Carelli V, Bose S et al. First application of extremely high-resolution magnetic resonance imaging to study microscopic features of normal and LHON human optic nerve. *Ophthalmology* 2002; **109**: 1085–1091.
65. Erickson RP. Leber's optic atrophy, a possible example of mitochondrial inheritance. *Am J Hum Genet* 1972; **24**: 348–349.
66. Chinnery PF, Brown DT, Andrews RM et al. The mitochondrial ND6 gene is a hot spot for mutations that cause Leber's hereditary optic neuropathy. *Brain* 2001; **124**: 209–218.
67. Valentino ML, Barboni P, Ghelli A et al. The ND1 gene of complex I is a mutational hot spot for Leber's hereditary optic neuropathy. *Ann Neurol* 2004; **56**: 631–641.
68. Torroni A, Petrozzi M, D'Urbano L et al. Haplotype and phylogenetic analyses suggest that one European-specific mtDNA background plays a role in the expression of Leber hereditary optic neuropathy by increasing the penetrance of the primary mutations 11778 and 14484. *Am J Hum*

Genet 1997; **60**: 1107–1121.

69. Carelli V, Vergani L, Bernazzi B et al. Respiratory function in cybrid cell lines carrying European mtDNA haplogroups: implications for Leber's hereditary optic neuropathy. *Biochim Biophys Acta* 2002; **1588**: 7–14.
70. Man PY, Howell N, Mackey DA et al. Mitochondrial DNA haplogroup distribution within Leber hereditary optic neuropathy pedigrees. *J Med Genet* 2004; 41: e41.
71. Bu XD, Rotter JI. X chromosome-linked and mitochondrial gene control of Leber hereditary optic neuropathy: evidence from segregation analysis for dependence on X chromosome inactivation. *Proc Natl Acad Sci USA* 1991; **88**: 8198–8202.
72. Carelli V, Giordano C, d'Amati G. Pathogenic expression of homoplasmic mtDNA mutations needs a complex nuclear-mitochondrial interaction. *Trends Genet* 2003; **19**: 257–262.
73. Bu X, Rotter JI. Leber hereditary optic neuropathy: estimation of number of embryonic precursor cells and disease threshold in heterozygous affected females at the X-linked locus. *Clin Genet* 1992; **42**: 143–148.
74. Carelli V, Wang K, Valentino ML et al. Segregation analysis of a large LHON pedigree is consistent with the existence of a nuclear modifying gene. *Invest Ophthalmol Vis Sci* 2003; ARVO Abstract #937.
75. Chen JD, Cox I, Denton MJ. Preliminary exclusion of an X-linked gene in Leber optic atrophy by linkage analysis. *Hum Genet* 1989; **82**: 203–207.
76. Carvalho MRS, Muller B, Rotzer E et al. Leber's hereditary optic neuroretinopathy and the X-chromosomal susceptibility factor: no linkage to DXS7. *Hum Hered* 1992; **42**: 316–320.
77. Chalmers RM, Davis MB, Sweeney MG et al. Evidence against an X-linked visual loss susceptibility locus in Leber hereditary optic neuropathy. *Am J Hum Genet* 1996; **59**: 103–108.
78. Pegoraro E, Carelli V, Zeviani M et al. X-inactivation pattern in female LHON (Leber's hereditary optic neuropathy) patients do not support a strong X-linked determinant. *Am J Med Genet* 1996; **61**: 356–362.
79. Oostra RJ, Kemp S, Bolhuis PA, Bleeker-Wagemakers EM. No evidence for 'skewed' inactivation of the X chromosome as cause of Leber's hereditary optic neuropathy in female carriers. *Hum Genet* 1996; **97**: 500–505.
80. Pegoraro E, Vettori A, Valentino ML et al. X-inactivation pattern in multiple tissues from two Leber's hereditary optic neuropathy (LHON) patients. *Am J Med Genet* 2003; **119**: 37–40.
81. Man PY, Brown DT, Wehnert MS et al. NDUFA-1 is not a nuclear modifier gene in Leber hereditary optic neuropathy. *Neurology* 2002; **58**: 1861–1862.
82. Borras C, Sastre J, Garcia-Sala D et al. Mitochondria from females exhibit higher antioxidant gene expression and lower oxidative damage than males. *Free Radic Biol Med* 2003; **34**: 546–552.
83. Sadun AA, Carelli V, Salomao SR et al. Extensive investigation of a large Brazilian pedigree of 11778/haplogroup J Leber hereditary optic neuropathy. *Am J Ophthalmol* 2003; **136**: 231–238.
84. Riordan-Eva P, Sanders MD, Govan GG et al. The clinical features of Leber's hereditary optic neuropathy defined by the presence of a pathogenic mitochondrial DNA mutation. *Brain* 1995; **118**: 319–337.
85. Redmill B, Mutamba A, Tandon M. Leber's hereditary optic neuropathy following trauma. *Eye* 2001; **15**: 544–547.
86. DuBois LG, Feldon SE. Evidence for metabolic trigger for Leber's hereditary optic neuropathy. A case report. *J Clin Neuroophthalmol* 1992; **12**: 15–16.
87. Dotti MT, Plewnia K, Cardaioli E et al. A case of ethambutol-induced optic neuropathy harbouring the primary mitochondrial LHON mutation at nt 11778. *J Neurol* 1998; **245**: 302–303.
88. De Marinis M. Optic neuropathy after treatment with anti-tuberculous drugs in a subject with Leber's hereditary optic neuropathy mutation. *J Neurol* 2001; **248**: 818–819.
89. Warner JE, Ries KM. Optic neuropathy in a patient with AIDS. *J Neuroophthalmol* 2001; **21**: 92–94.
90. Mackey DA, Fingert JH, Luzhansky JZ et al. Leber's hereditary optic neuropathy triggered by antiretroviral therapy for human immunodeficiency virus. *Eye* 2003; **17**: 312–317.
91. Tsao K, Aitken PA, Johns DR. Smoking as an aetiological factor in a pedigree with Leber's hereditary optic neuropathy. *Br J Ophthalmol* 1999; **83**: 577–581.
92. Brown MD. The enigmatic relationship between mitochondrial dysfunction and Leber's hereditary

optic neuropathy. *J Neurol Sci* 1999; **165**: 1–5.

93. Smith KJ, Kapoor R, Felts PA. Demyelination: the role of reactive oxygen and nitrogen species. *Brain Pathol* 1999; **9**: 69–92.
94. Larsson N-G, Andersen O, Holme E et al. Leber's hereditary optic neuropathy and complex I deficiency in muscle. *Ann Neurol* 1991; **30**: 701–708.
95. Ross-Cisneros FN, Win PH, Carelli V, Sadun AA. Vascular abnormalities in optic nerves from two cases of Leber's hereditary optic neuropathy. *Invest Ophthalmol Vis Sci* 2001; ARVO Abstract #3361.
96. Kjer P. Infantile optic atrophy with dominant mode of inheritance: a clinical and genetic study of 19 Danish families. *Acta Ophthalmol Scand* 1959; **37**: 1–146.
97. Jacobson DM, Stone EM. Difficulty differentiating Leber's from dominant optic neuropathy in a patient with remote visual loss. *J Clin Neuroophthalmol* 1991; **11**: 152–157.
98. Votruba M, Thiselton D, Bhattacharya SS. Optic disc morphology of patients with OPA1 autosomal dominant optic atrophy. *Br J Ophthalmol* 2003; **87**: 48–53.
99. Johnston PB, Gaster RN, Smith VC, Tripathi RC. A clinicopathologic study of autosomal dominant optic atrophy. *Am J Ophthalmol* 1979; **88**: 868–875.
100. Kjer P, Jensen OA, Klinken L. Histopathology of eye, optic nerve and brain in a case of dominant optic atrophy. *Acta Ophthalmol* (Copenh) 1983; **61**: 300–312.
101. Eiberg H, Kjer B, Kjer P, Rosenberg T. Dominant optic atrophy (OPA1) mapped to chromosome 3q region. I. Linkage analysis. *Hum Mol Genet* 1994; **3**: 977–980.
102. Kerrison JB, Arnould VJ, Ferraz Sallum JM et al. Genetic heterogeneity of dominant optic atrophy, Kjer type: Identification of a second locus on chromosome 18q12.2–12.3. *Arch Ophthalmol* 1999; **117**: 805–810.
103. Barbet F, Hakiki S, Orssaud C. A third locus for dominant optic atrophy on chromosome 22q. *J Med Genet* 2005; 42: e1.
104. Ozden S, Duzcan F, Wollnik B. Progressive autosomal dominant optic atrophy and sensorineural hearing loss in a Turkish family. *Ophthalmic Genet* 2002; **23**: 9–36.
105. Alexander C, Votruba M, Pesch UEA. *OPA1*, encoding a dynamin-related GTPase, is mutated in autosomal dominant optic atrophy linked to choromosome 3q28. *Nat Genet* 2000; **26**: 211–215.
106. Delettre C, Lenaers G, Griffoin J-M et al. Nuclear gene *OPA1*, encoding a mitochondrial dynamin-related protein, is mutated in dominant optic atrophy. *Nat Genet* 2000; **26**: 207–210.
107. Pesch UEA, Leo-Kottler B, Mayer S et al. *OPA1* mutations in patients with autosomal dominant optic atrophy and evidence for semi-dominant inheritance. *Hum Mol Genet* 2001; **10**: 1359–1368.
108. Toomes C, Marchbank NJ, Mackey DA et al. Spectrum, frequency and penetrance of *OPA1* mutations in dominant optic atrophy. *Hum Mol Genet* 2001; **10**: 1369–1378.
109. Delettre C, Griffoin J-M, Kaplan J et al. Mutation spectrum and splicing variants in the *OPA1* gene. *Hum Genet* 2001; **109**: 584–591.
110. Thiselton DL, Alexander C, Taanman J-W et al. A comprehensive survey of mutations in the *OPA1* gene in patients with autosomal dominant optic atrophy. *Invest Ophthalmol Vis Sci* 2002; **43**: 1715–1724.
111. Delettre C, Lenaers G, Pelloquin L et al. *OPA1* (Kjer type) dominant optic atrophy: a novel mitochondrial disease. *Mol Genet Metab* 2002; **5**: 97–107.
112. Amati-Bonneau P, Odent S, Derrien C et al. The association of autosomal dominant optic atrophy and moderate deafness may be due to the R445H mutation in the *OPA1* gene. *Am J Ophthalmol* 2003; **136**: 1170–1171.
113. Payne M, Yang Z, Katz BJ et al. Dominant optic atrophy, sensorineural hearing loss, ptosis, and ophthalmoplegia: a syndrome caused by a missense mutation in *OPA1*. *Am J Ophthalmol* 2004; **138**: 749–755.
114. Olichon A, Emorine LJ, Descoins E et al. The human dynamin-related protein *OPA1* is anchored to the mitochondrial inner membrane facing the inner-membrane space. *FEBS Lett* 2002; **523**: 171–176.
115. Olichon A, Baricault L, Gas N et al. Loss of *OPA1* perturbates the mitochondrial inner membrane structure and integrity, leading to cytochrome c release and apoptosis. *J Biol Chem* 2003; **278**: 7743–7746.
116. Chinnery PF, Howell N, Lightowlers RN, Turnbull DM. Molecular pathology of MELAS and MERRF. The relationship between mutation load and clinical phenotypes. *Brain* 1997; **120**:

1713–1721.
117. Rummelt V, Folberg R, Ionasescu V et al. Ocular pathology of MELAS syndrome with mitochondrial DNA nucleotide 3243 point mutation. *Ophthalmology* 1993; **100**: 1757–1766.
118. Chang TS, Johns DR, Walker D et al. Ocular clinicopathologic study of the mitochondrial encephalomyopathy overlap syndromes. *Arch Ophthalmol* 1993; **111**: 1254–1262.
119. Hwang JM, Park HW, Kim SJ. Optic neuropathy associated with mitochondrial $tRNA^{[Leu(UUR)]\ A3243G}$ mutation. *Ophthalmic Genet* 1997; **18**: 101–105.
120. Cavanagh JB, Harding BN. Pathogenic factors underlying the lesions in Leigh's disease. Tissue responses to cellular energy deprivation and their clinico-pathological consequences. *Brain* 1994; **117**: 1357–1376.
121. Hayashi N, Geraghty MT, Green WR. Ocular histopathologic study of a patient with the T 8993-G point mutation in Leigh's syndrome. *Ophthalmology* 2000; **107**: 1397–1402.
122. Carroll WM, Kriss A, Baraitser M et al. The incidence and nature of visual pathway involvement in Friedreich's ataxia. *Brain* 1980; **103**: 413–434.
123. Anikster Y, Kleta R, Shaag A et al. Type III 3-methylglutaconic aciduria (optic atrophy plus syndrome, or Costeff optic atrophy syndrome): identification of the *OPA3* gene and its founder mutation in Iraqi Jews. *Am J Hum Genet* 2001; **69**: 1218–1224.
124. Jin H, May M, Tranebjaerg L et al. A novel X-linked gene, *DDP*, shows mutations in families with deafness (DFN-1), dystonia, mental deficiency and blindness. *Nat Genet* 1996; **14**: 177–180.
125. Taylor RW, Birch-Machin MA, Schaefer J et al. Deficiency of complex II of the mitochondrial respiratory chain in late-onset optic atrophy and ataxia. *Ann Neurol* 1996; **39**: 224–232.
126. Birch-Machin MA, Taylor RW, Cochran B et al. Late-onset optic atrophy, ataxia, and myopathy associated with a mutation of a complex II gene. *Ann Neurol* 2000; **48**: 330–335.
127. Rigoli L, Salpietro DC, Caruso RA et al. Mitochondrial DNA mutation at np 3243 in a family with maternally inherited diabetes mellitus. *Acta Diabetol* 1999; **36**: 163–167.
128. Pulkes T, Eunson L, Patterson V et al. The mitochondrial DNA G13513A transition in ND5 is associated with a LHON/MELAS overlap syndrome and may be a frequent cause of MELAS. *Ann Neurol* 1999; **46**: 916–919.
129. Corona P, Antozzi C, Carrara F et al. A novel mtDNA mutation in the ND5 subunit of complex I in two MELAS patients. *Ann Neurol* 2001; **49**: 106–110.
130. Liolitsa D, Rahman S, Benton S et al. Is the mitochondrial complex I ND5 gene a hot-spot for MELAS causing mutations? *Ann Neurol* 2003; **53**: 128–132.
131. Chol M, Lebon S, Benit P et al. The mitochondrial DNA G13513A MELAS mutation in the NADH dehydrogenase 5 gene is a frequent cause of Leigh-like syndrome with isolated complex I deficiency. *J Med Genet* 2003; **40**: 188–191.
132. Kirby DM, Boneh A, Chow CW et al. Low mutant load of mitochondrial DNA G13513A mutation can cause Leigh's disease. *Ann Neurol* 2003; **54**: 473–478.
133. Jun AS, Brown MD, Wallace DC. A mitochondrial DNA mutation at nucleotide pair 14459 of the NADH dehydrogenase subunit 6 gene associated with maternally inherited Leber hereditary optic neuropathy and dystonia. *Proc Natl Acad Sci USA* 1994; **91**: 6206–6210.
134. Shoffner JM, Brown MD, Stugard C et al. Leber's hereditary optic neuropathy plus dystonia is caused by a mitochondrial DNA point mutation. *Ann Neurol* 1995; **38**: 163–169.
135. Kirby DM, Kahler SG, Freckmann ML et al. Leigh disease caused by the mitochondrial DNA G14459A mutation in unrelated families. *Ann Neurol* 2000; **48**: 102–104.
136. Blakely EL, de Silva R, King A et al. LHON/MELAS overlap syndrome associated with a mitochondrial *MTND1* gene mutation. *Eur J Hum Genet* 2005; **13**: 623–627.
137. Funalot B, Reynier P, Vighetto A et al. Leigh-like encephalopathy complicating Leber's hereditary optic neuropathy. *Ann Neurol* 2002; **52**: 374–377.
138. Carelli V, Sadun AA. Optic neuropathy in LHON and Leigh syndrome: a common pathogenic mechanism? *Ophthalmology* 2001; **108**: 1172–1173.
139. Hasegawa H, Matsuoka T, Goto Y, Nonaka I. Strongly succinate dehydrogenase-reactive blood vessels in muscles from patients with mitochondrial myopathy, encephalopathy, lactic acidosis, and

stroke-like episodes. *Ann Neurol* 1991; **29**: 601–605.
140. Bruno C, Martinuzzi A, Tang Y et al. A stop-codon mutation in the human mtDNA cytochrome *c* oxidase I gene disrupts the functional structure of complex IV. *Am J Hum Genet* 1999; **65**: 611–620.
141. Rotig A, Cormier V, Chatelain P et al. Deletion of mitochondrial DNA in a case of early-onset diabetes mellitus, optic atrophy, and deafness (Wolfram syndrome, MI 222300). *J Clin Invest* 1993; **91**: 1095–1098.
142. Harding AE. Classification of the hereditary ataxias and paraplegias. *Lancet* 1983; **1**: 1151–1155.
143. Campuzano V, Montermini L, Molto MD et al. Friedreich's ataxia: autosomal recessive disease caused by an intronic GAA triplet repeat expansion. *Science* 1996; **271**: 1423–1427.
144. Givre SJ, Wall M, Kardon RH. Visual loss and recovery in a patient with Friedreich ataxia. *J Neuro-Ophthalmol* 2000; **20**: 229–233.
145. Fortuna F, Barboni P, Liguori R et al. Characterization of optic neuropathy in Friedreich ataxia. *Neurology* 2005; **64**(Suppl 1): S01003.
146. Giacchetti M, Monticelli A, De Biase I et al. Mitochondrial DNA haplogroups influence the Friedreich's ataxia phenotype. *J Med Genet* 2004; **41**: 293–295.
147. Rotig A, de Lonlay P, Chretien D et al. Aconitase and mitochondrial iron-sulphur protein deficiency in Friedreich ataxia. *Nat Genet* 1997; **17**: 215–217.
148. Ouahchi K, Arita M, Kayden H et al. Ataxia with isolated vitamin E deficiency is caused by mutations in the α-tocopherol transfer protein. *Nat Genet* 1995; **9**: 141–145.
149. Lodi R, Rinaldi R, Gaddi A et al. Brain and skeletal muscle bioenergetic failure in familial hypobetalipoproteinemia. *J Neurol Neurosurg Psychiatry* 1997; **62**: 574–580.
150. Costeff H, Gadoth N, Apter N et al. A familial syndrome of infantile optic atrophy, movement disorder, and spastic paraplegia. *Neurology* 1989; **39**: 595–597.
151. Kleta R, Skovby F, Christensen E et al. 3-Methylglutaconic aciduria type III in a non-Iraqi-Jewish kindred: clinical and molecular findings. *Mol Genet Metab* 2002; **76**: 201–206.
152. Reynier P, Amati-Bonneau P, Verny C et al. OPA3 gene mutations responsible for autosomal dominant optic atrophy and cataract. *J Med Genet* 2004; **41**: e110.
153. Roesch K, Curran SP, Tranebjaerg L, Koehler CM. Human deafness dystonia syndrome is caused by a defect in assembly of the DDP1/TIMM8a-TIMM13 complex. *Hum Mol Genet* 2002; **11**: 477–486.
154. Tranebjaerg L, Hamel BC, Gabreels FJ et al. A de novo missense mutation in a critical domain of the X-linked DDP gene causes the typical deafness-dystonia-optic atrophy syndrome. *Eur J Hum Genet* 2000; **8**: 464–467.
155. Tranebjaerg L, Jensen PK, Van Ghelue M et al. Neuronal cell death in the visual cortex is a prominent feature of the X-linked recessive mitochondrial deafness-dystonia syndrome caused by mutations in the TIMM8a gene. *Ophthalmic Genet* 2001; **22**: 207–223.
156. Binder J, Hofmann S, Kreisel S et al. Clinical and molecular findings in a patient with a novel mutation in the deafness-dystonia peptide (DDP1) gene. *Brain* 2003; **126**: 1814–1820.
157. Roesch K, Hynds PJ, Varga R et al. The calcium-binding aspartate/glutamate carriers, citrin and aralar1, are new substrates for the DDP1/TIMM8a-TIMM13 complex. *Hum Mol Genet* 2004; **13**: 2101–2111.
158. Atorino L, Silvestri L, Koppen M et al. Loss of m-AAA protease in mitochondria causes complex I deficiency and increased sensitivity to oxidative stress in hereditary spastic paraplegia. *J Cell Biol* 2003; **163**: 777–787.
159. Ferreirinha F, Quattrini A, Pirozzi M et al. Axonal degeneration in paraplegin-deficient mice is associated with abnormal mitochondria and impairment of axonal transport. *J Clin Invest* 2004; **113**: 231–242.
160. Rizzo III JF, Lessell S. Tobacco amblyopia. *Am J Ophthalmol* 1993; **116**: 84–87.
161. Sadun AA, Martone JF, Reyes L et al. Epidemic of optic neuropathy in Cuba. *JAMA* 1994; **271**: 663–664.
162. Miller NR. Retrobulbar toxic and deficiency optic neuropathies. In: Miller NR, ed. *Walsh and Hoyt's Clinical Neuro-ophthalmology*. 4th ed. Vol 1. Baltimore: Williams and Wilkins, 1982; 289–307.
163. Harley RD, Huang NN, Macri CH, Green WR. Optic neuritis and optic atrophy following chloramphenicol in cystic fibrosis patients. *Trans Am Acad*

Ophthalmol and Otolaryngol 1970; **74**: 1011–1031.

164. Alvarez KL, Krop LC. Ethambutol induced ocular toxicity revisited. *Ann Pharmacother* 1993; **27**: 102–103.
165. Sobel RS, Yanuzi RA. Optic nerve toxicity: a classification in retinal and choroidal manifestations of systemic disease. In: *Retinal amd Choroidal Manifestations of Disease* Singerman LJ, Jampol LM, eds. Baltimore: Williams and Wilkins 1991; 226–250.
166. Victor M, Dreyfus PM. Tobacco-alcohol amblyopia. *Arch Ophthal* 1965; **74**: 649–657.
167. Smiddy WE, Green WR. Nutritional amblyopia. A histopathological study with retrospective clinical correlation. *Graefe's Arch Clin Exp Ophthalmol* 1987; **225**: 321–324.
168. Solberg Y, Rosner M, Belkin M. The association between cigarette smoking and ocular diseases. *Surv Ophthalmol* 1998; **42**: 535–547.
169. Pryor WA, Arbour NC, Upham B, Church DF. The inhibitory effect of extracts of cigarette tar on electron transport of mitochondria and submitochondrial particles. *Free Radic Biol Med* 1992; **12**: 365–372.
170. Ballinger SW, Bouder TG, Davis GS et al. Mitochondrial genome damage associated with cigarette smoking. *Cancer Res* 1996; **56**: 5692–5697.
171. Kennedy JR, Elliot AM. Cigarette smoke: the effect of residue on mitochondrial structure. *Science* 1970; **168**: 1097–1098.
172. Cullom ME, Heher KL, Miller NR et al. Leber's hereditary optic neuropathy masquerading as tobacco-alcohol amblyopia. *Arch Ophthalmol* 1993; **111**: 1482–1485.
173. Sadun AA, Martone JF, Muci-Mendoza R et al. Epidemic optic neuropathy in Cuba: eye findings. *Arch Ophthalmol* 1994; **112**: 691–699.
174. Plant GT, Mtanda AT, Arden GB, Johnson GJ. An epidemic of optic neuropathy in Tanzania: characterization of the visual disorder and associated peripheral neuropathy. *J Neurol Sci* 1997; **145**: 127–140.
175. Lee E, Burger S, Shah J et al. Linezolid-associated toxic optic neuropathy: a report of 2 cases. *Clin Infect Dis* 2003; **37**: 1389–1391.
176. Palenzuela L, Hahn NM, Nelson RP Jr et al. Does linezolid cause lactic acidosis by inhibiting mitochondrial protein synthesis? *Clin Infect Dis* 2005; **40**: e113–116.
177. Lin AH, Murray RW, Vidmar TJ, Marotti KR. The oxazolidinone eperezolid binds to the 50S ribosomal subunit and competes with binding of chloramphenicol and lincomycin. *Antimicrob Agents Chemother* 1997; **41**: 2127–2131.
178. Shiraki H. Neuropathy due to intoxication with anti-tuberculous drugs from neuropathological viewpoint. *Adv Neurol Sci* 1973; **17**: 120–.
179. Pavlakis SG, Phillips PC, DiMauro S. Mitochondrial myopathy, encephalopathy, lactic acidosis, and strokelike episodes: a distinctive clinical syndrome. *Ann Neurol* 1984; **16**: 481–488.
180. Holt IJ, Harding AE, Petty RK, Morgan-Hughes JA. A new mitochondrial disease associated with mitochondrial DNA heteroplasmy. *Am J Hum Genet* 1990; **46**: 428–433.
181. Kearns TP. External ophthalmoplegia, pigmentary degeneration of the retina, and cardiomyopathy: a newly recognized syndrome. *Tr Am Ophth Soc* 1965; **63**: 559–625.
182. Eagle RC Jr, Hedges TR, Yanoff M. The atypical pigmentary retinopathy of Kearns-Sayre syndrome. A light and electron microscopic study. *Ophthalmology* 1982; **89**: 1433–1440.
183. McKechnie NM, King M, Lee WR. Retinal pathology in the Kearns-Sayre syndrome. *Br J Ophthalmol* 1985; **69**: 63–75.
184. Isashiki Y, Nakagawa M, Ohba N et al. Retinal manifestations in mitochondrial diseases associated with mitochondrial DNA mutation. *Acta Ophthalmol Scand* 1998; **76**: 6–13.
185. Hirano M, Pavlakis SG. Mitochondrial myopathy, encephalopathy, lactic acidosis, and strokelike episodes (MELAS): current concepts. *J Child Neurol* 1994; **9**: 4–13.
186. Goto Y, Nonaka I, Horai S. A mutation in the $tRNA^{Leu(UUR)}$ gene associated with the MELAS subgroup of mitochondrial encephalomyopathies. *Nature* 1990; **348**: 651–653.
187. MITOMAP: A Human Mitochondrial Genome Database. http://www.mitomap.org, 2005.
188. Sue CM, Mitchell P, Crimmins DS et al. Pigmentary retinopathy associated with the mitochondrial DNA 3243 point mutation. *Neurology* 1997; **49**: 1013–1017.
189. Smith PR, Bain SC, Good PA et al. Pigmentary retinal dystrophy and the syndrome of maternally

inherited diabetes and deafness caused by the mitochondrial DNA 3243 tRNA(Leu) A to G mutation. *Ophthalmology* 1999; **106**: 1101–1108.
190. Latvala T, Mustonen E, Uusitalo R, Majamaa K. Pigmentary retinopathy in patients with the MELAS mutation 3243A→G in mitochondrial DNA. *Graefes Arch Clin Exp Ophthalmol* 2002; **240**: 795–801.
191. Uziel G, Moroni I, Lamantea E et al. Mitochondrial disease associated with the T8993G mutation of the mitochondrial ATPase 6 gene: a clinical, biochemical and molecular study in six families. *J Neurol Neurosurg Psychiatry* 1997; **63**: 16–22.
192. de Vries DD, van Engelen BG, Gabreels FJ et al. A second missense mutation in the mitochondrial ATPase 6 gene in Leigh's syndrome. *Ann Neurol* 1993; **34**: 410–412.
193. Tatuch Y, Christodoulou J, Feigenbaum A et al. Heteroplasmic mtDNA mutation (T→G) at 8993 can cause Leigh disease when the percentage of abnormal mtDNA is high. *Am J Hum Genet* 1992; **50**: 852–858.
194. Carelli V, Baracca A, Barogi S et al. Biochemical-clinical correlation in patients with different loads of the mitochondrial DNA T8993G mutation. *Arch Neurol* 2002; **59**: 264–270.
195. Ortiz RG, Newman NJ, Shoffner JM et al. Variable retinal and neurologic manifestations in patients harboring the mitochondrial DNA 8993 mutation. *Arch Ophthalmol* 1993; **111**: 1525–1530.
196. Chowers I, Lerman-Sagie T, Elpeleg ON et al. Cone and rod dysfunction in the NARP syndrome. *Br J Ophthalmol* 1999; **83**: 190–193.
197. Kerrison JB, Biousse V, Newman NJ. Retinopathy of NARP syndrome. *Arch Ophthalmol* 2000; **118**: 298–299.
198. Porto FB, Mack G, Sterboul MJ et al. Isolated late-onset cone-rod dystrophy revealing a familial neurogenic muscle weakness, ataxia, and retinitis pigmentosa syndrome with the T8993G mitochondrial mutation. *Am J Ophthalmol* 2001; **132**: 935–937.
199. Yamada T, Hayasaka S, Hongo K, Kubota H. Retinal dystrophy in a Japanese boy harboring the mitochondrial DNA T8993G mutation. *Jpn J Ophthalmol* 2002; **46**: 460–462.
200. Adachi M, Torii J, Volk BW et al. Electron microscopic and enzyme histochemical studies of cerebellum, ocular and skeletal muscles in chronic progressive ophthalmoplegia with cerebellar ataxia. *Acta Neuropathol* (Berl) 1973; **23**: 300–312.
201. Ringel SP, Wilson WB, Barden MT. Extraocular muscle biopsy in chronic progressive external ophthalmoplegia. *Ann Neurol* 1979; **6**: 326–339.
202. Matsuoka T, Goto Y, Nonaka I. 'All-or-none' cytochrome c oxidase positivity in mitochondria in chronic progressive external ophthalmoplegia: an ultrastructural-cytochemical study. *Muscle Nerve* 1993; **16**: 206–209.
203. Carta A, D'Adda T, Carrara F, Zeviani M. Ultrastructural analysis of extraocular muscle in chronic progressive external ophthalmoplegia. *Arch Ophthalmol* 2000; **118**: 1441–1445.
204. Moraes CT, DiMauro S, Zeviani M et al. Mitochondrial DNA deletions in progressive external ophthalmoplegia and Kearns-Sayre syndrome. *N Engl J Med* 1989; **320**: 1293–1299.
205. Laforet P, Lombes A, Eymard B et al. Chronic progressive external ophthalmoplegia with ragged-red fibers: clinical, morphological and genetic investigations in 43 patients. *Neuromuscul Disord* 1995; **5**: 399–413.
206. Moraes CT, Ciacci F, Bonilla E et al. Two novel pathogenic mitochondrial DNA mutations affecting organelle number and protein synthesis. Is the $tRNA^{Leu(UUR)}$ gene an etiologic hot spot? *J Clin Invest* 1993; **92**: 2906–2915.
207. Silvestri G, Servidei S, Rana M et al. A novel mitochondrial DNA point mutation in the tRNA(Ile) gene is associated with progressive external ophthalmoplegia. *Biochem Biophys Res Commun* 1996; **220**: 623–627.
208. Zeviani M, Servidei S, Gellera C et al. An autosomal dominant disorder with multiple deletions of mitochondrial DNA starting at the D-loop region. *Nature* 1989; **339**: 309–311.
209. Zeviani M, Bresolin N, Gellera C et al. Nucleus-driven multiple large-scale deletions of the human mitochondrial genome: a new autosomal dominant disease. *Am J Hum Genet* 1990; **47**: 904–914.
210. Suomalainen A, Majander A, Haltia M et al. Multiple deletions of mitochondrial DNA in several tissues of a patient with severe retarded depression and familial progressive external ophthalmoplegia. *J Clin Invest* 1992; **90**: 61–66.
211. Suomalainen A, Kaukonen J, Amati P et al. An autosomal locus predisposing to deletions of

mitochondrial DNA. *Nat Genet* 1995; **9**: 146–151.

212. Kaukonen J, Zeviani M, Comi GP et al. A third locus predisposing to multiple deletions of mtDNA in autosomal dominant progressive external ophthalmoplegia. *Am J Hum Genet* 1999; **65**: 256–261.
213. Van Goethem G, Dermaut B, Lofgren A et al. Mutation of *POLG* is associated with progressive external ophthalmoplegia characterized by mtDNA deletions. *Nat Genet* 2001; **28**: 211–212.
214. Kaukonen J, Juselius JK, Tiranti V et al. Role of adenine nucleotide translocator 1 in mtDNA maintenance. *Science* 2000; **289**: 782–785.
215. Spelbrink JN, Li FY, Tiranti V et al. Human mitochondrial DNA deletions associated with mutations in the gene encoding Twinkle, a phage T7 gene 4-like protein localized in mitochondria. *Nat Genet* 2001; **28**: 223–231.
216. Lamantea E, Tiranti V, Bordoni A et al. Mutations of mitochondrial DNA polymerase γ are a frequent cause of autosomal dominant or recessive progressive external ophthalmoplegia. *Ann Neurol* 2002; **52**: 211–219.
217. Agostino A, Valletta L, Chinnery PF et al. Mutations of *ANT1*, *Twinkle*, and *POLG1* in sporadic progressive external ophthalmoplegia (PEO). *Neurology* 2003; **60**: 1354–1356.
218. Van Goethem G, Martin JJ, Dermaut B et al. Recessive *POLG* mutations presenting with sensory and ataxic neuropathy in compound heterozygote patients with progressive external ophthalmoplegia. *Neuromuscul Disord* 2003; **13**: 133–142.
219. Mancuso M, Filosto M, Bellan M et al. POLG mutations causing ophthalmoplegia, sensorimotor polyneuropathy, ataxia, and deafness. *Neurology* 2004; **62**: 316–318.
220. Luoma P, Melberg A, Rinne JO et al. Parkinsonism, premature menopause, and mitochondrial DNA polymerase gamma mutations: clinical and molecular genetic study. *Lancet* 2004; **364**: 875–882.
221. Melberg A, Lundberg PO, Henriksson KG et al. Muscle-nerve involvement in autosomal dominant progressive external ophthalmoplegia with hypogonadism. *Muscle Nerve* 1996; **19**: 751–757.
222. Filosto M, Mancuso M, Nishigaki Y et al. Clinical and genetic heterogeneity in progressive external ophthalmoplegia due to mutations in polymerase γ. *Arch Neurol* 2003; **60**: 1279–1284.
223. Hirano M, Silvestri G, Blake DM et al. Mitochondrial neurogastrointestinal encephalomyopathy (MNGIE): clinical, biochemical, and genetic features of an autosomal recessive mitochondrial disorder. *Neurology* 1994; **44**: 721–727.
224. Nishino I, Spinazzola A, Papadimitriou A et al. Mitochondrial neurogastrointestinal encephalomyopathy: an autosomal recessive disorder due to thymidine phosphorylase mutations. *Ann Neurol* 2000; **47**: 792–800.
225. Nishino I, Spinazzola A, Hirano M. Thymidine phosphorylase gene mutations in MNGIE, a human mitochondrial disorder. *Science* 1999; **283**: 689–692.
226. Hirano M, Nishigaki Y, Marti R. Mitochondrial neurogastrointestinal encephalomyopathy (MNGIE): a disease of two genomes. *Neurologist* 2004; **10**: 8–17.
227. Montagna P, Plazzi G, Cortelli P et al. Abnormal lactate after effort in healthy carriers of Leber's hereditary optic neuropathy. *J Neurol Neurosurg Psych* 1995; **58**: 640–641.
228. Cortelli P, Montagna P, Avoni P et al. Leber's hereditary optic neuropathy: genetic, biochemical, and phosphorus magnetic resonance spectroscopy study in an Italian family. *Neurology* 1991; **41**: 1211–1215.
229. Barbiroli B, Montagna P, Cortelli P et al. Defective brain and muscle energy metabolism shown by in vivo ^{31}P magnetic resonance spectroscopy in nonaffected carriers of 11778 mtDNA mutation. *Neurology* 1995; **45**: 1364–1369.
230. Cortelli P, Montagna P, Pierangeli G et al. Clinical and brain bioenergetics improvement with idebenone in a patient with Leber's hereditary optic neuropathy: a clinical and ^{31}P-MRS study. *J Neurol Sci* 1997; **148**: 25–31.
231. Schuman JS, Hee MR, Puliafito CA et al. Quantification of nerve fiber layer thickness in normal and glaucomatous eyes using optical coherence tomography. *Arch Ophthalmol* 1995; **113**: 586–596.
232. Schuman JS, Pedut-Kloizman T, Hertzmark E et al. Reproducibility of nerve fiber layer thickness measurements using optical coherence tomography. *Ophthalmology* 1996; **103**: 1889–1898.
233. Blumenthal EZ, Williams JM, Weinreb RN et al. Reproducibility of nerve fiber layer thickness measurements by use of optical coherence

tomography. *Ophthalmology* 2000; **107**: 2278–2282.
234. Carpineto P, Ciancaglini M, Zuppardi E et al. Reliability of nerve fiber layer thickness measurements using optical coherence tomography in normal and glaucomatous eyes. *Ophthalmology* 2003; **110**: 190–195.
235. Kanamori A, Nakamura M, Escano MF et al. Evaluation of the glaucomatous damage on retinal nerve fiber layer thickness measured by optical coherence tomography. *Am J Ophthalmol* 2003; **135**: 513–520.
236. Hoh ST, Greenfield DS, Mistlberger A et al. Optical coherence tomography and scanning laser polarimetry in normal, ocular hypertensive, and glaucomatous eyes. *Am J Ophthalmol* 2000; **129**: 129–135.
237. Guedes V, Schuman JS, Hertzmark E et al. Optical coherence tomography measurement of macular and nerve fiber layer thickness in normal and glaucomatous human eyes. *Ophthalmology* 2003; **110**: 177–189.
238. Barboni P, Savini G, Valentino ML et al. Retinal nerve fiber layer evaluation by optical coherence tomography in Leber's hereditary optic neuropathy. *Ophthalmology* 2005; **112**: 120–126.
239. Savini G, Barboni P, Valentino ML et al. Retinal nerve fiber layer evaluation by optical coherence tomography in unaffected carriers with Leber's hereditary optic neuropathy mutations. *Ophthalmology* 2005; **112**: 127–131.
240. Kerrison JB. Latent, acute, and chronic Leber's hereditary optic neuropathy. *Ophthalmology* 2005; **112**: 1–2.
241. Chinnery PF, Howell N, Andrews RM, Turnbull DM. Clinical mitochondrial genetics. *J Med Genet* 1999; **36**: 425–436.
242. Chinnery PF, Schon EA. Mitochondria. *J Neurol Neurosurg Psychiatry* 2003; **74**: 1188–1199.
243. Smeitink J, van den Heuvel L, DiMauro S. The genetics and pathology of oxidative phosphorylation. *Nat Rev Genet* 2001; **2**: 342–352.
244. DiMauro S, Schon EA. Mitochondrial respiratory-chain diseases. *N Engl J Med* 2003; **348**: 2656–2668.
245. King MP, Attardi G. Human cells lacking mtDNA: repopulation with exogenous mitochondria by complementation. *Science* 1989; **246**: 500–503.
246. King MP, Attardi G. Isolation of human cell lines lacking mitochondrial DNA. *Methods Enzymol* 1996; **264**: 304–313.
247. King MP, Koga Y, Davidson M, Schon EA. Defects in mitochondrial protein synthesis and respiratory chain activity segregate with the tRNA$^{Leu(UUR)}$ mutation associated with mitochondrial myopathy, encephalopathy, lactic acidosis, and strokelike episodes. *Mol Cell Biol* 1992; **12**: 480–490.
248. Barrientos A, Moraes CT. Simultaneous transfer of mitochondrial DNA and single chromosomes in somatic cells: a novel approach for the study of defects in nuclear-mitochondrial communication. *Hum Mol Genet* 1998; **7**: 1801–1808.
249. Tiranti V, Hoertnagel K, Carrozzo R et al. Mutations of *SURF-1* in Leigh disease associated with cytochrome *c* oxidase deficiency. *Am J Hum Genet* 1998; **63**: 1609–1621.
250. Zhu Z, Yao J, Johns T et al. *SURF1*, encoding a factor involved in the biogenesis of cytochrome c oxidase, is mutated in Leigh syndrome. *Nat Genet* 1998; **20**: 337–343.
251. Mootha VK, Lepage P, Miller K et al. Identification of a gene causing human cytochrome *c* oxidase deficiency by integrative genomics. *Proc Natl Acad Sci USA* 2003; **100**: 605–610.
252. Tiranti V, D'Adamo P, Briem E et al. Ethylmalonic encephalopathy is caused by mutations in *ETHE1*, a gene encoding a mitochondrial matrix protein. *Am J Hum Genet* 2004; **74**: 239–252.
253. DiMauro S, Mancuso M, Naini A. Mitochondrial encephalomyopathies: therapeutic approach. *Ann NY Acad Sci* 2004; **1011**: 232–245.
254. Van Maldergem L, Trijbels F, DiMauro S et al. Coenzyme Q-responsive Leigh's encephalopathy in two sisters. *Ann Neurol* 2002; **52**: 750–754.
255. Harding AE, Sweeney MG, Govan GG, Riordan-Eva P. Pedigree analysis in Leber hereditary optic neuropathy families with a pathogenic mtDNA mutation. *Am J Hum Genet* 1995; **57**: 77–86.
256. Macmillan C, Kirkham T, Fu K et al. Pedigree analysis of French Canadian families with T14484C Leber's herditary optic neuropathy. *Neurology* 1998; **50**: 417–422.
257. Howell N, Xu M, Halvorson S et al. A heteroplasmic LHON family: tissue distribution and trans-

mission of the 11778 mutation. *Am J Hum Genet* 1994; **55**: 203–206.
258. Mashima Y, Hiida Y, Oguchi Y. Remission of Leber's hereditary optic neuropathy with idebenone. *Lancet* 1992; **340**: 368–369.
259. Cortelli P, Montagna P, Pierangeli G et al. Clinical and brain bioenergetics improvement with idebenone in a patient with Leber's hereditary optic neuropathy. A clinical and ^{31}P-MRS study. *J Neurol Sci* 1997; **148**: 25–31.
260. Carelli V, Ghelli A, Cevoli S et al. Idebenone therapy in Leber's hereditary optic neuropathy: report of six cases. *Neurology* 1998; 50: A4.
261. Mashima Y, Kigasawa K, Wakakura M, Oguchi Y. Do idebenone and vitamin therapy shorten the time to achieve visual recovery in Leber hereditary optic neuropathy? *J Neuroophthalmol* 2000; **20**: 166–170.
262. Geromel V, Darin N, Chretien D et al. Coenzyme Q(10) and idebenone in the therapy of respiratory chain diseases: rationale and comparative benefits. *Mol Genet Metab* 2002; **77**: 21–30.
263. Wheeler L, WoldeMussie E, Lai R. Role of alpha-2 agonists in neuroprotection. *Surv Ophthalmol* 2003; **48**: 47–51.
264. Newman NJ. Prophylaxis for second eye involvement in Leber's hereditary optic neuropathy: a multicenter trial of topical brimonidine purite. *Neurology* 2005; **64**: A1.
265. Manfredi G, Fu J, Ojaimi J et al. Rescue of a deficiency in ATP synthesis by transfer of *MTATP6*, a mitochondrial DNA-encoded gene, to the nucleus. *Nat Genet* 2002; **30**: 394–399.
266. Guy J, Qi X, Pallotti F et al. Rescue of a mitochondrial deficiency causing Leber hereditary optic neuropathy. *Ann Neurol* 2002; **52**: 534–542.
267. Oca-Cossio J, Kenyon L, Hao H, Moraes CT. Limitations of allotopic expression of mitochondrial genes in mammalian cells. *Genetics* 2003; **165**: 707–720.
268. Srivastava S, Moraes CT. Manipulating mitochondrial DNA heteroplasmy by a mitochondrially targeted restriction endonuclease. *Hum Mol Genet* 2001; **10**: 3093–3099.
269. Tanaka M, Borgeld HJ, Zhang J et al. Gene therapy for mitochondrial disease by delivering restriction endonuclease *SmaI* into mitochondria. *J Biomed Sci* 2002; **9**: 534–541.
270. Mootha VK, Bunkenborg J, Olsen JV et al. Integrated analysis of protein composition, tissue diversity, and gene regulation in mouse mitochondria. *Cell* 2003; **115**: 629–640.
271. Ravagnan L, Roumier T, Kroemer G. Mitochondria, the killer organelles and their weapons. *J Cell Physiol* 2002; **192**: 131–137.
272. Hirano M. Transmitochondrial mice: proof of principle and promises. *Proc Natl Acad Sci USA* 2001; **98**: 401–403.
273. Wallace DC. Mouse models for mitochondrial disease. *Am J Med Genet* 2001; **106**: 71–93.
274. Sligh JE, Levy SE, Waymire KG et al. Maternal germ-line transmission of mutant mtDNAs from embryonic stem cell-derived chimeric mice. *Proc Natl Acad Sci USA* 2000; **97**: 14461–14466.
275. Sandbach JM, Coscun PE, Grossniklaus HE et al. Ocular pathology in mitochondrial superoxide dismutase (Sod2)-deficient mice. *Invest Ophthalmol Vis Sci* 2001; **42**: 2173–2178.
276. Biousse V, Pardue MT, Wallace DC, Newman NJ. The eyes of mito-mouse: mouse models of mitochondrial disease. *J Neuro-ophthalmol* 2002; **22**: 279–285.
277. Sadun A. Acquired mitochondrial impairment as a cause of optic nerve disease. *Trans Am Ophthalmol Soc* 1998; **96**: 881–923.
278. Zhang X, Jones D, Gonzalez-Lima F. Mouse model of optic neuropathy caused by mitochondrial complex I dysfunction. *Neurosci Lett* 2002; **326**: 97–100.
279. Qi X, Lewin AS, Hauswirth WW, Guy J. Optic neuropathy induced by reductions in mitochondrial superoxide dismutase. *Invest Ophthalmol Vis Sci* 2003; **44**: 1088–1096.
280. Qi X, Lewin AS, Hauswirth WW, Guy J. Suppression of complex I gene expression induces optic neuropathy. *Ann Neurol* 2003; **53**: 198–205.
281. Qi X, Lewin AS, Sun L et al. SOD2 gene transfer protects against optic neuropathy induced by deficiency of complex I. *Ann Neurol* 2004; **56**: 182–191.
282. Cho KS, Yang L, Lu B et al. Re-establishing the regenerative potential of central nervous system

6

Mitochondrial gastroenterology

Laurence Bindoff

Background

Mitochondrial dysfunction can affect any and indeed all systems of the body and the gastrointestinal tract is no exception. This chapter will deal with gastroenterological disease induced by dysfunction of the mitochondrial respiratory chain (MRC), the final common pathway for energy production in all eukaryotic cells. The MRC can be affected by genetic defects arising in one of two different genomes as well as by exogenous influences such as drugs. While energy production remains their single most important function, mitochondria perform many other functions, some of which are tissue-specific. In general, tissues with the highest energy requirement are those most frequently affected by MRC dysfunction and those in which dysfunction causes the most profound (for the patient) and obvious disease, for example the brain, retina and skeletal muscle.[1] Based on symptoms, however, the gastrointestinal tract[2] is frequently involved, but also frequently overlooked, such that it remains a largely unexplored area for mitochondrial physicians.[3]

I will define the gastrointestinal system as comprising the organs of digestion from the oral cavity to the rectum, including teeth and muscles of mastications gastrointestinal tract, liver and exocrine pancrea, (Figure 6.1). Disorders resulting from endocrine pancreatic dysfunction are covered elsewhere.

The gastrointestinal tract

The adult gastrointestinal tract (GIT) is a tube approximately 9 meters long comprising a smooth muscle wall and a mucous membrane lining. It has its own intrinsic nervous system (called the enteric nervous system) but it is also innervated by both parasympathetic and sympathetic components of the autonomic nervous system. The motor component of the intrinsic nervous system is concerned primarily with peristalsis. While it has a high degree of autonomy, it can also be modulated by the autonomic nervous system; parasympathetic nerves increase and sympathetic nerves decrease motility. The striated muscles of the oral cavity, the muscles of mastication, and those in the upper part of the esophagus and in the anal sphincter are controlled by other parts of the nervous system and are under voluntary control.

Major functions of the gastrointestinal tract include the digestion of food, with uptake of nutrients and other factors essential for growth and maintenance of homeostasis, and the excretion of unwanted by-products. The process of digestion begins with mechanical disruption of food in the oral cavity, a process that is dependent on striated muscle activity, the teeth and the production of fluid by the salivary glands. Further disruption, enzymatic digestion, secretions from both liver and exocrine pancreas, and uptake of nutrients/co-factors take place in the small bowel.

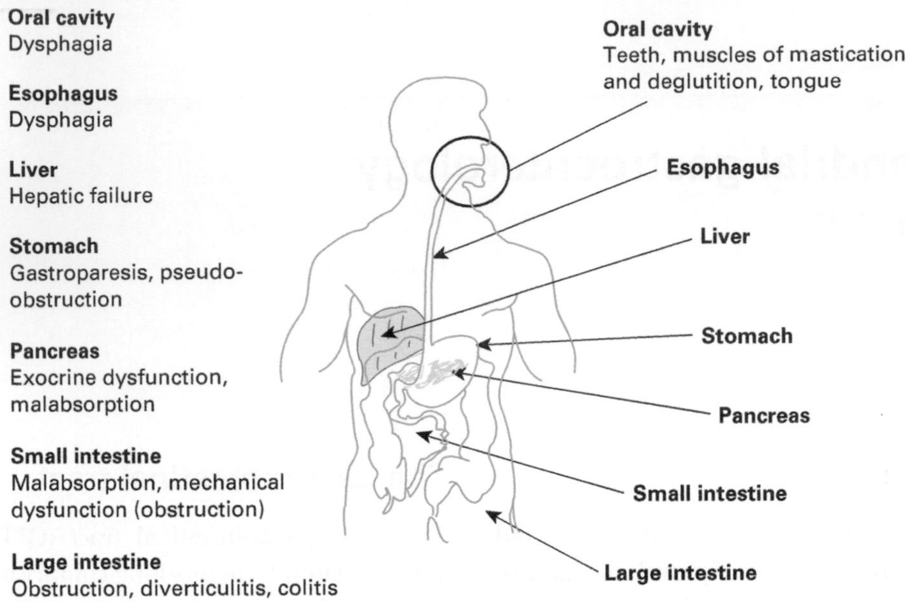

Figure 6.1 The gastrointestinal system. The parts of the GI system that are discussed are shown on the right hand side of the figure. On the opposite side are some of the potential problems that arise

Absorption of nutrients and control of fluid balance occur in the large bowel.

At the simplest level, we know that MRC dysfunction leads to inadequate energy production. Hence, processes most dependent on energy, such as gastric motility, are most likely to be affected. It is rare for gastrointestinal disease to be the sole or first manifestation of MRC disease, although this is sometimes exemplified by failure to thrive in children or cachexia in adults. Mitochondrial gastrointestinal dysfunction occurs most often in the context of disease affecting many systems. It is possible, therefore, to approach the question of gastrointestinal dysfunction in MRC disease by focusing either on the symptoms and their cause (a problem-based approach) or by looking at specific mitochondrial diseases and their gastroenterological manifestations. Both approaches are valid and valuable.

A detailed and careful clinical history is a prerequisite to any subsequent analysis. Gastrointestinal symptoms may occur at any stage, and patients may already have known MRC disease. Table 6.1 lists gastroenterological symptoms commonly encountered in patients with known MRC disease and gives potential causes. This list is not exhaustive and is not meant to suggest that symptoms such as dysphagia and vomiting by themselves raise the suspicion of MRC disease. There are no formal figures for prevalence, but experience tells us that gastrointestinal symptoms, such as these, are common. Presentation will differ depending on age. The symptoms listed in Table 6.1 are typically seen in children and adults. Infants have a very different repertoire. Table 6.2 lists the gastrointestinal features found in infants and is taken from a review of 300 cases.[4] Table 6.3 reverses the perspective and looks at which gastrointestinal features have been reported with various types of mitochondrial disease.

Since skeletal muscle is commonly involved in mitochondrial disease, dysphagia may result from weakness or premature fatigue of voluntary muscles involved in chewing or deglutition. Proper

Table 6.1 Gastroenterological symptoms that occur with mitochondrial respiratory chain disease

Problem	Potential cause
Dysphagia	• Incomplete chewing due to i. Poor dentition ii. Weak jaw muscles • Bulbar weakness or incoordination due to: i. Pyramidal disease, i.e. pseudobulbar palsy ii. Cerebellar disease • Cricopharyngeal dysfunction (achalasia)
Nausea and vomiting	• Abnormal motility/pseudo-obstruction i. Gastroparesis ii. Small intestinal dysmotility • Lactic acidosis • CNS disease affecting the autonomic nervous system: i. Brainstem (dorsal motor nucleus – vagus) ii. Spinal cord iii. Vestibular
Abdominal pain/discomfort	• Abnormal motility • Lactic acidosis • Diverticular disease • Colitis
Diarrhea	• Abnormal motility • Lactic acidosis • Malabsorption
Undernutrition/failure to thrive	• Malabsorption i. Energy defect ii. Bacterial overgrowth iii. Villous atrophy • Abnormal motility • Anorexia i. Secondary to nausea/vomiting or pain ii. Due to brain disease

mastication of food is essential to form a food bolus, such that dental disease may also contribute to the problem. Difficulty swallowing may reflect disease involving the brain, particularly the brain stem, and esophageal dysmotility may lead to dysphagia by not allowing food to pass from the hypopharynx to the upper esophagus. Clinical evaluation will often help define the site at which the problem arises, but radiological examination of the upper gastrointestinal tract (GIT) will often be required. Dysphagia is described in many different MRC disorders

Table 6.2 Gastroenterological manifestations of MRC disease in the very young[4]

Case #	Age of onset	Gastroenterological manifestation	MRC defect
1	3 wk.	FTT, VA	Complex II (H)
3	1 month	FTT	Complex I (Ly)
7	Neonatal	Duodenal atresia, duplication of the choledochus, agenesis of gallbladder	Complex I (Li)
10	Neonatal	Liver failure, thrombocytopenia	Complexes I+IV (Li)
11	3 month	CHARGE	Complex IV (M)
18	Neonatal	Growth failure, gut involvement	Quinone deficiency (Ly)
19	Neonatal	Pearson (antenatal fetal hydrops)	Complexes I+IV (Ly)

Case # refers to the case in the article cited. FTT=failure to thrive; VA=villous atrophy; CHARGE=Coloboma, Heart anomaly, choanal Atresia, Retardation, Genital and Ear anomalies; MRC defect gives the respiratory chain complex(es) affected and the tissue in which the abnormality occurred. H=Heart; Ly=lymphocytes; Li=liver; M=muscle.

including CPEO due to single mtDNA deletions and other syndromes caused by point mutations of mtDNA, such as MELAS. It is also seen with nuclear gene defects, such as those affecting polymerase γ and thymidine phosphorylase, both of which cause CPEO with multiple mtDNA deletions and mtDNA depletion.

Nausea is a non-specific symptom that may occur with or without vomiting. It is common among patients with all forms of mitochondrial disease, but the cause can be difficult to define. Subjective feelings of nausea and indeed vomiting may be associated with disorders of equilibrium, for example caused by disease affecting the vestibular system. Lesions of the brain, particularly the brain stem, are a common feature of Leigh syndrome, but may also occur in other mitochondrial disorders having a major encephalopathic element. Lastly, it appears that lactic acidosis itself can induce gastric stasis and indeed dysmotility of the stomach and small intestine. This can cause nausea, vomiting, bloating and a feeling of premature fullness.

Abdominal pain is a variable symptom amongst patients with MRC disease. It can range from griping/cramp-like pain to a constant discomfort and it arises most often because of altered GIT motility. For example, gastric or upper intestinal stasis may cause pseudo-obstruction. Pseudo-obstruction caused by failure of peristalsis, the propulsion of food along the gastrointestinal tract, may be due to direct involvement of the bowel muscle or of the intrinsic nervous system. Defects of gut motility have been recorded in several mitochondrial disorders both caused by mtDNA point mutations such as MELAS, and by nuclear gene defects, such as MNGIE (these are discussed below). Elevated lactate causes nausea, vomiting, and probably impairs gastric emptying. Since vagal efferents (parasympathetic nervous system) increase gut peristaltic activity, damage to this system, for example within the dorsal nucleus of the vagus, may be one cause of dysmotility syndromes.

Manifestations of MRC disease involving the large bowel are also recognized. Diverticulitis, possibly resulting from dysmotility, is described in MNGIE. Ischemic and other forms of colitis are described in patients with abdominal pain associated with a variety of different mitochondrial disorders, including MELAS, other point mutations

Table 6.3 Gastrointestinal symptoms reported with specific MRC disorders. The list is not exhaustive but gives a sample of syndromes reported with which type of MRC defect*

Gastrointestinal manifestation	Secondary to	Type of MRC defect
Dysphagia	Cricopharyngeal achalasia	Single detetion (KSS, PEO)
Abnormal motility	Neuromuscular involvement	MNGIE MELAS/A3243G Single mtDNA deletion
	Lactic acidosis	MNGIE MELAS/A3243G Leigh syndrome Any mtDNA defect
	Brainstem disease	Leigh syndrome MELAS/A3243G
Autonomic involvement	Secondary to diabetes	Any mtDNA defect, particularly MELAS/A3243G and mtDNA duplication
	Secondary to generalized neuropathy	Potentially any
Mucosal involvement	Villous atrophy	MELAS/A3243G Single deletion
Cyclical vomiting	Possibly due to stasis	MELAS/A3243G Single deletion
Hepatic involvement	mtDNA depletion	Deoxyguanosine kinase POLG
	Unknown	SCO1
	Secondary	Drugs (AIDS treatment), valproate
Failure to thrive	In children Cachexia in adult	Any mitochondrial defect. Think of MNGIE (look for ophthalmoplegia)

*MNGIE = mitochondrial neurogastrointestinal encephalomyopathy; MELAS = mitochondrial, encephalopathy, lactic acidosis and stroke-like episode; SCO1 = Assembly protein for cytochrome oxidase; POLG = polymerase gamma.

and single mtDNA deletions. There are no systematic data about the occurrence of these manifestations in mitochondrial disease: therefore, it is difficult to know whether these reflect true disease associations or just chance, as diverticulitis and non-specific inflammation are not uncommon.

Another common feature of MRC disease is undernutrition or failure to thrive; patients, both children and adults, are often small and thin. Failure to thrive may be due to one or more of a large number of causes, both within the gut and outside. It may also reflect the generalized defect in energy production. Whilst often used to explain failure to thrive, malabsorption in patients with MRC has rarely been documented. In addition, such patients may have anorexia due to disease within the central nervous system, e.g. encephalopathy, and nausea and vomiting secondary to whatever cause may also impair the appetite. Vitamin deficiency, possibly of dietary origin, has been recorded and the presence of bowel stasis (with or without diverticular disease) exposes the patient to the risk of bacterial overgrowth. Whether the energy defect associated with MRC dysfunction affects mucosal transport is unknown, but it is reasonable to suppose that this occurs. Lastly, endocrine dysfunction (other than diabetes mellitus) is not uncommon amongst patients with MRC disease, particularly those with single deletions and the Kearns–Sayre syndrome (KSS).

Investigation of patients with gastrointestinal symptoms and known MRC disease is no different than in patients with any other cause of gastrointestinal dysfunction. The clinical history defines the symptoms and directs the investigations required. For example, dysphagia necessitates a careful analysis of the stage at which swallowing difficulties occur. Is it with transfer of the food bolus back toward the upper esophagus or later? Are there symptoms of aspiration? Imaging is often required and this can be direct, e.g. endoscopy, or indirect, using contrast (videofluoroscopy). The same holds for symptoms suggesting obstruction, such as nausea, postprandial discomfort, vomiting, weight loss, and malnutrition. For a comprehensive review of symptoms and methods of investigation readers are referred to standard gastroenterological texts (including reference 5). The key question here is whether the patient has recognized MRC disease. If not, what feature should prompt us to consider this cause for the patient's symptoms? Table 6.4 gives some potential clues to the presence of mitochondrial disease, but cannot be considered exhaustive.

The liver

Liver dysfunction occurs with several mitochondrial defects[6] but especially in childhood disorders associated with mtDNA depletion,[7] defects of the COX assembly gene *SCO1*[8] and Alpers syndrome. Isolated liver dysfunction is rare, but the combination of liver disease with CNS or – less commonly – renal or hematological disease, suggests that the disorder is due to MRC dysfunction. Clearly, encephalopathy may also be secondary to hepatic insufficiency. In these cases, symptoms usually fluctuate or resolve dependent on the status of the liver.

The consequences of liver dysfunction are variable and there are no features, clinical or histological, that are specific for MRC disease. Manifestations range from vomiting and failure to thrive to coagulation defects. Since lactate is metabolized to glucose in the liver through gluconeogenesis, both profound lactic acidosis and hypoglycemia are potential consequences of liver dysfunction. Both are features of MRC-related liver disease. Death due to liver failure is recorded in patients with MRC disease (e.g. Alpers disease, see later), but in some cases death is precipitated by the coincidental use of sodium valproate. This drug can certainly induce liver failure and there are good theoretical reasons why it should be avoided in patients with suspected or proven MRC disease. Whether it is indeed the primary etiological factor in causing liver failure in children with MRC disorders remains to be proven.

Mitochondrial DNA depletion

The quantitative loss of mtDNA (depletion), was identified in the early 1990s and one of the first cases described had liver failure.[9] Subsequently, many more patients have been identified, in whom hepatic disease is a frequent manifestation, but myopathy and central nervous system disease are also found. Histological studies of the liver show fatty infiltration and cirrhosis.[10] Until recently, the genetic causes of this disorder were unknown. Autosomal recessive inheritance dictated that the causal gene was nuclear and confirmation came recently with the identification of mutations in the deoxyguanosine kinase (*DGUOK*)[11] and in the polymerase γ (*POLG*) genes.[12] Interestingly, mutations in the thymidine kinase (*TK2*) gene cause mtDNA depletion with a predominantly muscle phenotype.[13] All three gene products are expressed in mitochondria and are involved in the salvage pathways for nucleotides, highlighting once again the importance of dNTP pools for the maintenance[14] and homeostasis of mtDNA (see also MNGIE below) (see Box 6.1).

Cytochrome oxidase defects

SCO1 is one of the proteins involved in the assembly of the terminal MRC complex, complex IV, cytochrome *c* oxidase[15] (others include Surf1,[16,17] SCO2,[18,19] COX10,[8] COX15,[20] LRPPRC,[21] and ETHE1[22]). Mutations in the *SCO1* gene were linked to a syndrome comprising hepatic failure, ketoacidosis, and encephalopathy.[8] The disorder is inherited as an autosomal recessive trait and as yet we know little about its incidence or prevalence. Moreover, as other COX assembly gene defects produce disease elsewhere in the body, it is not clear whether SCO1 defects will remain specifically linked to liver disease.

Alpers syndrome

The combination of liver failure, epilepsy and developmental delay with neuronal loss is often called Alpers (or Alpers–Huttenlocher) syndrome (AHS).[6] How many children with this combination of features have MRC defects is as yet unknown,[23] but at least two different mitochondrial defects have been identified. One child had mutation in the cytochrome *c* oxidase II mtDNA gene.[24] The second mitochondrial defect – a much more common cause of AHS – involves the mitochondrial DNA polymerase γ.[12,25,26] These children have Alpers and depletion of mtDNA.

Secondary liver disease

Whilst the discussion has concentrated thus far on inherited mitochondrial disorders, acquired disorders must not be forgotten. One major example is the mtDNA depletion that results from treatment of AIDS with nucleoside analog reverse transcriptase inhibitors (NRTIs).[27] Treatment regimens now use combinations of NRTIs together with protease inhibitors. Recognized side effects of the NRTIs include myopathy, neuropathy, pancreatitis, bone marrow toxicity, hepatic toxicity and lactic acidosis; laboratory studies have shown that one of these drugs, azidothymidine (AZT), causes depletion of mitochondrial DNA in cultured cells and it is likely that all NRTIs have similar toxic effects on mitochondria. Among patients treated with NRTIs, lactic acidosis is common although rarely life-threatening. Symptoms include nausea and vomiting, abdominal discomfort, weight loss and fatigue.[28,29] Rarely, liver steatosis occurs. Whether these GI symptoms are related to elevated lactic acid levels, to direct mitochondrial toxicity of NRTIs (e.g. causing mtDNA depletion), to secondary effects of treatment, or to the underlying disease is not yet known. The similarity between these symptoms and those arising from primary mitochondrial disorders suggests, however, that they share a common etiology.

The exocrine pancreas

While involvement of the endocrine pancreas is common in MRC disease of whatever cause, the exocrine pancreas appears less frequently affected. Dysfunction of the exocrine pancreas and failure to

Box 6.1 Mitochondrial nucleotide pools

The synthesis of mtDNA requires the four nucleotides – dA, dC, dG, and dT – as raw materials. Where do they come from? It turns out that mitochondrial dNTP pools are regulated independently of the dNTP pools in the nucleus. The key difference is that mitochondria contain nucleoside salvage pathways for the synthesis of all four species. The nucleosides enter the organelle from the cytosol via a transporter, most likely the equilibrative nucleoside transporter (ENT1). Once inside, a mitochondrion-specific deoxyguanosine kinase (dGK) phosphorylates the purine nucleosides (dA and dG), while a mitochondrion-specifc thymidine kinase (TK2) phosphorylates the pyrimidines (dC and dT); 5′(3′)-deoxyribonucleotidase (dNT2) dephosphorylates the pyrimidines. The nucleosides are converted to nucleotides by presumed nucleoside monophosphate kinases (e.g. adenylate kinases [AKs] and UMP-CMP kinase [UCK]) and diphosphate kinases (NME4 and NME6; both proteins are bound to succinyl-CoA synthetase subunit β [SUCLA2], a TCA enzyme). The nucleotides are then incorporated into mtDNA by the mitochondrion-specific DNA polymerase, called polymerase γ (POLG).

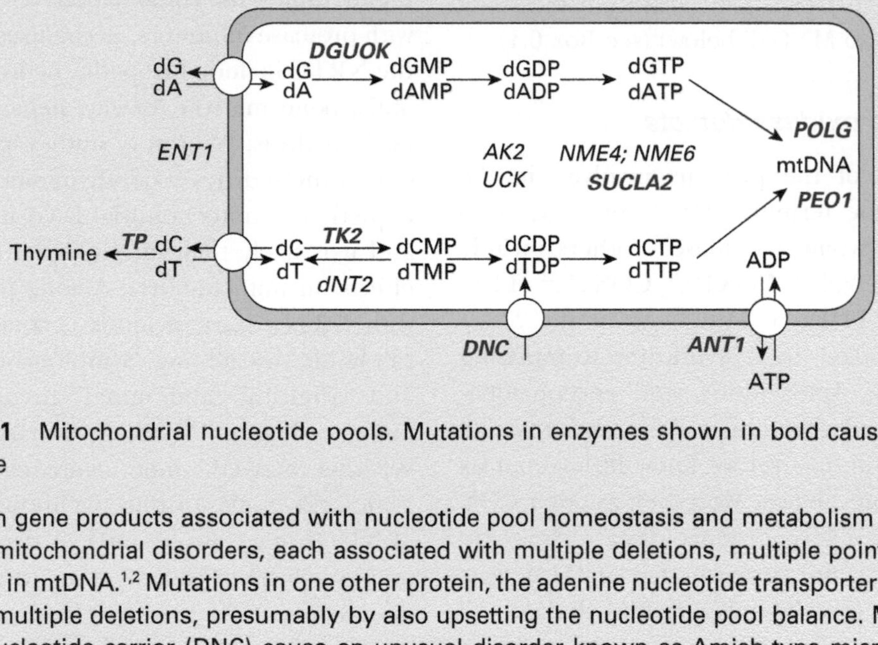

Figure B6.1.1 Mitochondrial nucleotide pools. Mutations in enzymes shown in bold cause mitochondrial disease

Mutations in gene products associated with nucleotide pool homeostasis and metabolism can cause a number of mitochondrial disorders, each associated with multiple deletions, multiple point mutations, or depletion in mtDNA.[1,2] Mutations in one other protein, the adenine nucleotide transporter (ANT1), can also cause multiple deletions, presumably by also upsetting the nucleotide pool balance. Mutations in the deoxynucleotide carrier (DNC) cause an unusual disorder known as Amish-type microencephaly. Note that mutations in thymidine phosphorylase (TP), which is not a mitochondrial protein, can also cause a mitochondrial disease – MNGIE – because alterations in the extra-mitochondrial nucleoside pools can have affects on the intra-mitochondrial pools, resulting in mtDNA mutations.[3]

References

1. Elpeleg O, Miller C, Hershkovitz E, Bitner-Glindzicz M et al. Deficiency of the ADP-forming succinyl-CoA synthase activity is associated with encephalomyopathy and mitochondrial DNA depletion. *Am J Hum Genet* 2005; **76**: 1081–1086.
2. Saada A. Deoxyribonucleotides and disorders of mitochondrial DNA integrity. *DNA Cell Biol* 2004; **23**: 797–806.
3. Marti R, Nishigaki Y, Vila MR, Hirano M. Alteration of nucleotide metabolism: a new mechanism for mitochondrial disorders. *Clin Chem Lab Med* 2003; **41**: 845–851.

secrete digestive enzymes leads to undernutrition or failure to thrive. These are common features of mitochondrial disease and ones that may have multiple causes. Malabsorption will prompt further investigation, including tests of exocrine pancreatic function, but these are seldom reported. Moreover, no studies have looked at exocrine pancreatic function in different MRC disorders. Postmortem studies of pancreas have shown various abnormalities, including the accumulation of degenerated mitochondria in a patient with the A3243G mutation and diabetes.[30]

The mitochondrial disorder classically linked with the exocrine pancreas is Pearson's (marrow-pancreas) syndrome.[31] Patients with this disorder develop refractory sideroblastic anemia with variable neutropenia and thrombocytopenia; bone marrow aspirates show vacuolation of both erythroid and myeloid precursors. Exocrine pancreas insufficiency manifests as failure to thrive, diarrhea, and malabsorption. Hepatic involvement[32] is frequent and in several children liver failure was the cause of death. Renal involvement is reported[32] and most children with this disorder have significant lactic acidosis. Muscle and CNS dysfunction appear less prominent than in other MRC disorders. Patients with this disorder usually succumb early, but some survive and go on to develop Kearns–Sayre syndrome (KSS, see later).

Pearson's syndrome is caused by a major rearrangement of mtDNA. In most cases, this is a single deletion,[33] but tandem duplication may also occur (Box 3.2).[34] It is not clear why, in one situation, a mtDNA rearrangement gives a predominantly neurological syndrome (i.e. KSS) and in another it causes bone marrow and pancreatic dysfunction. Rearrangements, such as those causing KSS are predominantly sporadic, although a recent multicenter study suggests that up to 20% may be inherited.[35] Whether it was single deletions or tandem duplications that were inherited was not addressed in this study.

Thus far, I have reviewed symptoms often encountered with known MRC disease. I would like to restate that gastrointestinal dysfunction is frequently overlooked, so the spectrum is likely to be wider. In addition, I have reported what is known, but it is likely that many, if not most, mitochondrial disorders are capable of producing similar features. As stated earlier, it is rare for gastroenterological features to be the primary manifestation of MRC disease. In Table 6.4, I have attempted to provide some clues to alert the physician to the presence of MRC discasc in patients presenting with gastroenterological disease and an as yet undetected mitochondrial defect. The take-home message behind this discussion is a reminder to us not to simply concentrate on 'our system'. Perhaps the most potent clue is ophthalmoplegia. This eye muscle disorder develops slowly and often without diplopia; even when quite profound, causing the patient to turn their head in order to maintain visual fixation, the patient may be unaware of it.

Specific mitochondrial diseases and their gastroenterological manifestations (Figure 6.2)

Mitochondrial neurogastrointestinal encephalomyopathy (MNGIE)

This fascinating condition is defined in large part by involvement of the gastrointestinal tract.[36] The disease can present from childhood to middle age and shows autosomal recessive inheritance. The gastrointestinal and neurological features of MNGIE are summarized in Table 6.5. In a series of 35 patients reported by Nishino and colleagues,[36] gastrointestinal symptoms were the presenting complaint in 55% of cases (10% of these having cachexia), although 100% of patients had gastrointestinal symptoms on direct questioning. Neurological manifestations, including ocular symptoms, symptoms related to

Table 6.4 Clues to the presence of MRC disease*

Feature	Comment
Ophthalmoplegia	Not always accompanied by symptoms such as diplopia! Mild ptosis may be the only indicator. Examine the eyes!
Mild compensated metabolic acidosis	A persistent mild acidosis not considered significant, e.g. bicarbonate of 16–19 mM
Glucose intolerance or frank diabetes in someone receiving parenteral nutrition	Seen in cases of e.g. MELAS/A3243G who have received parenteral nutrition for intestinal obstruction
Acidosis (lactate) provoked by intravenous glucose infusion	
More than one system involvement, e.g. failure to thrive and cortical disease (epilepsy, mental retardation)	There can be many reasons for involvement of several systems, not just MRC disease, however, mitochondrial disease is much more common than once realized.[73] One could provide several more: epilepsy and liver disease (Alpers); diabetes and deafness
Asymptomatic basal ganglia calcification	Often seen in KSS, which may present with non-neurological features
I could also suggest that we look more carefully at our diabetic patients admitted with coma	A known disease (i.e. diabetes) often prevents further thought; e.g. diabetes as the sole manifestation. This is taken to be the cause of whatever happens despite the absence of good evidence. Seen in patients with MELAS/A3243G

*It is not possible to give a complete inventory of everything that might suggest a MRC defect. The examples given come from personal experience and earlier reviews of clinical features that suggested the diagnosis of MRC disease in a cohort of 50 patients.[72] Refer to text for more detailed discussion.

peripheral neuropathy and hearing impairment, were the presenting complaint in 49% of cases. In this series, all patients had ptosis, ophthalmoplegia and signs of peripheral neuropathy when examined, but there are reports of patients who do not have ocular findings at presentation.[37] Interestingly, dementia appears not to be a problem despite the radiological presence of leukoencephalopathy. Lactic acid levels were elevated in more than 60% and, when examined, skeletal muscle biopsy was always abnormal, showing ragged-red fibers (RRF) and loss of cytochrome oxidase activity (100%). Lack of muscle involvement – though reported – is rare.[38]

The predominant gastrointestinal defect appears to be dysmotility, almost certainly due to a disturbance in the muscle component of the gut wall, although these patients do have a neuropathy and autonomic involvement cannot be excluded. Patients develop delayed gastric emptying, pseudo-obstruction and even pharyngeal and esophageal motility problems. Despite the presence of GI dysfunction, and in some cases cachexia, vitamin E, vitamin B12 and folate, when measured, were

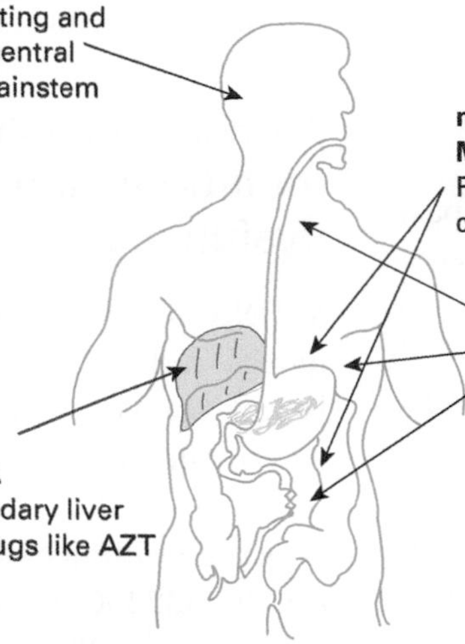

Figure 6.2 Where specific mitochondrial diseases affect the GI system. FTT=failure to thrive; POLG=mitochondrial DNA polymerase gamma; Sco1=cytochrome *c* oxidase assembly gene; AZT=azidothymidine

Table 6.5 Gastrointestinal symptoms and findings in patients with MNGIE*

Symptoms	Signs/findings
Borborygmi	Diverticulosis
Abdominal pain/ discomfort	Pseudo-obstruction
Early satiety	Gastroparesis
Nausea and vomiting	Hepatic dysfunction
Dysphagia	Cachexia
Diarrhea	Failure to thrive
Weight loss	

*Adapted from the information given by Nishino et al.[65]

normal, except in one case, who had a marginally low vitamin E level.

In the series of Nishino,[36] the cause of death was recorded for nine patients. Peritonitis secondary to intestinal rupture occurred in two, aspiration pneumonia in two, post-colostomy complication in one, and esophageal bleeding secondary to cirrhosis in one. Pathological studies of the bowel have shown variable results, including decreased number of smooth muscle cells,[39] visceral neuropathy,[40] and infiltration of the bowel (scleroderma-like).[41]

MNGIE is a recessive trait due to mutations in the thymidine phosphorylase (*TP*) gene.[36] Clinical diagnosis is supported by muscle biopsy findings of a mitochondrial defect (COX-negative RRF) and by analysis of mitochondrial DNA showing multiple mtDNA deletions, mtDNA depletion, or both.[42] Definitive diagnosis is achieved by identifying elevated thymidine in urine or blood, and decreased TP activity in buffy coat or in cultured cells such as fibroblasts. Mutational analysis confirms the diagnosis. As yet, there is no specific treatment for thymidine phosphorylase deficiency. Treatment of the bowel symptoms and malnutrition follows the same general principles as with other causes and will be reviewed later.

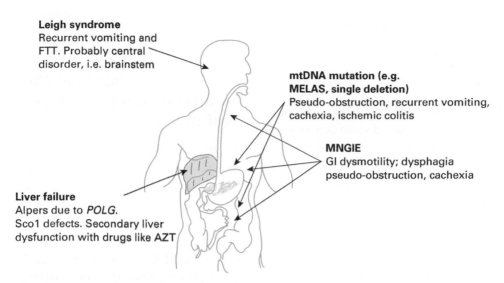

Other examples of nuclear gene defects impairing mtDNA homeostasis include the mitochondrial DNA polymerase (polymerase γ, POLG)[43,44] and the adenine nucleotide translocator.[45] Gastrointestinal dysfunction is also a feature of *POLG* mutations with dysphagia, cachexia[46] and chronic diarrhea reported.[44]

Leigh syndrome

Leigh syndrome (LS) is a generic term encompassing a group of disorders with diverse genetic etiology. The condition begins at or soon after birth, usually following a disease-free interval, although presentation up to and including young adult life is recorded.[47] These children develop a progressive disorder, with seizures, abnormal movements, mental retardation, ataxia, and optic atrophy or retinal disease. Gastrointestinal dysfunction is a major feature of LS. Poor feeding with poor sucking and recurrent vomiting, together with failure to thrive are common in babies having this syndrome from whatever cause.[47] The immediate cause of gastrointestinal dysfunction is not clear. As these children develop necrotic lesions in the basal ganglia, the brainstem, and the spinal cord, it is possible that there is disruption of the autonomic supply to the gastrointestinal tract (e.g. dorsal motor nucleus of the vagus). The presence of respiratory symptoms, such as irregular breathing and bouts of apnea and hyperventilation supports this possibility. These children also have lactic acidosis (again irrespective of cause) and some have a neuropathy.

Various genetic defects cause LS. Mutations of mtDNA, including those at position 8993 in the *ATP6* gene[48] as well as a mutation in *ND5*,[49] are important causes of what is often called maternal inherited Leigh syndrome (MILS). LS can also be due to defects in nuclear genes, such as *SURF1*,[16,50] a COX assembly gene, genes encoding subunits of complex I or complex II,[51,52] or components of the pyruvate dehydrogenase complex.[53]

Whatever the genetic or biochemical deficit, the condition is defined neuropathologically by its characteristic symmetrical involvement of the brain, particularly basal ganglia, and brainstem. There is a subacute necrotizing encephalopathy, and imaging studies reflect these findings by showing symmetrical changes in the basal ganglia.[54]

Primary mitochondrial DNA mutations and gastrointestinal dysfunction

MtDNA mutations, including single-base substitutions and single deletions, are numerically the largest source of MRC disease, particularly in adults, and to date more than 100 mutations are recorded.[55] While certain mutations are usually associated with stereotypical clinical manifestations, e.g. the A3243G mutation with MELAS, and single deletions with PEO, this phenotypic consistency is not typical. The same mutation can produce different phenotypes, e.g. the A3243G can produce MELAS, diabetes and deafness, or PEO, and, conversely, different mutations can produce the same phenotype (there are about a dozen different mtDNA mutations capable of producing the MELAS phenotype). The implications for our discussion of gastroenterological dysfunction are, therefore, that which is said about one type of mutation may equally well apply to others, or indeed all.

Mitochondrial encephalopathy, lactic acidosis and stroke-like episodes (MELAS)

The commonest cause of this syndrome is the A3243G mutation[56] in the $tRNA^{Leu(UUR)}$ mtDNA gene, although many other mtDNA mutations produce this phenotype.[55] Patients with this mutation and whatever clinical phenotype are frequently short and thin; diabetes mellitus is a common feature. GIT dysfunction as the major clinical manifestation is also recorded and includes pseudo-obstruction,[57,58] recurrent vomiting, diarrhea with cachexia,[59] and even ischemic colitis.[60] Interestingly, some patients had the A3243G mtDNA mutations in the affected organ, namely the gastrointestinal tract, whereas others did not.[61] In the absence of diabetic complications, the presumption is that in these cases the defect is within the central nervous system. MtDNA mutations other than the A3243G can cause gastrointestinal disease, although in most cases the GI features are part of a multisystem disorder. For example, mutations in the mitochondrial tRNAs for tryptophan[62] or lysine[63] can both cause neuro-gastrointestinal syndromes.

Single deletions of mtDNA

The distinction between single and multiple mtDNA deletions helps to differentiate primary mutations of the mitochondrial genome (single deletion/duplication) from nuclear genetic defects (multiple deletions). Single rearrangements most often cause PEO or Kearns–Sayre syndrome (KSS) and, in KSS, undernutrition and features of malnutrition are common. However, both disorders are dominated by neurological features, and do not present with gastrointestinal dysfunction. Nevertheless, dysphagia is common in patients with PEO and there are studies that suggest this is due to cricopharyngeal achalasia.[64] Enteropathy with villous atrophy is also well-recognized in patients with mtDNA rearrangements,[65] and cyclical vomiting[66] and pseudo-obstruction have also been described.

Management

Whilst self-evident, accurate diagnosis is a vital step to provide information about prognosis and possible complications.[67] Diabetes, including presymptomatic glucose intolerance, is a case in point; this should be identified and treated appropriately. Avoiding known mitochondrial toxins is important. Antibiotics such as tetracycline that disrupts intramitochondrial protein synthesis, ciprafloxacin that depletes mtDNA, and aminoglycoside that may cause deafness in sensitive individuals (those carrying a mutation in the 12S rRNA) should be avoided. There are theoretical grounds for avoiding sodium valproate since it may poison fatty acid oxidation and precipitate liver failure. Aerobic exercise is important. How much exercise is difficult to know but several studies point to clear benefits for the patient.[68]

General measures

Nutrition is an important area for any patient with chronic illness. A balanced diet with all the essential nutrients and vitamins is essential. In those individuals with signs of undernutrition or failure to thrive, careful examination of the potential causes is mandatory. Anorexia may be due to CNS disease, e.g. encephalopathy or epilepsy, or lactic acidosis. Vomiting and abdominal discomfort may reflect gastric stasis (pseudo-obstruction). Malabsorption may be present. The underlying defects must be identified before specific treatments can be instituted.

Swallowing is a complex process that can be disrupted at several levels from the oral cavity to the stomach. The reflex activity we call swallowing is controlled by 'swallowing' centers in the medulla oblongata and a total of 30 paired muscles are involved in the process.[5] Dysphagia is common in many forms of MRC disease, particularly those with myopathy such as KSS or CPEO. Videofluoroscopy and pressure studies in KSS suggest that the lesion lies at the level of the pharynx[69] and cricopharyngeal achalasia has been identified.[64] Cricopharyngeal myotomy may help these individuals, although no controlled trials of surgical treatment have been conducted. Proper assessment by qualified personnel is important, and simple measures, such as changing the type of food from solid to liquid may help when surgical intervention is deemed inappropriate.

Whether a clear cause for the dysphagia is identified or not, it is important to make sure that patients receive adequate caloric intake as well as essential vitamins and nutrients. It is also important to consider early intervention before undernutrition becomes an established pattern.

Since these patients have chronic disorders, any intervention will necessarily be long-term. For this reason, intravenous feeding is inappropriate. Enteral feeding is the preferred route and there are different options, including nasogastric feeding, percutaneous gastrostomy, or jejunostomy. A discussion of the advantages and disadvantages of each type of device is unnecessary here (see the discussion in reference 5) and in part will depend on the local expertise. Nasogastric tubes, however, have to be replaced often and appear in most studies to increase the risk of aspiration.

The type and amount of calories given will depend on age and level of activity. Since the defect in these patients lies in the terminal part of energy metabolism, there are no theoretical advantages to choosing one form of calorie, e.g. carbohydrate, over another, such as fat. In the absence of frank diabetes or glucose intolerance, I suggest a balanced diet and allow the dietician to prescribe the composition best suited to the patient's needs. Special requirements, such as pancreatic enzymes for those with exocrine pancreatic insufficiency will, of course, be added to the mixture.

The question of growth retardation in children is an interesting and difficult one. Indeed, many patients with mtDNA disease are small in stature. It is unclear how much this is due to calorie starvation, how much is secondary to the energy defect itself, and how much is hormonal, for example due to growth hormone deficiency. The need for adequate and timely nutritional support cannot be overemphasized. Currently, we have no method of replenishing energy stores. Growth hormone deficiency is seen particularly in KSS, but also in MELAS, and the question is whether we should treat these patients with growth hormone. As far as I am aware, there are no studies (controlled or otherwise) to help us answer this riddle and even case reports are sparse. In one study,[70] a patient with MERRF was given growth hormone to treat weight loss and muscle wasting. The patient's exercise capacity improved but there was no change in body composition.

Theoretically, increasing cellular activity to foster growth could precipitate metabolic problems in the presence of energy depletion. These should manifest systemically and could be monitored in a child receiving growth hormone. Much would depend on how many tissues are affected and on the degree of energy/mitochondrial dysfunction. The issue of whether a larger individual (i.e. more sick cells) would respond better than a smaller one is outside the scope of this chapter.

Lastly, is there a place for transplantation for liver failure due to MRC disease? As far as I can see, this question has been addressed only in children, and then not in a controlled study. In ten patients (five from one article and a further five taken from other publications)[71] in which liver transplantation was performed for delayed liver failure (coming on after 2 months), Dubern and colleagues describe mixed results, depending on whether or not extra-hepatic disease was also present. Five of the children survived and were reported doing well, while one had moderate muscular involvement 4–24 months after transplantation. The article suggests a thorough examination for evidence of extra-hepatic involvement, including imaging of the brain and muscle biopsy. In the presence of isolated liver failure, there may indeed be a place for transplantation.

Acknowledgments

I would like to thank Esther Downham for reading through the manuscript.

References

1. Chinnery PF, Schon EA. Mitochondria. *J Neurol Neurosurg Psychiatry* 2003; **74**: 1188–1199.
2. Gillis LA, Sokol RJ. Gastrointestinal manifestations of mitochondrial disease. *Gastroent Clin North Amer* 2003; **32**: 1–29.
3. Munnich A, Rustin P. Clinical spectrum and diagnosis of mitochondrial disorders. *Am. J Med Genet* 2001; **106**: 4–17.

4. von Kleist-Retzow JC, Cormier-Daire V, Viot G et al. Antenatal manifestations of mitochondrial respiratory chain deficiency. *J Pediatr* 2003; **143**: 208–212.
5. Quigley M, Pfeiffer RF. *Neuro-gastroenterology*. Philadelphia: Butterworth-Heinemann, 2004.
6. Morris AAM. Mitochondrial respiratory chain disorders and the liver. *Liver* 1999; **19**: 357–368.
7. Moraes CT, Shanske S, Tritschler HJ et al. MtDNA depletion with variable tissue expression: A novel genetic abnormality in mitochondrial diseases. *Am J Hum Genet* 1991; **48**: 492–501.
8. Valnot I, Osmond S, Gigarel N et al. Mutations of the *SCO1* gene in mitochondrial cytochrome *c* oxidase deficiency with neonatal-onset hepatic failure and encephalopathy. *Am J Hum Genet* 2000; **67**: 1104–1109.
9. Moraes CT, Zeviani M, Schon EA et al. Mitochondrial DNA deletion in a girl with features of Kearns–Sayre and Lowe syndromes: An example of phenotypic mimicry? *Am J Med Genet* 1991; **41**: 301–305.
10. Mandel H, Hartman C, Berkowitz D et al. The hepatic mitochondrial DNA depletion syndrome: Ultrastructural changes in liver biopsies. *Hepatology* 2001; **34**: 776–784.
11. Mandel H, Szargel R, Labay V et al. The deoxyguanosine kinase gene is mutated in individuals with depleted hepatocerebral mitochondrial DNA. *Nature Genet* 2001; **29**: 337–341.
12. Naviaux RK, Nguyen KV. *POLG* mutations associated with Alpers' syndrome and mitochondrial DNA depletion. *Ann Neurol* 2004; **55**: 706–712.
13. Saada A, Shaag A, Mandel H et al. Mutant mitochondrial thymidine kinase in mitochondrial DNA depletion myopathy. *Nature Genet* 2001; **29**: 342–344.
14. Saada A, Shaag A, Elpeleg O. mtDNA depletion myopathy: elucidation of the tissue specificity in the mitochondrial thymidine kinase (TK2) deficiency. *Mol Genet Metab* 2003; **79**: 1–5.
15. Shoubridge EA. Cytochrome *c* oxidase deficiency. *Am J Med Genet* 2001; **106**: 46–52.
16. Zhu Z, Yao J, Johns T et al. *SURF1*, encoding a factor involved in the biogenesis of cytochrome *c* oxidase, is mutated in Leigh syndrome. *Nature Genet* 1998; **20**: 337–343.
17. Tiranti V, Jaksch M, Hofmann S et al. Loss-of-function mutations of *SURF-1* are specifically associated with Leigh syndrome with cytochrome c oxidase deficiency. *Ann Neurol* 1999; **46**: 161–166.
18. Papadopoulou LC, Sue CM, Davidson MM et al. Fatal infantile cardioencephalomyopathy with COX deficiency and mutations in *SCO2*, a COX assembly gene. *Nature Genet* 1999; **23**: 333–337.
19. Jaksch M, Ogilvie I, Yao J et al. Mutations in *SCO2* are associated with a distinct form of hypertrophic cardiomyopathy and cytochrome *c* oxidase deficiency. *Hum Mol Genet* 2000; **9**: 795–801.
20. Antonicka H, Leary SC, Guercin G-H et al. Mutations in *COX10* result in a defect in mitochondrial heme A biosynthesis and account for multiple, early-onset clinical phenotypes associated with isolated COX deficiency. *Hum Mol Genet* 2003; **12**: 2693–2702.
21. Xu Z, Jung C, Higgins C et al. Mitochondrial degeneration in amyotrophic lateral sclerosis. *J Bioenerg Biomembr* 2004; **36**: 395–399.
22. Tiranti V, D'Adamo P, Briem E et al. Ethylmalonic encephalopathy is caused by mutations in *ETHE1*, a gene encoding a mitochondrial matrix protein. *Am J Hum Genet* 2004; **74**: 239–252.
23. Rasmussen M, Sanengen T, Skullerud K et al. Evidence that Alpers-Huttenlocher syndrome could be a mitochondrial disease. *J Child Neurol* 2000; **15**: 473–477.
24. Uusimaa J, Finnila S, Vainionpaa L et al. A mutation in mitochondrial DNA-encoded cytochrome *c* oxidase II gene in a child with Alpers-Huttenlocher-like disease. *Pediatrics* 2003; **111**: e262–e268.
25. Ferrari G, Lamantea E, Donati A et al. Infantile hepatocerebral syndromes associated with mutations in the mitochondrial DNA polymerase-γA. *Brain* 2005; **128**(4): 723–731.
26. Davidzon G, Mancuso M, Ferraris S et al. *POLG* mutations and Alpers syndrome. *Ann Neurol* 2005; **57**: 921–924.
27. Morris AAM, Carr A. HIV nucleoside analogues: new adverse effects on mitochondria? *Lancet* 1999; **354**: 1046–1047.
28. John M, Moore CB, James IR et al. Chronic hyperlactatemia in HIV-infected patients taking antiretroviral therapy. *AIDS* 2001; **15**: 795–797.
29. Gerard Y, Maulin L, Yazdanpanah Y et al. Symptomatic hyperlactatemia: an emerging complication of antiretroviral therapy. *AIDS* 2000; **14**: 2723–2730.
30. Onishi H, Hanihara T, Sugiyama N et al. Pancreatic exocrine dysfunction associated with mitochondrial

tRNA(Leu)(UUR) mutation. *J Med Genet* 1998; **35**: 255–257.
31. Pearson HA, Lobel JS, Kocoshis SA et al. A new syndrome of refractory sideroblastic anemia with vacuolization of marrow precursors and exocrine pancreatic dysfunction. *J Pediatr* 1979; **95**: 976–984.
32. Rötig A, Bourgeron T, Chretien D et al. Spectrum of mitochondrial DNA rearrangements in the Pearson marrow-pancreas syndrome. *Hum Mol Genet* 1995; **4**: 1327–1330.
33. Rotig A, Cormier V, Blanche S et al. Pearson's marrow-pancreas syndrome. A multisystem mitochondrial disorder in infancy. *J Clin Invest* 1990; **86**: 1601–1608.
34. Superti-Furga A, Schoenle E, Tuchschmidt P et al. Pearson marrow-pancreas syndrome with insulin-dependent diabetes, progressive renal tubulopathy, organic aciduria and elevated fetal haemoglobin caused by deletion and duplication of mitochondrial DNA. *Eur J Pediatr* 1993; **152**: 44–50.
35. Chinnery PF, DiMauro S, Shanske S et al. Risk of developing a mitochondrial DNA deletion disorder. *Lancet* 2004; **364**: 592–595.
36. Nishino I, Spinazzola A, Hirano M. Thymidine phosphorylase gene mutations in MNGIE, a human mitochondrial disorder. *Science* 1999; **283**: 689–692.
37. Bedlack RS, Vu TH, Hammans S et al. MNGIE neuropathy: five cases mimicking chronic inflammatory demyelinating polyneuropathy. *Muscle Nerve* 2004; **29**: 364–368.
38. Szigeti K, Wong LJ, Perng CL et al. MNGIE with lack of skeletal muscle involvement and a novel *TP* splice site mutation. *J Med Genet* 2004; **41**: 125–129.
39. Anuras S, Mitros F, Nowak T et al. A familial visceral myopathy with external ophthalmoplegia and autosomal recessive transmission. *Gastroenterology* 1983; **84**: 346–353.
40. Simon LT, Horoupian DS, Dorfman LJ et al. Polyneuropathy, ophthalmoplegia, leukoencephalopathy, and intestinal pseudo-obstruction: POLIP syndrome. *Ann Neurol* 1990; **28**: 349–360.
41. Bardosi A, Creutzfeldt W, DiMauro S et al. Myo-, neuro-, gastrointestinal encephalopathy (MNGIE syndrome) due to partial deficiency of cytochrome-c-oxidase. A new mitochondrial multisystem disorder. *Acta Neuropathol* 1987; **74**: 248–258.
42. Nishino I, Spinazzola A, Hirano M. MNGIE: from nuclear DNA to mitochondrial DNA. *Neuromusc Disord* 2001; **11**: 7–10.
43. Van Goethem G, Dermaut B, Lofgren A et al. Mutation of *POLG* is associated with progressive external ophthalmoplegia characterized by mtDNA deletions. *Nature Genet* 2001; **28**: 211–212.
44. Winterthun S, Ferrari G, He L et al. Autosomal recessive mitochondrial ataxic syndrome due to mitochondrial polymerase gamma mutations. *Neurology* 2005; **64**: 1204–1208.
45. Kaukonen J, Juselius JK, Tiranti V et al. Role of adenine nucleotide translocator 1 in mtDNA maintenance. *Science* 2000; **289**: 782–785.
46. Lamantea E, Tiranti V, Bordoni A et al. Mutations of mitochondrial DNA polymerase γA are a frequent cause of autosomal dominant or recessive progressive external ophthalmoplegia. *Ann Neurol* 2002; **52**: 211–219.
47. van Erven PM, Cillessen JP, Eekhoff EM et al. Leigh syndrome, a mitochondrial encephalo(myo)pathy. A review of the literature. *Clin Neurol Neurosurg* 1987; **89**: 217–230.
48. Uziel G, Moroni I, Lamantea E et al. The mitochondrial disease associated with the T8993G mutation of mitochondrial ATPase 6 gene: a clinical, biochemical, and molecular study in six families. *J Neurol Neurosurg Psychiat* 1997; **63**: 16–22.
49. Chol M, Lebon S, Benit P et al. The mitochondrial DNA G13513A MELAS mutation in the NADH dehydrogenase 5 gene is a frequent cause of Leigh-like syndrome with isolated complex I deficiency. *J Med Genet* 2003; **40**: 188–191.
50. Tiranti V, Hoertnagel K, Carrozzo R et al. Mutations of *SURF-1* in Leigh disease associated with cytochrome c oxidase deficiency. *Am J Hum Genet* 1998; **63**: 1609–1621.
51. Smeitink JAM, Sengers RCA, Trijbels F, Van den Heuvel B. Human NADH:ubiquinone oxidoreductase. *J Bioenerg Biomembr* 2001; **33**: 250–266.
52. Bourgeron T, Rustin P, Chretien D et al. Mutation of a nuclear succinate dehydrogenase gene results in mitochondrial respiratory chain deficiency. *Nature Genet* 1995; **11**: 144–149.
53. Wijburg FA, Barth PG, Bindoff L et al. Leigh syndrome associated with a deficiency of the pyruvate dehydrogenase complex: results of treatment with a ketogenic diet. *Neuropediatrics* 1992; **23**: 147–152.
54. Leigh D. Subacute necrotizing encephalomyelopathy in an infant. *J Neurol Neurosurg Psychiat* 1951; **14**: 216–221.

55. Mitomap. MITOMAP: A human mitochondrial genome database. http://www.mitomap.org. 2003
56. Goto Y, Nonaka I, Horai S. A mutation in the $\mathrm{tRNA}^{\mathrm{Leu(UUR)}}$ gene associated with the MELAS subgroup of mitochondrial encephalomyopathies. *Nature* 1990; **348**: 651–653.
57. Shimotake T, Furukawa T, Inoue K et al. Familial occurrence of intestinal obstruction in children with the syndrome of mitochondrial encephalomyopathy, lactic acidosis, and strokelike episodes (MELAS). *J Pediatr Surg* 1998; **33**: 1837–1839.
58. Campos Y, Lorenzo G, Martin MA et al. A mitochondrial $\mathrm{tRNA}^{\mathrm{Lys}}$ gene mutation (T8316C) in a patient with mitochondrial myopathy, lactic acidosis, and stroke-like episodes. *Neuromusc Disord* 2000; **10**: 493–496.
59. Kishimoto M, Hashiramoto M, Kanda F et al. Mitochondrial DNA mutations in a diabetic patient with gastrointestinal symptoms. *Lancet* 1995; **345**: 452.
60. Hess J, Burkhard P, Morris M et al. Ischaemic colitis due to mitochondrial cytopathy [letter]. *Lancet* 1995; **346**: 189–190.
61. Chinnery PF, Jones S, Sviland L et al. Mitochondrial enteropathy: the primary pathology may not be within the gastrointestinal tract. *Gut* 2001; **48**: 121–124.
62. Maniura-Weber K, Taylor RW, Johnson MA et al. A novel point mutation in the mitochondrial $\mathrm{tRNA}^{\mathrm{Trp}}$ gene produces a neurogastrointestinal syndrome. *Eur J Hum Genet* 2004; **12**: 509–512.
63. Verma A, Piccoli DA, Bonilla E et al. A novel mitochondrial G8313A mutation associated with prominent initial gastrointestinal symptoms and progressive encephaloneuropathy. *Pediatr Res* 1997; **42**: 448–454.
64. Kornblum C, Broicher R, Walther E et al. Cricopharyngeal achalasia is a common cause of dysphagia in patients with mtDNA deletions. *Neurology* 2001; **56**: 1409–1412.
65. Nishino I, Spinazzola A, Papadimitriou A et al. Mitochondrial neurogastrointestinal encephalomyopathy: an autosomal recessive disorder due to thymidine phosphorylase mutations. *Ann Neurol* 2000; **47**: 792–800.
65. Cormier-Daire V, Bonnefont J-P, Rustin P et al. Mitochondrial DNA rearrangements with onset as chronic diarrhea with villous atrophy. *J Pediatr* 1994; **124**: 63–70.
66. Boles RG, Chun N, Senadheera D, Wond L-J. Cyclical vomiting syndrome and mitochondrial DNA mutations. *Lancet* 1997; **350**: 1299–1300.
67. Bindoff L. Treatment of mitochondrial disorders: practical and theoretical issues. *Eur J Pediatr Neurol* 1999; **3**: 201–208.
68. Taivassalo T, Haller RG. Implications of exercise training in mtDNA defects – use or lose it? *Biochim Biophys Acta* 2004; **1659**: 221–231.
69. Katsanos KH, Nastos D, Noussias V et al. Manometric study in Kearns-Sayre syndrome. *Dis Esophagus* 2001; **14**: 63–66.
70. Carroll PV, Umpleby AM, Albany E et al. Growth hormone therapy may benefit protein metabolism in mitochondrial encephalomyopathy. *Clin Endocrinol* 1997; **47**: 113–117.
71. Dubern B, Broue P, Dubuisson C et al. Orthotopic liver transplantation for mitochondrial respiratory chain disorders: a study of 5 children. *Transplantation* 2001; **71**: 633–637.
72. Jackson MJ, Schaefer JA, Johnson MA et al. Presentation and clinical investigation of mitochondrial respiratory chain disease. A study of 51 patients. *Brain* 1995; **118**: 339–357.
73. Chinnery PF, Wardell TM, Singh-Kler R et al. The epidemiology of pathogenic mitochondrial DNA mutations. *Ann Neurol* 2000; **48**: 188–193.

7

Mitochondrial otology

Patrick F Chinnery and Timothy D Griffiths

Introduction

Impaired hearing is a common feature of mitochondrial disease,[1,2] often remaining undetected for many years and overshadowed by more acute or physically disabling aspects of a multisystem disorder.[3] However, unlike many other complications of mitochondrial dysfunction, hearing impairment often responds well to treatment.[4] Physicians should therefore keep the auditory system at the front of their mind each time they see a new patient with suspected mitochondrial disease, or when they review patients with an established diagnosis. Laboratory investigations should be used to detect sub-clinical hearing loss, leading to appropriate treatment as soon as it becomes a significant problem. In this chapter, we will review the auditory system, clinical audiological investigation, and discuss the different ways that hearing impairment can present in mitochondrial disorders.

A deeper understanding of mitochondrial otopathology has important implications, providing unique insight into disease mechanisms that are likely to have broader relevance for other mitochondrial disorders. For example, clinical and genetic studies of families transmitting the 1555A→G mitochondrial DNA (mtDNA) mutation demonstrate the way that specific environmental factors can interact with the mitochondrion and cause disease (aminoglycoside sensitivity), and point towards a complex interaction between nuclear and mitochondrial genomes. Although mitochondrial dysfunction may also play an important part in much more common causes of deafness (including age-related hearing loss, or presbyacusis,[5,6] and hair-cell survival after toxin and noise-induced auditory damage[7]), this lies beyond the scope of this chapter.

The auditory system

The first stage of the auditory system is the cochlea where incoming sound energy is converted to a neural code in the auditory nerve. Sound creates a traveling wave along the basilar membrane where the position of the peak of the wave is dependent on the frequency of the incoming sound. Figure 7.1 shows a cross-section through the organ of Corti in the cochlea. The traveling wave displaces the stereocilia at the apex of the inner hair cells, leading to membrane depolarization, which in turn results in neural impulses in the corresponding branch of the auditory nerve. The transduction process is not determined by the passive mechanical properties of the cochlear partition alone. The outer hair cells contract and change the stiffness of the cochlear partition.[8,9] The resulting tuning with respect to frequency is greater than would be explained by the passive mechanical properties of the cochlea. Both inner and outer hair cells are rich in mitochondria, as is the stria vascularis, responsible for

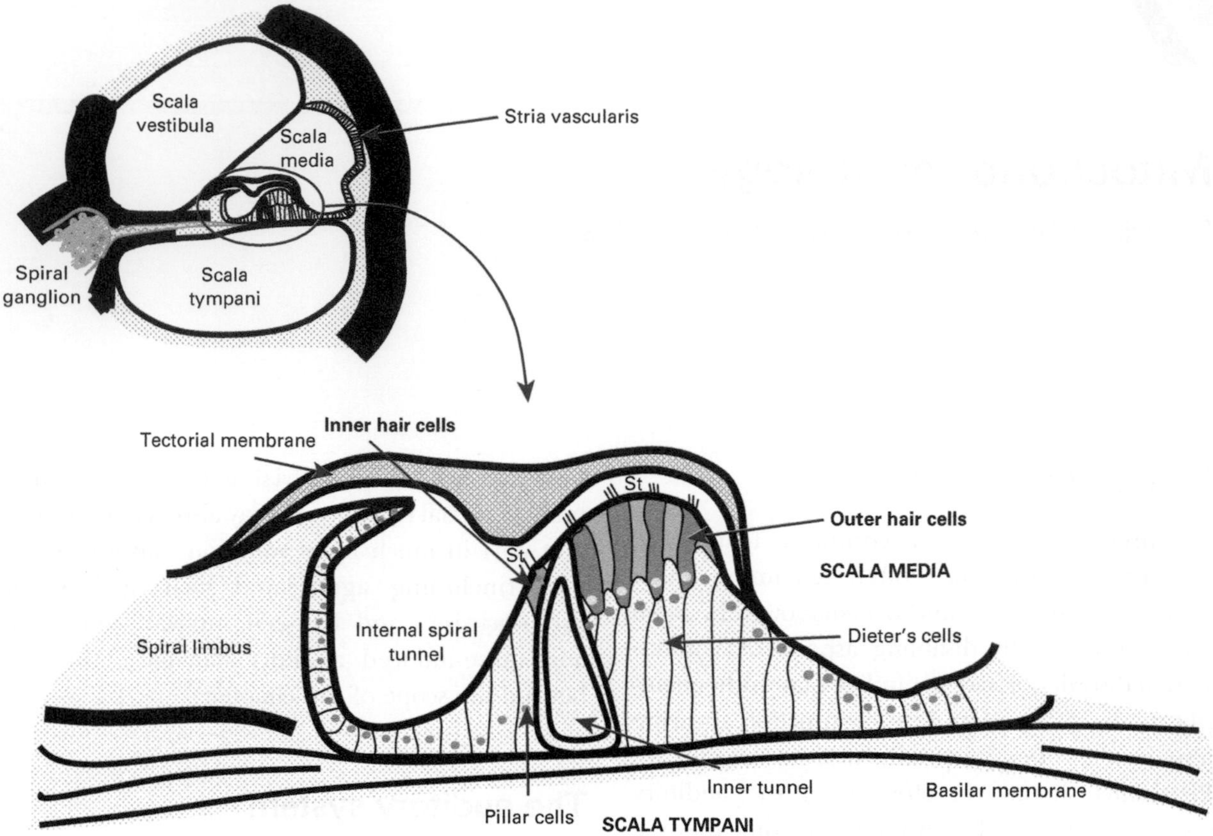

Figure 7.1 Cross-section of the cochlea (with thanks to Dr Steve Durham). St = stereocilia

generating the endolymphatic potential upon which the transduction process depends.

The central auditory pathway connects the cochlear nuclei, the first synapses of the auditory nerve in the brainstem, with the auditory cortices in the superior temporal plane. This pathway carries out further processing of sound information to allow the extraction of auditory features and the analysis of patterns in the time and frequency domains.[10] A more detailed account of the central pathway is beyond the scope of this review.

Normal hearing is therefore dependent upon the integrated function of a number of highly energy-dependent components. In the cochlea, the stria vascularis maintains the ionic gradients necessary for sound transduction and the complex interaction between inner and outer hair cells.[11] These components are highly metabolically active,[12,13] and it is likely that a respiratory chain defect and the attendant relative deficiency of intracellular ATP would impair the function of both the stria and the hair cells,[14] ultimately leading to cell death, possibly through apoptosis.[15] Likewise, neurons within the spiral ganglion and auditory nerve, brainstem nuclei and their connections within the mid-brain, and auditory cortical neurons are all energy-dependent with high rates of basal neuronal firing. In mammals, *all* of these components are post-mitotic, including the stria vascularis and hair cells.[16] These characteristics render them particularly vulnerable to the effects of mitochondrial DNA (mtDNA) mutations, which tend to accumulate in post-mitotic tissues throughout

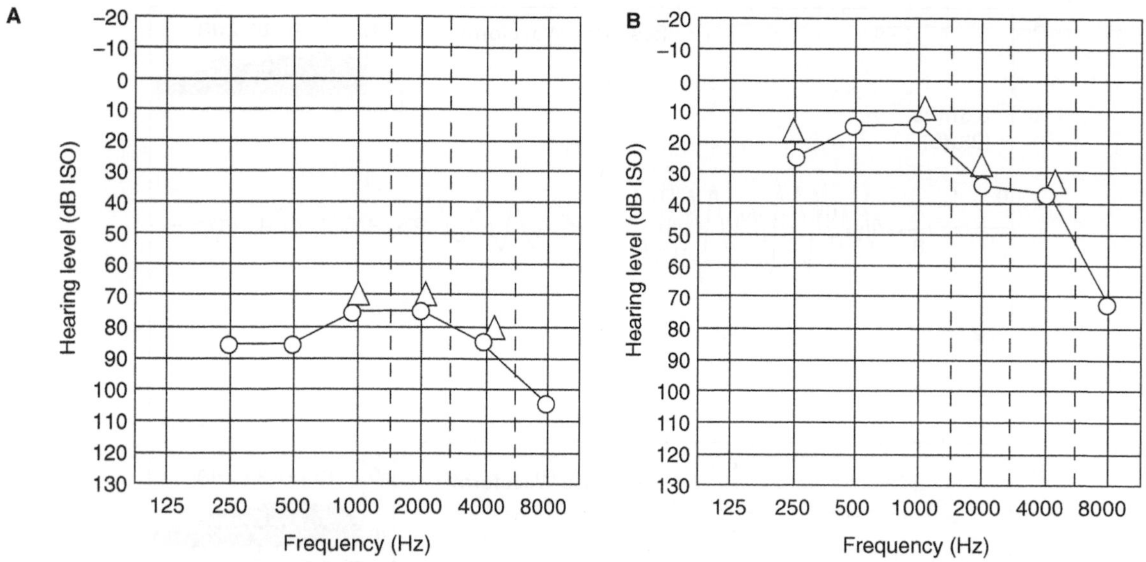

Figure 7.2 Pure tone audiograms showing: (**A**) severe hearing loss across all frequencies in a 44-year-old male harboring the mtDNA 3243A→G $tRNA^{Leu(UUR)}$ mutation; and (**B**) high-frequency hearing loss in a 56-year-old male with Kearns–Sayre syndrome due to a single 4.7-kb deletion of mtDNA. Open circles = air conduction, open triangles = bone conduction. dB = decibel hearing loss, ISO = international standards organization. Reproduced with permission from Oxford University Press, *Brain* 2000; **123**: 82–92

life in patients with heteroplasmic mtDNA disorders.[17]

Clinical investigation of the auditory system

Mitochondrial disorders are often characterized by cochlear deafness, which can be evaluated using the pure tone audiogram as a standard clinical tool (Figure 7.2). Deafness is not just a straightforward loss of transduction at the inner hair cell, and can actually be modeled as having two components that are associated with dysfunction of the inner and outer hair cells.[18] The separate assessment of inner and outer hair cell function requires more sophisticated psychophysical techniques (see below). Otoacoustic emissions[19] are measurements of sounds produced by the cochlea itself and depend upon the active mechanism described above (Figure 7.3).

Beyond the cochlea, the function of the auditory nerve and ascending pathway can be assessed using brainstem evoked electroencephalogram (EEG) potentials measured in response to sound clicks (Figure 7.4). Waves I and II of the brainstem potential arise from the auditory nerve, whilst waves III to V arise from central brainstem structures below the inferior colliculus in the tectum. Structural imaging using magnetic resonance imaging allows identification of lesions within the ascending auditory pathway (Figure 7.5). The detailed assessment of central auditory pathologies is further described in reference 20.

In the future, functional magnetic resonance imaging and magnetoencephalography may develop into clinical tools for the assessment of central auditory processing.[21] At the moment, these are primarily research tools.

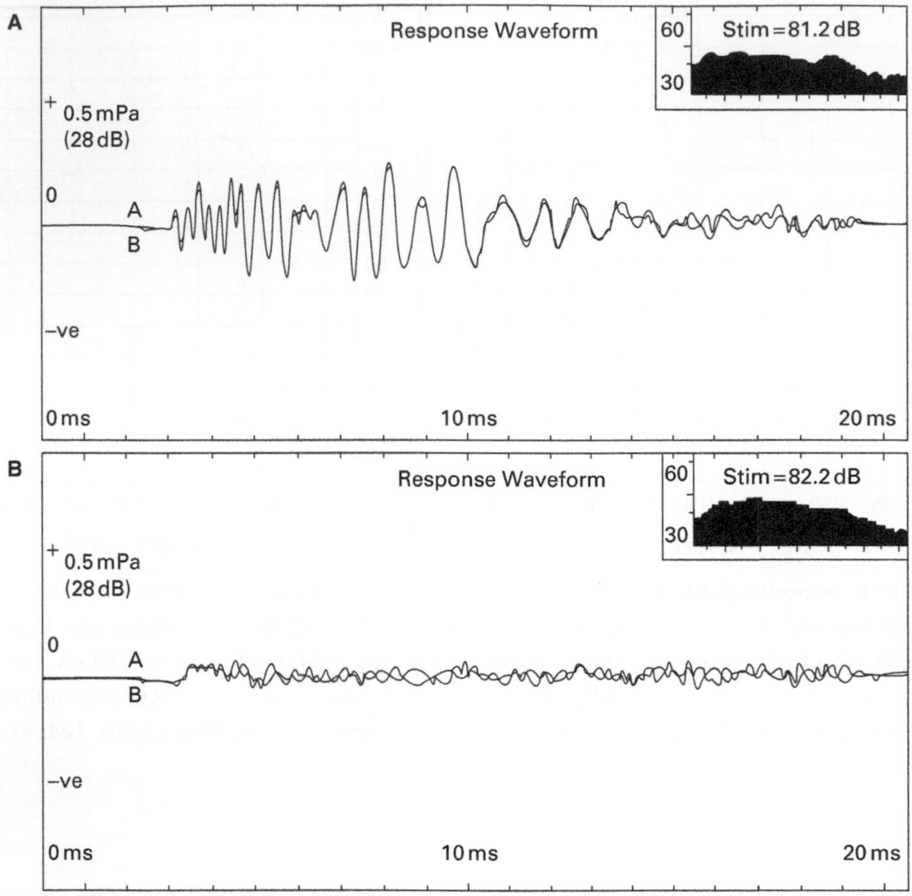

Figure 7.3 Otoacoustic emissions: (**A**) present in a normal individual; and (**B**) absent in a 48-year-old female harboring the mtDNA 3243A→G $tRNA^{Leu(UUR)}$ mutation. Reproduced with permission from Oxford University Press, *Brain* 2000; **123**: 82–92

Mitochondrial otopathology

The pathological examination of the inner ear is technically demanding, highly specialized, and only possible post-mortem. There have therefore only been a few detailed pathological studies of the auditory system in patients with mitochondrial disease. Although important, these studies provide limited insight because the tissue was examined many years after the onset of hearing impairment, only leaving passing clues as to the primary pathological event. Pathological changes were severe in a girl with Kearns–Sayre syndrome, with almost complete absence of the organ of Corti, a reduction of 60–70% of cells in the spiral ganglion, and almost complete degeneration of nerve fibers in the bony spiral lamina[22,23] (see Table 7.1 for a summary of the Kearns–Sayre syndrome). In a middle-aged patient with diabetes and deafness due to the 3243A→G mtDNA $tRNA^{Leu(UUR)}$ gene mutation, the stria vascularis was markedly atrophic throughout the whole cochlea, and there was a profound loss of outer hair cells (OHCs). Intriguingly, the inner hair cells and supporting cells were minimally affected, along with Reissner's membrane. In the

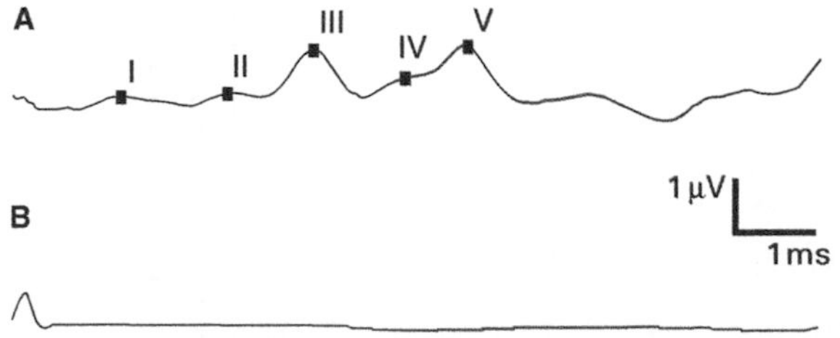

Figure 7.4 Brain stem evoked responses: (**A**) normal response from a 33-year-old male harboring a single 4-kb deletion of mtDNA; and (**B**) absent response in a 39-year-old female with severe hearing loss harboring the mtDNA 3243A→G tRNA$^{Leu(UUR)}$ mutation. Signal averaged response for the left ear due to alternate compression and rarefaction clicks at 8 Hz. Offline filtering was carried out using a pass band of 100 Hz to 3 kHz. Reproduced with permission from Oxford University Press, *Brain* 2000; **123**: 82–92

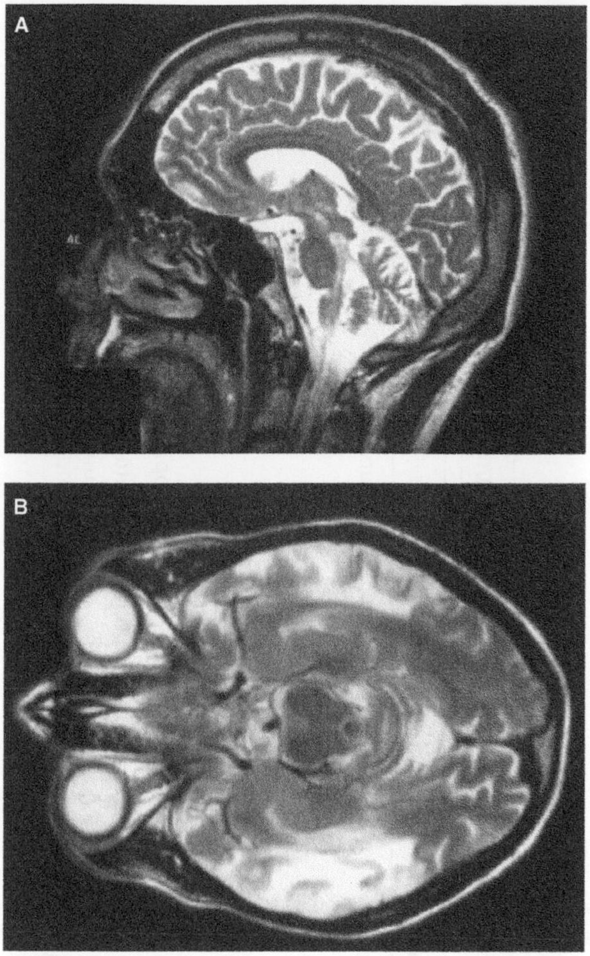

Figure 7.5 MRI imaging. (**A**) Midline T2-weighted fast spin echo (FSE) image. Abnormal high signal is noted extending bilaterally from the medulla through the midbrain in a 30-year-old male with the Kearns–Sayre syndrome due to a single 7 kb deletion of mtDNA. (**B**) Axial T_2-weighted FSE image at the level of the midbrain showing generalized atrophy with bilateral temporal lobe infarction in a 39-year-old female with the mtDNA 3243A→G tRNA$^{Leu(UUR)}$ mutation. Reproduced with permission from Oxford University Press, *Brain* 2000; **123**: 82–92

spiral ganglion, the neurons corresponding to the basal cochlea were preferentially affected.[23] By contrast, post-mortem examination of the inner ear in a patient with a loss-of-function mutation in the nuclear gene *DDP1/TIMM8a* which affects mitochondrial protein import (see Table 7.1, and below), showed near complete loss of the spiral ganglion cells and both central and peripheral processes, but striking preservation of the organ of Corti, hair cells and stria vascularis.[24] Thus, the pathological features in at least one nuclear genetic mitochondrial disorder are almost the mirror image of those in two mtDNA disorders, although all are thought to cause a defect of ATP production by the respiratory chain. The reason for this discrepancy must therefore lie elsewhere.

The clinical phenotype of mitochondrial deafness: a clue to the pathophysiology

Physiological and psychophysical studies of the auditory system in patients with mitochondrial disease do provide insight into the underlying pathology. Hearing loss is usually peripheral (due to cochlear or auditory nerve dysfunction), but in patients with a multisystem mitochondrial

Table 7.1 Hearing impairment in mitochondrial disease – genotype and phenotype

Category		Syndrome	Principal associated features	Molecular defect	Inheritance
Syndromic	Multi-systemic	KSS	PEO, ptosis, ataxia, pigmentary retinopathy, heart block	mtDNA deletion	S
		CPEO	+/– Proximal limb weakness	mtDNA deletion or point mutation	S or M
		MELAS	Seizures, encephalopathy, stroke-like episodes, diabetes mellitus, cardiomyopathy	mtDNA 3243A→G	M
		Leigh syndrome	Relapsing encephalopathy, ataxia, cardiomyopathy, hepatic failure	Nuclear or mtDNA	M or AR
		Encephalomyopathy	Myopathy, diabetes, encephalopathy, ataxia	mtDNA 14709T→C	M
	Oligosyndromic	MIDD	Diabetes mellitus	mtDNA 3243A→G	M
		MIDD	Diabetes mellitus	mtDNA 8296A→G	M
		MDD	Dystonia, cortical blindness, paranoid delusions	*TIMM8A*	XLR
Non-syndromic (isolated)	Aminoglycoside-induced	D		mtDNA 1555A→G	M
	Non-aminoglycoside-induced	D		mtDNA 1555A→G	M
		D		mtDNA 3243A→G	M
		D		mtDNA 7445A→G	M
		D		mtDNA 7472insC	M
		D		mtDNA 7511T→C	M

AR = autosomal recessive; CPEO = chronic progressive external ophthalmoplegia; D = isolated (non-syndromic) deafness; KSS = Kearns–Sayre syndrome; MELAS = mitochondrial encephalomyopathy with lactic acidosis and stroke-like episodes; MIDD = maternally inherited diabetes and deafness; M = maternal inheritance; S = sporadic; XLR = X-linked recessive.

disorder, the auditory system may be affected at the brain stem, midbrain or at a higher level in the auditory cortex.

The peripheral hearing loss typically affects high frequencies first, followed by intermediate frequencies, and finally involving low frequencies and causing the typical 'flat' audiogram seen in a severely deaf individual (Figure 7.2).[3,25,26] The preferential involvement of high frequencies corresponds to the pathological features in a patient with 3243A→G reported by Yamasoba et al.[23] and may be related to the relatively high energy requirements of the basal cochlea. The vast majority of patients with mitochondrial deafness have absent otoacoustic emissions (Figure 7.3), providing strong evidence that the cochlea is the component most sensitive to mitochondrial dysfunction.[3,26–28]

Recently developed psychophysical techniques make it is possible to tease out the various components of the cochlea in vivo.[29,30] Techniques are available for the estimation of inner hair cell death, and for the assessment of auditory filter widths, which are dependent on active mechanisms involving the outer hair cells. Using this approach, Griffiths et al. studied 11 patients harboring the 3243A→G mutation, and showed evidence of both inner and outer hair cell dysfunction in mitochondrial deafness.[31] The inner hair cell dysfunction preferentially involved the basal (high-frequency) cochlea and was apparent even in patients with mild hearing loss detected by speech and pure tone audiometry, while outer hair cell dysfunction was noted in some patients with near-normal hearing. This study identified selective deficits over specific frequency ranges, providing evidence against a generalized effect of the metabolic deficit on the stria vascularis, and in favor of a specific effect on the hair cells themselves. In terms of the specific hair cells affected, the technique for assessment of inner hair cell dysfunction in this study actually measures cell death, as opposed to the technique for the assessment of outer hair cell dysfunction, which can detect a more subtle impairment. It is not possible, therefore, to make any categorical statement about the relative effect on hair cell types, although both are affected by the process. These findings correspond to the pathological features noted postmortem in patients with 3243A→G,[23] but contrast with the autopsy findings in other mitochondrial disorders,[24] thus illustrating the different cochlear mechanisms involved in different mitochondrial disorders.

Detailed physiological studies of centrally mediated mitochondrial deafness are usually not possible because the severe peripheral component prevents physiological stimuli from reaching the brainstem pathways (Figure 7.4). High-resolution structural imaging can be helpful in this context, demonstrating high signal on T2-weighted imaging within the brainstem and involving the central auditory pathways and the auditory cortex (Figure 7.5).

Mitochondrial otopathology: the relationship between genotype and phenotype

Hearing impairment is common in patients with mitochondrial disorders, affecting over half of all cases at some time in the course of the disease.[3,32] Although the final common pathway for the hearing loss is thought to involve ATP deficiency secondary to a biochemical defect of the respiratory chain, the clinical presentation of mitochondrial deafness varies considerably – both in terms of associated clinical features and of natural history. These factors have a profound impact on clinical management as will be discussed in the next section.

The spectrum of mitochondrial hearing loss is summarized in Table 7.1. In some patients, deafness is only part of a multisystem disorder, often involving the central nervous system, neuromuscular system or endocrine organs. In severe

Box 7.1 Transcription of mitochondrial DNA

Transcription of human mtDNA is 'prokaryotic-like'. Instead of transcribing each of the 37 genes separately, as would be the case for transcription of nuclear genes, two giant 16-kb polycistronic precursor transcripts are synthesized, one encoded by the L-strand and the other by the H-strand.[1] There are two closely spaced promoters, both located within the D-loop, controlling transcription of the respective heavy- and light-strands (HSP and LSP; see Figure B7.1.1). Most of the 37 genes – both rRNAs, 14 tRNAs, and 12 of the 13 polypeptide-coding genes – are encoded by the H-strand (meaning that they have the same sequence as the L-strand); only eight tRNAs and one mRNA (ND6) are encoded by the L-strand. It is thought that the tRNAs, which 'punctuate' the genes around the circle, are excised precisely from the precursor RNAs, thereby releasing not only the tRNAs, but the flanking rRNAs and mRNAs as well.[2] Following cleavage, the 3′ termini of the mRNAs are polyadenylated and the tRNAs acquire certain base modifications and additions. OH and OL are origins of replication of the heavy and light strands, respectively, in the Clayton model (see Box 3.1).

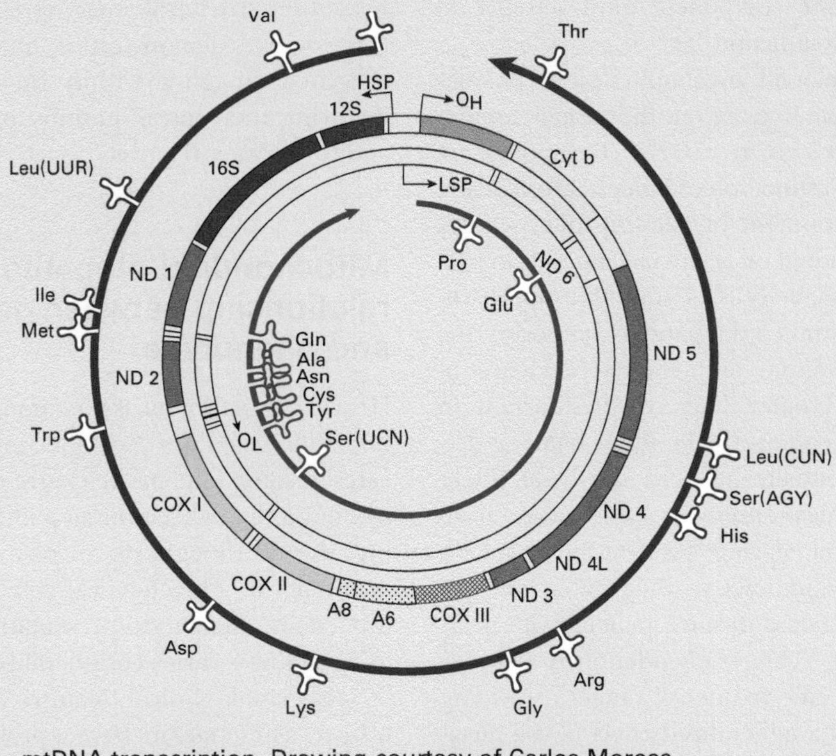

Figure B7.1.1 mtDNA transcription. Drawing courtesy of Carlos Moraes

References

1. Gaspari M, Larsson NG, Gustafsson CM. The transcription machinery in mammalian mitochondria. *Biochim Biophys Acta* 2004; **1659**: 148–152.
2. Attardi G, Chomyn A, King MP et al. Regulation of mitochondrial gene expression in mammalian cells. *Biochem Soc Trans* 1990; **18**: 509–513.

multisystem disease, such as Kearns–Sayre syndrome, deafness often follows other neurological features such as ataxia, ptosis and external ophthalmoplegia,[33] whereas it may be the presenting feature of other multisystem disorders such as mitochondrial encephalomyopathy with lactic acidosis and stroke-like episodes (MELAS).[34] Deafness may also be prominent in patients with oligosyndromic disease, such as X-linked deafness dystonia,[35] or maternally inherited diabetes and deafness.[36] By contrast, there are also a number of 'pure' mitochondrial deafness disorders, the most common probably being maternally inherited deafness due to the 1555A→G mtDNA mutation, which also causes aminoglycoside-induced deafness.[37,38] The 3243A→G mtDNA tRNA Leu$^{(UUR)}$ mutation also causes a pure deafness phenotype in some families, and a number of mutations in the mtDNA tRNA$^{Ser(UCN)}$ gene also appear to cause isolated maternally inherited deafness.[39–41] All of these molecular defects cause respiratory chain defects with ATP deficiency, and it is not totally clear why the clinical phenotype can vary so much from mutation to mutation. Although the tissue distribution of mutated mtDNA could explain some of the differences (see Chapter 1), this is not the case for 1555A→G and some of the tRNA$^{Ser(UCN)}$ mutations, which are homoplasmic in all tissue studied. Tissue homoplasmy is a particular characteristic of organ-specific pathogenic mtDNA mutations (see discussion in reference 42), and environmental factors appear to be particularly important under these circumstances. In the following sections we will consider the genotype and phenotype of four different mitochondrial deafness syndromes to illustrate these principles.

The mtDNA 3243A→G Leu$^{(UUR)}$ tRNA gene mutation

The mtDNA 3243A→G Leu$^{(UUR)}$ tRNA gene mutation was first described in a patient with mitochondrial encephalomyopathy with lactic acidosis and stroke-like episodes (MELAS), a severe multisystem neurological disorder associated with cardiomyopathy and deafness.[43] It therefore came as a surprise that the same gene defect was identified in a large multigenerational Dutch pedigree segregating with a more limited phenotype – isolated diabetes and deafness.[36] It is now well-recognized that 3243A→G can cause deafness in isolation, although the coexistence of diabetes and maternal inheritance greatly increases the likelihood of this specific disorder when seen in the clinic.[44] Typically, deafness begins in late teenage years or early adult life and is slowly progressive. The natural history has been well documented in Finnish pedigrees.[45] Although a slow relentless decline is the most common course, acute unilateral or bilateral deterioration is also well-recognized, sometimes occurring spontaneously, and sometimes in association with intercurrent febrile illnesses.[3,26,28] In patients with additional neurological and cardiac features, irreversible hearing loss can accompany acute encephalopathic episodes, suggesting a common mechanism involving acute metabolic compromise.

The 3243A→G mutation affects almost every aspect of Leu$^{(UUR)}$ tRNA function.[46] The mutation is predicted to affect tRNA folding, which alters RNA processing, tRNA stability, aminoacylation, base modification and, possibly, the way the tRNA interacts with the ribosome.[46] The 3243A→G mutation is invariably heteroplasmic in affected individuals.[47] In vitro studies using 143B osteosarcoma and A549 lung carcinoma-derived cybrids have shown that the mutation is highly recessive in cell culture. The cybrids only express a biochemical defect when the proportion of mutated mtDNA exceeds 90%, resulting in a marked decrease in intramitochondrial protein synthesis and reduction in cellular oxygen consumption.[48] These effects appear to be particularly severe in cell lines with a relative depletion of total mtDNA.[49] The percentage of mutated mtDNA (mutation load) also appears to be important clinically. In humans, the auditory transduction apparatus is largely composed of post-mitotic (non-dividing) cells. Although it is not possible to study cochlear mutation load in vivo, the percentage level of 3243A→G can be measured in other post-mitotic tissues such as skeletal muscle. The degree of hearing loss correlates well with the mutation load in skeletal muscle,[3] and the progressive nature of the hearing loss may be related to the accumulation of mutated mtDNA within the cochlea. Although this appears to be the general trend, there are clear exceptions to the rule. In one patient with 3243A→G, severe hearing loss was associated with low levels of mutated mtDNA in skeletal muscle.[50] This may occur because of unequal segregation of mutated mtDNA among different tissues during early development, so that occasionally, by chance, high levels are present in the cochlear precursors, and lower levels in skeletal muscle precursor cells.

Although the percentage of mutated mtDNA undoubtedly contributes to the clinical variability seen among patients, this does not provide the whole explanation. It is currently not known why certain maternal pedigrees transmitting 3243A→G tend to develop a pure deafness-diabetes phenotype, whereas others only show ptosis and external ophthalmoplegia, and yet others are affected by the severe multisystem MELAS phenotype.[51] Additional genetic factors are likely to be important, but have yet to be identified.

The mtDNA 1555A→G 12S rRNA gene mutation

The 1555A→G 12S rRNA gene mutation was first described in an Arab-Israeli pedigree with maternally inherited deafness.[37] Most of the affected individuals had a severe and profound sensorineural deafness which began during infancy, but the disorder presented in adult life in some individuals. Subsequent work showed that the 1555A→G mutation also predisposed to aminoglycoside-induced deafness.[37] The mutation makes the human rRNA more like the bacterial rRNA in the region critically important for aminoglycoside sensitivity.[37,52] The 1555A→G mutation was detected in 27% of Spaniards with familial deafness,[38] where it has occurred multiple times in different genetic backgrounds.[53] In Japan, 1555A→G was detected in 3% of all patients with sensorineural deafness attending a hospital outpatient clinic, and 30% of them had a history of aminoglycoside exposure.[54]

With hindsight, the clinical phenotype of the original Arab-Israeli family was unusual. The 1555A→G mutation generally causes late-onset, slowly progressive sensorineural deafness, which, like other forms of mitochondrial deafness, initially affects high frequencies.[55] Typically, the hearing loss is spontaneous and slowly progressive, but acute deterioration is well documented in patients exposed to aminoglycosides such as streptomycin and gentamycin.

Differences in the clinical phenotype are matched in vitro. Cell lines from affected individuals show impaired growth on galactose medium, which selects for respiratory chain function.[56] Cell lines from affected individuals also show more marked growth impairment than cell lines established from unaffected individuals harboring the same homoplasmic mtDNA mutation.[57] However, when mitochondria from these cell lines are transferred to a different nuclear background (143B osteosarcoma cell cybrids), all express growth impairment, irrespective of the growth performance of the parental cell line.[57] These observations highlight the importance of the background nuclear genotype in the phenotypic expression of this disorder in vitro. Segregation analysis in 1555A→G families provides further evidence of a nuclear genetic modifier locus, which appears to be inherited as an autosomal recessive trait. There is clear evidence of a nuclear–mitochondrial interaction in a mouse model of deafness,[58] and there have been various attempts to identify the functional genetic variants in humans, including extensive screening of candidate genes.[59] Recent genetic mapping studies point towards a locus on chromosome 8,[60] and there is preliminary evidence that a polymorphic variant in the untranslated region of the human transcription factor B1M gene (*TFB1M*) may modulate the phenotype.[61]

The mtDNA tRNA Ser$^{(UCN)}$ gene mutations

A number of different point mutations in the mtDNA tRNA Ser$^{(UCN)}$ gene cause progressive, bilateral sensorineural deafness.[39–41] The phenotype is similar to the deafness seen in patients with 1555A→G, but there is no evidence of aminoglycoside sensitivity with these mutations. In the cases described so far, the 7511T→C mutation causes isolated non-syndromic deafness,[40] but other mutations in the same gene are sometimes associated with additional features. For example, the 7445A→G mutation also causes palmoplantar keratoderma,[39] and the 7472insC mutation has been described in a patient with a complex neurological phenotype.[41]

The molecular pathology of the 7445A→G mutation has been well described. This mutation affects pre-tRNA processing,[62] causing a reduction in the steady-state tRNA level and a mild translational defect. The severity of the translational defect is worse in cell lines from patients from severely affected families, suggesting that additional mitochondrial or nuclear genetic factors modify the biochemical and clinical phenotype.[62] The mutation also involves the *COXI* stop codon, but no effect on *COXI* mRNA has been observed. The mutation does, however, affect steady-state levels of the *ND6* mRNA which, like the tRNA Ser$^{(UCN)}$ gene, is also encoded by the mtDNA light (L) strand, suggesting indirectly that the *ND6* and tRNA Ser$^{(UCN)}$ transcripts are generated by the same common pathway. By contrast, the 7472insC mutation is associated with a similar reduction in the steady-state tRNA level and an extremely subtle effect on protein synthesis, but no effect on *ND6* mRNA levels.[63] This may partly explain differences in the clinical phenotype associated with different mutations of this small tRNA gene.

X-linked deafness-dystonia (Mohr–Tranebjaerg syndrome)

X-linked recessive deafness and dystonia (Mohr–Tranebjaerg syndrome, MTS/DFN1, MIM 304700) is characterized by adult-onset generalized dystonia associated with progressive sensorineural deafness, and, sometimes, with cortical blindness, bulbar muscle dysfunction (predominantly dysphagia), and psychiatric features (paranoia).[35] Although the disorder is an X-linked recessive trait, females do show clinical features with late onset and mild deafness-dystonia phenotype, probably related to the skewed Lyonization (X-inactivation) that has been documented in this disorder.[64]

Most patients have either frame-shift or deletion mutations in a gene coding for an 11-kDa protein DDP-1/TIMM8a located on chromosome Xq21.3–Xq22.[65] These mutations prevent the correct assembly of the DDP1/TIMM8a–TIMM13 complex, leading to a reduction in the level of Tim23p in the inner mitochondrial membrane.[66] Tim23p mediates the import of nuclear-encoded mitochondrial proteins into the mitochondrial matrix. It is therefore thought that DDP1/TIMM8a mutations cause disease through ATP deficiency due to impaired mitochondrial protein import. It is currently unclear why this apparently essential protein should cause such a tissue specific disorder with a characteristic pathological phenotype (see above), but there are clinical similarities with mtDNA-related disorders, such as the optic atrophy/dystonia phenotype seen in some patients with the 14459G→A mtDNA *ND6* mutation.[67,68] As already noted, the cochlear pathology of this mitochondrial disorder is strikingly different from other

Box 7.2 Translation of mitochondrial mRNAs

Translation of mitochondrial mRNAs[1] takes place on mitochondrial ribosomes, which are made up of the mtDNA-encoded 12S and 16S ribosomal RNAs (rRNAs) plus approximately 90 ribosomal proteins (~50 in the large ribosomal subunit and ~40 in the small subunit), all of which are imported into the organelle from the cytosol.

Human mitochondria have their own genetic code, which differs from the 'universal' code at four of the 64 triplet positions (AUA specifies methionine instead of isoleucine; UGA specifies tryptophan instead of 'stop'; and AGA and AGG specify 'stop' instead of arginine) (Figure B7.2.1). These changes guarantee that only mtDNA-encoded messages can be translated faithfully. Conversely, mitochondrial sequences that entered the nucleus and integrated into nuclear DNA (there are about 1000 of these 'mitochondrial pseudogenes' in nuclear DNA), even if transcribed, would not be able to be translated correctly on cytoplasmic ribosomes.

UUU	F	Phe	UCU	S	Ser	UAU	Y	Tyr	UGU	C	Cys
UUC	F	Phe	UCC	S	Ser	UAC	Y	Tyr	UGC	C	Cys
UUA	L	Leu	UCA	S	Ser	UAA	*	Ter	**UGA**	*****	**Ter→Trp**
UUG	L	Leu	UCG	S	Ser	UAG	*	Ter	UGG	W	Trp
CUU	L	Leu	CCU	P	Pro	CAU	H	His	CGU	R	Arg
CUC	L	Leu	CCC	P	Pro	CAC	H	His	CGC	R	Arg
CUA	L	Leu	CCA	P	Pro	CAA	Q	Gln	CGA	R	Arg
CUG	L	Leu	CCG	P	Pro	CAG	Q	Gln	CGG	R	Arg
AUU	I	Ile	ACU	T	Thr	AAU	N	Asn	AGU	S	Ser
AUC	I	Ile	ACC	T	Thr	AAC	N	Asn	AGC	S	Ser
AUA	**I**	**Ile→Met**	ACA	T	Thr	AAA	K	Lys	**AGA**	**R**	**Arg→Ter**
AUG	M	Met	ACG	T	Thr	AAG	K	Lys	**AGG**	**R**	**Arg→Ter**
GUU	V	Val	GCU	A	Ala	GAU	D	Asp	GGU	G	Gly
GUC	V	Val	GCC	A	Ala	GAC	D	Asp	GGC	G	Gly
GUA	V	Val	GCA	A	Ala	GAA	E	Glu	GGA	G	Gly
GUG	V	Val	GCG	A	Ala	GAG	E	Glu	GGG	G	Gly

Figure B7.2.1 The mitochondrial genetic code. Changes from the nuclear code are in bold

In human mitochondria, the initiation codon for translation (AUG or AUA, both specifying methionine) is located at the very beginning of the mature message (i.e. there is little or no 5′-untranslated region). In this case, it is unclear how the ribosome recognizes and binds to the message. The downstream, 3′, end of the message is also short. The last amino acid-specifying codon is usually located within one or two nucleotides of the end of the message, and the messages often end with a U or a UA. Addition of a poly(A) tail to the mRNA converts the final U or UA to UAA, which is a translational termination codon. Two mRNAs contain a pair of 'overlapping' messages, that is, one contiguous piece of mRNA specifies two different polypeptides, with the 3′ end of the first message overlapping the 5′ end of the adjacent message. In both cases, the pair of polypeptides belong to the same respiratory complex: one message encodes subunits ND4 and ND4L of complex I, while the other encodes subunits 6 and 8 of complex V.

Reference

1. Taanman JW. The mitochondrial genome: structure, transcription, translation and replication. *Biochim Biophys Acta* 1999; **1410**: 103–123.

mitochondrial diseases (see above), indicating that ATP depletion cannot be the only mechanism involved in these diseases.

Managing hearing impairment in mitochondrial disorders

Although it may seem obvious, identifying and characterizing the hearing loss is the key to managing patients with mitochondrial deafness. Many patients do not complain of hearing deficit, either because this may be overshadowed by other features of the disease (such as recurrent seizures, dementia or poor glycemic control), or because they see it as a trivial component of their very complex disorder.[3] Pure tone speech audiometry can demonstrate a clinically significant deficit in the absence of overt symptoms,[3] and the disability associated with the hearing impairment may only become apparent after successful amplification with a hearing aid. In most patients, the primary deficit is cochlear and responds well to amplification. Simple single or binaural amplification may be adequate for a number of years or even decades, although anecdotally we have found that digital aids are more effective than the more conventional analog aids that are routinely supplied by state-funded health services.

There are a number of potential explanations for a poor response to amplification. It is important to consider additional pathology, either due to the same mitochondrial defect affecting a different component of the auditory system such as the brainstem and connections, or due to a coincidental middle-ear disease. It is also important to ask about tinnitus, as masking may improve auditory function. The deficit may, however, be too severe to respond well (for example, see Figure 7.2B). Severe deterioration can occur acutely, particularly in patients with the 3243A→G mutation[3,26] (possibly through acute metabolic compromise) and patients with 1555A→G (related to aminoglycoside exposure).[37] In patients with 3243A→G, psychophysical studies have shown the presence of 'dead regions' of cochlea in the high-frequency range,[31] which are unlikely to respond to amplification. Patients with a severe binaural defect that does not respond well to amplification should be considered for cochlear implantation.

Since the first recorded cochlear implant in a patient with Kearns–Sayre syndrome,[69] many patients have successfully received implants (1555A→G,[70] 3243A→G,[26,71,72] and other mtDNA mutations[73]). In many ways, patients with mitochondrial disease are 'ideal' recipients of a cochlear implant because the hearing loss develops well after speech development, and often in isolation (as in patients with diabetes and deafness due to 3243A→G, or non-syndromic deafness due to 1555A→G). A recent systematic review of the literature (March 2003) identified 12 detailed descriptions of patients with mitochondrial sensorineural deafness who had cochlear implants.[74] All 12 cases had profound post-lingual deafness. The age of onset of the deafness and the age at surgery varied, but 58% were able to converse on the telephone following the procedure, and the remainder had good open-set speech recognition. There were no reported complications. The procedure should, however, only be undertaken with caution, and we encourage the ear surgeon to discuss the issue with a physician experienced in mitochondrial disorders. It is also important to look carefully for systemic features of mitochondrial disease in all but the most straightforward of cases. The implantation procedure requires a general anesthetic and takes a number of hours. It is essential that the anesthetist be aware of co-morbid features, including asymptomatic cardiomyopathy, impaired glucose tolerance, lactic acidemia, or neuromuscular ventilatory weakness.[75,76] Even before embarking on the complex and intensive work-up prior to surgery, it is important to consider the natural history of the disorder in the individual patient. This can be extremely unpredictable, particularly in patients with 3243A→G, and there are anecdotal reports of exacerbation of an otherwise quiescent encephalopathy following surgical procedures. Cognitive impairment, hidden by severe deafness, may limit the auditory rehabilitation after successful surgery, and it may not be prudent to invest in a cochlear implant in a patient with a very poor prognosis from the outset.

Despite these cautionary words, there is little doubt that cochlear implantation has a dramatic and significant impact on the disability associated with mitochondrial disorders, providing the patient is well-selected and carefully screened for potential complications.

Conclusions

Hearing impairment is a common feature of mitochondrial disease, either in isolation, or as part of a complex multisystem disorder, with the cochlea bearing the brunt of the pathology. Ultimately, all forms of mitochondrial deafness arise through a respiratory chain defect causing ATP depletion, but it is not clear why hearing should be preferentially affected in some mitochondrial disorders and not in others, nor why the cochlear pathology can vary between different disorders. This issue is not unique to mitochondrial otology, and is a recurring theme throughout this book. Further investigation of the auditory system may provide some answers to these fundamental questions of mitochondrial pathology. There is clear evidence of a major environmental influence in some forms of mitochondrial deafness, and the interaction between nuclear and mitochondrial genes appears to be important. Addressing these issues is therefore likely to have much broader implications for our understanding of the pathophysiology of mitochondrial medicine.

From the clinical viewpoint, hearing loss is arguably the most rewarding feature to treat in mitochondrial disease – both for the physician and for the patient, where a simple hearing aid or cochlear implant can have a dramatic effect on personal and family life.

Acknowledgments

The authors are both Wellcome Trust Senior Fellows in Clinical Science.

References

1. Leonard JV, Schapira AH. Mitochondrial respiratory chain disorders I: mitochondrial DNA defects. *Lancet* 2000; **355**(9200): 299–304.
2. McFarland R, Taylor RW, Chinnery PF et al. A novel sporadic mutation in cytochrome *c* oxidase subunit II as a cause of rhabdomyolysis. *Neuromuscul Disord* 2004; **14**(2): 162–166.
3. Chinnery PF, Elliot C, Green GR et al. The spectrum of hearing loss due to mitochondrial DNA defects. *Brain* 2000; **123**: 74–81.
4. Chinnery PF, Bindoff LA. 116th ENMC international workshop: the treatment of mitochondrial disorders, 14th–16th March 2003, Naarden, The Netherlands. *Neuromuscul Disord* 2003; **13**(9): 757–764.
5. Keithley EM, Harris B, Desai K et al. Mitochondrial cytochrome oxidase immunolabeling in aged human temporal bones. *Hear Res* 2001; **157**(1–2): 93–99.
6. Pickles JO. Mutation in mitochondrial DNA as a cause of presbyacusis. *Audiol Neurotol* 2004; **9**(1): 23–33.
7. Hyde GE, Rubel EW. Mitochondrial role in hair cell survival after injury. *Otolargygol Head Neck Surg* 1995; **113**: 530–540.
8. Dallos P. The active cochlea. *J Neurosci* 1992; **12**(12): 4575–4585.
9. Nobili R, Mammano F, Ashmore J. How well do we understand the cochlea? *Trends Neurosci* 1998; **21**(4): 159–167.
10. Griffiths TD, Warren JD. What is an auditory object? *Nature Neurosci Rev* 2004; **5**: 887–892.
11. Dallos P, Evans BN. High-frequency motility of outer hair cells and the cochlear amplifier. *Science* 1995; **267**(5206): 2006–2009.
12. Thalmann I, Marcus NY, Thalmann R. Adenine nucleotides of the stria vascularis. *Arch Otorhinolaryngol* 1979; **224**(1–2): 89–95.

13. Wada J, Paloheimo S, Thalmann I et al. Maintenance of cochlear function with artificial oxygen carriers. *Laryngoscope* 1979; **89**(9 Pt 1): 1457–1473.
14. Cortopassi G, Hutchin T. A molecular and cellular hypothesis for aminoglycoside-indiced deafness. *Hearing Res* 1994; **78**: 27–30.
15. Wallace DC. Mitochondrial diseases in mouse and man. *Science* 1999; **283**: 1482–1488.
16. Fernandez C, Hinojosa R. Postnatal development of endocochlear potential and stria vascularis in the cat. *Acta Otolaryngol* 1974; **78**(3–4): 173–186.
17. Schon EA, Bonilla E, DiMauro S. Mitochondrial DNA mutations and pathogenesis. *J Bioenerget Biomemb* 1997; **29**: 131–149.
18. Moore BCJ, Glasberg BR. A model of loudness perception applied to cochlear hearing loss. *Auditory Neurosci* 1997; **3**: 289–311.
19. Kemp DT. Stimulated otacoustic emissions from within the human auditory system. *J Acoustic Society Am* 1978; **64**: 1386–1391.
20. Griffiths TD. Central auditory pathologies. *Br Med Bull* 2002; **63**: 107–120.
21. Griffiths TD. Functional Imaging of Pitch Processing. In: Plack CJ, Oxenham AJ, eds. *Pitch: Neural Coding and Perception*. New York: Springer Verlag, 2005.
22. Lindsay JR, Hinojosa R. Histopathologic features of the inner ear associated with Kearns-Sayre syndrome. *Arch Otolaryngol* 1976; **102**(12): 747–752.
23. Yamasoba T, Tsukuda K, Oka Y et al. Cochlear histopathology associated with mitochondrial transfer $RNA^{Leu(UUR)}$ gene mutation. *Neurology* 1999; **52**(8): 1705–1707.
24. Merchant SN, McKenna MJ, Nadol JB, Jr., et al. Temporal bone histopathologic and genetic studies in Mohr-Tranebjaerg syndrome (DFN-1). *Otol Neurotol* 2001; **22**(4): 506–511.
25. Elverland HH, Torbergsen T. Audiologic findings in a family with mitochondrial disorder. *Am J Otology* 1991; **12**: 459–465.
26. Sue CM, Lipsett LJ, Crimmins DS et al. Cochlear origin of hearing loss in MELAS syndrome. *Ann Neurol* 1998; **43**: 350–359.
27. Yamasoba T, Oka Y, Tsukuda K et al. Auditory findings in patients with maternally inherited diabetes and deafness harboring a point mutation in the mitochondrial transfer $RNA^{Leu(UUR)}$ gene. *Laryngoscope* 1996; **106**: 49–53.
28. Oshima T, Ueda N, Ikeda K et al. Bilateral sensorineural hearing loss associated with the point mutation in mitochondrial genome. *Laryngoscope* 1996; **106**: 43–48.
29. Moore BC, Vickers DA, Plack CJ, Oxenham AJ. Inter-relationship between different psychoacoustic measures assumed to be related to the cochlear active mechanism. *J Acoust Soc Am* 1999; **106**(5): 2761–2778.
30. Moore BC, Huss M, Vickers DA et al. A test for the diagnosis of dead regions in the cochlea. *Br J Audiol* 2000; **34**(4): 205–224.
31. Griffiths TD, Blakemore S, Elliott C et al. Psychophysical evaluation of cochlear hair cell damage due to the A3243G mitochondrial DNA mutation. *J Assoc Res Otolaryngol* 2001; **2**(2): 172–179.
32. Chinnery P, Howell N, Lightowlers R, Turnbull D. Molecular pathology of MELAS and MERRF: the relationship between mutation load and clinical phenotype. *Brain* 1997; **120**: 1713–1721.
33. Zeviani M, Moraes CT, DiMauro S et al. Deletions of mitochondrial DNA in Kearns-Sayre syndrome. *Neurology* 1988; **38**(9): 1339–1346.
34. Hirano M, Ricci E, Koenigsberger MR et al. MELAS: an original case and clinical criteria for diagnosis. *Neuromuscul Disord* 1992; **2**(2): 125–135.
35. Tranebjaerg L, Schwartz C, Eriksen H et al. A new X linked recessive deafness syndrome with blindness, dystonia, fractures, and mental deficiency is linked to Xq22. *J Med Genet* 1995; **32**(4): 257–263.
36. van den Ouweland JWM, Lemkes HHPJ, Ruitenbeek K. Mutation in mitochondrial $tRNA^{Leu(UUR)}$ gene in a large pedigree with maternally transmitted type II diabetes mellitus and deafness. *Nat Genet* 1992; **1**: 368–371.
37. Prezant TR, Agapian JV, Bohlman MC et al. Mitochondrial ribosomal RNA mutations associated with both antibiotic-induced and non-syndromic deafness. *Nat Genet* 1993; **4**: 289–294.
38. Estivill X, Govea N, Barcelo A et al. Familial progressive sensorineural deafness is mainly due to the mtDNA A1555G mutation and is enhanced by treatment with aminoglycosides. *Am J Hum Genet* 1998; **62**: 27–35.
39. Reid FM, Vernham GA, Jacobs HT. A novel mitochondrial point mutation in a maternal pedigree with sensorineural deafness. *Hum Mutat* 1994; **3**: 243–247.

40. Sue CM, Tanji K, Hadjigeorgiou G et al. Maternally inherited hearing loss in a large kindred with a novel T7511C mutation in the mitochondrial DNA $tRNA^{Ser(UCN)}$ gene. *Neurology* 1999; **52**(9): 1905–1908.
41. Verhoeven K, Ensink RJ, Tiranti V et al. Hearing impairment and neurological dysfunction associated with a mutation in the mitochondrial $tRNA^{Ser(UCN)}$ gene. *Eur J Hum Genet* 1999; **7**(1): 45–51.
42. Carelli V, Giordano C, d'Amati G. Pathogenic expression of homoplasmic mtDNA mutations needs a complex nuclear-mitochondrial interaction. *Trends Genet* 2003; **19**(5): 257–262.
43. Goto Y, Nonaka I, Horai S. A mutation in the $tRNA^{Leu(UUR)}$ gene associated with the MELAS subgroup of mitochondrial encephalomyopathies. *Nature* 1990; **348**(6302): 651–653.
44. Majamaa K, Moilanen JS, Uimonen S et al. Epidemiology of A3243G, the mutation for mitochondrial encephalomyopathy, lactic acidosis, and strokelike episodes: prevalence of the mutation in an adult population. *Am J Hum Genet* 1998; **63**: 447–454.
45. Uimonen S, Moilanen JS, Sorri M et al. Hearing impairment in patients with 3243A→G mtDNA mutation: phenotype and rate of progression. *Hum Genet* 2001; **108**(4): 284–289.
46. Jacobs HT, Holt IJ. The np 3243 MELAS mutation: damned if you aminoacylate, damned if you don't. *Hum Mol Genet* 2000; **9**(4): 463–465.
47. Ciafaloni E, Ricci E, Shanske S et al. MELAS: clinical features, biochemistry, and molecular genetics. *Ann Neurol* 1992; **31**(4): 391–398.
48. Chomyn A, Martinuzzi A, Yoneda M et al. MELAS mutation in mtDNA binding site for transcription termination factor causes defects in protein synthesis and in respiration but no change in levels of upstream and downstream mature transcripts. *Proc Natl Acad Sci USA* 1992; **89**(10): 4221–4225.
49. Bentlage HACM, Attardi G. Relationship of genotype to phenotype in fibroblast-derived transmitochondrial cell lines carrying the 3243 mutation associated with MELAS encephalomyopathy: shift towards mutant genotype and role of mtDNA copy number. *Hum Mol Genet* 1996; **5**: 197–205.
50. Mancuso M, Filosto M, Forli F et al. A nonsyndromic hearing loss caused by very low levels of the mtDNA A3243G mutation. *Acta Neurol Scand* 2004; **110**(1): 72–74.
51. Petruzzella V, Moraes CT, Sano MC et al. Extremely high levels of mutant mtDNAs co-localize with cytochrome c oxidase-negative ragged-red fibers in patients harboring a point mutation at nt 3243. *Hum Mol Genet* 1994; **3**(3): 449–454.
52. Hamasaki K, Rando RR. Specific binding of aminoglycosides to a human rRNA construct based on a DNA polymorphism which causes aminoglycoside-induced deafness. *Biochemistry* 1997; **36**(40): 12323–12328.
53. Torroni A, Cruciani F, Rengo C et al. The A1555G mutation in the 12S rRNA gene of human mtDNA: recurrent origins and founder events in families affected by sensorineural deafness. *Am J Hum Genet* 1999; **65**(5): 1349–1358.
54. Usami S, Abe S, Akita J et al. Prevalence of mitochondrial gene mutations among hearing impaired patients. *J Med Genet* 2000; **37**(1): 38–40.
55. Usami S, Abe S, Kasai M et al. Genetic and clinical features of sensorineural hearing loss associated with the 1555 mitochondrial mutation. *Laryngoscope* 1997; **107**(4): 483–490.
56. Inoue K, Takai D, Soejima A et al. Mutant mtDNA at 1555 A to G in 12S rRNA gene and hypersusceptibility of mitochondrial translation to streptomycin can be co-transferred to ρ 0 HeLa cells. *Biochem Biophys Res Commun* 1996; **223**(3): 496–501.
57. Guan MX, Fischel-Ghodsian N, Attardi G. Nuclear background determines biochemical phenotype in the deafness-associated mitochondrial 12S rRNA mutation. *Hum Mol Genet* 2001; **10**(6): 573–580.
58. Johnson KR, Zheng QY, Bykhovskaya Y et al. A nuclear-mitochondrial DNA interaction affecting hearing impairment in mice. *Nat Genet* 2001; **27**(2): 191–194.
59. Jacobs HT. Pathological mutations. In: Holt I, ed. *Genetics of Mitochondrial Diseases*. Oxford: Oxford University Press, 2004: 138–139.
60. Bykhovskaya Y, Yang H, Taylor K et al. Modifier locus for mitochondrial DNA disease: linkage and linkage disequilibrium mapping of a nuclear modifier gene for maternally inherited deafness. *Genet Med* 2001; **3**(3): 177–180.
61. Bykhovskaya Y, Mengesha E, Wang D et al. Human mitochondrial transcription factor B1 as a modifier gene for hearing loss associated with the mitochondrial A1555G mutation. *Mol Genet Metab* 2004; **82**(1): 27–32.

62. Guan MX, Enriquez JA, Fischel-Ghodsian N et al. The deafness-associated mitochondrial DNA mutation at position 7445, which affects $tRNA^{Ser(UCN)}$ precursor processing, has long-range effects on NADH dehydrogenase subunit ND6 gene expression. *Mol Cell Biol* 1998; **18**(10): 5868–5879.
63. Toompuu M, Tiranti V, Zeviani M, Jacobs HT. Molecular phenotype of the np 7472 deafness-associated mitochondrial mutation in osteosarcoma cell cybrids. *Hum Mol Genet* 1999; **8**(12): 2275–2283.
64. Plenge RM, Tranebjaerg L, Jensen PK et al. Evidence that mutations in the X-linked *DDP* gene cause incompletely penetrant and variable skewed X inactivation. *Am J Hum Genet* 1999; **64**(3): 759–767.
65. Tranebjaerg L, Hamel BC, Gabreels FJ et al. A *de novo* missense mutation in a critical domain of the X-linked DDP gene causes the typical deafness-dystonia-optic atrophy syndrome. *Eur J Hum Genet* 2000; **8**(6): 464–467.
66. Roesch K, Curran SP, Tranebjaerg L, Koehler CM. Human deafness dystonia syndrome is caused by a defect in assembly of the DDP1/TIMM8a-TIMM13 complex. *Hum Mol Genet* 2002; **11**(5): 477–486.
67. Jun AS, Brown MD, Wallace DC. A mitochondrial DNA mutation at nucleotide pair 14459 of the NADH dehydrogenase subunit 6 gene associated with maternally inherited Leber hereditary optic neuropathy and dystonia. *Proc Natl Acad Sci USA* 1994; **91**(13): 6206–6210.
68. Wallace DC, Murdock DG. Mitochondria and dystonia: the movement disorder connection? *Proc Natl Acad Sci USA* 1999; **96**(5): 1817–1819.
69. Yamaguchi T, Himi T, Harabuchi Y et al. Cochlear implantation in a patient with mitochondrial disease – Kearns-Sayre syndrome: a case report. *Adv Otorhinolaryngol* 1997; **52**: 321–323.
70. Tono T, Ushisako Y, Kiyomizu K et al. Cochlear implantation in a patient with profound hearing loss with the A1555G mitochondrial mutation. *Am J Otol* 1998; **19**(6): 754–757.
71. Rosenthal EL, Kileny PR, Boerst A, Telian SA. Successful cochlear implantation in a patient with MELAS syndrome. *Am J Otol* 1999; **20**(2): 187–190; discussion 190–191.
72. Yasumura S, Aso S, Fujisaka M, Watanabe Y. Cochlear implantation in a patient with mitochondrial encephalopathy, lactic acidosis and stroke-like episodes syndrome. *Acta Otolaryngol* 2003; **123**(1): 55–58.
73. Counter PR, Hilton MP, Webster D et al. Cochlear implantation of a patient with a previously undescribed mitochondrial DNA defect. *J Laryngol Otol* 2001; **115**(9): 730–732.
74. Sinnathuray AR, Raut V, Awa A et al. A review of cochlear implantation in mitochondrial sensorineural hearing loss. *Otol Neurotol* 2003; **24**(3): 418–426.
75. Thompson VA, Wahr JA. Anesthetic considerations in patients presenting with mitochondrial myopathy, encephalopathy, lactic acidosis, and stroke-like episodes (MELAS) syndrome. *Anesth Analg* 1997; **85**(6): 1404–1406.
76. Chinnery PF, Turnbull DM. Mitochondrial medicine. *Q J Med* 1997; **90**: 657–666.

8

Mitochondrial endocrinology

Maria A Yialamas, Leif C Groop, and Vamsi K Mootha

Introduction

It can be argued that the first mitochondrial disease ever described was initially evaluated in an endocrine clinic. In 1962, Rolf Luft reported the case of a young woman who suffered from euthyroid hypermetabolism.[1] Biochemical and ultrastructural studies were suggestive of a defect in the coupling efficiency of this patient's mitochondria. While the molecular etiology of 'Luft disease' is still not known today, this initial case report sparked the creation of 'mitochondrial medicine.'

There appears to be an ever-expanding role for the mitochondrion in both rare and common human diseases. Key cellular processes, such as oxidative phosphorylation, apoptosis, steroid and lipid biosynthesis, and intermediary metabolism, are situated in this organelle, linking it to virtually all organ systems. Evolutionary and genetic studies suggest that environmental factors, such as climate and food supply, may have shaped the pattern of mitochondrial DNA haplotypes across the world, contributing to the spectrum of common human diseases observed today.[2] Although mitochondrial dysfunction, resulting from mutations in mtDNA or nuclear DNA, has traditionally been associated with encephalomyopathy, it is now clear that virtually all organ systems can be affected.

Endocrine dysfunction appears to be a very common manifestation of mitochondrial disease. Chinnery and Turnbull have gone so far as to suggest that diabetes may be the most common mtDNA disease phenotype.[3] A recent survey of patients with documented respiratory chain disease reported that following the nervous system, the endocrine system is most frequently affected in these patients. In fact, nearly 50% of these patients had some form of endocrine dysfunction.[4] Clinicians caring for patients with mitochondrial disease need to become increasingly aware of its endocrine manifestations, since most of the disorders are treatable. When endocrine organ involvement is suspected, referral to an endocrinologist may help in guiding the diagnosis and treatment. Improvement of the endocrine disorder may also have benefit to other affected systems.

Here we review the various endocrine disorders that can arise in mitochondrial diseases, with a special focus on diabetes.

Mitochondria and diabetes

Diabetes represents a collection of diseases characterized by chronic hyperglycemia, and is one of the leading causes of cardiovascular disease, stroke, limb loss, blindness, and renal failure.[5] Diabetes mellitus is characterized and defined by hyperglycemia. Current American Diabetes Association criteria for the diagnosis include either a fasting blood glucose > 126 mg/dL or a random glucose > 200 mg/dL on two occasions. An oral glucose tolerance test can also be used to establish the diagnosis with a 2-hour glucose value greater than 200 mg/dL.[6] Maintenance of normal glucose homeostasis requires the action of a glucose sensor in the pancreatic β-cell that detects increases in circulating glucose and converts this signal into increased insulin secretion. Increased insulin then suppresses glucose output from the liver and promotes glucose uptake in peripheral tissues such as skeletal muscle and adipose tissue.

Diabetes can result from an impaired secretion of insulin by the β-cell, as well as by a loss of its action (termed insulin resistance) in peripheral tissues, such as skeletal muscle, fat and liver. It has long been known that increased insulin resistance can eventually lead to decline in function of the pancreatic β-cell. Likewise, an impaired secretion of insulin can result in hyperglycemia, eventually leading to peripheral insulin resistance. This dynamic relationship often makes it difficult to pinpoint the primary event leading to diabetes. Diabetes is the prototypical complex disease, as many genes (individually and in combination) and environmental factors (e.g., diet, exercise, drugs) can contribute to its heritability, age of onset, and severity.[7]

Recent studies have suggested that the mitochondrion may lie at the heart of all forms of non-immune diabetes.[8–12] The hypothesis that either inherited or acquired mitochondrial dysfunction may underlie all forms of diabetes may help unify a number of observations gleaned through genetics, clinical medicine, epidemiology, and pharmacology. This idea would also be consistent with the thrifty gene hypothesis,[13] which states that genotypes which were selected for during times of food or water scarcity may be detrimental during times of food surplus. In this section, we review the clinical features of mitochondrial diabetes, due to mutations in mtDNA, as well as some evidence supporting the notion that this organelle may underlie all forms of non-immune diabetes.

Mitochondrial diabetes due to variation in mtDNA

By general consensus mtDNA mutations cause approximately 1.5% of cases of diabetes in Europe, and perhaps as much as 5% of diabetes in East Asia, particularly in Japan.[14]

Clinically, mitochondrial diabetes typically presents as an unremarkable form of diabetes, sometime between 22 and 35 years of age, between the peak ages of onset for type 1 diabetes and type 2 diabetes or maturity-onset diabetes of the young (MODY).[15] The disorder is maternally inherited and can be characterized by a defect in insulin secretion or, occasionally, by insulin resistance. Interestingly, the majority of these patients are thin (BMI < 25 kg/m^2). Although most eventually require insulin therapy, ketoacidosis is rare and these patients rarely, if ever, exhibit circulating glutamic acid decarboxylase (GAD) antibodies.[16] Mitochondrial diabetes can be accompanied by other disorders, such as cardiomyopathy, short stature, and central or peripheral nervous system involvement, including sensorineural deafness, myopathy, encephalopathy, visual failure (retinitis pigmentosa, optic atrophy), stroke, seizures, and dementia.[14,17]

Proof of the mitochondrial origin of this form of diabetes stems from genetic analysis. The diagnosis is usually made by genetic demonstration of mtDNA mutations in PCR-amplified DNA from peripheral blood leukocytes (PBL) or preferably buccal mucosal cells. The level of heteroplasmy can sometimes be low in PBL cells and has a tendency to decline with aging, which can make the diagnosis difficult. In a very large fraction of patients with mitochondrial diabetes, there are heteroplasmic mutations that can often be detected in the mtDNA, particularly in genes encoding tRNAs (Figure 8.1). The mutation load can be quite low in patients with mitochondrial diabetes, and there does not appear to be a strong

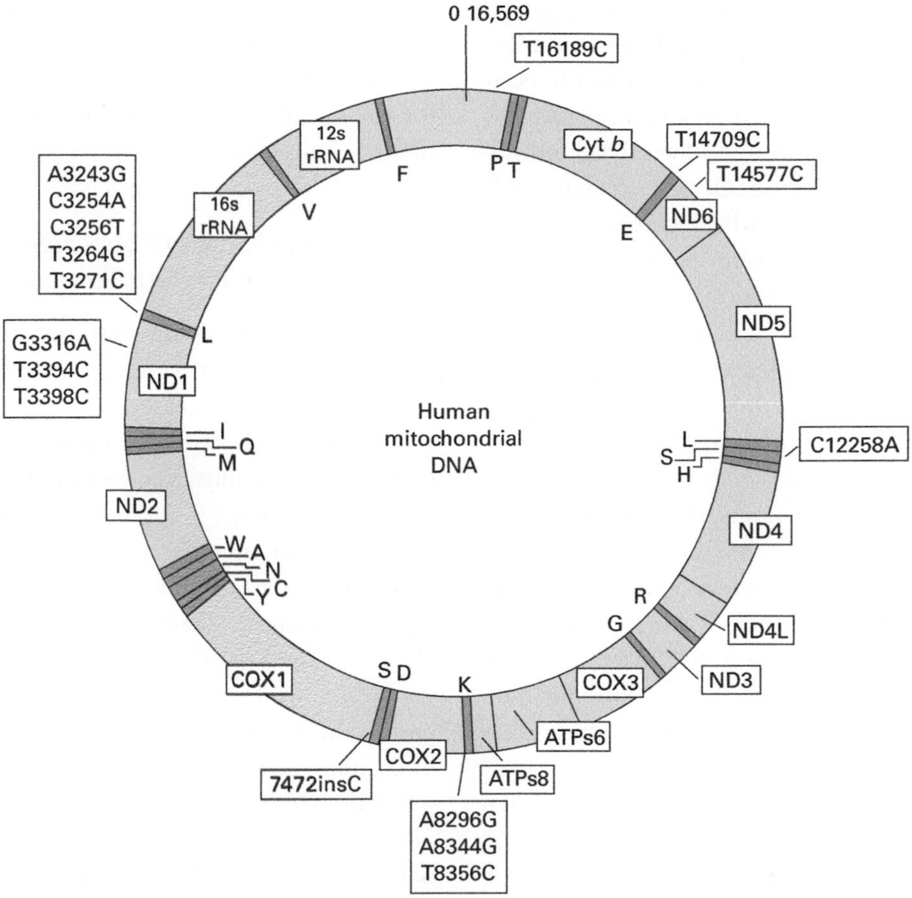

Figure 8.1 The human mitochondrial DNA (mtDNA) and mtDNA mutations associated with diabetes. (Modified from Maechler and Wollheim, *Nature* 2001.[21])

relationship between the level of heteroplasmy in circulating cells and the severity of the disease.[18] However, the age of onset of diabetes may be correlated to the level of heteroplasmy.[14]

The leucyl-tRNA^{UUR} substitution of A for G at nucleotide 3243 (A3243G), traditionally associated with mitochondrial myopathy, encephalopathy, lactic acidosis, and stroke-like episodes (MELAS), seems to be particularly associated with diabetes, and is the causative lesion in a distinct syndrome known as maternally inherited diabetes and deafness (MIDD).[19] At least seven other mtDNA mutations (Figure 8.1), particularly in tRNA genes of the mitochondrion, can be associated with diabetes, although A3243G appears to be the most common.[20,21] mtDNA deletions can also be associated with diabetes.[22]

MIDD is characterized by diabetes as well as by a neurosensory hearing loss (as reflected by a reduced perception of high-tone frequencies > 5 kHz) that typically precedes diabetes. Other co-morbidities have also been reported, including gastrointestinal abnormalities (e.g. dysmotility), cardiomyopathy, renal dysfunction, and macular pattern dystrophy.[16,23,24] Diabetes or impaired glucose tolerance associated with the A3243G mutation becomes clinically manifest in the early 30s. A study of Dutch individuals with the A3243G mutation revealed that by age 70 nearly all individuals have impaired glucose tolerance or diabetes.[18]

Patients with mitochondrial diabetes may or may not initially be insulin-requiring, and can initially be treated with sulfonylurea agents or thiazolidinediones (TZDs). These patients can also be treated with metformin, although this is discouraged given the theoretical risk of lactic acidosis. Insulin treatment is typically required as the disease progresses.

A major unanswered question is how mutations in mtDNA, particularly in the leucyl-tRNA^{UUR} gene, can give rise to diabetes. Defects in insulin production as well as insulin resistance have been reported in patients with A3243G-associated diabetes.[18] Most studies to date suggest that the A3243G mutation initially gives rise to islet cell dysfunction and an initial defect in insulin secretion.[20,25,26]

In vitro studies have suggested that a high fraction of heteroplasmy can result in decreased oxidative phosphorylation (OXPHOS) capacity in cybrid cell lines.[27] The A3243G mutation itself is believed to result in dimerization of leucyl-tRNA^{UUR} and decreased aminoacylation.[28] The precise biochemical consequences are not known but in cybrid cells (see Box 5.1) it appears that accumulation of the mutation leads to decreased oxygen consumption and ATP production. In islet cells, this may have the consequence of lowering the ATP/ ADP ratio, which could lead to decreased insulin secretion. In addition, alterations in the electron transport chain may give rise to increased reactive oxygen species (ROS), which may lead to increased apoptosis and further decline of islet cell function. This hypothesis is consistent with the age-dependent decline in β-cell function observed with the A3243G-mutation, and is consistent with post-mortem studies, which have demonstrated decreased islet cell mass in β-cells as well as in the glucagon producing α-cells in patients with the mutation.[29] The simultaneous loss of glucagon may account for the fact that these patients rarely suffer from diabetic ketoacidosis (DKA).

Mendelian disorders characterized by mitochondrial dysfunction and diabetes

It is worthwhile noting that several Mendelian disorders associated with mitochondrial dysfunction often exhibit diabetes.

Wolfram syndrome (also known as DIDMOAD, or diabetes insipidus, diabetes mellitus, optic atrophy, and deafness) is an autosomal recessive disorder due to mutations in the *WFS1* gene on chromosome 4. The disorder is characterized by type 1 diabetes in association with optic atrophy. *WFS1* encodes a transmembrane protein called wolframin, which appears to be localized to the ER and to the mitochondrion, perhaps as a regulator of cellular calcium.[30]

Friedreich's ataxia is an autosomal recessive neurodegenerative disease characterized by cerebellar ataxia, dysarthria, nystagmus, and cardiomyopathy. About 20% of patients with this disease also develop insulin resistance sometime during their lifetime. The disease is associated with an expanded trinucleotide repeat in the frataxin gene, whose gene product is a mitochondrial protein directing iron–sulfur-cluster assembly.

Patients with familial amyotrophic lateral sclerosis (ALS) often have mutations in genes encoding ROS scavenging enzymes of the cell. In a number of small studies it has been shown that these patients suffer from impaired glucose tolerance and diabetes mellitus.[31]

Finally, Huntington's disease is another disorder that is characterized by degeneration of the basal ganglia as well as by chorea and dementia. In humans and in mouse models, diabetes mellitus is frequently seen. These patients typically have insulin deficiency, but later, they also develop measurable insulin resistance.[32] While the exact function of huntingtin is still not known, recent work has suggested that the mutant protein may interfere with mitochondrial bioenergetics.

Mitochondrial contribution to the common form of diabetes

Based on the above studies, it is clear that mutations in mtDNA or in nuclear genes encoding mitochondrial proteins can give rise to syndromes that can be characterized, in part, by diabetes. However, there is mounting evidence that even type 2 diabetes may stem from defects in mitochondrial function. It has long been appreciated that the inheritance of type 2 diabetes shows an excess of maternal transmission[33,34] – this could be due to intrauterine effects, imprinting, or possibly involvement of mtDNA. The two hallmark features of the common form of diabetes, impaired insulin secretion and reduced insulin action (insulin resistance), may have mitochondrial etiologies. Here, we review the evidence suggesting mitochondrial involvement in both of these key processes.

Mitochondria and β-cell function

Blood glucose is carefully regulated by insulin secretion from pancreatic β-cells (Figure 8.2). Glucose equilibrates across the plasma membrane and is phosphorylated by glucokinase to produce glucose-6-phosphate. This step regulates the rate of glycolysis and the production of pyruvate. When blood glucose levels are high, the level of glycolysis in the β-cell is high. Pyruvate then enters the TCA cycle, situated in the mitochondrion, which produces NADH and FADH. These reducing equivalents then drive the electron transport chain, producing ATP. The increased ATP/ADP ratio causes the closure of the plasma membrane K_{ATP} channels, allowing the opening of voltage-sensitive Ca^{2+} channels, similar to those found in other excitable cells. The increase in calcium then causes the release of insulin-containing secretory granules.

Hence, mitochondrial metabolism is able to directly link plasma glucose levels with insulin release, a process known as metabolism–secretion coupling. Several decades ago it was established that mitochondrial dysfunction results in impaired glucose-stimulated insulin secretion. Lowering oxygen levels and poisoning the electron transport chain with inhibitors can block this response. Cells in which mtDNA has been depleted, ρ^0 cells, are viable but exhibit impaired insulin secretion. Interestingly, agents that raise calcium are still able to induce insulin release in such cells, suggesting that the defect is in the mitochondrion. In fact, replenishment of the cells with mtDNA restores glucose-induced insulin release.[35]

Genetic studies in mice, too, have clearly shown that β-cell dysfunction can result from mitochondrial dysfunction. Tfam knockout mice, in which the mitochondrial transcription factor Tfam has been disrupted, exhibit a diabetic phenotype, and the islets exhibit decreased OXPHOS activity and glucose-induced insulin secretion.[36]

Mitochondrial ROS generation and scavenging may serve as a link between organelle dysfunction and β-cell demise. Excess glucose and lipids, which can lead to increased ROS, are known to be toxic to β-cells.[37] It is believed that the β-cell guards against this possibility through uncoupling protein 2 (UCP2), an inner membrane mitochondrial protein that can dissipate the proton motive force and that is activated by superoxide. Genetic and environmental factors may result in increased β-cell ROS generation, which may lead to cellular apoptosis and loss of β-cell mass.

Insulin resistance and mitochondria

For years, it has been appreciated that insulin resistance in skeletal muscle, fat, and liver is one of the hallmark features of diabetes. In high-risk individuals, deposition of fat in muscle and liver

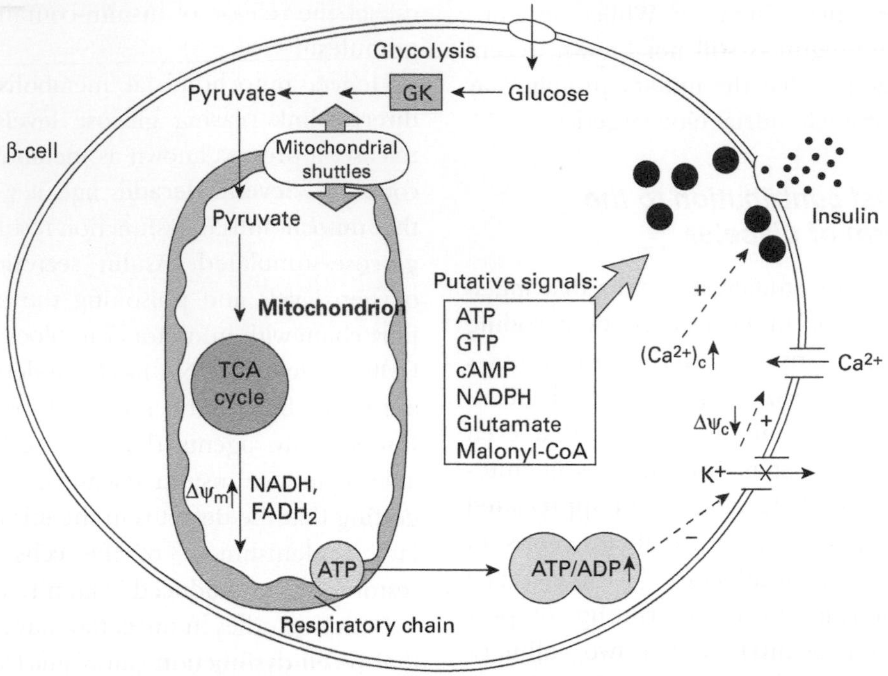

Figure 8.2 Role of mitochondria in β-cell function. The mitochondrion plays a central role in linking metabolism to insulin secretion. Glucose enters the pancreatic β-cell and is metabolized to pyruvate via cytosolic glycolysis. Via the mitochondrial oxidative phosphorylation (OXPHOS) system, pyruvate is oxidized to generate ATP from ADP. This results in a net increase in the cytosolic ATP/ADP ratio, which closes the K_{ATP} channels and depolarizes the β-cell. Depolarization then activates voltage-gated calcium channels which allow calcium influx into the β-cell, leading to the secretion of insulin granules. (Modified from Maechler and Wollheim, *Nature* 2001.[21])

precedes insulin resistance as the first detectable feature of the disease.[12,38] While a number of pathways have been implicated in cellular or animal models of insulin resistance, none of these pathways has been shown to be consistently altered in the common form of diabetes.

Several recent genomic approaches have pointed to impaired mitochondrial biogenesis (Figure 8.3) as a common feature underlying insulin resistance.[8,9,39] These studies used DNA microarrays (see Box 8.1) to profile the skeletal muscle of individuals with varying levels of insulin resistance and independently reached the conclusion that in individuals with diabetes, there is a reduced expression of the nuclear genes encoding mitochondrial proteins, in particular, those encoding components of oxidative phosphorylation. Mootha et al. showed that in Northern Europeans the expression of OXPHOS genes is reduced not only in diabetics, but also in individuals with impaired glucose tolerance.[8] Moreover, the expression of OXPHOS genes is highly correlated with VO_2max in all individuals, which has previously been shown to be an extremely strong marker of insulin sensitivity. Patti et al. examined Mexican Americans and showed that the expression of OXPHOS genes is also reduced in the muscle of healthy, first-degree relatives of individuals with type 2 diabetes.[9] Both of these studies hence suggest that reduced OXPHOS expression is a

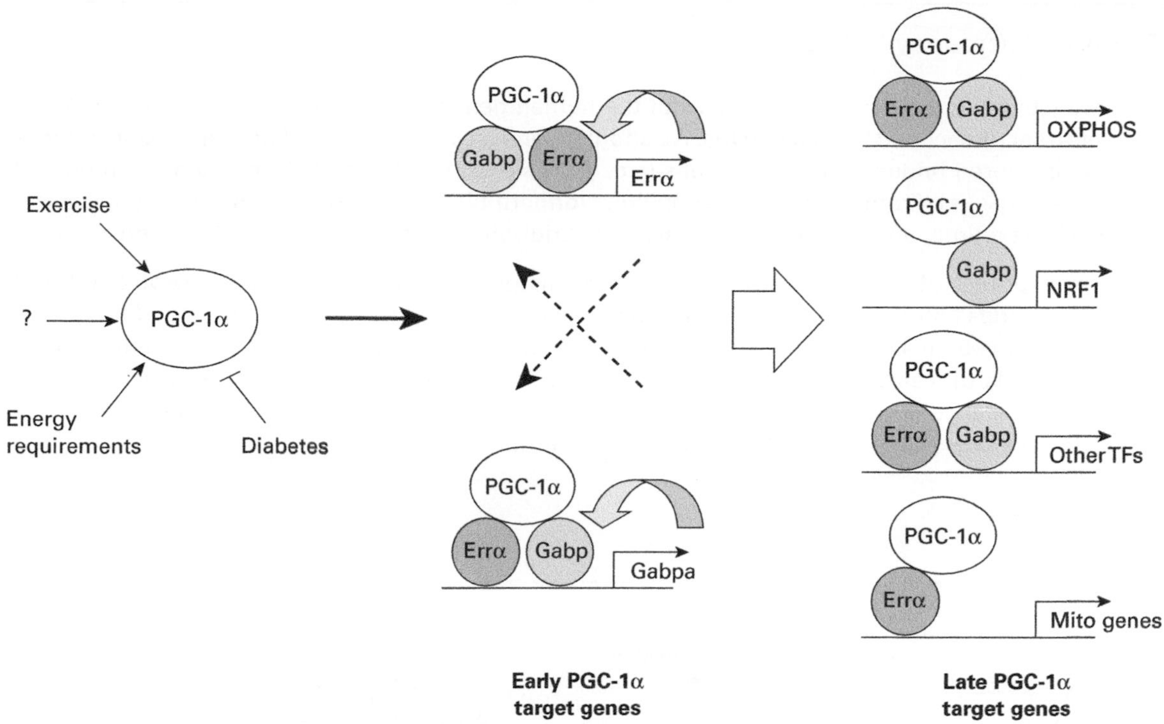

Figure 8.3 Overview of mitochondrial biogenesis. The transcriptional co-activator PGC-1α is a key regulator whose expression levels are controlled by cold, adrenergic inputs, exercise, nutrient status, and diabetes. As PGC-1α levels rise, it partners with the transcription factors ERRα and GABPA/B to co-activate these transcription factors via a double-positive feedback loop. Together, these three factors then partner to stimulate the transcription of a number of genes, including nuclear-encoded members of OXPHOS and other mitochondrial proteins.[40] In addition, this circuit leads to the stable rise of nuclear NRF-1, a transcription factor which is involved in the regulation of the mitochondrial transcription factor TFAM, which is imported into the mitochondrion to promote mtDNA replication.[74] PGC-1 = peroxisome proliferator-activated receptor-γ co-activator 1, ERRα = estrogen related receptor alpha; GABP = GA binding protein A; NRF1 = nuclear respiratory factor-1

phenotype appearing relatively early in the development of type 2 diabetes.

Mootha et al. further showed that observed changes appear to lie downstream of the transcriptional co-activator PGC-1α, which has been shown to be a master regulator of mitochondrial biogenesis. Because the expression of PGC-1α is also reduced in these patients, it appears that in the common form of diabetes, in Northern Europeans as well as in Mexican Americans, there is a PGC-1α-dependent decrease in mitochondrial biogenesis. A recent study has further dissected the pathway of mitochondrial biogenesis and suggests that the orphan nuclear receptor ERRα, the ETS transcription factor GABPA/B, and PGC-1α may form a regulatory switch that lies upstream of NRF1 and other transcription factors mediating mitochondrial biogenesis[40] – this regulatory circuit may represent a novel target for antidiabetic medications.

Functional studies using very different approaches have also suggested that reduced OXPHOS

Box 8.1 Microarray technology

The availability of the complete sequence of the human genome means that, in principle, we know the entire set of encoded human mRNAs. We should therefore be able to ask if the expression of these mRNAs is altered under various conditions (e.g. glucose-rich vs glucose-free medium, or in normal vs diseased tissue). From a practical standpoint, Northern blot analysis can examine only a handful of mRNAs at a time, and the various subtractive hybridization methods in use are time consuming.

The development of DNA microarrays, also known as gene chips, has solved this problem. Short oligonucleotides (20–50 nt in length), each with a defined and unique sequence corresponding to each mRNA, is arrayed on a grid (Figure B8.1.1).[1] The grid is about the size of a postage stamp, but can contain thousands of 'cells,' each with an oligonucleotide representing one specific gene or mRNA. In a modification of this method, hundreds of full-length cDNAs representing individual mRNAs are 'spotted' on a glass slide and are analyzed in a similar manner.[2]

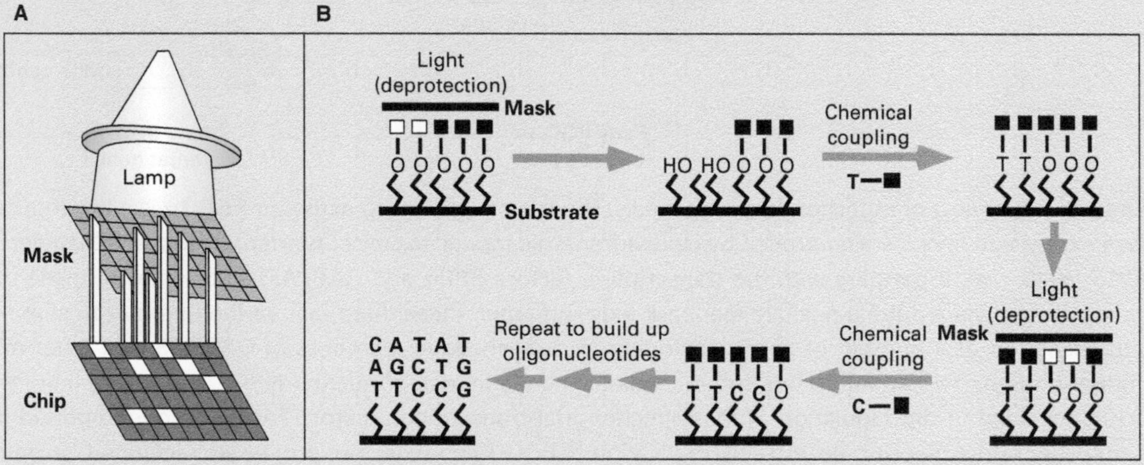

Figure B8.1.1 Microarray technology. **(A)** Using microlithography to make a chip. **(B)** The nucleotide sequence on the array is 'built up' in a series of light-catalyzed steps that successively protect and deprotect the nucleotides in a controlled manner. Adapted from Reference 1 with permission.

The chip is 'queried' by hybridizing fluorescently labeled cDNAs derived from mRNAs from the two sources under comparison (e.g. red cDNA probes from mRNA derived from normal tissue and green probes from diseased tissue mRNA), and comparing the colored signals derived from each source (Figure B8.1.2). Thus, one can determine in a single experiment which genes are up-regulated (i.e. red signal predominates), which are down-regulated (i.e. green signal predominates), and which are unchanged (both red and green signals are equal in intensity, giving a yellow signal).

Microarray analysis can also be used to develop 'functional maps,' in which each mRNA is a node in a network, with mRNAs 'pointing' towards or away from other mRNAs, depending on whether they are upstream or downstream of each other in a pathway.[3]

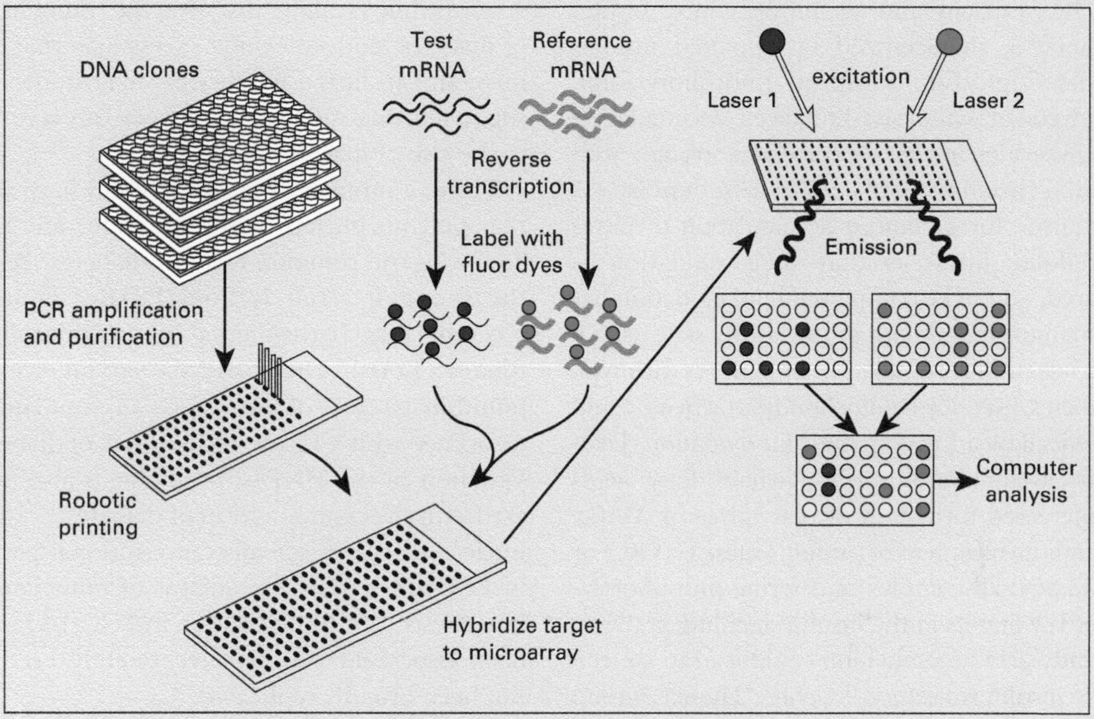

Figure B8.1.2 Microarray analysis. Adapted from reference 2, with permission

References

1. Lipshutz RJ, Fodor SP, GingerasTR, Lockhart DJ. High density synthetic oligonucleotide arrays. *Nat Genet* 1999; **21**: 20–24.
2. Duggan DJ, Bittner M, Chen Y et al. Expression profiling using cDNA microarrays. *Nat Genet* 1999; **21**: 10–14.
3. Tong AH, Drees B, Nardelli G et al. A combined experimental and computational strategy to define protein interaction networks for peptide recognition modules. *Science* 2002; **295**: 321–324.

activity in muscle may represent a signature feature of diabetes. Kelley and colleagues have examined skeletal muscle from individuals with impaired glucose tolerance as well as diabetes and found altered mitochondrial morphology as well as OXPHOS activity.[12] Petersen and Shulman have used in vivo ^{31}P-NMR-based measurements of OXPHOS activity to demonstrate that diabetic individuals have reduced ATP synthetic capacities. Moreover, they showed that the healthy first-degree relatives of individuals with DM2 also have reduced OXPHOS activity.[11] These functional studies complement the genomic studies and further establish reduced mitochondrial biogenesis as a feature of diabetes.

The mechanism by which reduced OXPHOS capacity is related to insulin resistance is currently not known. Specifically, we do not know whether a common signal leads simultaneously to reduced OXPHOS expression and insulin resistance, or whether there is a causal relationship between OXPHOS capacity and insulin resistance. Insulin resistance is characterized by impaired insulin-stimulated glucose transport, phosphorylation, and glycogen synthesis. Enhanced accumulation of triglycerides in muscle correlates strongly with impaired insulin-stimulated glucose uptake. A prerequisite for enhanced accumulation of intramyocellular lipids is that their oxidation is impaired, and in fact, impaired lipid oxidation has been demonstrated both in the fasting state as well as during insulin stimulation in patients with type 2 diabetes. Reduced mitochondrial activity could theoretically lead to impaired fat oxidation, leading to accumulation of long-chain fatty acids and increased formation of diacylglycerol (DAG). Through involvement of protein kinase C (PKC) or the IKkβ/NFkβ complex and serine phosphorylation of key targets in the insulin signaling pathway, such fatty acid accumulation could lead to skeletal muscle insulin resistance.[41] George Thomas' group has recently shown that the signaling molecule S6 kinase (S6K), an integrator of nutrient sensing, signaling, and protein synthesis, may play a key role in integrating nutrient levels with mitochondrial biogenesis and insulin receptor activity.[42]

Mitochondrial dysfunction in diabetes: cause or consequence?

The question still unanswered is whether inherited or acquired mitochondrial dysfunction represents the cause or the consequence of type 2 diabetes. Functional, epidemiological, and clinical studies favor the causal hypothesis.

First, the decreased expression of PGC-1α and OXPHOS genes is seen already in individuals with impaired glucose tolerance or in healthy first-degree relatives of patients with type 2 diabetes.[8,9] Also, first-degree relatives of patients with type 2 diabetes show impaired ATP synthesis in skeletal muscle as measured by NMR spectroscopy.[11]

Second, from an epidemiological standpoint, it is worthwhile recalling that even the common form of diabetes tends to exhibit excess maternal transmission.[34] In fact, a number of small studies have suggested that mtDNA haplotypes can contribute to the risk of diabetes.[43]

Third, a number of genetic studies have shown that polymorphisms in several genes are associated with the common form of diabetes. Perhaps the strongest result is from PPAR-γ, a nuclear receptor that is the target of the thiazolidinediones (TZDs). The Pro12Ala variant, which is found in 10–15% of the Caucasian population, is associated with a 15% decreased risk of diabetes.[44] Variation in the HNF4α promoter is also associated with the common form of diabetes.[45,46] These nuclear receptors are all transcriptional partners of PGC-1α, a master regulator of mitochondrial biogenesis.[47] In fact, variation in PGC-1α has also been associated with diabetes, though these have not been broadly replicated.[48]

Finally, clinical and pharmacologic studies strongly support the notion that mitochondrial biogenesis can contribute to diabetes. It has long been appreciated that the best non-pharmacologic intervention for improving insulin resistance is exercise. The recent Diabetes Prevention Program Trial in patients with type 2 diabetes confirmed that exercise was the most effective way to prevent diabetes in those with impaired glucose tolerance.[49] Exercise is known to increase mitochondrial biogenesis in skeletal muscle and concomitantly improve total body VO_2max, which is itself a marker for insulin resistance. The TZDs represent a category of drugs that improve insulin resistance. Recent studies have shown that they serve as a synthetic agonist for the nuclear hormone receptor PPARγ, and one of the effects is to increase mitochondrial biogenesis in fat and possibly in muscle.[50] Recent studies have also shown that high intake of caffeine can reduce one's lifetime risk of developing diabetes,[51] and caffeine has been shown in vitro to increase mitochondrial biogenesis.[52] In addition, the lipodystrophy seen in patients with human immunodeficiency virus infection appears to be due to the mitochondrial toxicity of highly active antiretroviral therapy.[53]

Taken together, there is biochemical, genetic, and clinical support for a key role for mitochondrial biogenesis in diabetes. Additional studies are needed to determine if and how mitochondrial diabetes resulting from mtDNA mutations may be related to the expression phenotype seen in the common form of the disease.

Other endocrine disorders in mitochondrial disease

Here, we review some of the other endocrine manifestations in patients with mtDNA disorders.

Short stature

Short stature is defined as a standing height more than two standard deviations below the mean for age and gender. Short stature may result from endocrine disease, systemic illness (e.g. chronic renal failure, malnutrition), or primary skeletal disorders (e.g. achondroplasia, *SHOX* haploinsufficiency). The endocrine causes of short stature include impaired growth hormone (GH) secretion or action, hypothyroidism, and glucocorticoid excess. Short stature is frequently seen in patients with mtDNA defects, with an estimated 35% of all such patients so affected.[4,54] It can be seen in patients with MELAS, myoclonus epilepsy and ragged-red fibers (MERRF), progressive external ophthalmoplegia (PEO), and Kearns–Sayre syndrome (KSS). Of note, short stature can also be seen in patients with mitochondrial diseases due to mutations in nuclear genes, as in Barth syndrome.[55]

The etiology of the short stature in mitochondrial disorders is varied. Matsuzaki et al. reported two girls with MELAS in whom they were able to establish a diagnosis of growth hormone-releasing hormone deficiency.[56] In another study, patients with the A3243G mutation underwent growth hormone provocation studies, which revealed deficient pituitary growth hormone secretion.[57] Quade and colleagues carefully evaluated 21 patients with PEO and found six of them had short stature, possibly secondary to growth hormone deficiency.[58] Last, more than one disorder can account for short stature in patients with mitochondrial disease as was demonstrated by a girl with MELAS with both growth hormone deficiency and central hypothyroidism.[59] Short stature is a common symptom of mitochondrial disease, whether due to mitochondrial or nuclear defects, and can be due to more than one etiology, the most common of which appears to be GH deficiency. Investigations into the clinical effectiveness of GH supplementation are limited. Although there is no established therapy for short stature in patients with mitochondrial disease, there are reports suggesting that in patients with documented GH deficiency, replacement therapy can have a benefit.[56,60]

Because of the prevalence of this disorder and the potential therapy available, critical evaluation of possible endocrine causes and therapies is needed.

Gonadal dysfunction

Patients with gonadal disorders can present with a variety of signs and symptoms. Males may present with cryptorchidism, lack of or delay in puberty, low libido, and erectile dysfunction. In females, the manifestations include delayed puberty, late menarche, primary or secondary amenorrhea, or oligomenorrhea. The etiology may be hypothalamic, pituitary, or gonadal (ovaries and testes) disease. Gonadal dysfunction appears to frequently accompany mtDNA-based disorders and has been described in patients with PEO, MELAS, and MERRF.[58,61]

In a study of 21 patients with PEO, Quade et al. found that 38% exhibited symptoms, physical examination signs, or laboratory evidence of a reproductive disorder.[58] Chen et al. reviewed six patients with MELAS and MERRF, and five had evidence of gonadal dysfunction either by history or physical examination.[61] Symptoms included delayed puberty, primary amenorrhea, or secondary amenorrhea in women and delayed puberty and erectile dysfunction in men. Gonadotropin levels and luteinizing hormone-releasing hormone stimulation testing suggest hypothalamic or pituitary dysfunction. In fact, an autopsy report of a patient with MELAS due to a mutation in mitochondrial $tRNA^{Leu(UUR)}$ revealed that the hypophysis had the highest level of heteroplasmy.[62]

In addition to the studies described above, there are a few case reports describing testosterone insufficiency in patients with mtDNA mutations.[63]

Because of the small number of studies to date, it is difficult to determine the actual prevalence of reproductive dysfunction in patients with mitochondrial disease as well as the site of the defect (hypothalamic, pituitary, or gonadal). No studies have systematically examined the safety and efficacy of testosterone or estrogen replacement therapy in patients with mitochondrial disease. It is interesting to postulate whether or not gonadal disorders have mitochondrial pathophysiologic correlates in the same manner as diabetes.

Other endocrine manifestations

A variety of other endocrine disorders have been described in case reports or small case series of mtDNA diseases. These endocrine disorders include hypoparathyroidism, thyroid disease (hypothyroidism or hyperthyroidism), and adrenal disease (adrenal insufficiency or hyperaldosteronism).

Hypoparathyroidism is characterized by deficient parathyroid hormone production. Symptoms can range from subclinical disease to paresthesias to seizures, depending on the degree of resulting hypocalcemia, Hypoparathyroidism has been described in patients with mitochondrial disorders, especially those with KSS and PEO.[64,65]

Hypothyroid symptoms include cold intolerance, fatigue, weight gain, coarse hair, and constipation. Hyperthyroid symptoms include heat intolerance, palpitations, weight loss, and diarrhea. Symptoms can be extremely mild to very severe depending on the degree of dysfunction. Thyroid dysfunction, both hypothyroidism and hyperthyroidism, has been reported in patients with mitochondrial disease[66,67] and was found in up to 17% of patients with respiratory chain dysfunction in one study.[4] It does not appear to be a feature of mtDNA disorders characterized by deletions.[54,58,68]

Symptoms of adrenal insufficiency include nausea, fatigue, weight loss, and orthostasis. Adrenal insufficiency has been described in patients with mitochondrial disease.[69–72] Hyperaldosteronism, which can present as hypertension, has also been described in patients with mitochondrial disease.[54,73] As with many of the other endocrinopathies, the actual prevalence of adrenal disease in these patients is not known.

Clinical evalution and treatment considerations

At present, we advocate that all clinicians caring for patients with mitochondrial disease be aware of the reported endocrinopathies that may appear in such patients. All patients should be assessed for possible diabetes, short stature, gonadal dysfunction, thyroid dysfunction, hypoparathyroidism, and adrenal insufficiency (Table 8.1).

An initial history and physical exam ought to explore these possible features. An initial history must include assessment for polydipsia, polyuria, and weight loss as initial signs of diabetes mellitus. Questions should be asked regarding regularity of menses in women and erectile function and libido in men. Symptoms of thyroid disease such as heat or cold intolerance, weight loss or gain, change in skin or hair texture, and constipation or diarrhea should be elicited. A diagnosis of hypoparathyroidism should be

Table 8.1 Endocrine manifestations in mitochondrial disorders

Endocrinopathy	Signs and symptoms	Screening tests
Diabetes	Polyuria, polydipsia, polyphagia, weight loss	Fasting blood sugar
Short stature	Short stature for gender and age	Plot height on growth chart: if 2 SD below mean: IGF-1, IGF-BP3, bone age, GH provocative testing
Hypogonadism	Poor development of secondary sexual characteristics, infertility, delayed puberty, amenorrhea	In men: morning total testosterone, LH, FSH In women: estradiol, LH, FSH
Hypoparathyroidism	Tetany, paresthesias, seizures, cramps	Calcium, albumin, phosphorus, parathyroid hormone (PTH)
Hypothyroidism	Weight gain, fatigue, cold intolerance, constipation, dry skin, hair loss, menstrual irregularities	Thyroid-stimulating hormone (TSH), free thyroxine (free T4)
Adrenal insufficiency	Orthostasis, fatigue, hyponatremia, hyperkalemia	Morning cortisol: if < 18 μg/dL, then cosyntropin stimulation test

SD = standard deviation; IGF-1 = insulin-like growth factor-1; IGF-BP3 = insulin-like growth factor binding protein 3; GH = growth hormone; LH = leutenizing hormone; FSH = follicle-stimulating hormone.

considered when patients describe muscle cramping or paresthesias.

Physical examination ought to include a careful height measurement, thyroid examination, assessment of secondary sexual characteristics, and assessment of Chvostsek's and Trousseau's signs.

An initial laboratory evaluation ought to include a fasting glucose level. In addition, calcium, albumin, phosphate, parathyroid hormone (PTH), thyroid-stimulating hormone (TSH) and free thyroxine (free T4) levels should be ordered to assess for hypoparathyroidism and thyroid disease. If gonadal dysfunction is suggested by the history or physical exam, follicle-stimulating hormone (FSH) and luteinizing hormone (LH) should be ordered in addition to an estradiol level in women and an early morning total testosterone level in men. If orthostasis, nausea, or unexplained weight loss are present, then the patients should be assessed for adrenal insufficiency with a morning cortisol or cosyntropin stimulation test. If any of the components of the history, physical, or screening endocrine labs are suggestive of diabetes, short stature, gonadal dysfunction, thyroid disease, hypoparathyroidism or adrenal insufficiency, we advocate early referral to an endocrinologist for careful diagnostic studies followed by treatment initiation (Table 8.1).

Treatment

For patients with mtDNA-based diabetes, it is likely that the mainstay of therapy will involve sulfonylureas, diet, and insulin therapy. We have found that these patients can also benefit from insulin sensitizers, in particular TZDs. Future studies may determine whether specific forms of disease may benefit from specific therapies. Because metformin has been associated with lactic acidosis in isolated cases, we currently prefer avoidance of this drug, especially in patients with MELAS. While carnitine, antioxidants and CoQ10 are often prescribed to patients with mtDNA disorders, there are no studies to date that provide convincing evidence that they improve diabetes.

With regard to the other endocrinopathies, hormone replacement of the deficient hormone(s) may be needed. Female and male patients diagnosed with reproductive disorders may require estrogen or testosterone replacement. Patients with hypothyroidism will need to be treated with thyroid hormone replacement, and patients with hypoparathyroidism may need calcium and vitamin D replacement.

Summary

It is clear that a variety of endocrinopathies accompany human mitochondrial diseases, those due to mtDNA mutations as well as those due to nuclear defects. Tremendous research has focused on the role of the mitochondria in various forms of diabetes. We anticipate that in the coming years, specific mechanistic links between this organelle and insulin deficiency and insulin resistance will be established.

In patients with mitochondrial disease, however, we are lacking careful and systematic studies of endocrine function. It is important that we first determine the frequency of endocrinopathies in patients with these disorders and how they manifest. In addition, studies are needed to determine the etiology of these endocrinopathies and may require careful frequent hormone blood sampling and/or stimulation testing. Last, the efficacy of current endocrine standard treatments must be assessed in these patients.

The potential psychological and physical benefits of hormonal replacement may prove to greatly improve mitochondrial patients' quality of life. Treating short stature and hypogonadism will help with social interactions. Thyroid hormone replacement can influence mitochondrial biogenesis and can directly impact mitochondrial energetics. Normalization of calcium may help with neurologic symptoms, including seizure control, and treatment of adrenal insufficiency may help with fatigue and orthostasis seen in patients. Because the endocrine system is so intimately linked to cellular energetics, careful evaluation and treatment of endocrine dysfunction in patients with mitochondrial disease is extremely important and should be pursued.

Acknowledgments

We thank David Holtzmann, Paul Boepple, Katherine Sims, and Corrine Welt for useful discussions and careful review of this chapter.

References

1. Luft R, Ikkos D, Palmieri G et al. A case of severe hypermetabolism of nonthyroid origin with a defect in the maintenance of mitochondrial respiratory control: a correlated clinical, biochemical, and morphological study. *J Clin Invest* 1962; **41**: 1776–1804.
2. Wallace DC, Ruiz-Pesini E, Mishmar D. mtDNA variation, climatic adaptation, degenerative diseases, and longevity. *Cold Spring Harb Symp Quant Biol* 2003; **68**: 479–486.
3. Chinnery PF, Turnbull DM. Mitochondrial medicine. *QJM* 1997; **90**(11): 657–667.
4. Finsterer J, Jarius C, Eichberger H. Phenotype variability in 130 adult patients with respiratory chain disorders. *J Inherit Metab Dis* 2001; **24**(5): 560–576.
5. Zimmet P. Globalization, coca-colonization and the chronic disease epidemic: can the Doomsday scenario be averted? *J Intern Med* 2000; **247**(3): 301–310.
6. American Diabetes Association Screening for type 2 diabetes. *Diabetes Care* 2004; **27** Suppl 1: S11–S14.
7. Florez JC, Hirschhorn JN, Altshuler D. The inherited basis of diabetes mellitus: implications for the genetic analysis of complex traits. *Ann Rev Genomics Hum Genet* 2003; **4**: 257–291.
8. Mootha VK, Lindgren CM, Eriksson KF et al. PGC-1α-responsive genes involved in oxidative

phosphorylation are coordinately downregulated in human diabetes. *Nat Genet* 2003; **34**(3): 267–273.
9. Patti ME, Butte AJ, Crunkhorn S et al. Coordinated reduction of genes of oxidative metabolism in humans with insulin resistance and diabetes: Potential role of *PGC1* and *NRF1*. *Proc Natl Acad Sci USA* 2003; **100**(14): 8466–8471.
10. Petersen KF, Befroy D, Dufour S et al. Mitochondrial dysfunction in the elderly: possible role in insulin resistance. *Science* 2003; **300**(5622): 1140–1142.
11. Petersen KF, Dufour S, Befroy D et al. Impaired mitochondrial activity in the insulin-resistant offspring of patients with type 2 diabetes. *N Engl J Med* 2004; **350**(7): 664–671.
12. Kelley DE, He J, Menshikova EV et al. Dysfunction of mitochondria in human skeletal muscle in type 2 diabetes. *Diabetes* 2002; **51**(10): 2944–2950.
13. Neel JV. Diabetes mellitus: a 'thrifty' genotype rendered detrimental by 'progress'? *Am J Hum Genet* 1962; **14**: 353–362.
14. Suzuki S, Oka Y, Kadowaki T et al. Clinical features of diabetes mellitus with the mitochondrial DNA 3243 (A-G) mutation in Japanese: maternal inheritance and mitochondria-related complications. *Diabetes Res Clin Pract* 2003; **59**(3): 207–217.
15. Hattersley AT. Diagnosis of maturity-onset diabetes of the young in the pediatric diabetes clinic. *J Pediatr Endocrinol Metab* 2000; **13** Suppl 6: 1411–1417.
16. Guillausseau PJ, Massin P, Dubois-LaForgue D et al. Maternally inherited diabetes and deafness: a multicenter study. *Ann Intern Med* 2001; **134**(9 Pt 1): 721–728.
17. Cervin C, Liljestrom B, Tuomi T et al. Cosegregation of MIDD and MODY in a pedigree: functional and clinical consequences. *Diabetes* 2004; **53**(7): 1894–1899.
18. Maassen JA, 'T Hart LM, Van Essen E et al. Mitochondrial diabetes: molecular mechanisms and clinical presentation. *Diabetes* 2004; **53** Suppl 1: S103–S109.
19. van den Ouweland JM, Lemkes HH, Ruitenbeek W et al. Mutation in mitochondrial $tRNA^{Leu(UUR)}$ gene in a large pedigree with maternally transmitted type II diabetes mellitus and deafness. *Nat Genet* 1992; **1**(5): 368–371.
20. Kadowaki T, Kadowaki H, Mori Y et al. A subtype of diabetes mellitus associated with a mutation of mitochondrial DNA. *N Engl J Med* 1994; **330**(14): 962–968.
21. Maechler P, Wollheim CB. Mitochondrial function in normal and diabetic β-cells. *Nature* 2001; **414**(6865): 807–812.
22. Ballinger SW, Shoffner JM, Hedaya EV et al. Maternally transmitted diabetes and deafness associated with a 10.4 kb mitochondrial DNA deletion. *Nat Genet* 1992; **1**(1): 11–15.
23. Ohkubo K, Yamano A, Nagashima M et al. Mitochondrial gene mutations in the $tRNA^{Leu(UUR)}$ region and diabetes: prevalence and clinical phenotypes in Japan. *Clin Chem* 2001; **47**(9): 1641–1648.
24. Jansen JJ, Maassen JA, van der Woude FJ et al. Mutation in mitochondrial $tRNA^{Leu(UUR)}$ gene associated with progressive kidney disease. *J Am Soc Nephrol* 1997; **8**(7): 1118–1124.
25. Kanamori A, Tanaka K, Umezawa S et al. Insulin resistance in mitochondrial gene mutation. *Diabetes Care* 1994; **17**(7): 778–779.
26. Velho G, Byrne MM, Clement K et al. Clinical phenotypes, insulin secretion, and insulin sensitivity in kindreds with maternally inherited diabetes and deafness due to mitochondrial $tRNALeu^{(UUR)}$ gene mutation. *Diabetes* 1996; **45**(4): 478–487.
27. Chomyn A, Enriquez JA, Micol V et al. The mitochondrial myopathy, encephalopathy, lactic acidosis, and stroke-like episode syndrome-associated human mitochondrial $tRNALeu^{(UUR)}$ mutation causes aminoacylation deficiency and concomitant reduced association of mRNA with ribosomes. *J Biol Chem* 2000; **275**(25): 19198–19209.
28. Wittenhagen LM, Kelley SO. Dimerization of a pathogenic human mitochondrial tRNA. *Nat Struct Biol* 2002; **9**(8): 586–590.
29. Kobayashi T, Nakanishi K, Nakase H et al. In situ characterization of islets in diabetes with a mitochondrial DNA mutation at nucleotide position 3243. *Diabetes* 1997; **46**(10): 1567–1571.
30. Smith CJ, Crock PA, King BR et al. Phenotype-genotype correlations in a series of wolfram syndrome families. *Diabetes Care* 2004; **27**(8): 2003–2009.
31. Reyes ET, Perurena OH, Festoff BW et al. Insulin resistance in amyotrophic lateral sclerosis. *J Neurol Sci* 1984; **63**(3): 317–324.
32. Andreassen OA, Dedeoglu A, Stanojevic V et al. Huntington's disease of the endocrine pancreas: insulin deficiency and diabetes mellitus due to

impaired insulin gene expression. *Neurobiol Dis* 2002; **11**(3): 410–424.
33. Dorner G, Mohnike A. Further evidence for a predominantly maternal transmission of maturity-onset type diabetes. *Endokrinologie* 1976; **68**(1): 121–124.
34. Alcolado JC, Alcolado R. Importance of maternal history of non-insulin dependent diabetic patients. *BMJ* 1991; **302**(6786): 1178–1180.
35. Soejima A, Inoue K, Takai D et al. Mitochondrial DNA is required for regulation of glucose-stimulated insulin secretion in a mouse pancreatic beta cell line, MIN6. *J Biol Chem* 1996; **271**(42): 26194–26199.
36. Silva JP, Kohler M, Graff C et al. Impaired insulin secretion and beta-cell loss in tissue-specific knock-out mice with mitochondrial diabetes. *Nat Genet* 2000; **26**(3): 336–340.
37. Bakker SJ, Gans RO, ter Maaten JC et al. The potential role of adenosine in the pathophysiology of the insulin resistance syndrome. *Atherosclerosis* 2001; **155**(2): 283–290.
38. Jacob S, Machann J, Rett K et al. Association of increased intramyocellular lipid content with insulin resistance in lean nondiabetic offspring of type 2 diabetic subjects. *Diabetes* 1999; **48**(5): 1113–1119.
39. Sreekumar R, Halvatsiotis P, Schimke JC et al. Gene expression profile in skeletal muscle of type 2 diabetes and the effect of insulin treatment. *Diabetes* 2002; **51**(6): 1913–1920.
40. Mootha VK, Handschin C, Arlow D et al. Errα and Gabpa/b specify PGC-1α-dependent oxidative phosphorylation gene expression that is altered in diabetic muscle. *Proc Natl Acad Sci USA* 2004; **101**(17): 6570–6575.
41. Kim JK, Fillmore JJ, Sunshine MJ et al. PKC-θ knockout mice are protected from fat-induced insulin resistance. *J Clin Invest* 2004; **114**(6): 823–827.
42. Um SH, Frigerio F, Watanabe M et al. Absence of S6K1 protects against age- and diet-induced obesity while enhancing insulin sensitivity. *Nature* 2004; **431**(7005): 200–205.
43. Poulton J, Luan J, Macaulay V et al. Type 2 diabetes is associated with a common mitochondrial variant: evidence from a population-based case-control study. *Hum Mol Genet* 2002; **11**(13): 1581–1583.
44. Altshuler D, Hirschhorn JN, Klannemark M et al. The common PPARγ Pro12Ala polymorphism is associated with decreased risk of type 2 diabetes. *Nat Genet* 2000; **26**(1): 76–80.
45. Silander K, Mohlke KL, Scott LJ et al. Genetic variation near the hepatocyte nuclear factor-4 alpha gene predicts susceptibility to type 2 diabetes. *Diabetes* 2004; **53**(4): 1141–1149.
46. Love-Gregory LD, Wasson J, Ma J et al. A common polymorphism in the upstream promoter region of the hepatocyte nuclear factor-4 alpha gene on chromosome 20q is associated with type 2 diabetes and appears to contribute to the evidence for linkage in an Ashkenazi Jewish population. *Diabetes* 2004; **53**(4): 1134–1140.
47. Puigserver P, Spiegelman BM. Peroxisome proliferator-activated receptor-γ coactivator 1α (PGC-1α): transcriptional coactivator and metabolic regulator. *Endocr Rev* 2003; **24**(1): 78–90.
48. Muller YL, Bogardus C, Beamer BA et al. A functional variant in the peroxisome proliferator-activated receptor γ2 promoter is associated with predictors of obesity and type 2 diabetes in Pima Indians. *Diabetes* 2003; **52**(7): 1864–1871.
49. Knowler WC, Barrett-Connor E, Fowler SE et al. Reduction in the incidence of type 2 diabetes with lifestyle intervention or metformin. *N Engl J Med* 2002; **346**(6): 393–403.
50. Wilson-Fritch L, Burkart A, Bell G et al. Mitochondrial biogenesis and remodeling during adipogenesis and in response to the insulin sensitizer rosiglitazone. *Mol Cell Biol* 2003; **23**(3): 1085–1094.
51. Tuomilehto J, Hu G, Bidel S et al. Coffee consumption and risk of type 2 diabetes mellitus among middle-aged Finnish men and women. *JAMA* 2004; **291**(10): 1213–1219.
52. Ojuka EO, Jones TE, Han DH et al. Raising Ca^{2+} in L6 myotubes mimics effects of exercise on mitochondrial biogenesis in muscle. *Faseb J* 2003; **17**(6): 675–681.
53. Brinkman K, Smeitink JA, Romijn JA et al. Mitochondrial toxicity induced by nucleoside-analogue reverse-transcriptase inhibitors is a key factor in the pathogenesis of antiretroviral-therapy-related lipodystrophy. *Lancet* 1999; **354**(9184): 1112–1115.
54. Harvey JN, Barnett D. Endocrine dysfunction in Kearns-Sayre syndrome. *Clin Endocrinol (Oxf)* 1992; **37**(1): 97–103.
55. Barth PG, Wanders RJ, Vreken P et al. X-linked cardioskeletal myopathy and neutropenia (Barth

syndrome) (MIM 302060). *J Inherit Metab Dis* 1999; **22**(4): 555–567.

56. Matsuzaki M, Izumi T, Shishikura K et al. Hypothalamic growth hormone deficiency and supplementary GH therapy in two patients with mitochondrial myopathy, encephalopathy, lactic acidosis and stroke-like episodes. *Neuropediatrics* 2002; **33**(5): 271–273.
57. Yorifuji T, Kawai M, Momoi T et al. Nephropathy and growth hormone deficiency in a patient with mitochondrial $tRNA^{Leu(UUR)}$ mutation. *J Med Genet* 1996; **33**(7): 621–622.
58. Quade A, Zierz S, Klingmuller D. Endocrine abnormalities in mitochondrial myopathy with external ophthalmoplegia. *Clin Investig* 1992; **70**(5): 396–402.
59. Balestri P, Grosso S. Endocrine disorders in two sisters affected by MELAS syndrome. *J Child Neurol* 2000; **15**(11): 755–758.
60. Egger J, Lake BD, Wilson J. Mitochondrial cytopathy. A multisystem disorder with ragged red fibres on muscle biopsy. *Arch Dis Child* 1981; **56**(10): 741–752.
61. Chen CM, Huang CC. Gonadal dysfunction in mitochondrial encephalomyopathies. *Eur Neurol* 1995; **35**(5): 281–286.
62. Shiraiwa N, Ishii A, Iwamoto H et al. Content of mutant mitochondrial DNA and organ dysfunction in a patient with a MELAS subgroup of mitochondrial encephalomyopathies. *J Neurol Sci* 1993; **120**(2): 174–179.
63. Nishigaki Y, Tadesse S, Bonilla E et al. A novel mitochondrial $tRNA^{Leu(UUR)}$ mutation in a patient with features of MERRF and Kearns-Sayre syndrome. *Neuromuscul Disord* 2003; **13**(4): 334–340.
64. Pellock JM, Behrens M, Lewis L et al. Kearns-Sayre syndrome and hypoparathyroidism. *Ann Neurol* 1978; **3**(5): 455–458.
65. Dewhurst AG, Hall D, Schwartz MS et al. Kearns-Sayre syndrome, hypoparathyroidism, and basal ganglia calcification. *J Neurol Neurosurg Psychiatry* 1986; **49**(11): 1323–1324.
66. Case records of the Massachusetts General Hospital. Weekly clinicopathological exercises. Case 34–1987. A 30-year-old woman with an ocular motility disturbance, myopathy, and hypocalcemia. *N Engl J Med* 1987; **317**(8): 493–501.
67. Yang CY, Lam HC, Lee HC et al. MELAS syndrome associated with diabetes mellitus and hyperthyroidism: a case report from Taiwan. *Clin Endocrinol (Oxf)* 1995; **43**(2): 235–239.
68. Danta G, Hilton RC, Lynch PG. Chronic progressive external ophthalmoplegia. *Brain* 1975; **98**(3): 473–492.
69. Bruno C, Minetti C, Tang Y et al. Primary adrenal insufficiency in a child with a mitochondrial DNA deletion. *J Inherit Metab Dis* 1998; **21**(2): 155–161.
70. Boles RG, Roe T, Senadheera D et al. Mitochondrial DNA deletion with Kearns-Sayre syndrome in a child with Addison disease. *Eur J Pediatr* 1998; **157**(8): 643–647.
71. Artuch R, Pavia C, Playan A et al. Multiple endocrine involvement in two pediatric patients with Kearns-Sayre syndrome. *Horm Res* 1998; **50**(2): 99–104.
72. Nicolino M, Ferlin T, Forest M et al. Identification of a large-scale mitochondrial deoxyribonucleic acid deletion in endocrinopathies and deafness: report of two unrelated cases with diabetes mellitus and adrenal insufficiency, respectively. *J Clin Endocrinol Metab* 1997; **82**(9): 3063–3067.
73. Park SB, Ma KT, Kook KH et al. Kearns-Sayre syndrome-3 case reports and review of clinical feature. *Yonsei Med J* 2004; **45**(4): 727–735.
74. Wu Z, Puigserver P, Andersson U et al. Mechanisms controlling mitochondrial biogenesis and respiration through the thermogenic co-activator PGC-1. *Cell* 1999; **98**: 115–124.

9

Mitochondrial nephrology

Agnès Rötig and Patrick Niaudet

The energy requirement of the nephron

One important function of the kidney is the reabsorption of 99% of the glomerular ultrafiltrate. Membranes are usually impermeable to ions, thus ion-motive pumps are needed to convert the energy derived from ATP hydrolysis into an electrochemical potential that can drive transport against a concentration gradient. The primary active transporter in kidney is the sodium-potassium adenosine triphosphatase (Na^+,K^+-ATPase). A secondary active transport system allows solutes to move along an electrochemical gradient without direct consumption of energy. This secondary transporter uses the potential energy stored in transmembrane ion gradient. Several ATP-driven solute pumps are involved in the primary active transport. The major classes of kidney ion-translocating ATPases are Na^+,K^+-ATPase, H^+,K^+-ATPase, Ca^{2+}-ATPase, and H^+-ATPase. These various ATPases are distributed along the nephron according to the demands for solute transport and the required metabolic machinery. The Na^+,K^+-ATPase couples the hydrolysis of one ATP molecule to the translocation of three Na^+ and two K^+ ions against their electrochemical gradients. In the renal medulla, this Na^+,K^+-ATPase uses approximately 10 000 ATP molecules per minute per enzyme molecule. This enzyme is an oligomeric membrane protein, the minimal functional unit being a heterodimer of α- and β-subunits. The principal isozyme in kidney is α1β1. The highest levels of Na^+,K^+-ATPase in kidney are in the medullary thick ascending limb of Henle's loop, in the cortical thick ascending limb of Henle's loop, and in the distal convoluted tubule (Figure 9.1). Ca^{2+}-ATPase activity is high in the distal convoluted tubule, whereas the vacuolar H^+-ATPase is present in proximal tubules, thick ascending limbs, distal convoluted tubules and intercalated cells of the collecting duct.[1]

The reabsorption of water and solutes requires a considerable amount of energy, which explains why the kidneys, whose weight represents less than 1% of the body mass, consume 10% of total body oxygen.[2] The energy, which is needed for solute and water reabsorption, comes from oxidative reactions that produce ATP. The mitochondrial oxidative phosphorylation accounts for 95% of the total ATP production in the kidney. There is considerable variability along the nephron in ion transport demand. In general, there is a strong correlation between active Na^+ transport, Na^+,K^+-ATPase, mitochondrial density, and cellular ATP content. This is, for example, the case of the medullary thick ascending limb of Henle's loop, whereas the inner medullary collecting duct, which carries out lower amounts of Na^+ transport, has fewer mitochondria and less Na^+,K^+-ATPase. In keeping with this, it was shown long ago that there is a functional

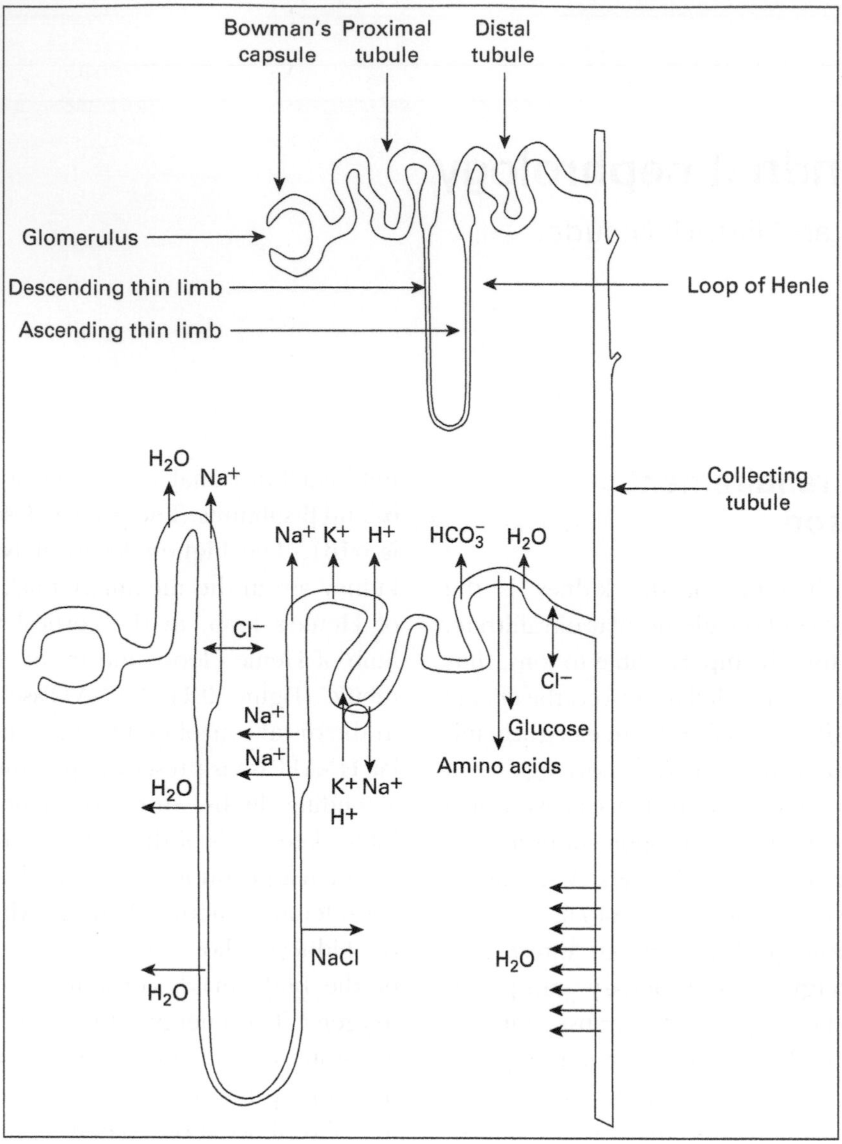

Figure 9.1 Schematic representation of nephron. The total length of a nephron is 20–44 mm

coupling between active Na^+ and K^+ transport and respiration.[3,4] ATP hydrolysis by Na^+,K^+-ATPase acts as a feedback signal to the mitochondria for the regulation of ATP synthesis.

In summary, ATP is essential to drive the sodium–potassium-ATPase pumps that generate the electrical gradient across proximal tubular epithelium and maintain a low concentration of sodium in the intracellular environment. All other absorptive functions, including those for sugar, phosphate, and amino acids are handled through co-transporters. Therefore, it is not surprising that the most frequent renal defect in mitochondrial diseases is a proximal tubulopathy.

Renal dysfunction in mitochondrial disorders

Tubulopathy

Renal disease has been reported more frequently in children than in adults. In children, the most frequent renal manifestation is proximal tubulopathy resulting in a more or less complete and severe form of DeToni–Debré–Fanconi syndrome.[5,6] The DeToni–Debré–Fanconi syndrome includes urinary losses of amino acids, glucose, proteins, phosphate, uric acid, calcium, bicarbonate, potassium, sodium, and water. The proximal tubulopathy is often moderate and several authors have reported isolated hyperaminoaciduria in the absence of clinical manifestations. Most patients, however, show plasma acidosis secondary to urinary bicarbonate losses, hypophosphatemia due to decreased phosphate reabsorption, hypercalciuria, glycosuria, and tubular proteinuria. Some patients may also develop growth retardation, rickets, or dehydration. Renal biopsy shows nonspecific anomalies of the tubular epithelium, with dilatations and obstructions by casts, dedifferentiation, or atrophy. Giant mitochondria are often observed. Extra-renal symptoms are always present and include myopathy, neurological symptoms, Pearson syndrome, diabetes mellitus, or cardiac problems. Most patients develop tubular symptoms before the age of 2 years and over 40% of them die during the first year of life. Several reported cases had neonatal onset.[7–9]

Tubular acidosis

Patients with mitochondrial disorder may also present with isolated proximal tubular acidosis and hypercalciuria,[10] or with signs of salt depletion and hypokalemic metabolic alkalosis compatible with Bartter's syndrome.[11,12] Katsanos et al. reported a patient with Kearns–Sayre syndrome, who had hypoparathyroidism and severe hypomagnesemia secondary to tubular dysfunction.[13]

Nephrotic syndrome

Children with mitochondrial cytopathies may present with steroid-resistant nephrotic syndrome and focal segmental glomerular sclerosis (FSGS).[14,15] Several authors have described children with the triad of steroid-resistant nephrotic syndrome, hypoparathyroidism, and sensorineural deafness.[15–21] The patients reported by Barakat had an autosomal recessive mode of inheritance and progressed to end-stage renal failure during early childhood.[16] Two sisters reported by Brun et al. had steroid-resistant FSGS,[15] but also myopathy, ophthalmoplegia, pigmentary retinopathy, and hypoparathyroidism. Hypoparathyroidism and sensorineural hearing loss have also been reported in association with renal tubular defects[22] or renal dysplasia.[23] These patients also had myopathy, ophthalmoplegia, pigmentary retinopathy, or hypoparathyroidism. Some patients progressed to end-stage renal failure. Finally, some patients with nephritic syndrome also presented with cardiomyopathy.[24]

Coenzyme Q_{10} deficiency was reported in two siblings with severe encephalopathy, nephrotic syndrome, and renal failure. As the in vitro addition of quinone to cultured fibroblasts stimulated respiration and enzyme activities, the patients were treated with oral ubidecarenone and improved dramatically.[25] Coenzyme Q_{10} deficiency caused encephalomyopathy and nephrotic syndrome in another family: this infant, the child of consanguineous parents, also responded dramatically to coenzyme Q_{10} supplementation.[26] A homozygous missense mutation in the *COQ2* gene has been identified in this family.[27]

Tubulointerstitial nephropathy

Tubulointerstitial nephropathy has been described in a few patients.[28–31] The clinical presentation is characterized by polyuria secondary to impaired urinary-concentrating ability and by progression to end-stage renal failure. Patients do not show proximal tubular defects. Histologically, renal biopsy shows diffuse interstitial fibrosis with tubular atrophy and sclerotic glomeruli within the area of interstitial fibrosis. These patients also had extra-renal symptoms: hearing loss and cardiomyopathy, myopathy and growth retardation, mental retardation and pigmentary retinopathy. The same clinical nephropathy may be seen in patients with nephronophthisis, which can be associated with retinitis pigmentosa and cerebral ataxia. The presence of medullary cysts on ultrasound examination and thickened tubular basement membranes on renal biopsy is suggestive of nephronophthisis. The patient reported by Szabolcs et al. with chronic tubulointerstitial nephropathy also had signs of Fanconi syndrome with glycosuria, proteinuria, and high fractional excretion of phosphate.[32]

Adult presentations

In adults, renal involvement has been reported with the A3243G-MELAS mtDNA mutation. Guéry et al. recently described renal symptoms in nine patients with this mutation. Renal lesions consisted of FSGS in two patients, tubulointerstitial nephropathy in three, and bilateral enlarged cystic kidneys in one.[33] In a retrospective study of seven patients with FSGS, Hotta et al. found the MELAS mutation in four women,[34] in whom proteinuria had been discovered during childhood by routine examination. Two of them developed diabetes mellitus and one hearing loss. Doleris et al. also reported four adult patients with FSGS and the MELAS mutation.[35] Altogether, 24 adult patients with mitochondrial cytopathy and renal involvement have been reported in the literature.[33–39] Females are four times more often affected than males. The first renal symptoms occur in early adulthood and are the initial manifestations of the disease in one third of cases. Proteinuria was accompanied by nephrotic syndrome in only one third of cases. None of the patients had signs of tubular dysfunction. Most patients progressed to end-stage renal failure at a median age of 33 years. Renal biopsy most often showed non-specific lesions, such as focal and segmental glomerular sclerosis. Electron microscopy sometimes showed abnormal mitochondria in podocytes. Some authors have described severe hyaline changes in the cytoplasm of smooth muscle cells in small arteries. Some patients had no evidence of focal or segmental glomerular sclerosis but only non-specific tubulo-interstitial lesions.

Diabetes mellitus developed in the majority of patients, but usually several years after the nephropathy had been discovered. A positive family history of diabetes mellitus is frequently reported, but renal biopsy does not show any signs of diabetic glomerulopathy. Hearing loss is also a common finding, which often precedes the onset of renal disease and diabetes mellitus. The association of deafness and hereditary glomerulopathy explains how a number of patients had been diagnosed as having Alport syndrome. It is important to keep in mind that patients with mitochondrial cytopathy do not have hematuria, which is a constant feature of Alport syndrome.

The A3243G mtDNA mutation has been associated with maternally inherited diabetes mellitus and deafness. The same mutation was found to occur in approximately 1% of diabetic patients in Europe and in Japan.[40,41] Interestingly, in a cohort of 54 French patients with type 2 diabetes mellitus and the mtDNA 3243 mutation, 28% also had renal disease, whereas the prevalence of diabetic retinopathy was only 8%, suggesting that the nephropathy was due to the mitochondrial cytopathy.[42] Iwasaki et al. found the mtDNA 3243 mutation in eight (5.9%) of 135 patients with diabetes mellitus and end-stage renal failure.[43] Five of the eight patients later developed symptoms of MELAS. The mutation was not found in any of the 92 control patients with end-stage renal failure but without diabetes mellitus.

Metabolic investigation of patients with renal dysfunction

A deficiency of the RC should alter the redox status in the plasma. Indeed, excess NADH due to RC deficiency increases the ketone body (β-OH butyrate/acetoacetate) molar ratio in the mitochondria as well as the lactate/pyruvate (L/P) molar ratio in the cytoplasm, with secondary elevation of blood lactate. For these reasons, screening for RC deficiencies includes the determination of lactate, pyruvate, ketone bodies and their molar ratios.

It should be stressed, however, that these metabolic abnormalities may not be present in patients with proximal tubulopathy because the impaired proximal tubular functions may lower blood lactate and increase urinary lactate. For this reason, normal plasma lactate does not rule out a mitochondrial disorder with proximal tubulopathy. In these cases, the clue to the diagnosis comes from the association with other related symptoms. Moreover, gas chromatography–mass spectrometry can detect high amounts of lactate and Krebs cycle intermediates in the urine.

Enzymologic investigations of patients with renal dysfunction

Measurements of RC function by polarography and spectrophotometry allow identifying the biochemical nature of the deficiency.[44] Polarography measures oxygen consumption by mitochondria in the presence of various oxidative substrates (see Box 9.1). The only limitation of this technique is that it requires fresh tissue: no polarographic studies are possible on frozen material. Spectrophotometric studies assess isolated or combined respiratory chain complexes using specific electron donors and acceptors. The question of what tissue should be investigated deserves particular attention. Ideally, the affected tissue is the one that should be studied. However, when the disease is expressed in difficult to access organs such as the kidney, accessible peripheral tissues should be extensively tested (including skeletal muscle, cultured skin fibroblasts, and circulating lymphocytes). Moreover, as renal disease is always associated with involvement of other tissues, as indicated by the coexistence of diabetes/deafness, myopathy, encephalopathy, or liver failure, the study of peripheral tissues is often informative, thus making a kidney biopsy unnecessary for enzymological studies of the RC. Whatever the affected organ, it is mandatory to take skin biopsies from patients for subsequent enzymological and genetic investigations on cultured fibroblasts, which is feasible even post-mortem.

RC analysis allows to identify the defective complex(es). No specific enzyme deficiency is associated with renal disease, but nephropathy is more frequently associated with complex III or with multiple RC deficiencies. This conclusion is based on the high incidence in nephropatic patients of (i) mitochondrial $tRNA^{Leu}$ mutation in adults,[33–39] (ii) large-scale mtDNA rearrangements;[29,32] and (iii) the *BCS1L* nuclear gene mutation in children[7] (see below). Ubiquinone deficiency is a rare cause of mitochondrial disorder, but the neonatal variant often includes renal involvement.[25]

Genetic bases of mitochondrial disorders with kidney involvement

Any mode of inheritance can be observed in mitochondrial diseases, whatever the clinical symptoms: autosomal recessive, dominant, X-linked, maternal, or sporadic.[45] Accordingly, mutations in both mitochondrial and nuclear genes have been identified in patients with mitochondrial disorder and renal involvement. However, the molecular definition of RC defects is complicated by the dual genetic control of RC proteins and by the high number of genes involved in the biogenesis

Box 9.1 Polarography

One of the classic ways of assessing mitochondrial function is by measuring oxygen consumption using an oxygen electrode, otherwise known as polarography. The underlying principle is that mitochondria consume oxygen at complex IV (cytochrome *c* oxidase, or COX) (Figure B9.1.1). Thus, problems with respiratory chain function in patient cells will be revealed as a decrease in oxygen consumption relative to that in control cells.

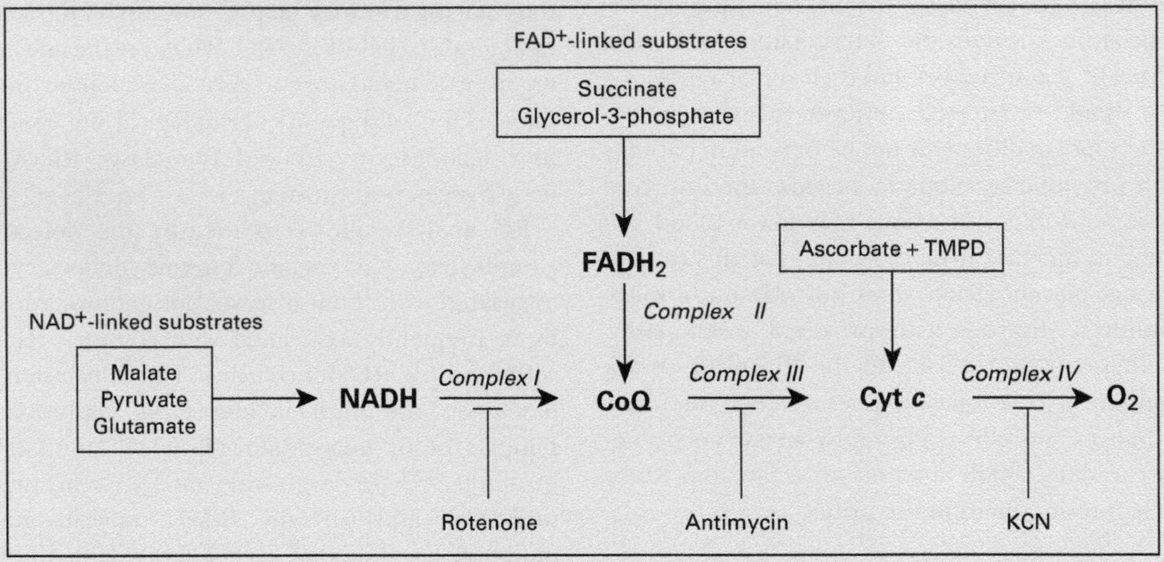

Figure B9.1.1 Oxygen consumption by the respiratory chain. O_2 is consumed in the final step, at complex IV. Some substrates for, and inhibitors of, the various respiratory complexes are shown. Ascorbate reduces tetramethylphenylenediamine (TMPD) to transfer electrons to cytochrome *c*. KCN, potassium cyanide

Polarography can be used to assess not only respiratory chain function but also the coupling of oxygen consumption to ATP synthesis. Since different substrates feed reducing equivalents (NADH, $FADH_2$) at different points in the chain (see Figure B9.1.1), adding specific substrates to the polarographic chamber can pinpoint which step in the chain is compromised, thus giving insight into the underlying genetic defect; the use of complex-specific respiratory chain inhibitors is similarly helpful (Figure B9.1.2A).[1] Alternatively, one can evaluate mitochondrial function based on the ability of the respiratory chain to generate ATP from ADP. In other words, one can add ADP to the cells and then ask if the rate of oxygen consumption (called state III) is increased relative to the 'resting' state rate obtained when ATP is added (called state IV) (Figure B9.1.2B).[2] Oligomycin, an inhibitor of ATP synthase, can also be used to assess the coupling of oxygen consumption to ATP synthesis.

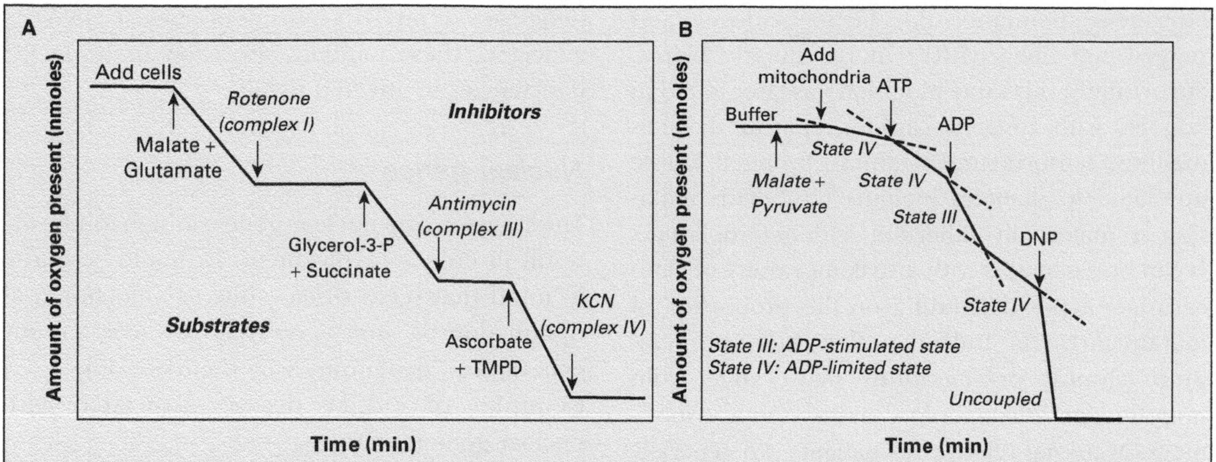

Figure B9.1.2 Polarography. (**A**) Idealized trace showing the effects of various respiratory chain inhibitors. Adapted from reference 1, with permission. (**B**) Idealized trace showing rates of oxygen consumption upon addition of ATP (ATP-limited state; shallower slope) or ADP (ATP-stimulated state; steeper slope). The difference in the state IV slopes before and after addition of ATP is due to the slight amount of ADP that is unavoidably present in most preparations of ATP. Addition of 2,4-dinitrophenol (DNP) punches holes in the inner membrane, thus dissipating the membrane potential and uncoupling oxygen consumption (and proton flow) from ATP synthesis: oxygen is consumed by complex IV but protons are not pumped across the inner membrane (i.e. uncoupled respiration). Adapted from reference 2, with permission

Polarography has been used extensively to screen patients (mainly in cells from muscle biopsies) for respiratory chain dysfunction, and has also been used as one measurement of mitochondrial function in transmitochondrial hybrid (cybrid) cells (see Box 5.1) containing patient mitochondria.

References

1. Hofhaus G, Shakeley RM, Attardi G. Use of polarography to detect respiration defects in cell cultures. *Methods Enzymol* 1996; **264**: 476–483.
2. Trounce IA, Kim YL, Jun AS, Wallace DC. Assessment of mitochondrial oxidative phosphorylation in patient muscle biopsies, lymphoblasts, and transmitochondrial cell lines. *Methods Enzymol* 1996; **264**: 484–509.

and assembly of the RC. Therefore, only in very few patients (10–15% in our experience) have etiological mutations been identified.

Mitochondrial DNA point mutations

The A3243G change in the $tRNA^{Leu}$ gene is one of the most common mtDNA point mutations resulting in impairment of mtDNA translation. This mutation was first associated with mitochondrial encephalomyopathy with lactic acidosis and stroke-like episodes (MELAS).[46] MELAS is characterized by onset in childhood of intermittent hemicranial headache, vomiting, proximal limb weakness, and recurrent neurological deficits resembling strokes (hemiparesis, cortical blindness, hemianopsia), lactic acidosis, and ragged red fibers (RRF) in the muscle biopsy. Surprisingly, this same mutation was later found in families with isolated cardiomyopathy, diabetes mellitus, sensorineural deafness, or renal failure unrelated to diabetes mellitus.[36,47–50] This mutation is maternally inherited and heteroplasmic. It can be associated with a striking variety of clinical phenotypes depending on the proportion of mutant mtDNAs. Indeed, within the same pedigree, clinical presentations may range from migraines and diabetes to a multisystemic involvement. Maternal relatives of patients are generally healthy as long as they have no more than 85% mutant mtDNA. Once the percentage of mutant mtDNA rises above this level, there are increasingly serious clinical manifestations, illustrating the sharp threshold of mtDNA mutations affecting protein synthesis.

Mitochondrial DNA large rearrangements

Large mtDNA rearrangements have been described in several patients with tubulopathy, chronic tubulointerstitial nephritis, or renal tubular dysfunction.[29,51] These deletions take away 2–10 kb of mtDNA and usually encompass several coding and tRNA genes. They are usually sporadic and probably occur de novo during oogenesis or in early development. The size and the location of these deletions are not related to the clinical symptoms or to the severity of the disease.[52–53]

Mitochondrial DNA depletion

This group of mtDNA diseases is characterized by a paucity of mtDNA copy numbers in one or more tissues. Cases of lethal infantile respiratory, muscle, liver, or kidney failure have been ascribed to mtDNA depletion, and are consistent with autosomal recessive inheritance.[54,55] In these patients, there is a marked (sometimes tissue-specific) deficiency of mtDNA but not of nuclear DNA. As expected, these patients also show multiple RC deficiencies in affected tissues.

Nuclear genes

Mutations in any nuclear gene could theoretically result in kidney involvement. It should be borne in mind that renal disease due to mitochondrial dysfunction is not very frequent (8% in our experience), explaining why there are only a few examples of kidney disease associated with nuclear gene mutations.

The *COX10* gene encodes heme A:farnesyl transferase, which catalyzes the first step in the conversion of protoheme to the heme A of cytochrome *c* oxidase (COX). Mutations in this gene have been identified in a child who presented with ataxia and growth failure at 18 months.[56] His neurological condition gradually worsened over the next 6 months. At 2 years of age, he had poor eye contact, severe muscle weakness, hypotonia, ataxia, ptosis, pyramidal syndrome, and status epilepticus. Blood and CSF lactate were elevated (3.8 and 3.1 mmol/L), and GC/MS detected urinary lactate and Krebs cycle intermediates. Increased levels of urinary amino acids were suggestive of a proximal tubulopathy. *COX10* mutations have been reported in two other patients, one with anemia and Leigh syndrome, the other with anemia, sensorineural deafness, and fatal infantile hypertrophic cardiomyopathy. Thus, so far there is no characteristic phenotype associated with *COX10* mutations. The yeast *BCS1* gene encodes a mitochondrial inner membrane protein of the AAA family, which chaperones the assembly of the Rieske iron–sulfur protein of complex III of the respiratory chain. *BCS1L*, the human homolog, is also involved in complex III assembly. Mutations of this gene have been identified in four families of Turkish origin: patients had liver failure, lactic acidosis, hepatocellular insufficiency, tubulopathy, encephalopathy, deafness, and blindness.[7] All the mutations were in highly conserved domains of the BCS1L protein and resulted in complex III deficiency.

It is likely that other nuclear genes causing renal disease will be identified because several consanguineous and/or multiplex families had multisystem involvement including renal disease, but the genetic defect (or defects) have not yet been identified.

References

1. Kone BC. The metabolic basis of solute transport. In: Brenner BM, ed. *The Kidney*. Philadelphia: Saunders, 2004: 231–308.
2. Segall L, Daly SE, Blostein R. Mechanistic basis for kinetic differences between the rat alpha 1, alpha 2, and alpha 3 isoforms of the Na,K-ATPase. *J Biol Chem* 2001; **276**: 31535–31541.
3. Whittam R. Active cation transport as a pace-maker of respiration. *Nature* 1961; **191**: 603–604.
4. Blond DM, Whittam R. The regulation of kidney respiration by sodium and potassium ions. *Biochem J* 1964; **92**: 158–167.
5. Campos Y, Garcia-Silva T, Barrionuevo CR et al. Mitochondrial DNA deletion in a patient with mitochondrial myopathy, lactic acidosis, and stroke-like episodes (MELAS) and Fanconi's syndrome. *Pediatr Neurol* 1995; **13**: 69–72.
6. Wang LC, Lee WT, Tsai WY et al. Mitochondrial cytopathy combined with Fanconi's syndrome. *Pediatr Neurol* 2000; **22**: 403–406.
7. de Lonlay P, Valnot I, Barrientos A et al. A mutant mitochondrial respiratory chain assembly protein causes complex III deficiency in patients with tubulopathy, encephalopathy and liver failure. *Nat Genet* 2001; **29**: 57–60.
8. Ning C, Kuhara T, Matsumoto I. Simultaneous metabolic profile studies of three patients with fatal infantile mitochondrial myopathy-de Toni-Fanconi-Debre syndrome by GC/MS. *Clin Chim Acta* 1996; **247**: 197–200.
9. Wendel U, Ruitenbeek W, Bentlage HA et al. Neonatal De Toni-Debre-Fanconi syndrome due to a defect in complex III of the respiratory chain. *Eur J Pediatr* 1995; **154**: 915–918.
10. Eviatar L, Shanske S, Gauthier B et al. Kearns-Sayre syndrome presenting as renal tubular acidosis. *Neurology* 1990; **40**: 1761–1763.
11. Goto Y, Itami N, Kajii N et al. Renal tubular involvement mimicking Bartter syndrome in a patient with Kearns-Sayre syndrome. *J Pediatr* 1990; **116**: 904–910.
12. Menegon LF, Amaral TN, Gontijo JA. Renal sodium handling study in an atypical case of Bartter's syndrome associated with mitochondriopathy and sensorineural blindness. *Ren Fail* 2004; **26**: 195–197.
13. Katsanos KH, Elisaf M, Bairaktari E et al. Severe hypomagnesemia and hypoparathyroidism in Kearns-Sayre syndrome. *Am J Nephrol* 2001; **21**: 150–153.
14. Niaudet P, Rötig A. The kidney in mitochondrial cytopathies. *Kidney Int* 1997; **51**: 1000–1007.
15. Brun P, Ogier de Baulny H, Peuchmaur M et al. Les atteintes rénales des cytopathies mitochondriales. In: *Journées Parisiennes de Pédiatrie*. Flammarion Médecine Sciences: Paris. 1994: 227–234.
16. Barakat AY, D'Albora JB, Martin MM et al. Familial nephrosis, nerve deafness, and hypoparathyroidism. *J Pediatr* 1977; **91**: 61–64.
17. Inui K, Fukushima H, Tsukamato H et al. Mitochondrial encephalomyopathies with the mutation of the $tRNA^{Leu(UUR)}$ gene. *J Pediatr* 1992; **120**: 62–66.
18. Yorifuji T, Kawai M, Momoi T et al. Nephropathy and growth hormone deficiency in a patient with mitochondrial $tRNA^{Leu(UUR)}$ mutation. *J Med Genet* 1996; **33**: 621–622.
19. Mochizuki H, Joh K, Kawame H et al. Mitochondrial encephalomyopathies preceded by de-Toni-Debre-Fanconi syndrome or focal segmental glomerulosclerosis. *Clin Nephrol* 1996; **46**: 347–352.
20. Cheong HI, Chae JH, Kim JS et al. Hereditary glomerulopathy associated with a mitochondrial $tRNA^{Leu}$ gene mutation. *Pediatr Nephrol* 1999; **13**: 477–480.
21. Hameed R, Raafat F, Ramani P et al. Mitochondrial cytopathy presenting with focal segmental glomerulosclerosis, hypoparathyroidism, sensorineural deafness, and progressive neurological disease. *Postgrad Med J* 2001; **77**: 523–526.
22. Shaw NJ, Haigh D, Lealmann GT et al. Autosomal recessive hypoparathyroidism with renal

insufficiency and developmental delay. *Arch Dis Child* 1999; **66**: 1191–1194.

23. Bilous RW, Murty G, Parkinson DB et al. Autosomal dominant familial hypoparathyroidism, sensorineural deafness, and renal dysplasia. *N Engl J Med* 1992; **327**: 1069–1074.
24. Goldenberg A, Huynh Ngoc L, Thouret MC et al. Respiratory chain deficiency presenting as congenital nephrotic syndrome. *Pediatr Nephrol* 2005; **20**: 465–469.
25. Rötig A, Appelkvist EL, Geromel V et al. Quinone-responsive multiple respiratory-chain dysfunction due to widespread coenzyme Q_{10} deficiency. *Lancet* 2000; **356**: 391–392.
26. Salviati L, Sacconi S, Murer L et al. Infantile encephalomyopathy and nephropathy with CoQ10 deficiency: a CoQ10-responsive condition. *Neurology* 2005; **65**: 606–608.
27. Quinzii C, Naini AB, Salviati L et al. A mutation in para-hydroxybenzoate: polyprenyl transferase *(COQ2)* causes primary coenzyme Q10 deficiency. *Am J Hum Genet* 2006; in press.
28. Donaldson MDC, Warner AA, Trompeter RS et al. Familial juvenile nephronophthisis, Jeune's syndrome, and associated disorders. *Arch Dis Child* 1985; **60**: 426–434.
29. Rötig A, Goutières F, Niaudet P et al. Deletion of mitochondrial DNA in patient with chronic tubulointerstitial nephritis. *J Pediatr* 1995; **126**: 597–601.
30. Tzen CY, Tsai JD, Wu TY et al. Tubulointerstitial nephritis associated with a novel mitochondrial point mutation. *Kidney Int* 2001; **59**: 846–854.
31. Zsurka G, Ormos J, Ivanyi B et al. Mitochondrial mutation as a probable causative factor in familial progressive tubulointerstitial nephritis. *Hum Genet* 1997; **99**: 484–487.
32. Szabolcs MJ, Seigle R, Shanske S et al. Mitochondrial DNA deletion: a cause of chronic tubulointerstitial nephropathy. Kidney Int 1994; **45**: 1388–1396.
33. Guéry B, Choukroun G, Noel LH et al. The spectrum of systemic involvement in adults presenting with renal lesion and mitochondrial $tRNA^{Leu}$ gene mutation. *J Am Soc Nephrol* 2003; **14**: 2099–2108.
34. Hotta O, Inoue CN, Miyabayashi S et al. Clinical and pathologic features of focal segmental glomerulosclerosis with mitochondrial $tRNA^{Leu(UUR)}$ gene mutation. *Kidney Int* 2001; **59**: 1236–1243.
35. Doleris LM, Hill GS, Chedin P et al. Focal segmental glomerulosclerosis associated with mitochondrial cytopathy. *Kidney Int* 2000; **58**: 1851–1858.
36. Jansen JJ, Maassen JA, van der Woude FJ et al. Mutation in mitochondrial $tRNA^{Leu(UUR)}$ gene associated with progressive kidney disease. *J Am Soc Nephrol* 1997; **8**: 1118–1124.
37. Kurogouchi F, Oguchi T, Mawatari E et al. A case of mitochondrial cytopathy with a typical point mutation for MELAS, presenting with severe focal-segmental glomerulosclerosis as main clinical manifestation. *Am J Nephrol* 1998; **18**: 551–556.
38. Nakamura S, Yoshinari M, Doi Y et al. Renal complications in patients with diabetes mellitus associated with an A to G mutation of mitochondrial DNA at the 3243 position of leucine tRNA. *Diabetes Res Clin Pract* 1999; **44**: 183–189.
39. Hirano M, Konishi K, Arata N et al. Renal complications in a patient with A-to-G mutation of mitochondrial DNA at the 3243 position of leucine tRNA. *Intern Med* 2002; **41**: 113–118.
40. Reardon W, Ross RJM, Sweeney MG et al. Diabetes mellitus associated with a pathogenic point mutation in mitochondrial DNA. *Lancet* 1992; **340**: 1376–1379.
41. Kadowaki H, Tobe K, Mori Y et al. Mitochondrial gene mutation in insulin-deficient type of diabetes mellitus. *Lancet* 1993; **341**: 893–894.
42. Guillausseau PJ, Massin P, Dubois-LaForgue D et al. Maternally inherited diabetes and deafness: a multicenter study. *Ann Intern Med* 2001; **134**: 721–728.
43. Iwasaki N, Babazono T, Tsuchiya K et al. Prevalence of A-to-G mutation at nucleotide 3243 of the mitochondrial $tRNA^{Leu(UUR)}$ gene in Japanese patients with diabetes mellitus and end stage renal disease. *J Hum Genet* 2001; **46**: 330–334.
44. Rustin P, Chretien D, Gérard B et al. Biochemical, molecular investigations in respiratory chain deficiencies. *Clin Chim Acta* 1994; **228**: 35–51.
45. Rötig A, Munnich A. Genetic features of mitochondrial respiratory chain disorders. *J Am Soc Nephrol* 2003; **14**: 2995–3007.
46. Goto Y, Nonaka I, Horai S. A mutation in the $tRNA^{Leu(UUR)}$ gene associated with the MELAS

subgroup of mitochondrial encephalomyopathies. *Nature* 1990; **348**: 651.
47. Mitomap http://www.mitomap.org/
48. Damian MS, Seibel P, Reichmann H et al. Clinical spectrum of the MELAS mutation in a large pedigree. *Acta Neurol Scand* 1995; **92**: 409.
49. Hsieh F, Gohh R, Dworkin L. Acute renal failure and the MELAS syndrome, a mitochondrial encephalomyopathy. *J Am Soc Nephrol* 1996; **7**: 647.
50. Manouvrier S, Rötig A, Hannebique G et al. Point mutation of the mitochondrial $tRNA^{Leu}$ gene (A 3243 G) in maternally inherited hypertrophic cardiomyopathy, diabetes mellitus, renal failure, and sensorineural deafness. *J Med Genet* 1995; **32**: 654–656.
51. Majander A, Suomalainen A, Vettenranta K et al. Congenital hypoplastic anemia, diabetes, and severe renal tubular dysfunction associated with a mitochondrial DNA deletion. *Pediatr Res* 1991; **30**: 327–330.
52. Holt IJ, Harding AE, Morgan-Hughes JA. Deletions of muscle mitochondrial DNA in mitochondrial myopathies: sequence analysis and possible mechanisms. *Nucleic Acids Res* 1989; **17**: 4465–4469.
53. Rötig A, Bourgeron T, Chretien D et al. Spectrum of mitochondrial DNA rearrangements in the Pearson marrow-pancreas syndrome. *Hum Mol Genet* 1995; **4**: 1327–1330.
54. Moraes CT, Shanske S, Tritschler HJ et al. mtDNA depletion with variable tissue expression – A novel genetic abnormality in mitochondrial diseases. *Am J Hum Genet* 1991; **48**: 492.
55. Carrozzo R, Bornstein B, Lucioli S et al. Mutation analysis in 16 patients with mtDNA depletion. *Hum Mutat* 2003; **21**: 453–454.
56. Valnot I, von Kleist-Retzow JC, Barrientos A et al. A mutation in the human heme A:farnesyltransferase gene (*COX10*) causes cytochrome c oxidase deficiency. *Hum Mol Genet* 2000; **9**: 1245–1249.

10

Mitochondrial hematology and oncology

Norbert Gattermann and Stefanie Zanssen

Hematology

Patients with mitochondrial DNA disorders usually do not present with hematological problems.[1] This is unlikely to be explained by random partitioning of mitochondria in early embryogenesis leading to a comparatively low proportion of mutant mtDNA in hematopoietic tissue. More likely explanations include the bone marrow's ability to expand and thus compensate for functional impairment, and its capability to select against cells containing genetically defective mitochondria (see below). However, bone marrow function can be drastically impaired when a mtDNA mutation is present in a sufficiently high percentage, as illustrated by Pearson syndrome.[2]

Pearson syndrome

Pearson's syndrome (PS) is a rare congenital disorder characterized by lactic acidosis, exocrine pancreatic insufficiency, and severe refractory anemia necessitating repeated blood transfusions. The anemia is usually accompanied by neutropenia and thrombocytopenia. The bone marrow shows dysplastic changes, including moderate numbers of ringed sideroblasts and prominent vacuolization of precursor cells. PS is caused by large deletions of mtDNA (Figure 10.1).[3,4] Most children with PS die before 3 years of age. Interestingly, those who survive become independent of blood transfusions (J Poulton, Oxford, and C Niemeyer, Freiburg, personal communication). Apparently, there is selection against hematopoietic stem cells harboring high percentages of deleted mtDNA molecules. High mutation loads of severe mtDNA defects, such as large deletions, seem to be incompatible with the accelerated stem cell proliferation required under conditions of hematopoietic stress. In such circumstances, random segregation together with selection pressure can 'purge' the bone marrow, at least to a certain extent. This is not possible in postmitotic tissues, as shown by survivors of PS, who go on to develop Kearns–Sayre syndrome,[5–7] dominated by cardiac and neurological problems (see Chapter 2).

Other mtDNA diseases

In patients who do not have PS but present in childhood or adolescence with mitochondrial myopathy due to large mtDNA deletions, blood cells usually have low mutation loads, even when the percentage of mutant mtDNA is high in skeletal muscle.[8,9] Again, this suggests selection against functionally important mtDNA deletions in the hematopoietic system.

Does this concept also apply to point mutations of mtDNA? The MELAS (mitochondrial

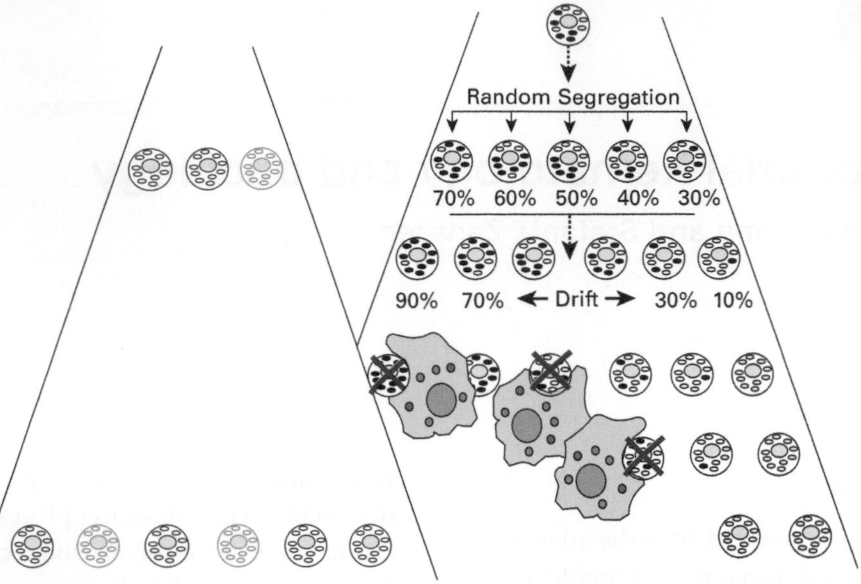

Figure 10.1 Random segregation of mitochondria (and mitochondrial DNA). Homoplasmic wildtype daughter cells (left). In the case of heteroplasmy (coexistence of wild-type and mutant mtDNA), random segregation creates daughter cells with different proportions of mutant mtDNA (right). This principle helps to explain intraclonal heterogeneity

encephalomyopathy, lactic acidosis, and stroke-like episodes) syndrome is caused by the A3243G point mutation in the mitochondrial $tRNA^{Leu(UUR)}$ gene. This mutation impairs mitochondrial protein synthesis, thereby leading to respiratory chain dysfunction. MELAS patients are not known to have ineffective hematopoiesis, probably because their leukocytes have consistently lower proportions of mutant mtDNA than skeletal muscle,[10] approximately 58% vs 84%.[11] In addition, the difference between blood and skeletal muscle increases with age, due to a progressive decline of mutant mtDNAs in blood.[12] This was shown by a study that compared paired blood DNA samples at intervals of 9–19 years in six MELAS patients: the proportions of mutant mtDNA declined in all cases by 12–29%.[13] In contrast, the proportion of mutant mtDNA usually increases in muscle.[14] These findings suggest that cells harboring pathogenic mtDNA point mutations are gradually selected out of the hematopoietic system, probably due to their impaired fitness to divide.

The selection pressure probably relates to the severity of the mitochondrial defect, which, in turn, depends both on the biochemical effects of the underlying mtDNA mutation and on the percentage of mutant mtDNAs in affected cells. If an mtDNA mutation is sufficiently benign to be tolerated by hematopoietic stem cells even at high levels of heteroplasmy, that mutation will not be cleared from the bone marrow.

Acquired idiopathic sideroblastic anemia

Of interest to hematologists, mitochondria are the site of heme synthesis. Therefore, mitochondrial dysfunction can impair hemoglobin production and cause anemia. mtDNA damage does not occur only in PS but can also explain the pathogenesis of acquired idiopathic sideroblastic anemia (AISA), a disorder included in the WHO classification of myelodysplastic syndromes[15] under the name of 'refractory anemia with ringed sideroblasts' (RARS). It is a clonal bone marrow disease arising from a multipotent hematopoietic stem cell. Red cell precursors show large abnormal iron granules surrounding the cell nucleus (hence the term 'ringed sideroblasts'),[1] which, on electron microscopy, correspond to mitochondria with massive iron accumulation in the matrix.

Clinical aspects

As in other myelodysplastic syndromes, the incidence of RARS is age-dependent, with most cases occurring after the age of 65. Crude annual incidence is about 1/100 000.[16] In patients whose morphological and functional changes in the bone marrow are restricted to the erythropoietic lineage, the risk of leukemic transformation is very low. However, if granulopoietic or megakaryopoietic precursors also show dysplastic changes, the cumulative risk of leukemic transformation is 11% 3 years after diagnosis.[17,18]

Diagnosis is established by bone marrow cytology, including iron staining. Ringed sideroblasts may be accompanied by other dysplastic changes. It is important to exclude reversible causes of sideroblastic anemia, such as alcoholism, chronic lead poisoning, or antituberculosis treatment with isoniazide. The diagnosis of a clonal bone marrow disease can be confirmed by detection of a clonal karyotype anomaly. While no chromosomal abnormalities are specifically associated with the sideroblastic phenotype, they apparently provide a growth advantage to the clone harboring the mitochondrial defect.

The only therapeutic approach, allogeneic stem cell transplantation, is rarely feasible because of the patient's advanced age. Combination therapy with the hematopoietic growth factors erythropoietin and G-CSF can substantially reduce apoptosis in bone marrow cells[13] and improve blood counts. Since inefficient erythropoiesis increases intestinal iron absorption and secondary hemosiderosis, which is aggravated by blood transfusions, patients also require iron chelation therapy.

Pathophysiology

In erythropoietic cells, large amounts of iron are imported into mitochondria for heme synthesis, and iron must be in the correct chemical form because ferrochelatase can utilize only ferrous iron (Fe^{2+}).[19] However, in sideroblastic anemia, iron accumulates in the ferric form (Fe^{3+}) and iron overload is attributed to failure by the mitochondrial respiratory chain (RC) to efficiently remove oxygen from the mitochondrial matrix.

Uncoupling protein-2 (Figure 10.2, bottom), which is expressed during erythroid differentiation, decreases the proton gradient across the inner mitochondrial membrane, which, in turn, stimulates RC activity in an attempt to preserve the gradient. The increased O_2 consumption creates a low-oxygen environment. By slowing down oxygen consumption, a respiratory chain defect (Figure 10.2, right) will leave more O_2 in the mitochondrial matrix. If iron, which crosses the inner mitochondrial membrane in the ferrous form, becomes reoxidized ($\rightarrow Fe^{3+}$) by the excess O_2, it will be rejected by ferrochelatase and will thus accumulate in the mitochondrial matrix.

Clonal mtDNA mutations have been discovered in the bone marrow of patients with AISA.[20–25] Mutations identified to date involve protein-coding genes (cytochrome *c* oxidase subunits I and II, cytochrome *b*, NADH dehydrogenase subunit 5, ATPase subunit 8), mitochondrial tRNA genes (tRNAs for Ala, Leu, Ser, Gly, Lys, Thr, Pro, Ile, Trp), and rRNA genes (16S-rRNA and 12S-rRNA). These mutations, which change conserved nucleotides/ amino acids, are not inherited but acquired in the bone marrow. They show heteroplasmy, i.e. coexistence of mutant and wild-type mtDNA, which is typical of DNA disorders.

Mitochondrial myopathy, lactic acidosis and sideroblastic anemia (MLASA)

MLASA (or MSA, mitochondrial myopathy and sideroblastic anemia) is a rare disease with

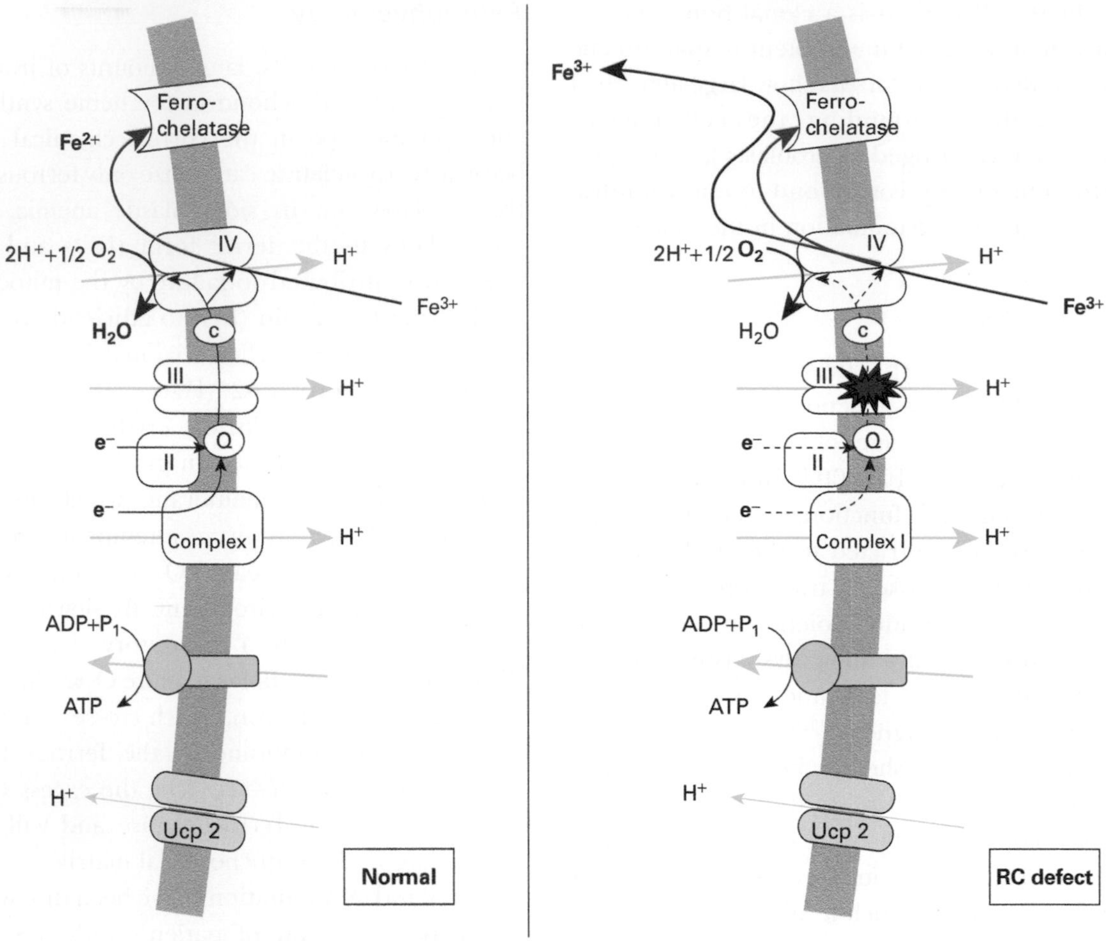

Figure 10.2 Schematic representation of iron transport, heme biosynthesis and its connection with the electron transport chain of the inner mitochondrial membrane. The gray band represents the inner mitochondrial membrane containing the respiratory chain complexes

autosomal recessive inheritance. The hallmark features include progessive exercise intolerance during childhood, onset of sideroblastic anemia around adolescence, basal lactic acidemia, and mitochondrial myopathy. Only a handful of cases have been reported.[26–28] The gene responsible for this disorder was mapped to chromosome 12q24.33,[29] and sequence analysis of the six genes in this region (as well as four putative genes with expression in bone marrow or muscle) identified a homozygous missense mutation in the pseudouridine synthase 1 gene (*PUS1*) in all patients with MLASA from two families. The mutation replaces a highly conserved amino acid, which is in the catalytic center of the protein, PUS1. The location of the protein is predicted to be mitochondrial on the basis of its amino acid composion. Indirect evidence suggests that pseudouridylation of human mitochondrial tRNAs requires PUS1p, and deficient pseudouridylation of tRNAs was proposed as the etiology of MLASA. Mitochondrial enzyme analysis revealed decreased activities of respiratory chain complexes containing mtDNA-encoded subunits, whereas the activities of two reference enzymes, succinate dehydrogenase and citrate synthase, were increased. It therefore appears that the nuclear defect in PUS1 translates into a problem with the mitochondrial translational machinery, a classical example of intergenomic communication defect (see Chapter 1). As in PS and RARS, in MLASA too erythropoiesis turns out to be particularly vulnerable to mitochondrial dysfunction. This is not surprising since heme synthesis, the major metabolic task of erythroblasts, is heavily dependent on mitochondrial activity.

Myelodysplastic syndromes

The WHO classification of myelodysplastic syndromes includes two acquired sideroblastic anemias with very different survival rate and risk of leukemic transformation. If dysplastic changes on cytomorphology are confined to the erythroid lineage, the disorder is designated 'refractory anemia with ringed sideroblasts' (RARS). If dysplastic changes affect granulocytopoiesis and/or megakaryopoiesis as well, the disorder is termed 'refractory cytopenia with multilineage dysplasia and ringed sideroblasts' (RCMD-RS). Other types of MDS may also show ringed sideroblasts in the bone marrow, but for ringed sideroblasts to be included in the designation of the disease, they must represent more than 15% of nucleated red cell precursors. Since mitochondrial iron overload is found not only in the two sideroblastic MDS types but, to a lesser degree, also in other myelodysplastic syndromes, mitochondrial dysfunction may represent a basic pathomechanism of MDS. Besides interfering with iron metabolism and heme synthesis, mitochondrial dysfunction may have broader implications for the hematopoietic system (see Figure 10.3).

ATP deficiency

In mammalian cells, there is a hierarchy of ATP-consuming processes,[30] and, if energy supply becomes inadequate, cells shut down their metabolic activities in a certain order. Synthesis of macromolecules, such as protein and RNA/DNA, is most sensitive to energy deprivation.[30] This may help to explain the dysfunction of bone marrow cells in MDS. A study of ineffective erythropoiesis in sideroblastic anemia,[31] showed accumulation of early polychromatic cells in G2 and of cells apparently arrested after a period in DNA synthesis. DNA synthesis was rarely seen in cells with pronounced siderotic deposits. Ultrastructural autoradiography later bolstered the concept that cells with large mitochondrial iron deposits become arrested in their progress through the cell cycle.[32] It was also shown that in erythroblasts, accumulation of iron-containing material within the mitochondria was frequently (but not invariably) associated with and possibly responsible for: (1) depression of RNA synthesis; and (2) even more marked depression of protein synthesis. Such impairment of macromolecule synthesis may partly explain the dysplastic phenotype of bone marrow cells in MDS.

ATP deficiency may also contribute to chromosomal instability. Since the mitotic spindle apparatus depends on ATP-consuming motor proteins, cells with inadequate ATP supply may have difficulty in correctly segregating chromosomes during mitosis. Notably, karyotype anomalies in MDS are characterized by losses or gains of whole chromosomes, or large deletions, rather than by specific translocations. In contrast, chromosomal instability is virtually absent in patients with erythroid sideroblastic anemia, in which only mild RC defect is proposed. In fact, these patients have the lowest frequency of karyotype anomalies, the lowest incidence of leukemic transformation, and the best survival.[17,18] In the case of more severe RC defects, impairment of ATP-dependent DNA repair mechanisms may be another pathway contributing to genomic instability. It has recently been shown that $CD34^+$ progenitors from MDS patients are more susceptible to induced oxidative DNA damage and have reduced DNA repair capacity than do healthy control subjects.[33]

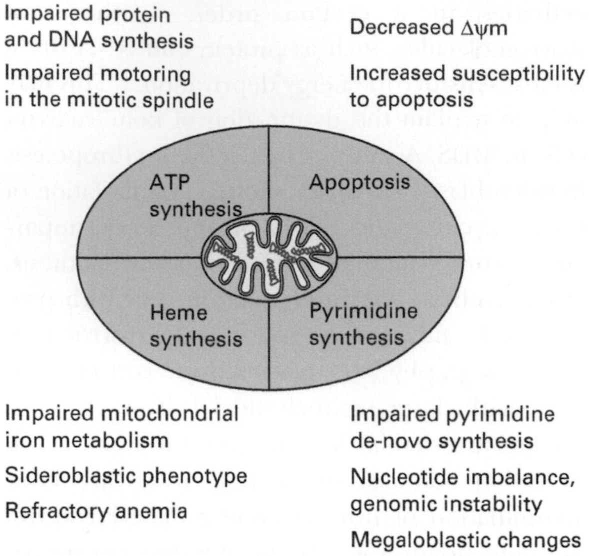

Figure 10.3 Pathways of mitochondrial defects for the hematopoietic system

Apoptosis

Although increased apoptosis of bone marrow cells is an important cause of ineffective hemopoiesis in MDS, it is not clear what triggers apoptosis. Intrinsic signals within the clonal cells may be at least as important as extrinsic apoptosis-inducing signals. Mitochondria play a central role as both regulators and effectors of apoptosis, and mitochondrial dysfunction can lead to necrotic and apoptotic cell death.[34] It is thus conceivable that mitochondrial defects predispose bone marrow cells to apoptosis. Hyperactivation of the mitochondria-caspase-9 pathway was seen in low-risk MDS and appears to be more important for the induction of apoptosis than the death receptor-caspase-8 pathway.[35] Apoptosis can be induced by specific mitochondrial respiratory chain inhibitors,[36] and mtDNA mutations may have similar consequences in MDS bone marrow cells.

While apoptosis is significantly increased in 'early' MDS types (< 10% blasts), it is comparable to normal controls in advanced MDS.[37,38] This does not contradict the concept that mitochondrial defects are more severe in advanced MDS because severe mitochondrial dysfunction may trigger genomic instability, and the consequent acquired chromosomal lesions may help the cells to escape apoptotic control.

Pyrimidine nucleotide synthesis

Dihydroorotate dehydrogenase (DHODH), an enzyme necessary for de novo pyrimidine nucleotide synthesis, is located in the inner mitochondrial membrane, where its function depends on its interaction with the respiratory chain. We have recently shown that inhibition of the respiratory chain impairs pyrimidine synthesis and thereby affects DNA precursor pool concentrations.[39] If cellular deoxyribonucleoside triphosphate levels are perturbed, a wide range of genetic events may follow due to aberrant DNA replication or repair.[40] In this way, mitochondrial dysfunction may again contribute to genomic instability. In addition, impaired pyrimidine nucleotide synthesis may help to explain the megaloblastic changes that are often found in MDS bone marrow cells.

Partial myeloperoxidase (MPO) defect is another cytomorphological feature of MDS that might be explained by mitochondrial dysfunction, because impaired mitochondrial heme synthesis will deprive MPO of its prosthetic group, i.e. heme.

A pathogenic role for mitochondrial dysfunction in myelodysplasia is also supported by the MDS-like effects of chloramphenicol, which suppresses mitochondrial protein synthesis via its direct action on the large ribosomal subunit of the organelle.

Interestingly, maturation of bone marrow cells in MDS is usually not arrested at any particular stage. In most cases, the MDS clone is capable of producing late-stage erythroblasts, even erythrocytes – as well as mature granulocytes and platelets – although many precursor cells die by apoptosis. The maturing cells display a variety of dysplastic and dysfunctional features. This sounds more like a 'sputtering engine' than a specific block in the maturational program. Considering that mitochondria are the powerhouses of the cell, it is tempting to speculate that myelodysplastic syndromes are in fact myeloproliferative disorders arising in a stem cell with a mitochondrial defect, which may be caused by mutations of mitochondrial DNA. In fact, we have identified mtDNA mutations in most patients with MDS analyzed (see reference 24 and unpublished data). mtDNA mutations have also been identified by Shin et al.[25]

Despite their possible contribution to MDS pathogenesis, mtDNA mutations alone cannot cause a myelodysplastic syndrome, or any other clonal bone marrow disease, because they are not likely to provide the cellular growth advantage that is necessary for clonal expansion. Any somatic mutation of mtDNA in the bone marrow is initially confined to the small clone consisting of the affected stem cell and its progeny. Therefore, in a polyclonal marrow, the mutation cannot do much harm to the hematopoietic system as a whole. Only if a stem cell carrying mutant mtDNA becomes transformed by additional nuclear DNA mutations, a clonal bone marrow can be established and clinical symptoms can occur (see Figure 10.4). Mitochondrial defects are likely to contribute to the phenotype of the clone, even if they are not instrumental in starting the clonal cellular proliferation.

Leukemia

He et al.[41] recently reported that approximately 40% of patients with acute or chronic leukemias have an acquired (somatic) point mutation of mtDNA in leukemic cells. Since the authors compared mtDNA from leukemic cells with mtDNA from buccal mucosa cells of the same patient, they were able to conclude that the altered mtDNA sequences in the bone marrow represented somatic mutations rather than inherited polymorphisms. Other workers compared mtDNA from clonal bone marrow disorders with mtDNA from healthy individuals,[25,42] but their results remain ambiguous because (1) sequence changes between patients and controls may simply reflect sequence variation within populations, and (2) bone marrow with clonal hematopoiesis cannot be compared with healthy polyclonal marrow. In clonal marrow, the mitochondrial genotype of a particular stem cell is amplified, whereas a healthy control sample contains mtDNA from many different stem cells. Though some of them may have acquired a mtDNA mutation, these mutations are not detectable by automated DNA sequencing, because they are present only in a small proportion of cells in the polyclonal marrow.

The mutations identified by He et al. are not necessarily important for leukemogenesis because there is mounting evidence that, as we grow older, the mitochondrial genome becomes mutated in the majority of our cells.[43–49] In highly proliferative tissues such as intestinal mucosa or bone marrow, mtDNA mutations occurring in differentiated cells are swiftly eliminated, because these cells have a short lifespan. In order to persist in a proliferative tissue, mtDNA mutations must occur in stem cells. As further explained in the Oncology section of this chapter, it has recently been shown that mtDNA mutations do occur in human stem cells, but it is unknown to what extent they contribute to tumor formation.

mtDNA amplification/circular dimer formation

Boultwood et al.[50] found that mtDNA was consistently amplified (2- to 50-fold) in the blast cells of acute myeloid leukemia (AML), as well as in chronic granulocytic leukemia (CGL) during blast crisis. In about half the patients, the increase in mtDNA/nuclear DNA ratio was more than eightfold. As a possible explanation, we suggested that incessant proliferation of transformed leukemic cells may strain mitochondrial biogenesis.[51] Electron microscopy showed that in myeloblastic leukemia mitochondria are less numerous and

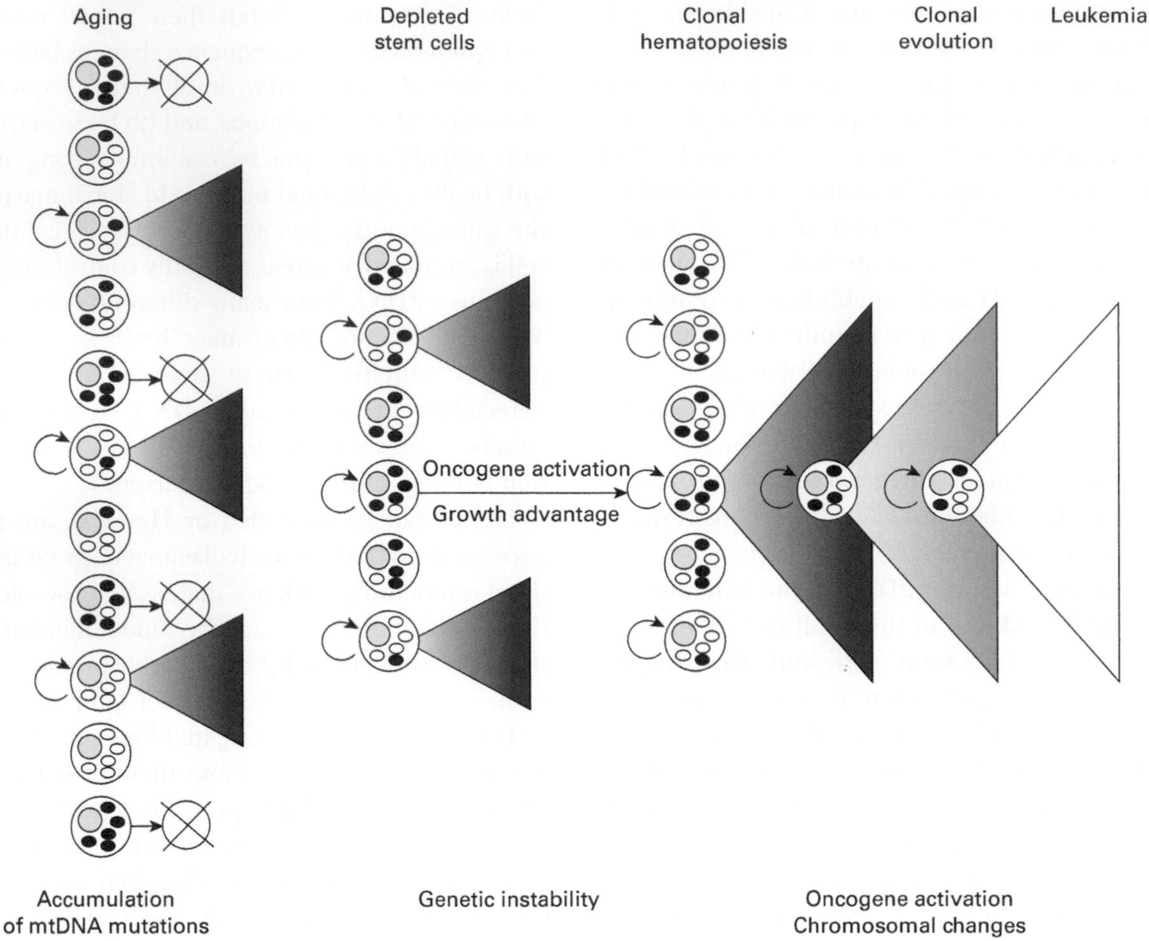

Figure 10.4 Schematic representation of MDS pathogenesis

smaller than in normal cells at the same stage of maturation.[52] Structural changes of mitochondria have also been observed.[52,53] It has also been shown that neoplastic transformation is associated with the coordinate induction of nuclear and mitochondrial oxidative phosphorylation (OXPHOS) genes. mtDNA transcript (mtRNA) levels are increased in viral and cellular oncogene-transformed rat fibroblasts, chick embryo fibroblasts, other human transformed cells, chemically induced hepatomas, and familial intestinal polyps (polyposis coli). OXPHOS gene up-regulation is probably a response to insufficient ATP production by mitochondria under circumstances of proliferative stress.[54] Amplification of mtDNA by AML cells may be a similar compensatory phenomenon, considering that an increased level of mtDNA usually reflects increased level of mtDNA transcription.[55]

Other workers observed circular dimers and complex catenated forms of mtDNA in acute leukemia,[56–58] and abnormal mtDNA length polymorphism consistent with gross abnormal dimer formation in myelodysplastic syndromes.[59] These findings may be linked to the amplification of mtDNA. Replication of human mtDNA is unusual, as its two strands are replicated from two distinct origins. DNA synthesis proceeds asymmetrically until it is completed on both strands, resulting in a catenated pair of circles (Box 3.1). The linked rings are broken and resealed to produce two daughter duplex mtDNAs. The whole process takes a relatively long time – about 2 hours. Under circumstances of continuous proliferative stress, mtDNA replication is increased, but the breaking and resealing of daughter strands of mtDNA, which requires the action of DNA topoisomerases, may not be able to accelerate to the same extent, thus leaving a significant proportion of replicated circular mtDNA strands interlinked. This failure may be due to ATP deficiency, considering that type II topoisomerases are ATP-dependent. If the phenomenon observed by Boultwood et al. mirrors the cell's attempt to cope, this effort may be severely hampered by the formation of catenated polymers, since steric considerations indicate that such complex forms of mtDNA are probably unsuitable for normal RNA synthesis. Therefore, a vicious circle may ensue, in which ATP depletion causes inadequate topo II activity and formation of mtDNA catenates, which in turn leads to impaired mtDNA transcription, disturbed mitochondrial protein synthesis, and further diminished ATP production.

Lymphoma

A marked shift from the predominant circular monomeric form of mtDNA to circles with twice the normal circumference, as well as multiple interlocking circles, was not only observed in acute leukemia but also in the leukemic phase of a poorly differentiated lymphocytic lymphoma.[60] The abnormal pattern was thought to reflect an intrinsic aberration in the processing of mtDNA, as it occurred in the absence of prior therapy with alkylating agents known to interact with DNA. However, there is no clear correlation between the neoplastic state of cells and the occurrence of complex forms of mtDNA, since the latter have also been observed in human B cells transformed by Epstein–Barr virus or phytohemagglutinin (PHA).[61] At lower frequency, complex forms of mtDNA were also found in lymphocytes isolated from donor blood.[62]

Chemotherapy-induced mtDNA mutations

Carew et al.[63] recently investigated the relationship between mtDNA mutations, reactive oxygen species (ROS) generation, and clinical outcomes in patients with chronic lymphocytic leukemia (CLL). Analysis of mtDNA from 20 CLL patients revealed that primary CLL cells from subjects exposed to chemotherapy had a significantly higher frequency of heteroplasmic mutations than did those from untreated patients. Overall, mtDNA mutations appeared to be associated with increased ROS generation. Patients refractory to conventional therapeutic agents tended to have higher mutation rates than patients who responded to treatment. The authors concluded that chemotherapy with certain DNA-damaging agents may cause mtDNA mutations, which initially appear heteroplasmic and are associated with increased ROS generation. They suggested that respiratory inefficiency resulting from mtDNA alterations may contribute to the elevated glycolytic activity (Warburg effect) and constitutive oxidative stress frequently observed in malignant cells. The increased ROS production could, in turn, lead to additional mutations in both nuclear DNA and mtDNA, contributing to genetic instability and disease progression. Because mitochondria play an essential role in apoptosis, the increase in ROS may also affect the sensitivity of cancer cells to chemotherapeutic agents. Previous studies indicated that ROS can stimulate cell proliferation and activate prosurvival transcription factors such as NF-κB.[64,65] Taking into consideration that many antiapoptotic proteins such as XIAP are under the transcriptional control of NF-κB, it is plausible that this effect could contribute to drug resistance and disease progression. On the other hand, the authors speculated that increased ROS generation may also provide a biochemical opportunity to preferentially kill cancer cells with novel anticancer agents that impose additional free radical stress to malignant cells.

Age-related accumulation of mtDNA mutations: impact on bone marrow function?

Age-related accumulation of somatic mtDNA rearrangements has been demonstrated in many tissues,[43] including bone marrow.[66] If somatic mtDNA mutations in cardiac muscle contribute to age-related heart failure, and hematopoietic stem cells also accumulate mtDNA mutations, why isn't age-related bone marrow failure a common cause of death?

Evidence has been presented that hematopoietic stem cells (HSC) are subject to aging.[67–69] Although they have the capacity to maintain hematopoiesis at steady-state, HSC populations in aged individuals may not always have the reserves necessary to respond to replicative stresses. The numbers of HSC and progenitor cells do not significantly decline in old age and, in some mouse strains, these numbers actually increase. The important effects of aging therefore may be on HSC quality rather than quantity. It is tempting to speculate that the quality of hematopoietic stem cells deteriorates as they acquire and preferentially amplify mtDNA mutations. Their differentiating progeny, which is more dependent on mitochondrial energy production, may suffer functional impairment or even apoptotic death, thus causing some degree of ineffective hematopoiesis. Nevertheless, the bone marrow appears to be able to compensate for deteriorating stem cell quality by driving more stem cells into the cycle. This kind of compensation is not possible in postmitotic tissue like heart muscle. However, continuously increased proliferation in the stem cell compartment may, in the long run, increase the risk of malignant transformation.

Oncology

A role for mitochondria in tumorigenesis was hypothesized over seven decades ago when biochemical studies showed that tumor cells have altered metabolic profiles and display high rates of glucose uptake and glycolysis, which was attributed to a primary defect in cell respiration.[70,71] Warburg and others suggested that cancer cells were due to heritable injuries to the mitochondria. This was disputed by Weinhouse,[72,73] who found that oxygen consumption was similar in tumor cells and in normal cells. However, later studies by Warburg, Burk and Schade[74] using pure cell suspensions, suggested that Weinhouse's studies may have resulted from the assessment of only a portion of the tumor cell population. Numerous studies carried out after Warburg's orginal observation have confirmed various defects of mitochondria in the cancer state. The problem is that of discriminating between changes induced by oncogenic agents elsewhere in the cell and changes primarily related to the onset of malignancy.

Regarding secondary mitochondrial changes, recent molecular studies of cancer have revealed that oncogenes and tumor-suppressor genes not only contribute to the growth and apoptotic phenotype of cancer cells, but may directly affect cellular energy metabolism.[75] The products of these genes alter the expression of transcription factors, which in turn regulate genes that encode metabolic enzymes and angiogenic factors. Because hypoxia is a key selective pressure on the progression of cancer cells, activation of HIF-1 (hypoxia-inducible transcription factor) and perhaps other transcription factors might play an important role in promoting the survival of cancer cells in adverse tumor microenvironments.

It is now widely held that a high glycolytic rate is not an invariable marker of the malignant state, whereas a reduced number of mitochondria is a more consistent observation.[76] Thus, the ratio between mitochondrial and glycolytic enzymes in cancer cells seems to be shifted in favor of glycolysis, and this is particularly so in rapidly growing tumors. Many tumor cells show both increased activity of hexokinase, the first enzyme involved in the commitment to glycolysis, and increased amount of hexokinase type II, which is bound to the outer mitochondrial membrane.[77–79] This enzyme appears to drive the process of glycolysis in tumor cells by providing both preferential access to mitochondrial-generated ATP, and protection against product inhibition by glucose-6-phosphatase.

Although increased aerobic glycolysis is probably not the fundamental defect in cancer, it has been speculated that metabolic changes related to mitochondrial function may confer an advantage in many different types of cancer, allowing tumor cells to grow, survive and invade.[75,76,80–88] In order to persist in the proliferating tumor cells, this advantage must be encoded by mitochondrial or nuclear genes.

mtDNA mutations

Interest in a primary role of mitochondria in tumorigenesis has been rekindled in recent years by the identification of somatic mtDNA mutations in many tumors and tumor cell lines.[89] These mutations include intragenic deletions, missense and chain-termination point mutations, and alterations of homopolymeric sequences that result in frameshift mutations. In principle, somatic mutations of mtDNA could contribute to neoplastic transformation by changing cellular energy capacities, modulating apoptosis, and increasing mitochondrial oxidative stress. Regarding oxidative stress, impairment of the mitochondrial respiratory chain results in increased production of $O_2^{\bullet-}$, which is converted to H_2O_2 by mitochondrial MnSOD. Mitochondrial H_2O_2 can diffuse to the cell nucleus, where it acts as a mitogen. Excessive mitochondrial generation of H_2O_2 can overwhelm the antioxidant defenses of the cytosol (catalase, glutathione peroxidase, and bilirubin) and cause DNA damage which, in turn, can lead to mutation, and thereby activation, of proto-oncogenes.[90] Increased ROS production is therefore a possible mitochondrial mutator phenotype, leading to further DNA damage and genetic instability.

Since many mtDNA mutations identified in solid tumors or clonal bone marrow disorders are either silent or mutations that change poorly conserved nucleotides or amino acids,[41,89] it seems excessive to claim that mtDNA mutations play an important role in carcinogenesis or leukemogenesis. On the other hand, it is also unjustified to claim that all mtDNA mutations are irrelevant. Why should mutations at well-conserved sites of mtDNA be innocent in tumor cells, while causing disease in non-malignant cells? Augenlicht and Heerdt[91] summarized the role of mtDNA mutations in tumorigenesis as follows: 'At this point, a reasonable, if broad speculation is that, among a high background of random mutations that provide no selective advantage, there are a smaller number of mutations that alter mitochondrial function and cell physiology in a manner that has significant effects of tumor development, or phenotype in one of several tumor-associated environments (for example, hypoxia, angiogenic insufficiency, or shift of metabolic phenotype). This is a scenario similar to that of tumors with defects in DNA repair: thousands of mutations accumulate in the nuclear genome, the vast majority of which are functionally and physiologically silent and overlay the few that have an impact on tumorigenesis. Unfortunately, there is still no way to identify the functionally important mutations'.

mtDNA mutations in stem cells?

It is now widely believed that most tumors arise in tissue-specific stem cells because differentiated cells generally do not have the self-renewal capacity that would allow them to originate a large tumor cell population. Considering that clonally expanded somatic mtDNA mutations have been identified in numerous human tumors (each probably originating in a stem cell), it would be interesting to know whether stem cells accumulate mtDNA mutations, and if so, at what rate.

The question is hard to answer because human stem cells are not accessible in sufficient quantity. Recently, this problem was elegantly solved by Taylor and coworkers, who studied colonic crypts as surrogate intestinal stem cells.[92] They analyzed microscopically the clonal population derived from one or two single cells – the stem cells – located at the base of each crypt. They reasoned that any mtDNA mutation found in the whole crypt must have been amplified from that very mutation in the stem cell itself. They further postulated that if a stem cell harbors an mtDNA mutation that disrupts mitochondrial respiratory chain function, and if that mutation expands (in the stem cell) to a level exceeding the threshold for dysfunction (typically >80% mutated mtDNA), then one ought to be able to observe both the dysfunction (by histochemical and/or biochemical means) and the mtDNA mutation (by genetic means) in the daughter population comprising the entire crypt. The authors examined normal colonic mucosa from 16 patients undergoing resection for colonic tumors, as well as colonoscopy biopsies from 12 individuals undergoing investigation of altered bowel function in which no pathology was found.

On serial transverse sections from individual crypts, two-color histochemistry was performed to detect simultaneously the enzymatic activities of cytochrome *c* oxidase (COX), which contains three subunits encoded by mtDNA, and succinate dehydrogenase (SDH), which contains no mitochondrial-encoded subunits. The incidence of COX-deficient colonic crypts showed a marked age-related increase, from an average of ~1% in persons around 40 years of age, to an average of ~15% in people around 80 years of age. The authors then performed PCR and mtDNA sequencing on the same crypts isolated by laser microdissection to search for somatic mutations that might correlate with the histochemistry. They found mtDNA mutations, mostly in COX-deficient crypts, and many, but not all, mutations were in COX or other protein-encoding genes. The few mutations found in COX-positive crypts were either neutral or in non-COX genes. Interestingly, some COX-deficient crypts had no mtDNA mutations; presumably these crypts had nuclear mutations affecting COX function. Altogether, there was a high mutational load in colonic stem cells. The complete mitochondrial genome was sequenced in 60 crypts, and 59 different mtDNA point mutations were detected, but many mtDNA mutations were probably not detected because automated DNA sequencing has a detection limit of about 30% heteroplasmy.

Since the mutations found in COX-deficient crypts predominantly affected protein-encoding genes and were very different from the spectrum seen in patients with mtDNA disease, the authors proposed that subunit mutations associated with more severe phenotypes are less compatible with transmission through the germline.

Taylor et al. not only established that mutations occur in colonic crypt stem cells, but also performed mathematical modeling to understand how frequently mtDNA mutations occur in these stem cells. Their analysis yielded a somatic mtDNA mutation rate in humans in vivo of $\sim 5 \times 10^{-5}$ mutations per genome per day. This corresponds to 1.10 mutations per site per million years, which is strikingly similar to pedigree-derived mtDNA substitution rates, and similar to the rate measured in cultured cells in vitro (2×10^{-8} mutations per site per cell division). The mutation rate is therefore substantially greater for mtDNA than for nuclear DNA (6×10^{-11} mutations per site per cell division).

The results obtained by Taylor et al. support a role for mtDNA mutations in the aging process. If a significant number of stem cells accumulate mutations, there will be a mixture of mutations within an individual, which may influence tissue function. The results also predict that many tumors will amplify an mtDNA mutation that was already present in the tumor stem cell. However, this work does not answer the question whether the presence of mtDNA mutations in tumors is purely coincidental or favored by some functional relations between mtDNA mutations and the developing tumor.

Is it all based on pure chance?

It is a longstanding debate whether selective amplification and fixation of a mutant mitochondrial genotype in single cells is solely based on random processes or promoted by preferential replication of mutant mtDNA over wild-type mtDNA. The problem can be simulated with computers. Elson et al.[93] developed a model of mtDNA replication in non-dividing cells. They showed that marked intracellular drift can occur in postmitotic cells during the span of human life. A single mutated mtDNA molecule may expand clonally to reach very high levels in the absence of any replicative advange. Coller et al.[94] focused on stem cells in proliferating tissues. By extensive computer modeling they demonstrated that there is sufficient opportunity for a stem cell (a potential tumor progenitor cell) to achieve homoplasmy through unbiased mtDNA replication and sorting during cell division. Their conclusions are supported by in vivo data. Single cell analysis of mtDNA in healthy human epithelial tissue revealed that the model correctly predicts the considerable observed frequency of homoplasmic mutant cells.[95] Therefore, random processes are sufficient to explain the incidence of homoplasmic mtDNA mutations in stem cells, and thus in human tumors. Chinnery et al.[96] recently proposed a model for the accumulation of mtDNA mutations in aging, cancer, and mitochondrial diseases, which is also based on random genetic drift as the most important mechanism. However, other mechanisms are not excluded.

Besides random processes, 'structural' and 'functional' mechanisms have been proposed to explain intracellular clonal expansion of mtDNA mutations.[97] The 'structural' mechanisms propose that preferential proliferation of the mutant species is based on properties of mutant DNA only, without any need to invoke the additional function of mutant tRNA or proteins coded by mtDNA. For example, deleted mtDNA molecules were hypothesized to proliferate faster because they are shorter.[98] This explanation is no longer accepted, because the entire mtDNA molecule is replicated in <90 minutes, which is much shorter than the time between replications. Alternatively, deletion/inactivation of some negative regulatory sequences may lead to a replicative advantage of mutant mtDNA.[99]

The 'functional' mechanisms assume that changes in function of mutant tRNA/protein(s) are essential for expansion. For example, there may be preferential survival of dysfunctional mitochondria bearing mutant DNA because decreased mitochondrial activity may reduce ROS-mediated damage and delay the removal of mutant organelles by mitochondrial turnover.[100] Alternatively, there may be a positive feedback loop stimulating synthesis of mtDNA in case of decreased ATP production.[99,101–104]

Such non-random processes cannot be dismissed, since single-cell analysis has revealed striking qualitative differences between the spectra of mtDNA mutations in proliferating epithelial cells on the one hand, and postmitotic cardiomyocytes on the other hand.[95] This finding would not be expected as a result of random processes. Instead, it suggests that the processes generating these mutations or the mechanisms driving them to homoplasmy are fundamentally different between the two tissues.

Detection of mtDNA mutations in tumors and bodily fluids

Recently, Penta et al.[89] reviewed all mtDNA alterations reported in hematological malignancies as well as solid tumors of the breast, colon, stomach, liver, kidney, bladder, head/neck, and lung. Two well-known papers on this topic come from the groups of Bert Vogelstein.[105,106] Polyak et al.[105] found somatic mutations of mtDNA in the majority of colorectal cancer cell lines and primary colorectal cancers. Fliss et al.[106] analyzed bladder cancers ($n=14$), head and neck tumors ($n=13$), and lung cancers ($n=14$). They amplified about 80% of the mitochondrial genome and compared it with normal mtDNA from the same patient, and thereby identified somatic mtDNA mutations in 64% of bladder cancers, 46% of head and neck tumors, and 43% of lung cancers. They also found that the mutant mtDNA was easily detected in the patients' bodily fluids. In patients who simultaneously carried a p53 mutation, the amount of mutant mtDNA fragments in the bodily fluids was 19–220 times that of mutant p53 DNA fragments. This finding, which was attributed to the high copy number of mtDNA in the tumor cells, suggested that mtDNA mutations are better suited than nuclear DNA mutations for the detection of tumor cells. The authors concluded that by virtue of their clonal nature and high copy number, mitochondrial mutations may provide a powerful molecular marker for non-invasive detection of cancer.

Further publications carry the same message.[107–110] For example, Jones et al.[109] found that the amount of mtDNA was six- to eight-fold higher in pancreatic carcinoma cells than in normal pancreatic cells. Again, this causes an increased mtDNA/nuclear DNA ratio, facilitating the detection of tumor-associated mtDNA mutations.

Mitochondrion as a novel target of anticancer chemotherapy

Costantini et al.[111] recently reviewed the possibility of targeting the mitochondrial permeability transition pore complex (PTPC) in order to overcome apoptosis resistance in anticancer chemotherapy. It is well established that apoptosis plays a pivotal role in tissue homeostasis and that inhibition of apoptosis may contribute to the transformation of cells or to the development of chemotherapy resistance. Mutations in apoptosis-regulatory genes (e.g. *p53*, *PTEN*, and *bcl-2* and its homologs) are involved in the pathogenesis of most human cancers. Similar mutations may also be involved in the development of chemoresistance.

In the process leading to physiologic or chemotherapy-induced apoptosis, mitochondrial membrane permeabilization is a critical event. The permeabilization event is, at least in part, under the control of the permeability transition pore complex. Oncoproteins from the Bcl-2 family and tumor suppressor proteins from the Bax family interact with PTPC to inhibit or facilitate membrane permeabilization. Conventional chemotherapeutic agents elicit mitochondrial permeabilization indirectly by induction of endogenous effectors that are involved in the physiologic control of apoptosis. However, an increasing number of experimental anticancer drugs, including lonidamine, arsenite, betulinic acid, CD437, and several amphiphatic cationic α-helical peptides, act directly on mitochondrial membranes and/or on the PTPC. Such agents may induce apoptosis in circumstances in which conventional drugs fail to act because endogenous apoptosis induction pathways, such as those involving p53, death receptors, or apical caspase activation, are disrupted. However, stabilization of the mitochondrial membrane by anti-apoptotic Bcl-2-like proteins reduces the cytotoxic potential of most of these drugs. Targeting of specific PTPC components may overcome this Bcl-2-mediated apoptosis inhibition. One strategy involves cross-linking of critical redox-sensitive thiol groups within the PTPC; another involves the use of ligands to the mitochondrial benzodiazepine receptor. Thus, the design of mitochondrion-targeted cytotoxic drugs may constitute a novel strategy for overcoming apoptosis resistance.

Mitochondrial enzymes in hereditary tumors

While the functional effects of mtDNA mutations in tumors remain to be proven, mutations in the

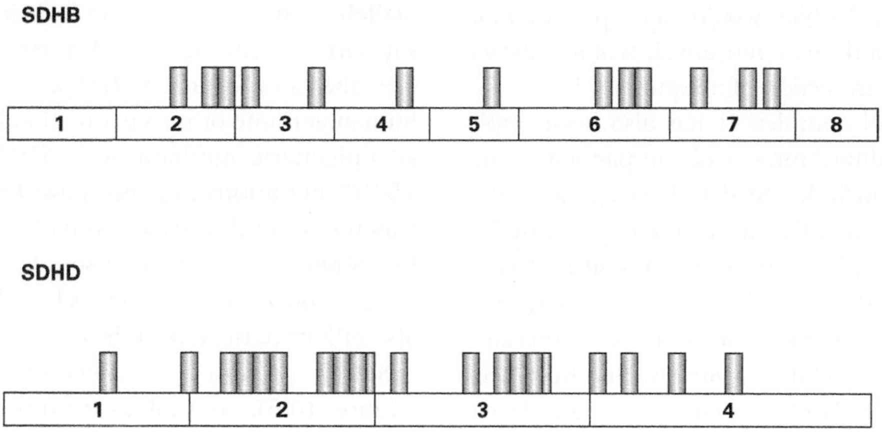

Figure 10.5 Schematic diagram of the SDHD and SDHB genes and germline heterozygous mutations found in pheochromocytoma and paraganglioma according to Eng et al.[114] The bar represents the length of the gene, which is subdivided into exons. The rectangles represent gene mutations.

nuclear genes encoding the mitochondrial enzymes succinate dehydrogenase (SDH) and fumarate hydrase (FH) have been shown to cause enzyme defects in neoplastic tissues. Mutations in SDH make individuals susceptible to pheochromocytoma and paraganglioma, and mutations in FH predispose to leiomyomatosis and renal cell carcinomas. Recently, the tumorigenic pathway of SDH deficiency has been documented.[112]

Succinate dehydrogenase deficiency in paraganglioma and pheochromocytoma

SDH (complex II of the respiratory chain) is involved both in the respiratory chain and in the Krebs cycle, where it converts succinate to fumarate and feeds electrons to the ubiquinone (UQ) pool. Complex II is a four-subunit enzyme that straddles the mitochondrial inner membrane. It is anchored to the membrane by the two membrane-spanning subunits cybL (cytochrome *b* large subunit encoded by SDHC) and cybS (cytochrome *b* small subunit encoded by SDHD). The extramembrane subunits SDHA and SDHB are both catalytic and face the mitochondrial matrix. SDHA is a flavoprotein and SDHB contains an iron–sulfur cluster. All four subunits are encoded by nuclear DNA (Figure 10.5).[113,114]

Mitochondrial pathology has been traditionally related to symptoms of the central nervous system,[115] such as seizures, encephalopathy, stroke-like episodes, migraines, and ataxia. Severe deficiency of complex II has been associated with neurodegenerative disorders, such as late-onset optic atrophy or Leigh syndrome (LS); LS is a subacute necrotizing encephalopathy of infancy (see Chapter 2).[116,117]

In LS patients with complex II deficiency, homozygous or compound heterozygous mutations have been found in the SDHA subunit of complex II.[118] These mutations inactivate the catalytic subunit and result in severe loss (up to 75%) of enzyme activity. Half of the reported mutations occur at the 3′ end of the gene, affecting the carboxy terminal end of the polypeptide, which comprises the catalytic core.[119]

The pathomechanism of neurodegeneration in Leigh syndrome is unknown. It has been hypothesized that impairment of oxidative phosphorylation may produce large quantities of reactive oxygen species (ROS),[114] which would cause peroxidation of the mitochondrial membrane, loss of membrane potential, and induction of apoptosis.

Deficiency of complex II has also been implicated in hereditary tumors of the paraganglionic system, which includes head and neck paraganglia, the adrenal medulla, and other paraganglia. Whereas most pheochromocytomas secrete catecholamines and lead to hypertensive crises, most paragangliomas of the head and neck region cause damage by encroaching on nerves. Head and neck paragangliomas (HNPs) are slow-growing and well-vascularized tumors.[120,121]

As reviewed by Baysal[122] approximately 10–50% of patients with HNPs and 10% of patients with pheochromocytomas have positive family histories. Most familial cases are caused by mutations in the SDH subunits *SDHB* and *SDHD* or by mutations in the von Hippel Lindau tumor suppressor gene (*VHL*). About 8% of sporadic pheochromocytoma and paraganglioma are also associated with mutations in *SDHB* and *SDHC*.[120,121] More recently, *SDHB* mutations have been also associated with renal cell carcinoma and papillary thyroid cancer[123] and *SDHD* mutations with colon cancer.[124]

Familiar paraganglioma are genetically heterogeneous and four loci have been identified so far: PGL1 (*SDHD*) maps to 11q23, PGL2 to 11q13.3, PGL3 (*SDHC*) to 1q21, and PGL4 (*SDHB*) to 1p36.1. Half of the mutations in the *SDHD* gene occur in exon 1 or 2 (Figure 10.5). Loss of either the SDHD or the SDHC anchor component in the mitochondrial inner membrane leads to decreased SDH catalytic activity.[125] Interestingly, mutations in the 5′ portion of the *SDHD* gene, which hinder assembly of the complex, are more commonly associated with pheochromocytoma, whereas mutations in the 3′ region of *SDHD*, which only affect catalytic activity, are more commonly associated with HNPs.[114]

SDHD might be maternally imprinted, because inheritance of this region follows paternal transmission exclusively. However, the finding of biallelic expression in some individuals does not support imprinting[126] and raises the question wheather a functional *SDHD* paralog exists in the human genome or if its expression is regulated by an epigenetic mechanism.[127] *SDHD* (as well as *SDHB*) mutations may not have full penetrance, leaving several at-risk individuals unaffected. Environmental conditions associated with increased oxygen concentration, such as low altitudes, might also influence the risk of developing these tumors.

SDHB (PGL4) mutations in exon 6 or 7 (Figure 10.5), as well as truncating mutations before residue 197, which binds the iron–sulfur moiety, are expected to prevent assembly of the catalytic unit. Coexistence of wild-type complexes and complexes lacking SDHB causes significant loss of enzyme activity.[128] To date, only one mutation has been described in the start codon of SDHC (PGL3) in three patients.[129]

Fumarase deficiency in hereditary leiomyomatosis and renal cell carcinoma

Fumarase hydratase (fumarase, FH) converts fumarate to malate in the Krebs cycle. FH is a monotetrameric enzyme which is present both in the mitochondrial matrix and in the cytosolic compartment, where it seems to be involved in amino acid metabolism. FH subunits include five α-helices and a lyase domain. The α helices from the four subunits form a superhelical structure in the core of the tetramer, which is the putative catalytic center. The lyase domain is also thought to be involved in catalytic activity.[130]

Mutations in the nuclear encoded FH gene are associated with two different conditions.[114] Homozygous or compound heterozygous germline mutations cause severe neurological dysfunction (gross developmental delay and death in the first decade) associated with complete loss of FH activity. Heterozygous germline mutations predispose to hereditary cutaneous and uterine leiomyomas as well as renal cell carcinomas (HLRCC). Nearly

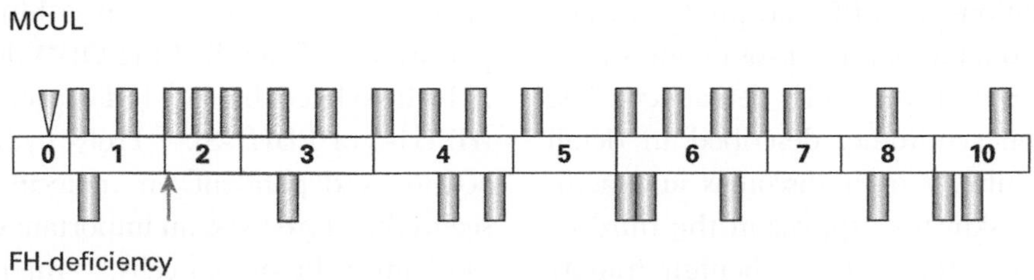

Figure 10.6 Schematic diagram of the FH gene and germline heterozygous mutations found in multiple cutaneous and uterine leiomyoma (MCUL) and in fumarase deficiency according to Alam et al.[132] The bar represents the length of the gene, which is subdivided into exons. Rectangles represent gene mutations, the arrowhead represents a whole gene deletion and the arrow represents a splice site mutation

Table 10.1 Inherited mitochondrial RCC syndromes with genodermatosis as a component

Syndrome	Skin affection	Histology of kidney cancer	Susceptibility gene
HLRCC	Leiomyoma	Papillary RCC Oncocytoma	FH
Birt–Hogg–Dube syndrome	Fibrofolliculoma	Chromophobe RCC Oncocytoma	Folliculin

80% of patients developed tumors in their thirties. Although papillary renal carcinoma[131] and tumors derived from the collecting duct system[132] such as oncocytomas are described as renal carcinomas, the overall risk to develop kidney cancer in families with leiomyoma appears to be low.[132]

Heterozygous mutations of the 5′ end of the FH gene appear to be associated with HLRCC, whereas mutations of the 3′ end are associated with FH-deficiency (with some overlap) (Figure 10.6). However, there is some overlap of phenotypes, as some carriers (recessive for FH deficiency) are predisposed to tumor development.[133] The spectrum of mutations includes missense and nonsense point mutations, microdeletions, and large-scale deletions encompassing the FH locus on 1q43. Loss of heterozygosity of the wild-type FH allele is present in nearly every tumor investigated so far. Common mutations seem to be N64T and G354R. Several mutations share a common haplotype, suggesting a founder effect. Interestingly, missense mutations, occurring very often at conserved sides of FH, lead to more severely reduced FH activity than truncating mutations.[132]

GENODERMATOSES IN HEREDITARY MITOCHONDRIAL KIDNEY CANCERS

At least two hereditary mitochondrial kidney cancer syndromes, HLRCC and Birt–Hogg–Dube syndrome, combine cancer with affections of the skin and therefore also belong to the group of genodermatoses (Table 10.1). Interestingly, in both genodermatosis–cancer syndromes the kidney tumors may show the histologic features of oncocytomas: cells replenished with pathologic mitochondria (see below).

Skin manifestations in HLRCC are predominantly multiple leiomyomata, but leiomyosarcomas have also been associated with FH deficiency. The Birt–Hogg–Dube syndrome, described in detail below, shows multiple trichodiscomas and acrochordons of the skin that appear in the third or fourth decade of life. Both are benign tumors of the hair apparatus and share the histology of follicular hamartomas.[134]

Model for tumorigenesis

The observation that homozygous loss-of-function germline mutations in *SDHA* or fumarate hydrase (*FH*) lead to neurodegeneration without cancer, whereas heterozygous germline mutations in *SDHB*, *SDHC* or *SDHD* genes or in the *FH* gene (see above) together with loss of heterozygosity of the wild-type allele lead to cancer is intriguing. However, heterozygous mutations in SDH or FH in non-tumor cells only reduce gene dosage and residual enzyme activities are enough for normal neuronal development, whereas homozygous mutations in these genes lead to a near-complete loss of enzyme activity in every cell, starving the developing nervous system of energy. Patients with LS or fumarase deficiency may die before the SDH- and FH-related tumors can develop.[114]

It has been proposed that mitochondrial dysfunction may be linked to carcinogenesis via apoptotic, ROS-mediated, or hypoxia-inducible factor (HIF)-mediated pathways.[113,114,122,135,136] The HIF pathway plays a pivotal role in the development of kidney cancers in von Hippel Lindau disease. The HIF is a heterodimer composed of an oxygen-inducible HIFα subunit and a HIFβ subunit. HIF is a transcription factor that induces transcription of hypoxia-inducible genes in the nucleus, leading to metastasis, angiogenesis, and cell proliferation. The von Hippel Lindau gene product (pVHL) binds to the oxygen-dependent degradation (ODD) domain of HIFα (in an oxygen-dependent manner) and targets it for steady degradation under normoxic conditions. This binding is only performed efficiently if the ODD domain of HIFα is hydroxylated by the HIFα-prolyl hydroxylases (HPH1-3 or PDH1-3).[137] Prolyl hydroxylase (PDH) activity is dependent on molecular oxygen and seems therefore to be an important oxygen-sensing mechanism in animal cells.[138] Interestingly, PDHs oxidize and decarboxylate α-ketoglutarate to succinate, using the metabolites of the Krebs cycle as cosubstrates during hydroxylation.[139] The cytoplasmic utilization of succinate is possible, because succinate can be transported – via the dicarboxylic acid translocator and the voltage-dependent anion channel – across the mitochondrial membranes into the cytoplasm. In hereditary pheochromocytoma, with the *SDHD* R22X mutation and loss of the remaining wild-type allele, the electron transfer activity of complex II is impaired and levels of HIF1α, HIF2α,/EPAS1, VEGF, and its receptor VEGR-R1 are increased.[125]

Selak and Gottlieb[112] were able to document experimentally a link between mitochondrial pathology and tumorigenesis (Figure 10.7). They showed that the HIF-mediated signaling pathway also plays a role in SDH deficiency and excluded the ROS-mediated pathway. Targeting SDHD with the RNA interference (RNAi) technique, they were able to reduce SDH activity to 50% and to increase succinate levels. The cytosolic succinate concentration had a profound effect on PDHs and, therefore, on the stabilization or degradation of HIF. They showed that HIF is stabilized, leading to transcription of its targets, including the proapoptotic BCL-2 family member BNIP3. HIFα is also known to target transcription of genes like growth-factor β (TGFβ), platelet-derived growth-factor-receptor β (PDGFβ), and a ligand for the epidermal growth factor receptor (EGFR). The oncogenetic effects of these genes lead to angiogenesis, metastasis, and tumor progression. Therefore, succinate may function as an intracellular messenger, which signals the mitochondrial metabolic/redox state via the cytosol to the nucleus. Succinate signaling may be

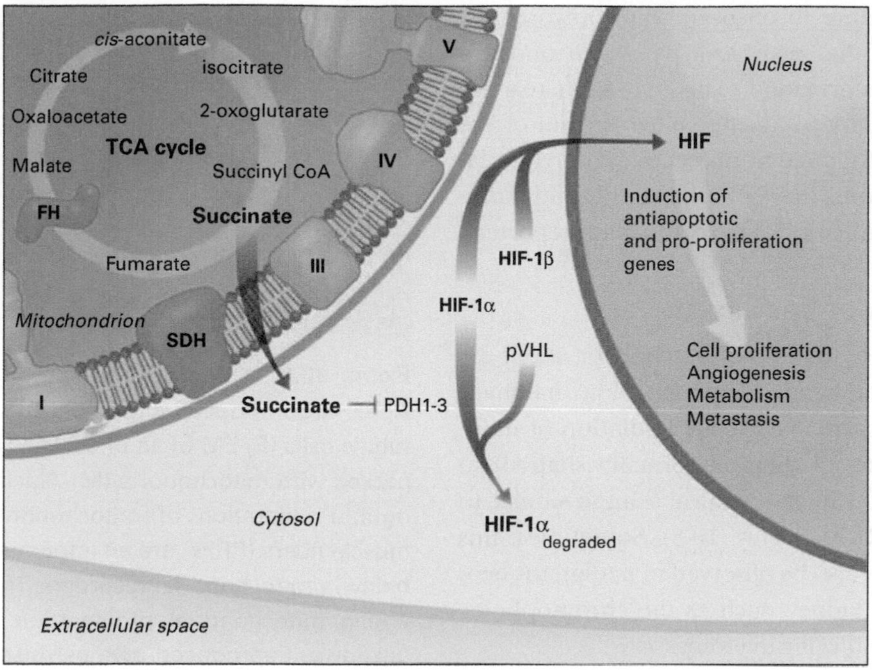

Figure 10.7 Schematic model for tumorigenesis depending on the succinate signaling pathway. Due to SDH inhibition, succinate accumulates intramitochondrially and is transported into the cytosol. Here, its high concentration inhibits the prolyl hydroxylases and thereby HIF-1α hydroxylation and degradation. HIF is now elevated and induces transcription of genes involved in tumor progression. (G. Maki, reproduced with permission from PLoS Medicine)

extended to the extracellular space, because it has recently been shown that succinate also binds to G-coupled receptor involved in the regulation of blood pressure.[140]

Recent reports of SDH deficiency in gastric and colorectal cancer[124] point towards a more general role of mitochondrial dysfunction in carcinogenesis. The additional role of SDH and succinate as intracellular redox status and oxygen sensors opens new avenues towards metabolic therapies for tumors. For example, chemical derivatives of α-ketoglutarate, which may overcome the product inhibition of prolyl hydroxylases by succinate, could induce the ubiquitination of HIF-1α and could thus be interesting candidates for treatment of tumors with SDH deficiency.

The pathomechanism for carcinogenesis described by Selak et al.[112] may also apply to tumors associated with FH deficiency because FH defects may also affect SDH through product inhibition, thus raising the succinate concentration (Figure 10.7). However this hypothesis still needs experimental support.

Mitochondrial pathology in sporadic oncocytomas

Pathology of oncocytoma

Oncocytomas are mostly benign tumors of the kidney, parathyroid, and salivary glands. Oncocytomas of the thyroid are also called Hurthle cell tumors. Oncocytes can occur ubiquitously (e.g. in the heart, leading to oncocytic cardiomyopathy), which implies that many cell types can undergo oncocytic transformation. This may be a reactive process secondary to functional exhaustion of the mitochondria followed by mitochondrial hyperplasia.[141] Oncocytoma may occur bilaterally and multifocally and familial cases have also been reported.

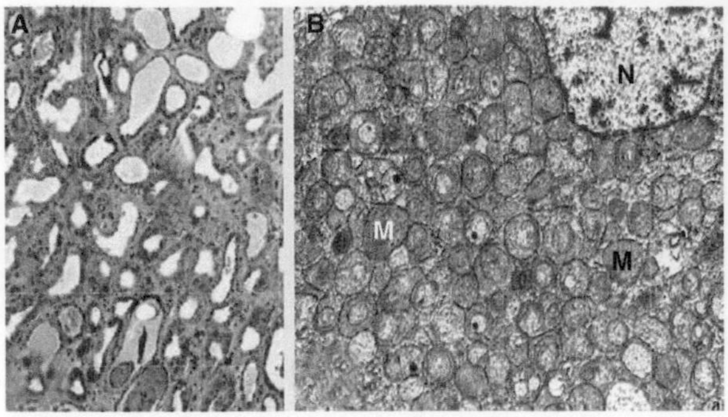

Figure 10.8 Kidney oncocytoma. **(A)** H&E stain. Note large red-staining oncocytic cells in renal tubule cells **(B)** EM of an oncocyte. The cytoplasm is packed with mitochondria (M). Nucleus (N) is at top right. Proliferation of mitochondria in individual muscle fibers (RRFs) are an important cause of morbidity in mitochondrial disorders. The signal(s) governing mitochondrial proliferation are completely unknown. Reproduced with permission of E Bonilla and EA Schon

ONCOCYTOMA OF THE KIDNEY

Oncocytomas of the kidney account for about 5% of all epithelial renal neoplasias. The hallmark of oncocytes is the massive accumulation of mitochondria (many of them abnormally shaped) in the cytoplasm, a morphological change similar to that seen in RRFs (Figure 10.8). Sometimes, this phenotype can also be observed in malignant neoplasms of the kidney, such as the chromophobic variants of renal cell carcinomas.

PATHOLOGY OF ONCOCYTOMA IN BIRT–HOGG–DUBE SYNDROME A familiar form of renal oncocytosis is the Birt–Hogg–Dube syndrome (BHD). Clinically, BHD is characterized by multiple hamartomas of the hair follicle, spontaneous pneumothorax, and renal cell tumors. Multiple oncocytomas may affect both kidneys. This syndrome supports the concept that oncocytoma may progress to chromophobe renal carcinomas, because in 50% of patients the tumors are, in fact, hybrids between oncocytomas and chromophobe renal cell carcinomas (RCCs). The spectrum of BHD kidney tumors further comprises 34% chromophobe RCCs, 5% oncocytoma, 10% clear cell RCC, and 2% papillary carcinoma of the kidney.[134,142] BHD is inherited as an autosomal dominant trait and is associated with mutations in the folliculin gene on chromosome 17q11.2. A hypermutable C_8 tract seems to represent a mutation hotspot in the folliculin gene.[143] BHD shows loss of heterozygosity as well as inactivation by somatic mutations of the second allele. So far, the BHD gene protein folliculin does not show homology to any known gene (family) and key functional domains have not been characterized. It is not clear if BHD patients have a predisposition to other malignancies, especially colorectal neoplasia. Folliculin mutations could not be found in sporadic oncocytoma and chromophobe RCCs.[144]

CYTOGENETICS OF RENAL ONCOCYTOMA Oncocytoma of the kidney can be divided karyotypically into three categories: (i) structural rearrangements involving 11q13.3; (ii) loss of chromosome 1 and of the Y chromosome; and (iii) no detectable chromosomal aberration.[145] Several reported translocations involving 1p36 raise the question of whether a tumor suppressor gene also involved in mitochondrial proliferation resides there. Rearrangements involving 11q13 include reciprocal translocations involving chromosomes 5,[146,147] 4, 9, and chromosome 11 itself.[141,145,148,149] In the group of patients without chromosomal alterations, mtDNA alterations have been described, including amplification of mtDNA and reduced mitochondrial transcripts.[150]

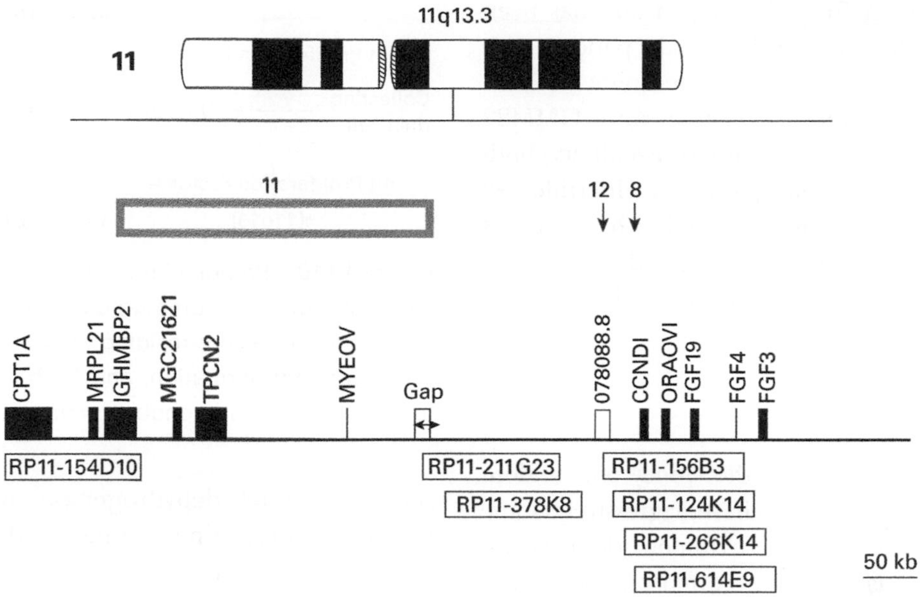

Figure 10.9 Schematic representation of the approximately 1-Mb genomic region encompassing the breakpoints in three oncocytomas with 11q13.3 rearrangements, based on the map of the human genome (http://genome.ucsc.edu; University of California, Santa Cruz). A fine mapping using regional BACs (white boxes below the line) revealed three breakpoints in close relationship to CCND1. The unfilled red box represents a predicted gene in the breakpoint area. The arrows indicate the approximate breakpoints in two cases and the gray-lined box represents the breakpoint area of another case

In an oncocytoma with an 11q13/5q35 reciprocal translocation, Sinke et al.[147] found that the breakpoint was within a region 400-kb centromeric to the cyclin D1 gene (*CCND1*; also called *BCL1*, for B-cell lymphoma1) on chromosome 11q13. In three oncocytomas with 11q13 rearrangements, using fluorescent in situ hybridization (FISH) with BAC clones harboring the above-mentioned 400-kb region, we also found that the 11q13 breakpoints were near the *CCND1 (BCL1)* gene (Figure 10.9). The rearrangement in one tumor consisted of a segmental duplication that included 11q13 and duplicated interesting mitochondrially related candidate genes such as *NADSYN1* and *UCP2/3*, which are distal to *CCND1*. A terminal deletion at 13q14.1 indicates that the mitochondrial gene *NDUFC2* may also be deleted.[151]

ONCOCYTOMA OF THE THYROID

Oncocytomas of the thyroid, also known as Huerthle cell tumors, may progress to Huerthle cell follicular carcinomas, which show a tendency to metastasize. The oxyphilic, mitochondria-rich Huerthle cells also occur in Huerthle cell follicular adenomas and Huerthle cell papillar carcinomas of the thyroid. The classification of oncocytoma as either adenoma or carcinoma uses the conventional criterion of vascular or capsular invasion as an indicator of malignancy. Huerthle cell carcinomas (HCC) have a higher frequency of loss of heterozygosity (LOH) on chromosome 17p13.3.[152] In HCC, the minimal critical region spans 411 kb and includes genes like *GEMIN4, CGI-150, NXN*, and *TIMM22*.[153] Recently, another gene, *HCCS1*, has been cloned from this region and has been shown to be mutated exclusively in patients with hepatocellular carcinoma. Interestingly, HCCS1 (a protein of unknown function) and TIMM22 (a member of the protein import machinery) both locate to mitochondria.[153] Familiar Huerthle cell tumors are consistently associated with alterations of chromosome 19p13.2,[154] where the presumed tumor suppressor gene *TCO* also resides.

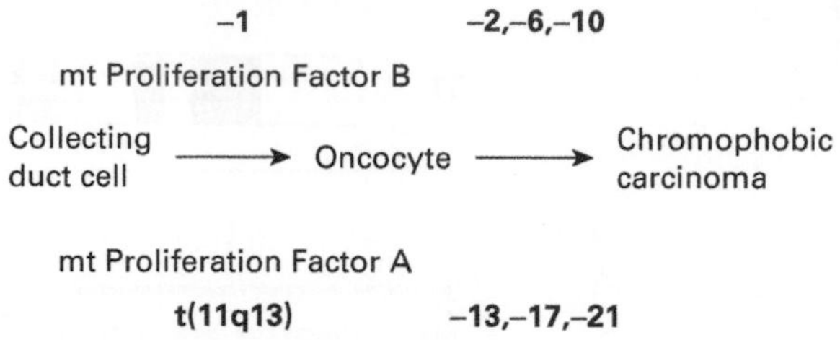

Figure 10.10 Proposed model for the oncocytoma/chromophobic carcinoma sequence in kidney tumors. Mitochondrial factors residing at 1p36 or 11q13 promote oncocyte formation, and further chromosome loss results in chromophobic carcinoma.

THE MALIGNANT POTENTIAL OF ONCOCYTOMA

Although oncocytomas of the kidney only seldom become malignant and behave aggressively, some reports indicate that these tumors do have an invasive potential.[155] However, morphological and immunohistochemical data point to a close relationship between oncocytoma and chromophobe renal carcinoma, both of which derive from the distal tubular epithelium. Hale's colloidal iron stain of chromophobe RCCs shows that the iron-positive vesicles in tumor cells actually represent abortive mitochondria. Progression from oncocytoma to chromophobe RCC has only been demonstrated morphologically in oncocytosis.[156,157] A genetic model for the adenoma/carcinoma sequence proposes that oncocytic adenomas first lose chromosomes 1 and Y, then also chromosomes 2, 6, 13, 17, and 21.[149,158] Mitochondrial factors encoded in the breakpoint regions of chromosomes 1p36 and 11q13, which are rich in mitochondrial genes, may contribute to the malignant transformation (Figure 10.10). To date, germline mutations in four genes, *VHL, MET, FH,* and folliculin (FLCN), have been identified in human renal tumors. Interestingly, in some patients with fumarase (FH) deficiency resulting in RCC, oncocytic–chromophobic hybrid tumors have also been found (personal communication, Dr Wendy Chung, Columbia University). Furthermore, expression profiling showed that chromophobe RCC and oncocytoma clustered in one class with the highest expression of mitochondrial genes, such as NADH dehydrogenase and fumarate hydratase, suggesting a functional relationship between these tumors.[159]

The malignant potential of Huerthle cell tumors is much higher than that of renal oncocytomas. Also, the mortality rate of oxyphilic carcinomas appears to be higher than that of other follicular thyroid carcinomas. The high prevalence of malignancy and the putative higher aggressivity of oncocytic carcinoma contrasts with the benign nature and low malignancy of most oxyphilic tumors in other organs.

Expression analysis of oncocytoma

The proliferation of mitochondria in oncocytomas is reflected by increased activities of respiratory chain complexes and increased mitochondrial biogenesis.[160] Expression profiling of oncocytomas reveals, as expected, up-regulation of many sequences related to mitochondrial biogenesis, cell proliferation, and oxidative metabolism,[161] such as glycolysis, Krebs cycle, and the respiratory chain (RC) (Box 8.1). Also up-regulated were genes involved in cell adhesion, cytoskeleton formation, cell cycle regulation, proteolysis, DNA repair, and transcription.[159] Cathepsin B was the most up-regulated nuclear gene in thyroid oncocytoma, together with *ZNF42, ADA, HINT1, IGF2R, DTR, CYBA, RPS18, MRLP49, MTND4, PRKDC,* and *POLD1*. Genes underexpressed in

Table 10.2 MtDNA, Citrate synthase and ATP synthesis in renal oncocytoma

Method	mtDNA	ΔmtDNA	CS	ATP synthesis	References
Enzyme activity			↑↑		181 172
Bioluminiscence				↓	164
Southern	↑↑	N			171 163

N, normal; ↑, increased; ↑↑, strongly increased; ↓, decreased.

thyroid oncocytomas are involved in various cellular processes, including lipid metabolism, inflammation, transcription, adhesion, signaling, and membrane structure (e.g. caveolin 1).[162]

Mitochondrial pathobiochemistry in oncocytoma

In all types of oncocytoma, the amount of mtDNA is higher than in control tissue,[163,164] but – when one considers the massive accumulation of mitochondria in oncocytic tissues – the number of mtDNA molecules per mitochondrion seems to be reduced. Gross alterations of mtDNA (e.g. the common deletion) were not found, nor were point mutations described thus far, except for polymorphic mtDNA C-tract alterations[165] and polymorphisms in restriction patterns (Table 10.2).[166,167]

Expression analysis of mitochondrial transcripts revealed decreased expression of *ND2, ND5, Cytb, ATPase 6/8*, and *12SRNA* in renal oncocytoma (Table 10.2).[168] The opposite was true for Huerthle cell tumors: all mitochondrial transcripts were generally up-regulated about two-fold.[162] In salivary gland oncocytomas, *ND2* and *ND5* transcripts were also up-regulated.[164,169] Interestingly, the steady-state level of nuclear mitochondrial gene transcripts, such as *ATPase synβ, GADPH*, and *ANT2* were generally elevated in oncocytomas. This suggests that a deficit of mitochondrial energy production may be compensated by a shift to glycolysis.[169]

Mitochondrial accumulation is reflected by the high citrate synthase activity of oncocytes (Table 10.2). Enzyme activities of respiratory chain (RC) complexes are also increased, except for complex I.[170–172] In particular, COX activity was seven-fold higher than in controls. Complex I is increased in thyroid oncocytoma,[164,169] but decreased in renal oncocytoma.[172] Western blots also showed a decreased amount of protein for complex I, whereas other RC complexes were increased in renal oncocytoma.[172] Immunohistochemistry revealed normal or slightly increased amounts of complexes I, II, IV, and V in renal and thyroid oncocytoma (Table 10.3).[173] Oxygen consumption was normal, but bioluminescence assays showed decreased ATP synthesis in thyroid oncocytoma (Table 10.2).[164]

Regulation and dysregulation of mitochondrial proliferation

The number of mitochondria can change in response to external stimuli. Nuclear respiratory factors 1 and 2 (NRF-1 and NRF-2)[174] are involved in the regulation of mitochondrial transcription and replication, and are themselves downstream of a newly discovered 'master regulator' of mitochondrial biogenesis, peroxisome proliferator-activated receptor gamma coactivator 1α (PGC-1α).[175–177] PGC-1 binds to the peroxisome proliferator activated receptor gamma (PPARγ), which belongs to the steroid hormone receptor family and is a

Table 10.3 Alterations of the RC complexes in renal oncocytoma

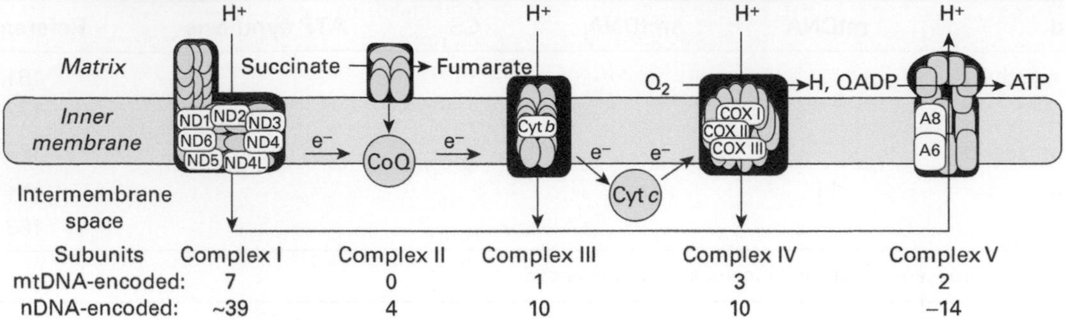

Method	Complex I	Complex II	Complex III	Complex IV	Complex V	References
Enzyme activity	↓	N or ↑	N or ↑	↑↑	N or ↑	172,181
2D-Page	↓	↑	↑	↑	↑	172,181
Northern	ND2↓ ND5↓		Cyt *b* ↓		ATPase 6/8↓	168,169
Immuno-HC		N		N	N	173

N, normal; ↑, increased; ↑↑, strongly increased; ↓, decreased.

regulator of brown fat development. Two other newly identified members of the PGC-1 family are PRC (PRC-1β related coactivator) and PGC-1β. All these coactivators interact with NRF-1 and NRF-2, which trans-activate a number of genes involved in mitochondrial functions, such as oxidative phosphorylation, protein import, and heme biosynthesis. They also mediate mitochondrial DNA (mtDNA) transcription and replication through two nuclear-encoded genes, mitochondrial transcription factor A (mtTFA), also known as TFAM or TF6, and mitochondrial transcription factor B (mtTFB).

Surprisingly, PPARγ is markedly reduced and PGC1α shows only a five-fold overexpression in thyroid oncocytomas, whereas TFAM and NRF were significantly overexpressed.[178] The gene encoding endothelial nitric oxide synthase (NOS3) is also overexpressed in oncocytic tumors,[161] and it has been shown that endogenous nitric oxide can trigger mitochondrial biogenesis through the induction of the PGC-1.[179]

The pathomechanism leading to mitochondrial proliferation is still far from known, although it was found that a non-mitochondrial cytosolic protein – neurotrophin-4 – was up-regulated specifically in RRFs.[180] A postulated uncoupling defect can now be excluded as the cause of mitochondrial proliferation because the expression of uncoupling proteins is not increased in renal oncocytomas and only slightly increased in thyroid oncocytomas.[164] In oncocytomas, increased mitochondrial biogenesis at the organelle level is clearly reflected by the increase in mitochondrial number and citrate synthase activity. However, relative to the huge number of organelles, mtDNA transcripts and mtDNA are decreased, consistent with the finding of decreased expression of TFAM.[164] The observed increased amount and activity of all RC complexes vis-à-vis the deficit in ATP production with a shift to glycolysis raises the question of whether induced mitochondrial biogenesis is a compensating mechanism for inefficient energy production.

An additional problem regards mitochondrial expression: is a nuclear factor involved in the maintenance of the mitochondrial transcriptome or proteome deficiency? This defect seems to be present in the oncocytoma's surrounding tissue and suggests that the culprit factor may have the additional ability to drive cells in the oncocytic tumor to transformation. The breakpoints in 11q13.3 near the oncogene *CCND1* hint to such a dual pathway in oncocytomas, namely cellular proliferation and mitochondrial proliferation. Dysregulation of *CCND1* expression is a reasonable explanation for the proliferation of cells in oncocytomas; one of the mitochondrial genes flanking *CCND1* may drive – perhaps in synergy with *CCND1* – the proliferation of mitochondria.[151]

References

1. Petty RKH, Harding AE, Morgan-Hughes JA. The clinical features of mitochondrial myopathy. *Brain* 1986; **109**: 915–938.
2. Pearson HA, Lobel JS, Kocoshis SA et al. A new syndrome of refractory sideroblastic anemia with vacuolization of marrow precursors and exocrine pancreatic dysfunction. *J Pediatr* 1979; **95**: 976–984.
3. Rötig A, Cormier V, Blanche S et al. Pearson's marrow-pancreas syndrome. A multisystem mitochondrial disorder in infancy. *J Clin Invest* 1990; **86**: 1601–1608.
4. Rötig A, Cormier V, Koll F et al. Site-specific deletions of the mitochondrial genome in the Pearson marrow-pancreas syndrome. *Genomics* 1991; **10**: 502–504.
5. McShane MA, Hammans SR, Sweeney M et al. Pearson syndrome and mitochondrial encephalomyopathy in a patient with a deletion of mtDNA. *Am J Hum Genet* 1991; **48**: 39–42.
6. Larsson NG, Holme E, Kristiansson B et al. Progressive increase of the mutated mitochondrial DNA fraction in Kearns-Sayre syndrome. *Pediatr Res* 1991; **28**: 131–133.
7. Nelson I, Bonne G, Degoul F et al. Kearns-Sayre syndrome with sideroblastic anemia: molecular investigations. *Neuropediatrics* 1992; **23**: 199–205.
8. Holt IJ, Harding AE, Cooper JM et al. Mitochondrial myopathies: clinical and biochemical features in 30 cases with major deletions of muscle mitochondrial DNA. *Ann Neurol* 1989; **26**: 699–708.
9. Moraes CT, DiMauro S, Zeviani M et al. Mitochondrial DNA deletions in progressive external ophthalmoplegia and Kearns-Sayre syndrome. *N Engl J Med* 1989; **320**: 1293–1299.
10. Ciafaloni E, Ricci E, Shanske S et al. MELAS: clinical features, biochemistry, and molecular genetics. *Ann Neurol* 1992; **31**: 391–398.
11. Goto Y-i, Horai S, Matsuoka T et al. Mitochondrial myopathy, encephalopathy, lactic acidosis, and stroke-like episodes (MELAS): a correlative study of the clinical features and mitochondrial DNA mutation. *Neurology* 1991; **42**: 545–550.
12. Poulton J, Morten K. Noninvasive diagnosis of the MELAS syndrome from blood DNA. *Ann Neurol* 1993; **34**: 116.
13. Rahman S, Poulton J, Marchington D, Suomalainen A. Decrease of 3243 A→G mtDNA mutation from blood in MELAS syndrome: a longitudinal study. *Am J Hum Genet* 2001; **68**: 238–240.
14. Holme E, Tulinius MH, Larsson N-G, Oldfors A. Inheritance and expression of mitochondrial DNA point mutations. *Biochim Biophys Acta* 1995; **1271**: 249–252.
15. Harris NL, Jaffe ES, Diebold J et al. World Health Organisation classification of neoplastic diseases of the hematopoietic and lymphoid tissues: report of the clinical advisory committee meeting—Airlie House, Virginia. *J Clin Oncol* 1999; **17**: 3835–3849.
16. Aul C, Gattermann N, Schneider W. Age-related incidence and other epidemiological aspects of myelodysplastic syndromes. *Br J Haematol* 1992; **82**: 358–367.
17. Gattermann N, Aul C, Schneider W. Two types of acquired idiopathic sideroblastic anaemia (AISA). *Br J Haematol* 1990; **74**: 45–52.
18. Germing U, Gattermann N, Aivado M et al. Two types of acquired idiopathic sideroblastic anaemia (AISA): a time-tested distinction. *Br J Haematol* 2000; **108**: 724–728.
19. Porra RJ, Jones OTG. Studies on ferrochelatase. *Biochem J* 1963; **87**: 181–192.
20. Gattermann N, Retzlaff S, Wang Y-L et al. A heteroplasmic point mutation of mitochondrial $tRNA^{Leu(CUN)}$ in non-lymphoid cell lineages from a patient with acquired idiopathic sideroblastic anaemia. *Br J Haematol* 1996; **93**: 845–855.

21. Gattermann N, Retzlaff S, Wang Y-L et al. Heteroplasmic point mutations of mitochondrial DNA affecting subunit I of cytochrome c oxidase in two patients with acquired idiopathic sideroblastic anemia. *Blood* 1997; **90**: 4961–4972.
22. Bröker S, Meunier B, Rich P et al. MtDNA mutations associated with sideroblastic anaemia cause a defect of mitochondrial cytochrome c oxidase. *Eur J Biochem* 1998; **258**: 132–138.
23. Wang Y-L, Choi H-K, Heinisch J et al. The MERRF mutation of mitochondrial DNA in the bone marrow of a patient with acquired idiopathic sideroblastic anemia. *Am J Hematol* 1999; **60**: 83–84.
24. Gattermann N. From sideroblastic anemia to the role of mitochondrial DNA mutations in myelodysplastic syndromes. *Leuk Res* 2000; **24**: 141–151.
25. Shin MG, Kajigaya S, Levin BC, Young NS. Mitochondrial DNA mutations in patients with myelodysplastic syndromes. *Blood* 2003; **101**: 3118–3125.
26. Rawles JM, Weller RO. Familial association of metabolic myopathy, lactic acidosis, and sideroblastic anemia. *Am J Med* 1974; **56**: 891–897.
27. Inbal A, Avissar NSM, Kuritzky A et al. Myopathy, lactic acidosis, and sideroblastic anemia: A new syndrome. *Am J Med Genet* 1995; **55**: 371–378.
28. Casas KA, Fischel-Ghodsian N. Mitochondrial myopathy and sideroblastic anemia. *Am J Med Genet* 2004; **125A**: 201–204.
29. Casas KA, Bykhovskaya Y, Mengesha E et al. Gene responsible for mitochondrial myopathy and sideroblastic anemia (MSA) maps to chromosome 12q24.33. *Am J Med Genet* 2004; **127A**: 44–49.
30. Buttgereit F, Brand MD. A hierarchy of ATP-consuming processes in mammalian cells. *Biochem J* 1995; **312**: 163–167.
31. Wickramasinghe SN, Chalmers DG, Cooper EH. A study of ineffective erythropoiesis in sideroblastic anaemia and erythraemic myelosis. *Cell Tissue Kinetics* 1968; **1**: 43–50.
32. Wickramasinghe SN, Hughes M. Capacity of ringed sideroblasts to synthesize nucleic acids and protein in patients with primary acquired sideroblastic anaemia. *Br J Haematol* 1978; **38**: 345–352.
33. van Duppen V, Raets V, Raeymaekers L et al. CD34+ progenitors from low-risk MDS patients are more susceptible to induced oxidative damage and have reduced DNA repair compared to healthy control subjects. *Blood* 2003; **102**(11): 916a.
34. Kroemer G, Reed JC. Mitochondrial control of cell death. *Nat Med* 2000; **6**: 513–519.
35. Tehranchi R, Fadeel B, Forsblom A-M et al. Evidence for a role of mitochondrial signaling in apoptosis in low-risk myelodysplastic syndromes. *Blood* 2001; **98**: 730a.
36. Wolvetang EJ, Johnson KL, Krauer K et al. Mitochondrial respiratory chain inhibitors induce apoptosis. *FEBS Lett* 1994; **339**: 40–44.
37. Parker JE, Fishlock KL, Mijovic J et al. 'Low-risk' myelodysplastic syndrome is associated with excessive apoptosis and an increased ratio of pro-versus anti-apoptotic bcl-2-related proteins. *Br J Haematol* 1998; **103**: 1075–1082.
38. Berger G, Hunault-Berger M, Rachieru P et al. Increased apoptosis in mononucleated cells but not CD34+ cells in blastic forms of myelodysplastic syndromes. *Hematol J* 2001; **2**: 87–96.
39. Gattermann N, Dadak M, Hofhaus G et al. Severe impairment of nucleotide synthesis through inhibition of mitochondrial respiration. *Nucleosides Nucleotides Nucl Acids* 2004; **23**(8–9): 1275–1279.
40. Kunz BA, Kohalmi SE, Kunkel TA et al. Deoxyribonucleoside triphosphate levels: A critical factor in the maintenance of genetic stability. *Mutat Res* 1994; **318**: 1–64.
41. He L, Luo L, Proctor SJ et al. Somatic mitochondrial DNA mutations in adult-onset leukaemia. *Leukemia* 2003; **17**(12): 2487–2491.
42. Ivanova R, Lepage V, Loste MN et al. Mitochondrial DNA sequence variation in human leukemic cells. *Int J Cancer* 1998; **76**: 495–498.
43. Wallace DC. Mitochondrial diseases in man and mouse. *Science* 1999; **283**: 1482–1488.
44. Cortopassi GA, Shibata DD, Soong N-W, Arnheim N. A pattern of accumulation of a somatic deletion of mitochondrial DNA in aging human tissues. *Proc Natl Acad Sci USA* 1992; **89**: 7370–7374.
45. Corral-Debrinski M, Shoffner JM, Lott MT, Wallace DC. Association of mitochondrial DNA damage with aging and coronary atherosclerotic heart disease. *Mutat Res* 1992; **275**: 169–180.
46. Kadenbach B, Munscher C, Frank V et al. Human ageing is associated with stochastic somatic mutations of mitochondrial DNA. *Mutat Res* 1995; **338**: 161–172.
47. Brierley EJ, Johnson MA, Lightowlers RN et al. Role of mitochondrial DNA mutations in human

aging: implications for the central nervous system and muscle. *Ann Neurol* 1998; **43**: 217–223.
48. Murdock DG, Christiacos NC, Wallace DC. The age-related accumulation of a mitochondrial DNA control region mutation in muscle, but not brain, detected by a sensitive PNA-directed PCR clamping based method. *Nucleic Acids Res* 2000; **28**: 4350–4355.
49. Coller HA, Bodyak ND, Khrapko K. Frequent intracellular clonal expansions of somatic mtDNA mutations. *Ann N Y Acad Sci* 2002; **959**: 434–447.
50. Boultwood J, Fidler C, Mills KI et al. Amplification of mitochondrial DNA in acute myeloid leukaemia. *Br J Haematol* 1996; **95**: 426–431.
51. Gattermann N, Aul C. Mitochondrial DNA amplification in AML: a hypothesis. *Br J Haematol* 1997; **97**: 242.
52. Bessis M. *Living Blood Cells and Their Ultrastructure*. Berlin, Heidelberg, New York: Springer-Verlag; 1973.
53. Schumacher HR, Szekely IE, Patel SB, Fisher DR. Leukemic mitochondria. I. Acute myeloblastic leukemia. *Am J Pathol* 1974; **74**: 71–82.
54. Torroni A, Stepien G, Hodge JA, Wallace DC. Neoplastic transformation is associated with coordinate induction of nuclear and cytoplasmic oxidative phosphorylation genes. *J Bio Chem* 1990; **265**: 20589–20593.
55. Attardi G. The human mitochondrial genetic system. In: DiMauro S, Wallace DC, eds. *Mitochondrial DNA in Human Pathology*. New York: Raven Press; 1993: 9–25.
56. Clayton DA, Vinograd J. Circular dimer and catenate forms of mitochondrial DNA in human leukaemic leukocytes. *Nature* 1967; **216**: 652–657.
57. Clayton DA, Vinograd J. Complex mitochondrial DNA in leukemic and normal human myeloid cells. *Proc Natl Acad Sci USA* 1969; **62**: 1077–1084.
58. Clayton DA, Smith CA. Complex mitochondrial DNA. *Int Rev Exp Pathol* 1975; **14**: 1–67.
59. Hatfill S, Kirby R. Abnormal mitochondrial DNA length polymorphism in patients with the myelodysplastic syndrome. *Blood* 1994; **84**: 314a.
60. Firkin FC, Clark-Walker GD. Abnormal mitochondrial DNA in acute leukemia and lymphoma. *Br J Haematol* 1979; **43**: 201–206.
61. Miguel A, Hernández-Yago J, Knecht E, Renau-Piqueras J. A comparative study of complex mitochondrial DNA in human lymphocytes transformed by Epstein-Barr virus and PHA. *Acta Haematologica* 1982; **68**: 96–104.
62. Christiansen G, Christiansen C, Zeuthen J. Complex forms of mitochondrial DNA in human B cells transformed by Epstein-Barr virus. *J Cancer Res Clin Oncol* 1983; **105**: 13–19.
63. Carew JS, Zhou Y, Alibar M et al. Mitochondrial DNA mutations in primary leukemia cells after chemotherapy: clinical significance and therapeutic implications. *Leukemia* 2003; **17**: 1437–1447.
64. Liu SL, Lin X, Shi DY et al. Reactive oxygen species stimulate human hepatoma cell proliferation via cross-talk between PI3K/PKB and JNK signaling pathways. *Arch Biochem Biophys* 2002; **406**: 173–182.
65. Haddad JJ. Redox regulation of pro-inflammatory cytokines and IκB-α/NF-κB nuclear translocation and activation. *Biochem Biophys Res Commun* 2002; **296**: 847–856.
66. Gattermann N, Berneburg M, Heinisch J et al. Detection of the ageing-associated 5-Kb deletion of mitochondrial DNA in blood and bone marrow of hematologically normal adults. Absence of the deletion in clonal bone marrow disorders. *Leukemia* 1995; **9**: 1704–1710.
67. Morrison SJ, Wandycz AM, Akashi K et al. The aging of hematopoietic stem cells. *Nat Med* 1996; **2**: 1011–1016.
68. Marley SB, Lewis JL, Davidson RJ et al. Evidence for a continuous decline in haematopoietic cell function from birth: application to evaluating bone marrow failure in children. *Br J Haematol* 1999; **106**: 162–166.
69. Geiger H, van Zant G. The aging of lympho-hematopoietic stem cells. *Nat Immunol* 2002; **3**: 329–333.
70. Warburg O. *Metabolism of Tumors*. London: Arnold Constable; 1930.
71. Warburg O. On the origin of cancer cells. *Science* 1956; **123**: 309–314.
72. Weinhouse S. Oxidative metabolism of neoplastic tissue. *Adv Cancer Res* 1955; **3**: 269–329.
73. Weinhouse S. On respiratory impairment in cancer cells. *Science* 1956; **124**: 267–269.
74. Burk D, Schade AL. On respiratory impairment in cancer cells. *Science* 1956; **124**: 270–272.
75. Dang CV, Semenza GL. Oncogenic alterations of metabolism. *Trends Biochem Sci* 1999; **24**: 68–72.

76. Pedersen PL. Tumor mitochondria and the bioenergetics of cancer cells. *Prog Exp Tumor Res* 1978; **22**: 190–274.
77. Arora KK, Parry DM, Pedersen PL. Hexokinase receptors: preferential enzyme binding in normal cells to nonmitochondrial sites and in transformed cells to mitochondrial sites. *J Bioenerget Biomem* 1992; **24**: 47–53.
78. Mathupala SP, Rempel A, Pedersen PL. Glucose catabolism in cancer cells. Isolation, sequence, and activity of the promoter for type II hexokinase. *J Bio Chem* 1995; **270**: 16918–16925.
79. Katabi MM, Chan HLB, Karp SE et al. Hexokinase type II: a novel tumor-specific promoter for gene-targeted therapy differentially expressed and regulated in human cancer cells. *Hum Gene Ther* 1999; **10**: 155–164.
80. Wilkie D, Egilsson V, Evans IH. Mitochondria in oncogenesis. *Lancet* 1975; **1**(7908): 697–698.
81. Carafoli E. Mitochondrial pathology: An overview. *Ann N Y Acad Sci* 1986; **488**: 1–18.
82. Shay JW, Werbin H. Are mitochondrial DNA mutations involved in the carcinogenic process? *Mutat Res* 1987; **186**: 149–160.
83. Richter C. Do mitochondrial DNA fragments promote cancer and aging? *FEBS Lett* 1988; **241**: 1–5.
84. Bandy B, Davison AJ. Mitochondrial mutations may increase oxidative stress: implications for carcinogenesis and ageing? *Free Radical Biol Med* 1990; **8**: 523–539.
85. Baggetto LG. Deviant energetic metabolism of glycolytic cancer cells. *Biochimie* 1992; **74**: 959–974.
86. Baggetto LG. Role of mitochondria in carcinogenesis. *Eur J Cancer* 1993; **29A**: 156–159.
87. Cavalli LR, Liang BC. Mutagenesis, tumorigenicity, and apoptosis: are the mitochondria involved? *Mutat Res* 2001; **398**: 19–26.
88. Neubert D, Hopfenmüller G, Fuchs G. Manifestation of carcinogenesis as a stochastic process on the basis of an altered mitochondrial genome. *Arch Toxicol* 1981; **48**: 89–125.
89. Penta JS, Johnson FM, Wachsman JT, Copeland WC. Mitochondrial DNA in human malignancy. *Mutat Res* 2001; **488**: 119–133.
90. Wallace DC. Mouse models for mitochondrial disease. *Am J Med Genet* (*Semin Med Genet*) 2001; **106**: 71–93.
91. Augenlicht LH, Heerdt BG. Mitochondria: integrators in tumorigenesis? *Nat Genet* 2001; **28**: 104–105.
92. Taylor RW, Barron MJ, Borthwick GM et al. Mitochondrial DNA mutations in human colonic crypt stem cells. *J Clin Invest* 2003; **112**: 1351–1360.
93. Elson JL, Samuels DC, Turnbull DM, Chinnery PF. Random intracellular drift explains the clonal expansion of mitochondrial mutations with age. *Am J Hum Genet* 2001; **68**: 802–806.
94. Coller HA, Khrapko K, Bodyak ND et al. High frequency of homoplasmic mitochondrial DNA mutations in human tumors can be explained without selection. *Nat Genet* 2001; **28**: 147–150.
95. Nekhaeva E, Bodyak ND, Kraytsberg Y et al. Clonally expanded mtDNA point mutations are abundant in individual cells of human tissues. *Proc Natl Acad Sci USA* 2002; **99**: 5521–5526.
96. Chinnery PF, Samuels DC, Elson JL, Turnbull DM. Accumulation of mitochondrial DNA mutations in ageing, cancer, and mitochondrial disease: is there a common mechanism? *Lancet* 2002; **360**: 1323–1325.
97. Kraytsberg Y, Nekhaeva E, Bodyak ND, Khrapko K. Mutation and intracellular clonal expansion of mitochondrial genomes: two synergistic components of the aging process? *Mech Ageing Dev* 2003; **124**: 49–53.
98. Wallace DC. Mitochondrial DNA mutations and neuromuscular disease. *Trends Genet* 1989; **5**: 9–13.
99. Shoubridge EA, Karpati G, Hastings KEM. Deletion mutants are functionally dominant over wild-type mitochondrial genomes in skeletal muscle fiber segments in mitochondrial disease. *Cell* 1990; **62**: 43–49.
100. de Grey AD. A proposed refinement of the mitochondrial free radical theory of ageing. *Bioessays* 1997; **19**: 161–166.
101. Chinnery PF, Samuels DC. Relaxed replication of mtDNA: a model with implications for the expression of disease. *Am J Hum Genet* 1999; **64**: 1158–1165.
102. Hofhaus G, Gattermann N. Mitochondria harbouring mutant mtDNA – a cuckoo in the nest? *Biol Chem* 1999; **380**: 871–877.
103. Haraguchi Y, Chung AB, Neill S, Wallace DC. OXBOX and REBOX, overlapping promotor elements of the mitochondrial F_0F_1-ATP synthase β subunit gene. *J Bio Chem* 1994; **269**: 9330–9334.
104. Coskun PE, Ruiz-Pesini E, Wallace DC. Control region mtDNA variants: Longevity, climatic

adaptation, and a forensic conundrum. *Proc Natl Acad Sci USA* 2003; **100**: 2174–2176.
105. Polyak K, Li Y, Zhu H et al. Somatic mutations of the mitochondrial genome in human colorectal tumours. *Nat Genet* 1998; **20**: 291–293.
106. Fliss MS, Usadel H, Cabalero OL et al. Facile detection of mitochondrial DNA mutations in tumors and bodily fluids. *Science* 2000; **287**: 2017–2019.
107. Jeronimo C, Nomoto S, Caballero OL et al. Mitochondrial mutations in early stage prostate cancer and bodily fluids. *Oncogene* 2001; **20**: 5195–5198.
108. Parrella P, Xiao Y, Fliss M et al. Detection of mitochondrial DNA mutations in primary breast cancer and fine-needle aspirates. *Cancer Res* 2001; **61**: 7623–7626.
109. Jones JB, Song JJ, Hempen PM et al. Detection of mitochondrial DNA mutations in pancreatic cancer offers a 'mass'-ive advantage over detection of nuclear DNA mutations. *Cancer Res* 2001; **61**: 1299–1304.
110. Okochi O, Hibi K, Uemura T et al. Detection of mitochondrial DNA alterations in the serum of hepatocellular carcinoma patients. *Clin Cancer Res* 2002; **8**: 2875–2878.
111. Costantini P, Jacotot E, Decaudin D, Kroemer G. Mitochondrion as a novel target of anticancer chemotherapy. *J Natl Cancer Inst* 2000; **92**: 1042–1053.
112. Selak MA, Armour SM, MacKenzie ED et al. Succinate links TCA cycle dysfunction to oncogenesis by inhibiting HIF-alpha prolyl hydroxylase. *Cancer Cell* 2005; **7**: 77–85.
113. Rustin P, Rotig A. Inborn errors of complex II – unusual human mitochondrial diseases. *Biochim Biophys Acta* 2002; **1553**: 117–122.
114. Eng C, Kiuru M, Fernandez MJ et al. A role for mitochondrial enzymes in inherited neoplasia and beyond. *Nat Rev Cancer* 2003; **3**: 193–202.
115. DiMauro S, Schon EA. Mitochondrial respiratory-chain diseases. *N Engl J Med* 2003; **348**: 2656–2668.
116. Leigh D. Subacute necrotizing encephalomyelopathy in an infant. *J Neurochem* 1951; **14**: 216–221.
117. DiMauro S, De Vivo DC. Genetic heterogeneity in Leigh syndrome. *Ann Neurol* 1996; **40**: 5–7.
118. Bourgeron T, Rustin P, Chretien D et al. Mutation of a nuclear succinate dehydrogenase gene results in mitochondrial respiratory chain deficiency. *Nat Genet* 1995; **11**: 144–149.
119. Parfait B, Chretien D, Rotig A et al. Compound heterozygous mutations in the flavoprotein gene of the respiratory chain complex II in a patient with Leigh syndrome. *Hum Genet* 2000; **106**: 236–243.
120. Baysal BE. Hereditary paraganglioma targets diverse paraganglia. *J Med Genet* 2002; **39**: 617–622.
121. Maher ER, Eng C. The pressure rises: update on the genetics of phaeochromocytoma. *Hum Mol Genet* 2002; **11**: 2347–2354.
122. Baysal BE. On the association of succinate dehydrogenase mutations with hereditary paraganglioma. *Trends Endocrinol Metab* 2003; **14**: 453–459.
123. Neumann HP, Pawlu C, Peczkowska M et al. Distinct clinical features of paraganglioma syndromes associated with SDHB and SDHD gene mutations. *JAMA* 2004; **292**: 943–951.
124. Habano W, Sugai T, Nakamura S et al. Reduced expression and loss of heterozygosity of the SDHD gene in colorectal and gastric cancer. *Oncol Rep* 2003; **10**: 1375–1380.
125. Gimenez-Roqueplo AP, Favier J, Rustin P et al. The R22X mutation of the SDHD gene in hereditary paraganglioma abolishes the enzymatic activity of complex II in the mitochondrial respiratory chain and activates the hypoxia pathway. *Am J Hum Genet* 2001; **69**: 1186–1197.
126. Baysal BE, Ferrell RE, Willett-Brozick JE et al. Mutations in SDHD, a mitochondrial complex II gene, in hereditary paraganglioma. *Science* 2000; **287**: 848–851.
127. Baysal BE. Genomic imprinting and environment in hereditary paraganglioma. *Am J Med Genet C Semin Med Genet* 2004; **129**: 85–90.
128. Gimenez-Roqueplo AP, Favier J, Rustin P et al. Functional consequences of a SDHB gene mutation in an apparently sporadic pheochromocytoma. *J Clin Endocrinol Metab* 2002; **87**: 4771–4774.
129. Niemann S, Muller U. Mutations in SDHC cause autosomal dominant paraganglioma, type 3. *Nat Genet* 2000; **26**: 268–270.
130. Teipel JW, Hill RL. The subunit interactions of fumarase. *J Biol Chem* 1971; **246**: 4859–4865.
131. Launonen V, Vierimaa O, Kiuru M et al. Inherited susceptibility to uterine leiomyomas and renal cell cancer. *Proc Natl Acad Sci USA* 2001; **98**: 3387–3392.
132. Alam NA, Rowan AJ, Wortham NC et al. Genetic and functional analyses of FH mutations in

multiple cutaneous and uterine leiomyomatosis, hereditary leiomyomatosis and renal cancer, and fumarate hydratase deficiency. *Hum Mol Genet* 2003; **12**: 1241–1252.

133. Tomlinson IP, Alam NA, Rowan AJ et al. Germline mutations in FH predispose to dominantly inherited uterine fibroids, skin leiomyomata and papillary renal cell cancer. *Nat Genet* 2002; **30**: 406–410.
134. Khoo SK, Giraud S, Kahnoski K et al. Clinical and genetic studies of Birt-Hogg-Dube syndrome. *J Med Genet* 2002; **39**: 906–912.
135. Linnartz B, Anglmayer R, Zanssen S. Comprehensive scanning of somatic mitochondrial DNA alterations in acute leukemia developing from myelodysplastic syndromes. *Cancer Res* 2004; **64**: 1966–1971.
136. Gattermann N. From sideroblastic anemia to the role of mitochondrial DNA mutations in myelodysplastic syndromes. *Leuk Res* 2000; **24**: 141–151.
137. Ivan M, Haberberger T, Gervasi DC et al. Biochemical purification and pharmacological inhibition of a mammalian prolyl hydroxylase acting on hypoxia-inducible factor. *Proc Natl Acad Sci USA* 2002; **99**: 13459–13464.
138. Schofield CJ, Ratcliffe PJ. Oxygen sensing by HIF hydroxylases. *Nat Rev Mol Cell Biol* 2004; **5**: 343–354.
139. Schofield CJ, Zhang Z. Structural and mechanistic studies on 2-oxoglutarate-dependent oxygenases and related enzymes. *Curr Opin Struct Biol* 1999; **9**: 722–731.
140. He W, Miao FJ, Lin DC et al. Citric acid cycle intermediates as ligands for orphan G-protein-coupled receptors. *Nature* 2004; **429**: 188–193.
141. Fuzesi L, Gunawan B, Braun S et al. Cytogenetic analysis of 11 renal oncocytomas: further evidence of structural rearrangements of 11q13 as a characteristic chromosomal anomaly. *Cancer Genet Cytogenet* 1998; **107**: 1–6.
142. Warren MB, Torres-Cabala CA, Turner ML et al. Expression of Birt-Hogg-Dube gene mRNA in normal and neoplastic human tissues. *Mod Pathol* 2004; **17**: 998–1011.
143. Nickerson ML, Warren MB, Toro JR et al. Mutations in a novel gene lead to kidney tumors, lung wall defects, and benign tumors of the hair follicle in patients with the Birt-Hogg-Dube syndrome. *Cancer Cell* 2002; **2**: 157–164.
144. Nagy A, Zoubakov D, Stupar Z et al. Lack of mutation of the folliculin gene in sporadic chromophobe renal cell carcinoma and renal oncocytoma. *Int J Cancer* 2004; **109**: 472–475.
145. Neuhaus C, Dijkhuizen T, van den Berg E et al. Involvement of the chromosomal region 11q13 in renal oncocytoma: case report and literature review. *Cancer Genet Cytogenet* 1997; **94**: 95–98.
146. van den Berg E, Dijkhuizen T, Storkel S et al. Chromosomal changes in renal oncocytomas. Evidence that t(5;11)(q35;q13) may characterize a second subgroup of oncocytomas. *Cancer Genet Cytogenet* 1995; **79**: 164–168.
147. Sinke RJ, Dijkhuizen T, Janssen B et al. Fine mapping of the human renal oncocytoma-associated translocation (5;11)(q35;q13) breakpoint. *Cancer Genet Cytogenet* 1997; **96**: 95–101.
148. Fuzesi L, Gunawan B, Braun S et al. Renal oncocytoma with a translocation t(9;11)(p23;q13). *J Urol* 1994; **152**: 471–472.
149. Dijkhuizen T, van den Berg E, Storkel S et al. Renal oncocytoma with t(5;12;11), der(1)1;8) and add(19): 'true' oncocytoma or chromophobe adenoma? *Int J Cancer* 1997; **73**: 521–524.
150. Tallini G. Oncocytic tumours. *Virchows Arch* 1998; **433**: 5–12.
151. Zanssen S, Gunawan B, Fuzesi L et al. Renal oncocytomas with rearrangements involving 11q13 contain breakpoints near CCND1. *Cancer Genet Cytogenet* 2004; **149**: 120–124.
152. Farrand K, Delahunt B, Wang XL et al. High resolution loss of heterozygosity mapping of 17p13 in thyroid cancer: Hurthle cell carcinomas exhibit a small 411-kilobase common region of allelic imbalance, probably containing a novel tumor suppressor gene. *J Clin Endocrinol Metab* 2002; **87**: 4715–4721.
153. Zhao X, Li J, He Y et al. A novel growth suppressor gene on chromosome 17p13.3 with a high frequency of mutation in human hepatocellular carcinoma. *Cancer Res* 2001; **61**: 7383–7387.
154. Harach HR, Lesueur F, Amati P et al. Histology of familial thyroid tumours linked to a gene mapping to chromosome 19p13.2. *J Pathol* 1999; **189**: 387–393.
155. Kovacs G, Szucs S, Eichner W et al. Renal oncocytoma. A cytogenetic and morphologic study. *Cancer* 1987; **59**: 2071–2077.
156. Al-Saleem T, Cairns P, Dulaimi EA et al. The genetics of renal oncocytosis: a possible model for

neoplastic progression. *Cancer Genet Cytogenet* 2004; **152**: 23–28.
157. Tickoo SK, Amin MB, Zarbo RJ. Colloidal iron staining in renal epithelial neoplasms, including chromophobe renal cell carcinoma: emphasis on technique and patterns of staining. *Am J Surg Pathol* 1998; **22**: 419–424.
158. van den Berg E, Dijkhuizen T, Oosterhuis JW et al. Cytogenetic classification of renal cell cancer. *Cancer Genet Cytogenet* 1997; **95**: 103–107.
159. Young AN, Amin MB, Moreno CS et al. Expression profiling of renal epithelial neoplasms: a method for tumor classification and discovery of diagnostic molecular markers. *Am J Pathol* 2001; **158**: 1639–1651.
160. Ebner D, Rodel G, Pavenstaedt I et al. Functional and molecular analysis of mitochondria in thyroid oncocytoma. *Virchows Arch B Cell Pathol Incl Mol Pathol* 1991; **60**: 139–144.
161. Baris O, Savagner F, Nasser V et al. Transcriptional profiling reveals coordinated upregulation of oxidative metabolism genes in thyroid oncocytic tumors. *J Clin Endocrinol Metab* 2004; **89**: 994–1005.
162. Jacques C, Baris O, Prunier-Mirebeau D et al. Two-step differential expression analysis reveals a new set of genes involved in thyroid oncocytic tumors. *J Clin Endocrinol Metab* 2005; **90**(4): 2314–2320.
163. Tallini G, Ladanyi M, Rosai J et al. Analysis of nuclear and mitochondrial DNA alterations in thyroid and renal oncocytic tumors. *Cytogenet Cell Genet* 1994; **66**: 253–259.
164. Savagner F, Chevrollier A, Loiseau D et al. Mitochondrial activity in XTC.UC1 cells derived from thyroid oncocytoma. *Thyroid* 2001; **11**: 327–333.
165. Capone RB, Ha PK, Westra WH et al. Oncocytic neoplasms of the parotid gland: a 16-year institutional review. *Otolaryngol Head Neck Surg* 2002; **126**: 657–662.
166. Brooks JD, Marshall FF, Isaacs WB et al. Absence of Hint1 restriction abnormalities in renal oncocytoma mitochondrial DNA. *Mol Urol* 1999; **3**: 1–3.
167. Welter C, Kovacs G, Seitz G et al. Alteration of mitochondrial DNA in human oncocytomas. *Genes Chromosomes Cancer* 1989; **1**: 79–82.
168. Faure Vigny H, Heddi A, Giraud S et al. Expression of oxidative phosphorylation genes in renal tumors and tumoral cell lines. *Mol Carcinog* 1996; **16**: 165–172.
169. Heddi A, Faure-Vigny H, Wallace DC et al. Coordinate expression of nuclear and mitochondrial genes involved in energy production in carcinoma and oncocytoma. *Biochim Biophys Acta* 1996; **1316**: 203–209.
170. Hunter VR, Pauly DF, Wolkowicz PE et al. Mitochondrial adenosine triphosphatase in the oxyphil cells of a renal oncocytoma. *Hum Pathol* 1990; **21**: 437–442.
171. Selvanayagam P, Rajaraman S. Detection of mitochondrial genome depletion by a novel cDNA in renal cell carcinoma. *Lab Invest* 1996; **74**: 592–599.
172. Simonnet H, Demont J, Pfeiffer K et al. Mitochondrial complex I is deficient in renal oncocytomas. *Carcinogenesis* 2003; **24**: 1461–1466.
173. Muller-Hocker J. Random cytochrome-C-oxidase deficiency of oxyphil cell nodules in the parathyroid gland. A mitochondrial cytopathy related to cell ageing? *Pathol Res Pract* 1992; **188**: 701–706.
174. Scarpulla RC. Nuclear control of respiratory chain expression in mammalian cells. *J Bioenerg Biomembr* 1997; **29**: 109–119.
175. Wu Z, Puigserver P, Andersson U et al. Mechanisms controlling mitochondrial biogenesis and respiration through the thermogenic coactivator PGC-1. *Cell* 1999; **98**: 115–124.
176. Knutti D, Kralli A. PGC-1, a versatile coactivator. *Trends Endocrinol Metab* 2001; **12**: 360–365.
177. Scarpulla RC. Nuclear activators and coactivators in mammalian mitochondrial biogenesis. *Biochim Biophys Acta* 2002; **1576**: 1–14.
178. Savagner F, Mirebeau D, Jacques C et al. PGC-1-related coactivator and targets are upregulated in thyroid oncocytoma. *Biochem Biophys Res Commun* 2003; **310**: 779–784.
179. Nisoli E, Falcone S, Tonello C et al. Mitochondrial biogenesis by NO yields functionally active mitochondria in mammals. *Proc Natl Acad Sci USA* 2004; **101**: 16507–66512.
180. Walker UA, Schon EA. Neurotrophin-4 is upregulated in ragged-red fibers associated with pathogenic mitochondrial DNA mutations. *Ann Neurol* 1998; **43**: 536–540.
181. Simmonet M, Alazard N, Pfeiffer K et al. Low mitochondrial respiratory chain content correlates with tumor aggressiveness in renal cell carcinoma. *Carcinogenesis* 2002; **23**: 759–768

11

Mitochondrial reproductive medicine

David R Thorburn

Introduction

Reproduction is an energy-requiring process, not only for the participants but also for their germ cells. Mitochondrial misbehavior could imperil many facets of the reproductive process, and it is interesting to first consider this from an evolutionary perspective. Sexual reproduction provides a mechanism whereby maternal and paternal nuclear genomes can recombine, allowing segregation of new haploid genomes into germ cells. This facilitates natural selection for advantageous mutations and against deleterious mutations (Box 11.1). In contrast, the mitochondrial DNA (mtDNA) genome is inherited maternally, providing little or no opportunity for recombination. Without recombination between maternal and paternal mtDNAs, transmission of mtDNA from mother to child is an asexual process.[1] This should lead to an accumulation of mildly deleterious mutations over generations[2] in a process known as Muller's ratchet.[3] Over many generations, the function of individual cells, organisms and, eventually, the species would be compromised. One would expect evolution to have acted on the reproductive system to develop mechanisms that prevent the gradual decline of mitochondrial function in future generations. Thus, it is not surprising that mitochondrial genes and nuclear genes encoding mitochondrial proteins play important roles in many aspects of reproductive medicine. This chapter describes the roles of mitochondrial function and genetics in male and female fertility, embryogenesis, follicular atresia, assisted reproduction technologies, and prevention of mitochondrial diseases.

Transmission of mitochondrial DNA between generations

A single somatic cell typically contains a few thousand copies of mtDNA, which represent about 1% of the cell's total DNA. However, germ cells show a remarkable difference in mtDNA copy number. In the mature mammalian oocyte the number of mtDNA copies is estimated to be between 100 000 and 300 000,[4–6] representing about half of the oocyte's total DNA content. In contrast, estimates of the mtDNA copy number in spermatozoa range from 50 to 700.[7,8] Despite what many textbooks state, paternal mitochondria do enter the egg at fertilization (Box 11.1).[9,10] Thus the fertilized egg contains a mixture of maternal and paternal mtDNA genomes, although the latter represent less than 1% of the mtDNA copies. Sheer weight of numbers though is not the only factor limiting transmission of paternal mtDNA to the fetus. Paternal mitochondria and mtDNA are usually eliminated early in embryogenesis.[11] This involves a process whereby certain mitochondrial proteins are ubiquitinated during spermatogenesis and subsequently recognized and destroyed by the egg's ubiquitin/proteasome-dependent proteolytic machinery after fertilization.[12,13]

A recent finding challenged the dogma that mtDNA is exclusively maternally inherited. A single patient was reported with mitochondrial myopathy caused by a de novo mtDNA mutation restricted to skeletal muscle. Extensive testing showed that the mutation had occurred in mtDNA inherited from his father,[14] which was abundant in skeletal muscle but not present in other tissues. This raised the possibility that other patients with mtDNA disease could also have inherited paternal mtDNA in affected tissues. Subsequent studies on 45 patients with sporadic mitochondrial myopathies, similar to the test case, showed no evidence of paternal mtDNA.[15,16] Paternal inheritance of mtDNA appears to be an extremely rare event and for practical medical purposes, transmission of mtDNA can be assumed to show virtually exclusive maternal inheritance (see Box 11.1).

In most individuals, mtDNA is homoplasmic, i.e. virtually all copies in all tissues have identical sequence. Many patients with mtDNA mutations show heteroplasmy, a mixture of mutant and wild-type sequences that can be present in different proportions in different tissues. Occasionally, healthy humans and other mammals are found to be heteroplasmic for two polymorphic variants of mtDNA, differing at a single nucleotide. Studies of heteroplasmic sheep, goats and cattle[17–19] showed that the offspring of heteroplasmic females can show dramatic variation in the proportions of the two mtDNA species. Rapid shifts in heteroplasmy also occur in humans[20–23] (Figure 11.1) but may not be a universal phenomenon for all mtDNA sequence variations or mutations in all families.[24,25]

Rapid shifts in heteroplasmy are not easily explained by a simple model in which two species of mtDNA, each present in thousands of copies, are distributed randomly to the offspring. This conundrum led to the concept of a mitochondrial bottleneck, whereby only a small number of mtDNA genomes are used as a template for replicating mtDNA in the next generation. The mechanism could rely on a simple reduction in the amount of mtDNA during early oogenesis,[26] or on selective replication of only a small subset of mtDNA molecules within a developing oocyte, or on a combination of these two mechanisms (Figure 11.2).[27,28]

Functionally, the mtDNA bottleneck may act to allow selection against deleterious mutations. Any new mutation in mtDNA will originally occur in a single mtDNA genome. If there were thousands of mtDNA genomes in each cell acting as templates for replication, it would most likely take many rounds of mtDNA replication and cell division for such a mutation to represent a substantial proportion of mtDNA in the cell or organism. In the absence of selection though, many such mutations could accumulate in small amounts, and Muller's ratchet would eventually impede mitochondrial function.[3] A germline bottleneck would result in rapid genetic drift. In most cases, this would lead to the loss of any mutations that were present in a small proportion of germ cell mtDNA. Occasionally though, the bottleneck will amplify a mutant genome to become the predominant species of mtDNA in the germ cell. Such a mechanism will expose the new mutation to the forces of natural selection operating at the level of the developing oocyte, embryo, or organism. In evolutionary terms, a germline bottleneck increases the efficacy of selection against deleterious mutations by increasing the variance in fitness among progeny.[29]

Factors other than the bottleneck, including selection against certain mutations, could operate during oogenesis. Neutral polymorphisms in mice and humans appear to be transmitted randomly between generations.[25,26] Some pathogenic mtDNA mutations appear to segregate faster than others and it has been suggested that there be selection in favor of the mutant allele.[30] However,

Box 11.1 Why is there maternal inheritance?

One of the arguments for the invention of sex is that mutations in a genome need not have deleterious consequences in the offspring, for the simple reason that the child's DNA is a mixture of two parental DNAs, and at least one allele from each parent will have a normally functioning gene. However, in haploid, asexually reproducing organisms, such as bacteria, a mutation in the parental cell is always transmitted to the two daughter cells, and, except for back mutation, is never eliminated. This, of course, is a recipe for disaster, because in such an organism mutations will accumulate relentlessly and irreversibly.

This phenomenon of maladaptation is known as 'Muller's ratchet':[1] in asexual haploids, if individuals with the *fewest* mutations (i.e. those in the best mutation class) do not reproduce, that loss of 'good' genes is irreversible, leaving those individuals in a poorer mutation class to predominate (i.e. the ratchet has turned). In the next generation, the next-best mutation class now becomes the best mutation class, and if they too do not reproduce (i.e. another turn of the ratchet), one can easily see how inexorably the population of poor-class individuals will ultimately predominate, presumably to the point where there are so many individuals with bad genes that the population becomes extinct.

Mitochondria are asexually reproducing organelles within a sexually reproducing host. Thus, Muller's rachet can also operate on mitochondria, when a population of mitochondria fails to pass on its 'best' mitochondria to a daughter cell.[2] In fact, there is *double* ratchet, one operating among the mitochondria in a single individual (e.g. the accumulation of deleted mtDNAs in a patient with Kearns–Sayre syndromely), and one operating among all the individuals in the population (e.g. the spread of the LHON mutation from a founder individual into a population).[2]

Given Muller's ratchet, we can now see why maternal inheritance (or more accurately uniparental inheritance, because some organisms, such as redwood trees, pass their mitochondria through the paternal line) evolved. If there were biparental inheritance of mitochondria, pathogenic mitochondrial mutations would eventually spread through the entire population through the combined actions of Muller's ratchet and simple genetic drift. Note that because of the threshold effect, the percent mutation (the level of heteroplasmy) in large numbers of individuals in the population could rise to extremely high levels (50–70% mutation) without having any pathological consequences. However, once sizeable numbers of individuals had ~70% mutated mtDNAs, one can easily see how the threshold could easily be crossed, giving rise to huge numbers of clinically affected individuals within a few generations, in effect wiping out the population.

Maternal inheritance, on the other hand, avoids extinction at the population level, but at the price of extinction within the maternal line. Put another way, founder mothers with, say, the MELAS mutation, will give rise to maternal pedigrees in which individuals die of MELAS, and as the mutation accumulates in the pedigree, at some point that lineage becomes extinct. However, because there is only maternal inheritance, the MELAS mutation has trouble spreading through the population, because all it takes to 'stop' the mutation is for a MELAS mother to have only boys, who can no longer pass on the mutation to their children. Moreover, MELAS girls with a high mutation load will have trouble reproducing simply due to the debilitating effects of the disease.

References

1. Muller HJ. The relation of recombination to mutational advance. *Mutat Res* 1964; **106**: 2–9.
2. Bergstrom CT, Pritchard J. Germline bottlenecks and the evolutionary maintenance of mitochondrial genomes. *Genetics* 1998; **149**: 2135–2146.

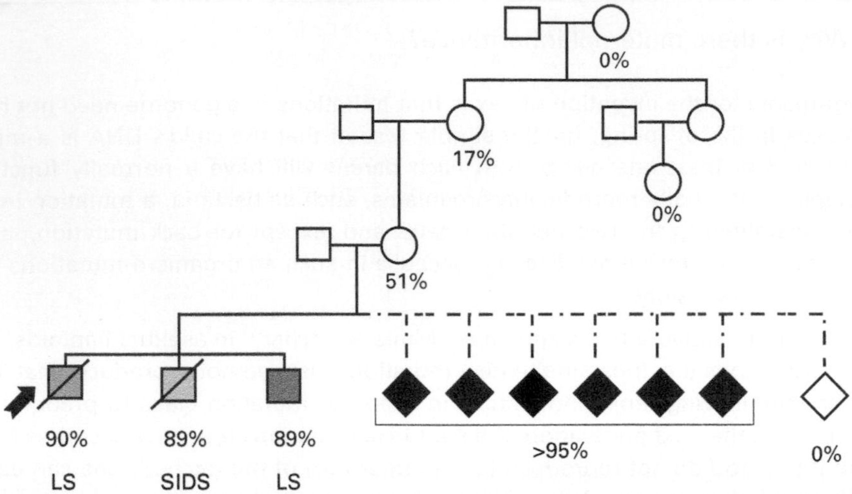

Figure 11.1 Heteroplasmic mutation loads in family members and oocytes of a family with the mitochondrial DNA T8993G mutation. The heteroplasmic mutant load of the mitochondrial DNA T8993G mutation is shown for the individuals tested and also for seven oocytes (depicted as diamonds) obtained by ovarian hyperstimulation in the family described by Blok et al.[23] LS, Leigh syndrome; SIDS, sudden infant death syndrome

analysis of human pedigrees with pathogenic mtDNA mutations is plagued by ascertainment bias, so this conclusion is controversial. The evidence of selection for or against mtDNA mutations during the reproductive cycle in humans will be discussed later.

Mitochondria and male fertility

Approximately one tenth of couples have fertility problems. This is due to male infertility in about 40% of cases, usually caused by a low number of sperm (oligozoospermia) or poorly motile sperm (asthenozoospermia).[31,32] Ejaculated sperm compete in a race to reach and fertilize the oocyte and pass on their nuclear genome. To be victorious, sperm must be able to oxidize sugars efficiently enough to provide the ATP that drives the flagellar motor. In oxidative phosphorylation (OXPHOS), electrons are transferred from substrates to oxygen, in the process generating a proton gradient – the mitochondrial membrane potential – that is used to power ATP synthesis.

So, what is the evidence that mitochondrial OXPHOS is an important determinant of sperm motility? Sperm motility declines rapidly with increasing concentration of OXPHOS inhibitors such as rotenone, antimycin A or potassium cyanide.[32] The chromosome X-encoded *PDHA1* gene, often implicated in mitochondrial energy generation disorders, has an autosomal homolog *PDHA2* in humans and mice showing testes-specific expression.[33] The likely evolutionary mechanism for this phenomenon is that the latter (haploid) stages of spermiogenesis require active transcription of essential bioenergetic genes and without an autosomal *PDHA* gene, motile chromosome Y-containing sperm either could not develop or could not compete with chromosome X-containing sperm.

Given these findings, mitochondrial dysfunction has long been considered a possible cause of male infertility[31] and numerous studies have

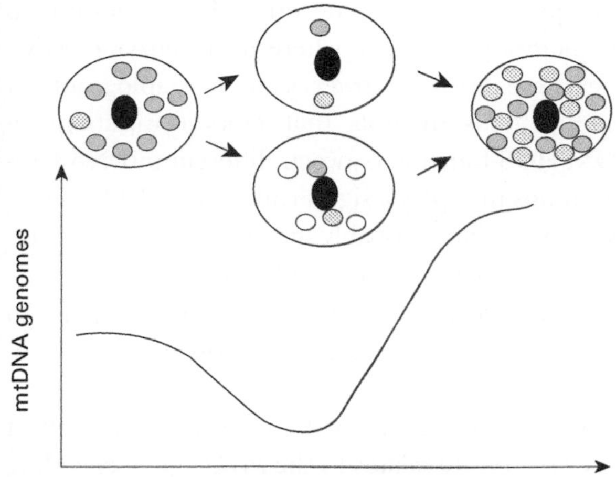

Figure 11.2 Diagrammatic representation of the mitochondrial DNA 'bottleneck', which occurs during the development of primordial germ cells into primary oocytes. The graph depicts an initial decline and subsequent expansion in the number of mtDNA genomes per cell and the schematic shows two possible mechanisms by which the bottleneck may occur. The left ellipse represents an early progenitor cell containing a mixture of mitochondria, of which 90% contain wild-type mtDNA (light gray) and 10% contain mutant mtDNA (speckled). The upper model suggests that rapid shifts in mtDNA heteroplasmic mutant load occur by a simple reduction to a very small number of mtDNA genomes, with any remaining genomes replicated to form the mtDNA pool of the developing oocyte. The lower model suggests that only a subset of the mtDNA genomes act as a template for mtDNA replication, while other mtDNA genomes (depicted in white) do not replicate and are lost by dilution during the subsequent expansion of mtDNA numbers

compared a range of mitochondrial features in sperm from fertile and infertile men as well as in motile sperm and in sperm with poor motility (Table 11.1). Sperm with poor motility have reportedly had decreased OXPHOS enzyme activities,[34,35] decreased mitochondrial membrane potential,[36–38] and an increased proportion of deleted mtDNA genomes.[39–41] While the first two findings seem consistent, the significance of the latter is unclear and there is disagreement about whether poorly motile sperm have a decreased amount of mtDNA[42] or an increased amount of mtDNA.[43] Recently, Marchetti and colleagues studied sperm from infertile patients enrolled in an in vitro fertilization (IVF) program and showed a correlation between the proportion of sperm with high mitochondrial membrane potential and high fertilization rates after IVF.[38] In all these studies that link mitochondrial abnormalities with abnormal sperm, it is unclear if the mitochondrial changes are a direct cause of sperm dysfunction or represent a mere association or a secondary response. There have been two reports of abnormal sperm motility in men with mitochondrial disorders[44,45] but again these could be

Table 11.1 Mitochondrial changes reported to be associated with decreased sperm motility

Mitochondrial parameter	Reference
Incubation with respiratory chain enzyme inhibitors	32
Decreased respiratory chain enzyme activities	34, 35
Decreased mitochondrial membrane potential	36–38
Increased proportion of deleted mtDNA	39–41
*Decreased amount of mtDNA	42
Increased mutant load of mtDNA A3243G mutation	47
mtDNA haplogroup T	32
**POLG* gene: lack of CAG_{10} allele	46

*Studies in which subsequent reports describe apparently conflicting data, as described in the text.

coincidental rather than causal. More recently, however, several studies have provided direct evidence that mtDNA 'fitness' and variants in a nuclear gene required for mtDNA replication can be primary genetic determinants of sperm dysmotility.[32,46,47]

Spiropoulos and colleagues studied sperm from a patient with a common pathogenic mtDNA mutation, the A3243G variant in the $tRNA^{Leu(UUR)}$ gene.[47] Like many other mtDNA mutations, the A3243G mutation is typically heteroplasmic and disease severity is largely determined by the proportion of mutant to wild-type mtDNA.[48] The heteroplasmic mutant load can vary between and within patient tissues and analysis of individual sperm showed that high levels of mutant mtDNA strongly correlated with low sperm motility.[47] This implies that the mtDNA mutation is directly causative of sperm dysmotility.

Pathogenic mutations in mtDNA are estimated to be present in at least 1 in 8000 individuals,[49] and while this may be a substantial underestimate, they appear to be too rare to be a common cause of male infertility. However, a study by Ruiz-Pesini and colleagues suggests that common mtDNA variants may also affect sperm motility. Individuals can be classified into different mtDNA haplogroups based on mtDNA sequence variants that arose and were fixed as populations dispersed and expanded out of Africa and into other continents. Ruiz-Pesini and colleagues assessed sperm features, mtDNA haplogroups, and OXPHOS enzyme activities in sperm from 545 men with fertility problems (Box 12.1).[32] Most of the mtDNA haplogroups showed no obvious difference in their prevalence in asthenozoospermic individuals versus non-asthenozoospermic individuals. However, the common mtDNA haplogroup H (present in 50% of their sample population) was significantly over-represented in non-asthenozoospermic individuals while haplogroup T (present in 6% of their sample population) was significantly over-represented in asthenozoospermic individuals. OXPHOS enzyme activities tended to be highest in sperm from haplogroup H and lowest in haplogroup T sperm, where mean enzyme activities were 20–30% lower than in haplogroup H sperm. This suggests that modest variations in OXPHOS function between different mtDNA haplogroups may play a significant role in determining sperm motility, probably in conjunction with other genetic and environmental factors.

In addition to mtDNA variants affecting sperm motility, it is possible that polymorphisms in nuclear OXPHOS genes could also play a role. To date, the only evidence that nuclear genes affect sperm motility relates to the *POLG* gene encoding the catalytic subunit of polymerase γ, responsible for replication of mtDNA. The *POLG* gene contains a CAG microsatellite repeat encoding a polyglutamine tract that is usually ten codons long. The CAG_{10} allele is found in different ethnic groups at an allele frequency of nearly 90% and is absent in only about 1% of individuals.[46] Analysis of *POLG* genotypes in different populations identified an association between absence of the common CAG_{10} allele and male infertility typified by a range of defects in sperm motility and morphology but not in sperm concentration.[46] A subsequent independent study of 1300 men confirmed the association between lack of the CAG_{10} allele and male infertility.[50] Surprisingly though, in this study lack of the CAG_{10} allele was not correlated with abnormal sperm motility or morphology, so the mechanism whereby the CAG_{10} allele compromises male fertility is still unclear. Another recent study failed to find any difference between the *POLG* genotypes of 195 infertile men and 190 normozoospermic controls.[51] Sperm count, motility, and morphology were comparable in carriers of the different genotypes, so the role of *POLG* variants in affecting male fertility remains uncertain.

Mitochondria and female fertility

The data described above support an important role for mitochondrial function in affecting male

Table 11.2 Evidence for and against mitochondria being key determinants of oocyte development, viability or functional competence

	References
Data supporting a major role for mitochondrial function	
IVF embryos less likely to have mtDNA deletions than oocytes	52
Oocyte mtDNA copy number lower in some infertile women	6, 53
Oocytes with higher ATP content have greater IVF developmental potential	54
Evolutionary role for atresia may be to select against oocytes with dysfunctional mitochondria	57
Data supporting a minor role for mitochondrial function	
Oocytes carrying pathogenic mtDNA mutations appear to develop normally	23, 24, 58
Children of mtDNA mutation carriers are equally likely to have an increase or decrease in mutation load	27
de novo mtDNA mutations are a common cause of mitochondrial disease	63–65

fertility. Given the large numbers of mitochondria in oocytes and the evolutionary importance of preventing accumulation of mutant mtDNA in the female germline, one may expect that mtDNA and OXPHOS function would play a critical role in oocyte development, viability, or functional competence. A range of data have been interpreted to support this view (Table 11.2).

- Approximately 50% of human oocytes contain deleted mtDNA genomes. Deletions represent a very small proportion of total oocyte mtDNA (<0.1%) and do not seem to change in amount with increasing age.[4,52] Analysis of IVF embryos found that a smaller proportion (~30%) contained deleted mtDNA, suggesting that oocytes lacking mtDNA deletions had greater developmental potential.[52]
- mtDNA content of individual oocytes can vary substantially between individuals and between oocytes from a single individual.[4,53] The average oocyte mtDNA copy number has been reported to be lower in women with idiopathic fertilization failure compared to women with normal fertilization or those with fertilization failure due to a sperm defect.[53] Similarly, oocyte mtDNA copy number was lower in women with ovarian insufficiency than in women with normal ovarian profiles or ovarian dystrophy.[6] Only the former group were characterized by poor quality of both oocytes and embryos.
- Van Blerkom and colleagues studied ATP content of mature human oocytes and developmental potential after uterine transfer of sibling embryos in 20 non-male factor IVF patients. They found that meiotic maturation occurs over a wide range of ATP contents, but that cohorts of oocytes with higher ATP contents showed a higher potential for continued embryogenesis and implantation.[54]
- Female germ cells are produced during fetal organogenesis: in humans, oocyte numbers peak at about 6×10^6 at 20 weeks of gestation, falling to about 2×10^6 at birth, 3×10^5 at puberty, 2.5×10^4 at 37 years and 1×10^3 at menopause.[55,56] This apparent wastage of germ cells, termed atresia, begs the question of whether it is an evolutionary mechanism of

quality control to ensure that only the best oocytes are ovulated. Krakauer and Mira[57] found a correlation between the size of the mtDNA bottleneck in various species and both the number of offspring and the proportion of ovarian follicles that undergo atresia. This led them to suggest that atresia was a developmental solution to remove oocytes containing mutant mtDNA genomes.

The observations above are consistent with the concept that mitochondrial function is a critical determinant of oocyte potential. However, as with much of the data on OXPHOS and sperm, many of these observations could be associations rather than causal links. An obvious way to test whether OXPHOS dysfunction is a critical determinant of oocyte potential is to consider data obtained from studies of women carrying heteroplasmic pathogenic mtDNA mutations. One might expect that primordial germ cells with high mtDNA mutant loads would be less likely to develop into primary oocytes than those with low mutant loads.

Three studies have reported levels of mutant mtDNA in human primary oocytes. Blok and colleagues studied seven oocytes from an asymptomatic woman carrying the mtDNA T8993G mutation,[23] who had had three children with Leigh syndrome or related mitochondrial disorders. Oocytes were obtained by ovarian hyperstimulation and oocyte retrieval. The woman had a mutant load in blood of 50%, and one of her oocytes contained undetectable mutant mtDNA while the other six had >95% mutation, in keeping with the mutant loads found in her three children (Figure 11.1). Marchington and colleagues studied 15 oocytes dissected from frozen ovary of a woman with Kearns–Sayre syndrome caused by mtDNA rearrangements.[58] The woman's mutant load was 22% in ovary, with individual oocytes ranging from 0% to 50% with a median level of 19%. Brown and colleagues studied 82 oocytes dissected from frozen ovary of an asymptomatic woman carrying the mtDNA A3243G mutation.[24] Mutant load in oocytes ranged from 0% to 45%, with a median level of 8% that was not significantly different from the mutant load of 18% in her skeletal muscle. It is apparent from these studies that atresia has not resulted in obvious loss of oocytes containing high mutant loads from the pool of primary oocytes. It is unclear if the mutant loads in the latter two studies were sufficiently high to cause biochemical dysfunction. However, the high mutant load of the T8993G mutation in six primary oocytes[23] is well above the threshold of ~70% where this mutation causes biochemical dysfunction and clinical disease.[59–62] If atresia does not result in preferential loss of oocytes with high mutant loads of the T8993G mutation, it seems very unlikely that it would act efficiently against oocytes with very small amounts of deleted mtDNA.

Given the small number of opportunities to study pathogenic mtDNA mutations in oocytes, it is also worth considering data on transmission of pathogenic mutations from heteroplasmic women to their children. If atresia led to preferential loss of oocytes with mutant mtDNA, or indeed if embryogenesis was highly dependent on mitochondrial function, one would predict that oocytes with lower mtDNA mutant loads were more likely to result in live-born children than oocytes with higher mtDNA mutant loads. The average mutant load in children of such women would therefore be expected to be lower than the mutant load found in the woman's somatic tissues. However, analysis of large numbers of maternal/child transmissions does not support this concept. Chinnery and colleagues studied all published reports on mother-to-child transmissions of six of the most common mtDNA point mutations.[27] Although it is difficult to completely exclude ascertainment biases in such reports, it was clear from the 338 cases documented that there was no strong evidence of selection for or against these mutations.

It is also worth noting that many patients with mtDNA point mutations appear to have de novo mutations that have amplified up to near-homoplasmy in a single generation. In perhaps a quarter of children with mitochondrial encephalopathies caused by mutations in mtDNA genes encoding subunits of complex V[63] and complex I[64,65] there is no detectable mutation nor symptoms in the mother or siblings. The most likely explanation is that such cases result from mtDNA mutations that slip through the mtDNA bottleneck and are amplified up to high levels in a very small proportion of the mother's oocytes. These oocytes clearly are not culled by atresia, have been successfully fertilized, undergone embryogenesis, and survived to term.

The data on transmission of pathogenic mtDNA point mutations argue that oocyte development and embryogenesis are actually remarkably tolerant of mitochondrial dysfunction. OXPHOS requirements in many fetal tissues appear to be much lower than in adult tissues since the activities of OXPHOS and related enzymes remain low until late gestation or after birth in brain,[66] muscle,[67] liver,[68,69] and kidney.[70] In the relatively anaerobic intrauterine environment,[56] fetal tissues can meet much of their energy demands through glycolysis,[71] and selective pressure on respiratory chain function in fetal tissues is likely to be weak. However, this does not mean that mitochondrial function is unimportant to the developing embryo and complete loss of mitochondrial OXPHOS function is not compatible with embryonic survival. Knockout mice with a profound deficiency of mtDNA (lacking a critical mtDNA transcription factor, Tfam),[72] cytochrome *c*[73] or the complex II SDHD subunit[74] give embryonic lethal phenotypes with fetal loss by mid-gestation. Despite the demonstration that rearranged mtDNA genomes can be transmitted to primary oocytes,[58] it is well recognized that mtDNA deletions are only very rarely transmitted from mother to child. A multicenter study recently reported on 40 women with an mtDNA rearrangement, who had had a total of 73 offspring.[75] Only three of these had clinical evidence of mitochondrial disease. The reason for this low recurrence is not clear, and may relate to uncertainty about when the original rearrangement occurred, that is during embryogenesis of the proband, their mother or their maternal grandmother.[75] Alternatively, it could be because a substantial mutant load of an mtDNA deletion causes too severe an OXPHOS defect to be compatible with development of a viable fetus.

The above studies on knockout mice show that extremely severe OXPHOS defects can cause spontaneous abortions in mice. This is also likely to be the case in humans for the most severe defects, so that these may never come to medical attention. It is not certain whether mutations known to cause disease in live-born children can also cause an increased rate of spontaneous abortions. This has been suggested for the mtDNA A3243G mutation[76] and for mutations in the *SCO2* gene causing complex IV deficiency.[77,78] However, this remains speculative because most of the miscarriages were not genotyped, so it is unclear if the association is causative or coincidental. There is no evidence for an excess of fetal deaths in large series of pedigrees with other mtDNA mutations (for example, see reference 63).

Assisted reproduction

Two assisted reproduction techniques have raised concerns about introduction of mtDNA at fertilization or into fertilized oocytes. These are intracytoplasmic sperm injection (ICSI) and ooplasmic transfer. ICSI is widely used for infertile couples, particularly for men with sperm immotility or low or absent sperm counts. It involves the injection of a single whole sperm, including the head, the midpiece containing mitochondria and tail into an oocyte. Two concerns have been raised,[79] firstly that this may bypass the mechanism by which paternal mtDNA is removed from the embryo, and secondly that it removes much of the selection against genes for male infertility. Sperm mtDNA, particularly from infertile men, may contain significant amounts of mutant mtDNA[39–41,80,81] and this could theoretically result in transmission of mutant sperm mtDNA that may ultimately lead to a child with mitochondrial disease. The estimates of mtDNA copy number in sperm and oocytes suggest that following ICSI, sperm could contribute ~0.05% of the total mtDNA content of the fertilized oocyte. A number of studies have investigated whether paternal mtDNA could be detected in children born following ICSI. No paternal mtDNA could be detected with a sensitivity ranging from 0.01% to 2% in blood of five to 27 newborns.[82] Using the more sensitive technique of solid phase mini-sequencing, no paternal mtDNA could be detected at a sensitivity of 0.001% in placenta, umbilical cord, blood, and buccal swabs of 11 children born following ICSI.[79] Thus, there is no evidence to suggest that paternal mtDNA is more likely to be transmitted to the developing fetus following ICSI than by normal fertilization. O'Connell and colleagues found that testicular sperm had fewer mtDNA deletions than epididymal sperm and recommended that testicular sperm should be preferred for ICSI in clinical treatment.[81] This would guard against the possibility that a small proportion of deleted mtDNA genomes from sperm could escape ubiquitin-dependent degradation in the fertilized oocyte and have a replicative advantage.

Ooplasmic transfer is a technique first described by Cohen and colleagues[83] in an attempt to improve the success rate of IVF in some infertile couples. The protocol aimed to rejuvenate the 'developmentally compromised oocytes' of older women with recurrent implantation failure by injecting them with a small proportion (5–15%) of cytoplasm from donor oocytes of young fertile women.[84] They subsequently reported the not-surprising result that some embryos, amniocytes, placenta, and fetal cord blood contained a mixture of donor and recipient mtDNA[85,86] and that mtDNA heteroplasmy could be detected in the blood of these children (Box 11.2).[84] This attracted wide media attention focused on the fact that these children have mitochondrial genetic material from two mothers. Apart from the ethical and legal questions raised by this issue, there has been ongoing debate about the efficacy and safety of the procedure.

Cohen and colleagues reported an apparently impressive rate of pregnancy in 40% of ooplasmic transfer procedures,[84] but the uncontrolled nature of the experiments meant that no firm conclusion could be drawn on whether the procedure itself was successful. If it does improve pregnancy rates, it is unclear whether this is due to the donor mitochondria, since early embryological development does not appear to be highly dependent on mitochondrial function.[87] If ooplasmic transfer is efficacious, the success may be due to one or more cytoplasmic RNAs, proteins, or small molecules introduced along with the mitochondria. It is possible that adding a small proportion of donor mitochondria may provide a 'kick start' to mitochondrial function. Developmentally arrested mouse two-cell embryos can re-initiate cleavage following injection of cytoplasm from a cycling two-cell embryo. Resumption of cleavage was accompanied by mitochondrial redistribution in the developing embryo[88] and perhaps the mitochondrial redistribution process is abnormal in oocytes from older women,[89] but such speculation awaits further data.

Two main concerns about safety of ooplasmic transfer have been raised. These are the potential for epigenetic modifications and the possibility that a heteroplasmic mixture of mtDNA from two maternal ancestors could result in some form of genomic incompatibility or instability. These concerns are highlighted by the report of two chromosomal abnormalities in clinical pregnancies following ooplasmic transfer.[90] Both involved 45,XO karyotypes, one ending in a spontaneous miscarriage in the first trimester and one detected

Box 11.2 Is Dolly a clone?

The cloning of Dolly the sheep in 1997 by Ian Wilmut and his colleagues in Scotland[1] raised many interesting questions, both technical and ethical. For mitochondriacs, there was one particular question of interest. In Wilmut's nuclear transfer method (Figure B11.2.1), a donor somatic cell was fused by electroporation with a recipient enucleated oocyte. During this whole-cell electrofusion, not only nucleus, but also the donor cytoplasm (including, of course, mitochondria), was transferred into the oocyte. For this reason, cloned animals created by electrofusion should contain mtDNAs from both the donor and recipient cytoplasms (i.e. they should be heteroplasmic).

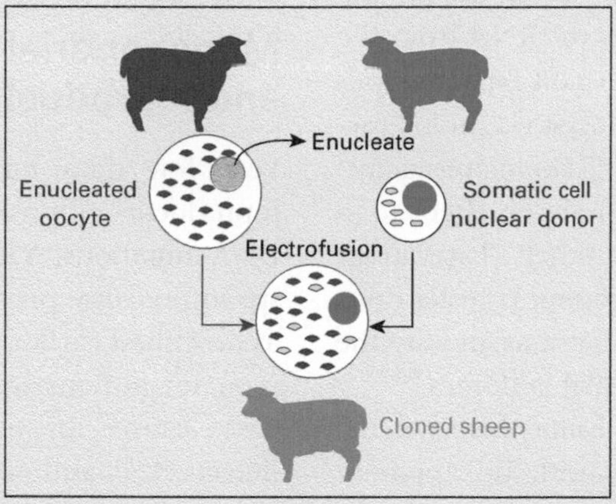

Figure B.11.2.1 How to clone a sheep. Drawing courtesy of Matthew Evans

Surprisingly, when the mtDNA of Dolly and nine other sheep derived by nuclear transfer was analyzed, the mtDNA was found to be derived exclusively from the recipient enucleated oocytes, with no detectable contribution from the somatic donor cells. Thus, Dolly and her siblings were, in fact, genetic chimeras, containing somatic cell-derived nuclear DNA but exclusively oocyte-derived mtDNA. In other words, Dolly was homoplasmic for the recipient cell mtDNA.

It turns out that the situation in sheep is apparently different than in other mammals, including humans. In cows cloned by electrofusion, for example, the cytoplasm was not exclusively derived from the donor cell, but rather was a mixture of donor somatic cell and recipient oocyte mtDNAs. In other words, the cows were heteroplasmic.

Humans, of course, have not been cloned – yet. Nevertheless, a reasonable guess as to whether the mtDNA from cloned humans would be homoplasmic or heteroplasmic can be deduced from the analysis of babies in which 'cytoplasmic transfer' was performed for therapeutic reasons. In this procedure, a small amount of cytoplasm (containing mitochondria) was transferred from a donor oocyte to a fertilized recipent oocyte. The resulting children were found to be heteroplasmic for both mtDNAs.[2] This implies that if humans were cloned, they, too, would likely be heteroplasmic.

References

1. Wilmut I, Schnieke AE, McWhir J et al. Viable offspring derived from fetal and adult mammalian cells. *Nature* 1997; **385**: 810–813.
2. Barritt JA, Brenner CA, Malter HE, Cohen J. Mitochondria in human offspring derived from ooplasmic transplantation. *Hum Reprod* 2001; **16**: 513–516.

by ultrasonography at 15 weeks and electively terminated. One of the 16 children born at that time following ooplasmic transfer developed pervasive developmental disorder, an autism-related disorder which occurs in up to one in 250 children.[90] These problems are not necessarily caused by the procedure but flag the need for serious consideration of safety issues.

The possibility of 'foreign' cytoplasm causing epigenetic effects was first suggested by the finding that transfer of ooplasm or oocyte RNA from the mouse mutant strain DDK to non-DDK oocytes prevents formation of the blastocyst via an interaction with the paternal genome.[91] The maternal factor in this process is specifically related to a mutation at the *Om* locus but other observations suggest wider potential for ooplasmic transfer causing epigenetic modifications that may modify the differential imprinting of parental genomes.[92,93]

Heteroplasmy for benign polymorphisms occurs in humans and other species with no apparent health concerns.[17–19] However, in these cases the two genomes differ at only a single nucleotide position, whereas mtDNA genomes derived from two unrelated individuals are likely to have multiple differences. Mouse models of heteroplasmy have been generated by several groups using ooplasmic transfer[26,27,94] or nuclear transfer.[95] Encouragingly, there have been no reports of ill health in these mice over ten or more generations. The proportions of the two mtDNA species are similar in all mouse tissues at birth, but, surprisingly, they then diverge, so that one of the mtDNA genomes may eventually replace the other.[96] The two mouse mtDNA genomes differ at 106 nucleotide positions, apparently resulting in postnatal selection for or against one mtDNA species in different tissues. This finding suggests that mtDNA genomes of different origin may function less well in some nuclear backgrounds. It is unclear if this has any health implications in humans, and it is disappointing that Cohen and colleagues have not published any analyses using methods with appropriate sensitivity to monitor heteroplasmy in children born after ooplasmic transfer, as discussed elsewhere.[87] More detailed studies of these children and further studies on animal models are needed before ooplasmic transfer can be recommended for widespread clinical use.[97,98] The US Food and Drug Administration stopped approvals for clinical applications of ooplasmic transfer in 2002 pending submission of properly constituted protocols.[56]

Mitochondrial disease and reproduction

Very few data have been published on the reproductive fitness of patients with mitochondrial DNA mutations. A few case reports have described sperm motility problems in some male patients, as described earlier. Hypogonadism is not uncommon in patients with severe mitochondrial diseases caused by mtDNA or nuclear OXPHOS defects,[99–101] and is discussed in more detail in Chapter 9. There are no data to suggest that healthy carriers of mtDNA mutations or nuclear OXPHOS defects are at increased risk of infertility. Large numbers of pedigrees have been reported in which women with low to moderate heteroplasmic mutant loads for many pathogenic mtDNA point mutations have had multiple children without apparent fertility problems. Moilanen and colleagues studied 32 female carriers of the mtDNA A3243G mutation and found they reproduced at the same rate as women in the general population.[102]

There is a major role for reproductive medicine in assisting the thousands of couples around the world who are at increased risk of having a child with a mitochondrial OXPHOS disorder due to a family history of mitochondrial disease. When considering reproductive options, it is useful to think of the proband as being in one of three separate groups: (i) having a known pathogenic mutation in a nuclear-encoded gene; (ii) having an OXPHOS enzyme defect in whom no pathogenic mutation has been identified; (iii) having a known pathogenic mutation in a mtDNA-encoded gene. The first group is no different to couples at risk for any other autosomal or X-linked genetic condition and can be offered prenatal diagnosis by direct mutation analysis of a chorionic villus sample (CVS) or amniocyte sample, IVF using donor gametes, or preimplantation genetic diagnosis (PGD) as appropriate. For couples in the second group, the genetic basis and recurrence risk are usually uncertain, except for specific examples where the enzyme defect, clinical presentation or family history imply a mode of inheritance. Reproductive options for this group vary depending on the details of their diagnosis but may include donor gametes or prenatal diagnosis by enzyme analysis of CVS or amniocytes, as discussed in more detail elsewhere.[28]

For couples at risk of transmitting a pathogenic mtDNA mutation, perhaps the most obvious and reliable method to avoid recurrence of mtDNA disease is IVF using donor oocytes and the partner's sperm (Figure 11.3). It would be highly inadvisable to use a maternal relative as the oocyte donor because she may carry oocytes with a high mutant load even though her blood may lack detectable mutant mtDNA. The two major limitations of this approach are (i) availability of donor oocytes, which restricts access to the procedure, and in some countries oocyte donation is illegal,[103] and (ii) personal or cultural views about the use of donor gametes or the desire for a child who is genetically related to both parents.

Until recently, prenatal diagnosis of mtDNA mutations was regarded as inadvisable. This was due to uncertainty about whether the mutant load of a heteroplasmic mtDNA mutation measured in CVS or amniocytes would be representative of other fetal tissues, whether it may change between analysis at 10–15 weeks' gestation and birth, and how to predict outcome based on a measured mutant load. More recently, this attitude has changed, particularly following an international workshop held in 1999.[104] Change has been driven by the long waiting lists for donor egg IVF and our improved understanding of mtDNA transmission derived from studies on heteroplasmic mouse models[26] and by detailed analyses of mtDNA transmission in families.[27,60]

There is now wide agreement that prenatal diagnosis by CVS analysis can be offered to women at low to moderate risk of transmitting the mtDNA T8993G or T8993C mutations,[104] and several such analyses have been reported.[105–109] These mutations are the easiest to consider because they show a particularly strong genotype/phenotype correlation, allowing the risk of an affected outcome to be predicted with reasonable accuracy based on the measured mutant load.[60] Significant limitations remain with this approach, particularly in predicting clinical outcome for a measured mutant load close to the pathogenic threshold of ~70% mutant mtDNA.[28] The recent description of recurrence risks for transmitting a mtDNA deletion[75] allows more informed consideration of prenatal diagnosis, and two such attempts have been described.[28,103]

Predicting outcome for other mtDNA point mutations is more problematic, as exemplified by the finding of an intermediate mutant load for a pregnancy at risk for the A3243G mutation.[110] Nonetheless, each case must be considered separately based on the mutation and the parents' attitudes[28] and it is likely that prenatal diagnosis will be used increasingly for mtDNA mutations, particularly in women who are at relatively low risk of having an affected child.

Increasing evidence suggests that PGD is also a logical option for women at risk of transmitting a mtDNA mutation.[28] PGD allows the preferential selection of unaffected embryos for transfer in order to establish a pregnancy (Figure 11.3), thus avoiding the need to terminate an already-established pregnancy. Although this selection could potentially be done by sampling either polar bodies or blastomeres, the latter approach is likely to be more reliable.[111] The high copy

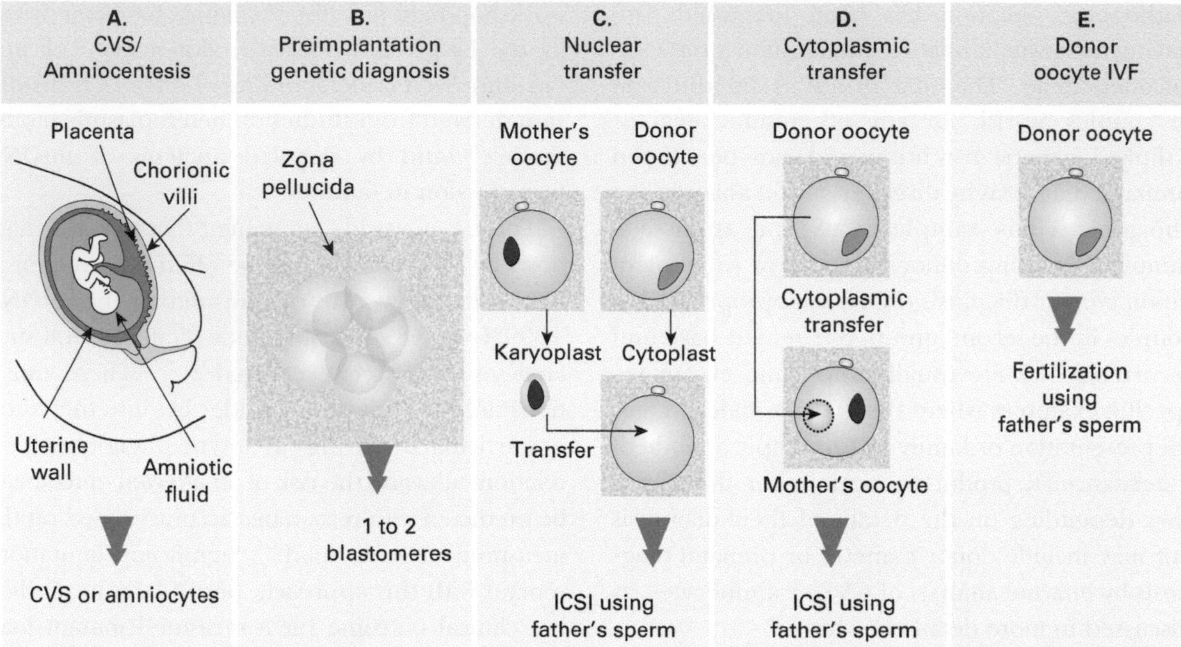

Genetic contribution of 'social' parents					
Nuclear genes:	M & F	M & F	M & F	M & F	Donor & F
mtDNA genes:	M	M	Donor (+ M?)	M (+ up to 1/3 Donor)	Donor

Figure 11.3 Current and future reproductive options for preventing transmission of mtDNA mutations. (**A**) Chorionic villus sampling (CVS) (at 10–13 weeks' gestation) or amniocentesis (at 15–18 weeks' gestation) can be performed to provide fetal cells for quantification of mutant mtDNA. If sufficient information is available for the particular mutation, then it may be possible to predict the risk of an affected outcome to enable the parents to decide whether to continue or terminate the pregnancy. (**B**) Preimplantation genetic diagnosis is most commonly performed by generating a number of eight-cell embryos using in vitro fertilization (IVF) of parental gametes, and then removing one or preferably two blastomeres for analysis. The mtDNA mutant load can be quantified, and only embryos with undetectable or very low amounts of mutant mtDNA would be regarded as suitable for implantation. (**C**) Nuclear transfer would involve the removal of the nucleus (and a thin rim of cytoplasm) from a mother's oocyte, and transfer of this nucleus to an enucleated donor oocyte, followed by fertilization using intracytoplasmic sperm injection (ICSI) and implantation; this procedure merits further research but currently could not be recommended for clinical use and is illegal in most countries. (**D**) Cytoplasmic transfer would involve the transfer of a proportion (perhaps a third) of the cytoplasm (containing mitochondria) from a donor oocyte into the cytoplasm of the mother's oocyte, followed by fertilization and implantation. For transfer of large cytoplasmic volumes, it may be preferable to first remove an equivalent volume of cytoplasm from the recipient mother's oocyte. As with nuclear transfer, this procedure merits further research but currently could not be recommended for clinical use. (**E**) Donor oocyte IVF uses a donor oocyte instead of the mother's oocyte, to eliminate the possibility of transmitting a familial mtDNA mutation. M, mother; F, father. Reproduced with permission from Thorburn and Dahl[28]

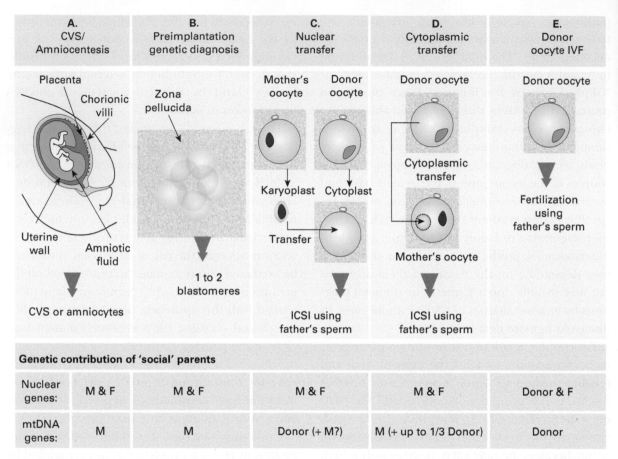

number of mtDNA (>10^4 copies per cell in an eight-cell embryo) means that mtDNA mutation analysis should be less prone to artefacts such as amplification failure and allele dropout that can complicate mutation analysis of nuclear gene defects in single cells. Like prenatal diagnosis, PGD for mtDNA mutations does have limitations. In some women, a large proportion of oocytes may have a substantial mutant load, in which case even multiple cycles of ovarian stimulation may not result in an unaffected embryo. An attractive feature of PGD for mtDNA mutations is that it may provide valuable information even if a successful unaffected pregnancy is not achieved. If most of the embryos tested have a substantial mtDNA mutant load, then oocyte donation is likely to be the only current option for ensuring an unaffected embryo. In contrast, if most of the embryos tested have undetectable mutant mtDNA, then the parents may opt for prenatal diagnosis in subsequent unassisted (natural) pregnancies. The first report of PGD for a mtDNA mutation was published recently.[112]

Each reproductive option for preventing transmission of mtDNA mutations has its own strengths and weaknesses, which are discussed in more detail elsewhere.[28] Each approach will suit some families but not others depending on the attitudes of the couple, influenced by cultural or religious traditions, to a number of issues. These include the use of donor gametes, pregnancy termination, risk of miscarriage, required degree of certainty, ability to tolerate the timeframe required for a result to be generated, the inconvenience and frequent need for multiple rounds of ovarian hyperstimulation in some IVF strategies, cost, and availability. In practice, many couples may try more than one reproductive option, depending on their experience with their first choice.

Acknowledgments

I thank numerous colleagues for their helpful discussions on this topic, including Drs H Dahl, S White, J Liebelt, A Boneh, L Wilton, R Jansen, S DiMauro, J Poulton, D Turnbull, P Chinnery, N Howell and E Shoubridge. This work was supported by grants from the National Health and Medical Research Council (NHMRC; Australia) and the Muscular Dystrophy Association; USA. David Thorburn is an NHMRC Senior Research Fellow.

References

1. Hoekstra RF. Evolutionary origin and consequences of uniparental mitochondrial inheritance. *Hum Reprod* 2000; **15**(Suppl 2): 102–11.
2. Muller HJ. The relation of recombination to mutational advance. *Mutat Res* 1964; **1**: 2–9.
3. Felsenstein J. The evolutionary advantage of recombination. *Genetics* 1974; **78**: 737–756.
4. Chen X, Prosser R, Simonetti S et al. Rearranged mitochondrial genomes are present in human oocytes. *Am J Hum Genet* 1995; **57**: 239–247.
5. Steuerwald N, Barritt JA, Adler R et al. Quantification of mtDNA in single oocytes, polar bodies and subcellular components by real-time rapid cycle fluorescence monitored PCR. *Zygote* 2000; **8**: 209–215.
6. May-Panloup P, Chretien MF, Jacques C et al. Low oocyte mitochondrial DNA content in ovarian insufficiency. *Hum Reprod* 2005; **20**: 593–597.
7. Jansen RP. Germline passage of mitochondria: quantitative considerations and possible embryological sequelae. *Hum Reprod* 2000; **15**(Suppl 2): 112–128.
8. Diez-Sanchez C, Ruiz-Pesini E, Lapena AC et al. Mitochondrial DNA content of human spermatozoa. *Biol Reprod* 2003; **68**: 180–185.
9. Gyllensten U, Wharton D, Josefsson A et al. Paternal inheritance of mitochondrial DNA in mice. *Nature* 1991; **352**: 255–257.
10. Ankel-Simons F, Cummins JM. Misconceptions about mitochondria and mammalian fertilization: implications for theories on human evolution. *Proc Nat Acad Sci USA* 1996; **93**: 13859–13863.
11. Cummins JM, Wakayama T, Yanagimachi R. Fate of microinjected sperm components in the mouse oocyte and embryo. *Zygote* 1997; **5**: 301–308.
12. Sutovsky P, Moreno RD, Ramalho-Santos J et al. Ubiquitinated sperm mitochondria, selective proteolysis, and the regulation of mitochondrial

inheritance in mammalian embryos. *Biol Reprod* 2000; **63**: 582–590.

13. Thompson WE, Ramalho-Santos J, Sutovsky P. Ubiquitination of prohibitin in mammalian sperm mitochondria: possible roles in the regulation of mitochondrial inheritance and sperm quality control. *Biol Reprod* 2003; **69**: 254–260.
14. Schwartz M, Vissing J. Paternal inheritance of mitochondrial DNA. *N Engl J Med* 2002; **347**: 576–580.
15. Filosto M, Mancuso M, Vives-Bauza C et al. Lack of paternal inheritance of muscle mitochondrial DNA in sporadic mitochondrial myopathies. *Ann Neurol* 2003; **54**: 524–526.
16. Taylor RW, McDonnell MT, Blakely EL et al. Genotypes from patients indicate no paternal mitochondrial DNA contribution. *Ann Neurol* 2003; **54**: 521–524.
17. Upholt WB, Dawid IB. Mapping of mitochondrial DNA of individual sheep and goats: rapid evolution in the D loop region. *Cell* 1977; **11**: 571–583.
18. Hauswirth WW, Laipis PJ. Mitochondrial DNA polymorphism in a maternal lineage of Holstein cows. *Proc Natl Acad Sci USA* 1982; **79**: 4686–4690.
19. Ashley MV, Laipis PJ, Hauswirth WW. Rapid segregation of heteroplasmic bovine mitochondria. *Nucleic Acids Res* 1989; **17**: 7325–7331.
20. Larsson NG, Tulinius MH, Holme E et al. Segregation and manifestations of the mtDNA tRNA(Lys) A→G(8344) mutation of Myoclonus Epilepsy and Ragged-Red Fibers (MERRF) syndrome. *Am J Hum Genet* 1992; **51**: 1201–1212.
21. Howell N, Xu M, Halvorson S et al. Heteroplasmic LHON family: Tissue distribution and transmission of the 11778 mutation. *Am J Hum Genet* 1994; **55**: 203–206.
22. Ghosh SS, Fahy E, Bodis-Wollner I et al. Longitudinal study of a heteroplasmic 3460 Leber hereditary optic neuropathy family by multiplexed primer-extension analysis and nucleotide sequencing. *Am J Hum Genet* 1996; **58**: 325–334.
23. Blok RB, Gook DA, Thorburn DR et al. Skewed segregation of the mtDNA nt8993 (T→G) mutation in human oocytes. *Am J Hum Genet* 1997; **60**: 1495–1501.
24. Brown DT, Samuels DC, Michael EM et al. Random genetic drift determines the level of mutant mtDNA in human primary oocytes. *Am J Hum Genet* 2001; **68**: 533–536.
25. Howell N, Halvorson S, Kubacka I et al. Mitochondrial gene segregation in mammals – Is the bottleneck always narrow? *Hum Genet* 1992; **90**: 117–120.
26. Jenuth JP, Peterson AC, Fu K et al. Random genetic drift in the female germline explains the rapid segregation of mammalian mitochondrial DNA. *Nat Genet* 1996; **14**: 146–151.
27. Chinnery PF, Thorburn DR, Samuels DC et al. The inheritance of mitochondrial DNA heteroplasmy: random drift, selection or both? *Trends Genet* 2000; **16**: 500–505.
28. Thorburn DR, Dahl HHM. Mitochondrial disorders: genetics, counseling, prenatal diagnosis and reproductive options. *Am J Med Genet (Semin Med Genet)* 2001; **106**: 102–114.
29. Bergstrom CT, Pritchard J. Germline bottlenecks and the evolutionary maintenance of mitochondrial genomes. *Genetics* 1998; **149**: 2135–2146.
30. Shoubridge EA. Mitochondrial DNA segregation in the developing embryo. *Hum Reprod* 2000; **15**(Suppl 2): 229–234.
31. Cummins JM, Jequier AM, Kan R. Molecular biology of human male infertility: links with aging, mitochondrial genetics, and oxidative stress? *Mol Reprod Dev* 1994; **37**: 345–362.
32. Ruiz-Pesini E, Lapena AC, Diez-Sanchez C et al. Human mtDNA haplogroups associated with high or reduced spermatozoa motility. *Am J Hum Genet* 2000; **67**: 682–696.
33. Brown RM, Dahl HH, Brown GK. Pyruvate dehydrogenase E1 alpha subunit genes in the mouse: mapping and comparison with human homologs. *Somat Cell Mol Genet* 1990; **16**: 487–492.
34. Ruiz-Pesini E, Diez C, Lapena AC et al. Correlation of sperm motility with mitochondrial enzymatic activities. *Clin Chem* 1998; **44**: 1616–1620.
35. Carra E, Sangiorgi D, Gattuccio F et al. Male infertility and mitochondrial DNA. *Biochem Biophys Res Commun* 2004; **322**: 333–339.
36. Kasai T, Ogawa K, Mizuno K et al. Relationship between sperm mitochondrial membrane potential, sperm motility, and fertility potential. *Asian J Androl* 2002; **4**: 97–103.
37. Wang X, Sharma RK, Gupta A et al. Alterations in mitochondria membrane potential and oxidative stress in infertile men: a prospective observational study. *Fertil Steril* 2003; **80**(Suppl 2): 844–850.

38. Marchetti C, Jouy N, Leroy-Martin B et al. Comparison of four fluorochromes for the detection of the inner mitochondrial membrane potential in human spermatozoa and their correlation with sperm motility. *Hum Reprod* 2004; **19**: 2267–2276.
39. Kao SH, Chao HT, Wei YH. Mitochondrial deoxyribonucleic acid 4977-bp deletion is associated with diminished fertility and motility of human sperm. *Biol Reprod* 1995; **52**: 729–736.
40. Kao SH, Chao HT, Wei YH. Multiple deletions of mitochondrial DNA are associated with the decline of motility and fertility of human spermatozoa. *Mol Hum Reprod* 1998; **4**: 657–666.
41. St John JC, Jokhi RP, Barratt CL. Men with oligoasthenoteratozoospermia harbour higher numbers of multiple mitochondrial DNA deletions in their spermatozoa, but individual deletions are not indicative of overall aetiology. *Mol Hum Reprod* 2001; **7**: 103–111.
42. Kao SH, Chao HT, Liu HW et al. Sperm mitochondrial DNA depletion in men with asthenospermia. *Fertil Steril* 2004; **82**: 66–73.
43. May-Panloup P, Chretien MF, Savagner F et al. Increased sperm mitochondrial DNA content in male infertility. *Hum Reprod* 2003; **18**: 550–556.
44. Folgero T, Bertheussen K, Lindal S et al. Mitochondrial disease and reduced sperm motility. *Hum Reprod* 1993; **8**: 1863–1868.
45. Lestienne P, Reynier P, Chretien MF et al. Oligoasthenospermia associated with multiple mitochondrial DNA rearrangements. *Mol Hum Reprod* 1997; **3**: 811–814.
46. Rovio AT, Marchington DR, Donat S et al. Mutations at the mitochondrial DNA polymerase (*POLG*) locus associated with male infertility. *Nat Genet* 2001; **29**: 261–262.
47. Spiropoulos J, Turnbull DM, Chinnery PF. Can mitochondrial DNA mutations cause sperm dysfunction? *Mol Hum Reprod* 2002; **8**: 719–721.
48. Chinnery PF, Howell N, Lightowlers RN et al. Molecular pathology of MELAS and MERRF. The relationship between mutation load and clinical phenotypes. *Brain* 1997; **120**: 1713–1721.
49. Chinnery PF, Johnson MA, Wardell TM et al. The epidemiology of pathogenic mitochondrial DNA mutations. *Ann Neurol* 2000; **48**: 188–193.
50. Jensen M, Leffers H, Petersen JH et al. Frequent polymorphism of the mitochondrial DNA polymerase gamma gene (POLG) in patients with normal spermiograms and unexplained subfertility. *Hum Reprod* 2004; **19**: 65–70.
51. Krausz C, Guarducci E, Becherini L et al. The clinical significance of the POLG gene polymorphism in male infertility. *J Clin Endocrinol Metab* 2004; **89**: 4292–4297.
52. Barritt JA, Brenner CA, Cohen J et al. Mitochondrial DNA rearrangements in human oocytes and embryos. *Mol Hum Reprod* 1999; **5**: 927–933.
53. Reynier P, May-Panloup P, Chretien MF et al. Mitochondrial DNA content affects the fertilizability of human oocytes. *Mol Hum Reprod* 2001; **7**: 425–429.
54. Van Blerkom J, Davis PW, Lee J. ATP content of human oocytes and developmental potential and outcome after in-vitro fertilization and embryo transfer. *Hum Reprod* 1995; **10**: 415–424.
55. Perez GI, Trbovich AM, Gosden RG et al. Mitochondria and the death of oocytes. *Nature* 2000; **403**: 500–501.
56. Jansen RP, Burton GJ. Mitochondrial dysfunction in reproduction. *Mitochondrion* 2004; **4**: 577–600.
57. Krakauer DC, Mira A. Mitochondria and germ-cell death. *Nature* 1999; **400**: 125–126.
58. Marchington DR, Macaulay V, Hartshorne GM et al. Evidence from human oocytes for a genetic bottleneck in an mtDNA disease. *Am J Hum Genet* 1998; **63**: 769–775.
59. Trounce I, Neill S, Wallace DC. Cytoplasmic transfer of the mtDNA nt 8993 T→G (*ATP6*) point mutation associated with Leigh syndrome into mtDNA-less cells demonstrates cosegregation with a decrease in state III respiration and ADP/O ratio. *Proc Natl Acad Sci USA* 1994; **91**: 8334–8338.
60. White SL, Collins VR, Wolfe R et al. Genetic counseling and prenatal diagnosis for the mitochondrial DNA mutations at nucleotide 8993. *Am J Hum Genet* 1999; **65**: 474–482.
61. Garcia JJ, Ogilvie I, Robinson BH et al. Structure, functioning, and assembly of the ATP synthase in cells from patients with the T8993G mitochondrial DNA mutation. Comparison with the enzyme in ρ^0 cells completely lacking mtDNA. *J Biol Chem* 2000; **275**: 11075–11081.
62. Mattiazzi M, Vijayvergiya C, Gajewski CD et al. The mtDNA T8993G (NARP) mutation results in an impairment of oxidative phosphorylation that can be improved by antioxidants. *Hum Mol Genet* 2004; **13**: 869–879.

63. White SL, Shanske S, McGill JJ et al. Mitochondrial DNA mutations at nucleotide 8993 show a lack of tissue- or age-related variation. *J Inherit Metab Dis* 1999; **22**: 899–914.
64. Lebon S, Chol M, Benit P et al. Recurrent de novo mitochondrial DNA mutations in respiratory chain deficiency. *J Med Genet* 2003; **40**: 896–899.
65. McFarland R, Kirby DM, Fowler KJ et al. de novo mutations in the mitochondrial *ND3* gene as a cause of infantile mitochondrial encephalopathy and complex I deficiency. *Ann Neurol* 2004; **55**: 58–64.
66. Takakubo F, Dahl HHM. Analysis of pyruvate dehydrogenase expression in embryonic mouse brain – localization and developmental regulation. *Brain Res Dev Brain Res* 1994; **77**: 63–76.
67. Sperl W, Sengers RC, Trijbels JM et al. Enzyme activities of the mitochondrial energy generating system in skeletal muscle tissue of preterm and fullterm neonates. *Ann Clin Biochem* 1992; **29**: 638–645.
68. Izquierdo JM, Luis AM, Cuezva JM. Postnatal mitochondrial differentiation in rat liver. Regulation by thyroid hormones of the β-subunit of the mitochondrial F_1-ATPase complex. *J Biol Chem* 1990; **265**: 9090–9097.
69. Valcarce C, Izquierdo JM, Chamorro M et al. Mammalian adaptation to extrauterine environment: mitochondrial functional impairment caused by prematurity. *Biochem J* 1994; **303**: 855–862.
70. Prieur B, Cordeau-Lossouarn L, Rotig A et al. Perinatal maturation of rat kidney mitochondria. *Biochem J* 1995; **305**: 675–680.
71. Cuezva JM, Ostronoff LK, Ricart J et al. Mitochondrial biogenesis in the liver during development and oncogenesis. *J Bioenerg Biomembr* 1997; **29**: 365–377.
72. Larsson NG, Wang J, Wilhelmsson H et al. Mitochondrial transcription factor A is necessary for mtDNA maintenance and embryogenesis in mice. *Nat Genet* 1998; **18**: 231–236.
73. Li K, Li Y, Shelton JM et al. Cytochrome c deficiency causes embryonic lethality and attenuates stress-induced apoptosis. *Cell* 2000; **101**: 389–399.
74. Piruat JI, Pintado CO, Ortega-Saenz P et al. The mitochondrial SDHD gene is required for early embryogenesis, and its partial deficiency results in persistent carotid body glomus cell activation with full responsiveness to hypoxia. *Mol Cell Biol* 2004; **24**: 10933–10940.
75. Chinnery PF, DiMauro S, Shanske S et al. Risk of developing a mitochondrial DNA deletion disorder. *Lancet* 2004; **364**: 592–596.
76. Yanagisawa K, Uchigata Y, Sanaka M et al. Mutation in the mitochondrial $tRNA^{Leu}$ at position 3243 and spontaneous abortions in Japanese women attending a clinic for diabetic pregnancies. *Diabetologia* 1995; **38**: 809–815.
77. Jaksch M, Ogilvie I, Yao J et al. Mutations in *SCO2* are associated with a distinct form of hypertrophic cardiomyopathy and cytochrome *c* oxidase deficiency. *Hum Mol Genet* 2000; **9**: 795–801.
78. Tay SK, Shanske S, Kaplan P et al. Association of mutations in *SCO2*, a cytochrome c oxidase assembly gene, with early fetal lethality. *Arch Neurol* 2004; **61**: 950–952.
79. Marchington DR, Scott Brown MS, Lamb VK et al. No evidence for paternal mtDNA transmission to offspring or extra-embryonic tissues after ICSI. *Mol Hum Reprod* 2002; **8**: 1046–1049.
80. Reynier P, Chretien MF, Savagner F et al. Long PCR analysis of human gamete mtDNA suggests defective mitochondrial maintenance in spermatozoa and supports the bottleneck theory for oocytes. *Biochem Biophys Res Commun* 1998; **252**: 373–377.
81. O'Connell M, McClure N, Lewis SE. Mitochondrial DNA deletions and nuclear DNA fragmentation in testicular and epididymal human sperm. *Hum Reprod* 2002; **17**: 1565–1570.
82. Danan C, Sternberg D, Van Steirteghem A et al. Evaluation of parental mitochondrial inheritance in neonates born after intracytoplasmic sperm injection. *Am J Hum Genet* 1999; **65**: 463–473.
83. Cohen J, Scott R, Schimmel T et al. Birth of infant after transfer of anucleate donor oocyte cytoplasm into recipient eggs. *Lancet* 1997; **350**: 186–187.
84. Barritt JA, Brenner CA, Malter HE et al. Mitochondria in human offspring derived from ooplasmic transplantation. *Hum Reprod* 2001; **16**: 513–516.
85. Barritt JA, Brenner CA, Willadsen S et al. Spontaneous and artificial changes in human ooplasmic mitochondria. *Hum Reprod* 2000; **15** (Suppl 2): 207–217.
86. Brenner CA, Barritt JA, Willadsen S et al. Mitochondrial DNA heteroplasmy after human ooplasmic transplantation. *Fertil Steril* 2000; **74**: 573–578.
87. Thorburn DR, Dahl HHM, Singh KK. The pros and cons of mitochondrial manipulation in the human germ line. *Mitochondrion* 2001; **1**: 123–127.

88. Muggleton-Harris AL, Brown JJ. Cytoplasmic factors influence mitochondrial reorganization and resumption of cleavage during culture of early mouse embryos. *Hum Reprod* 1988; **3**: 1020–1028.
89. Van Blerkom J, Davis P, Alexander S. Differential mitochondrial distribution in human pronuclear embryos leads to disproportionate inheritance between blastomeres: relationship to microtubular organization, ATP content and competence. *Hum Reprod* 2000; **15**: 2621–2633.
90. Barritt JA, Brenner CA, Malter HE et al. Rebuttal: interooplasmic transfers in humans. *Reprod Biomed Online* 2001; **3**: 47–48.
91. Renard JP, Baldacci P, Richoux-Duranthon V et al. A maternal factor affecting mouse blastocyst formation. *Development* 1994; **120**: 797–802.
92. Hawes SM, Sapienza C, Latham KE. Ooplasmic donation in humans: the potential for epigenic modifications. *Hum Reprod* 2002; **17**: 850–852.
93. Hiendleder S, Prelle K, Bruggerhoff K et al. Nuclear-cytoplasmic interactions affect in utero developmental capacity, phenotype, and cellular metabolism of bovine nuclear transfer fetuses. *Biol Reprod* 2004; **70**: 1196–1205.
94. Laipis PJ. Construction of heteroplasmic mice containing two mitochondrial DNA genotypes by micromanipulation of single-cell embryos. *Methods Enzymol* 1996; **264**: 345–357.
95. Meirelles FV, Smith LC. Mitochondrial genotype segregation in a mouse heteroplasmic lineage produced by embryonic karyoplast transplantation. *Genetics* 1997; **145**: 445–451.
96. Jenuth JP, Peterson AC, Shoubridge EA. Tissue-specific selection for different mtDNA genotypes in heteroplasmic mice. *Nat Genet* 1997; **16**: 93–95.
97. Templeton A. Ooplasmic transfer – proceed with care. *N Engl J Med* 2002; **346**: 773–775.
98. St John JC, Lloyd RE, Bowles EJ et al. The consequences of nuclear transfer for mammalian foetal development and offspring survival. A mitochondrial DNA perspective. *Reproduction* 2004; **127**: 631–641.
99. Harvey JN, Barnett D. Endocrine dysfunction in Kearns-Sayre syndrome – Case report and review. *Clin Endocrinol* 1992; **37**: 97–104.
100. Chen CM, Huang CC. Gonadal dysfunction in mitochondrial encephalomyopathies. *Eur Neurol* 1995; **35**: 281–286.
101. Gironi M, Lamperti C, Nemni R et al. Late-onset cerebellar ataxia with hypogonadism and muscle coenzyme Q10 deficiency. *Neurology* 2004; **62**: 818–820.
102. Moilanen JS, Majamaa K. Relative fitness of carriers of the mitochondrial DNA mutation 3243A>G. *Eur J Hum Genet* 2001; **9**: 59–62.
103. Graff C, Wredenberg A, Silva JP et al. Complex genetic counselling and prenatal analysis in a woman with external ophthalmoplegia and deleted mtDNA. *Prenat Diagn* 2000; **20**: 426–531.
104. Poulton J, Turnbull DM. 74th ENMC international workshop: mitochondrial diseases 19–20 November 1999, Naarden, the Netherlands. *Neuromuscul Disord* 2000; **10**: 460–462.
105. Harding AE, Holt IJ, Sweeney MG et al. Prenatal diagnosis of mitochondrial DNA(8993 T-G) disease. *Am J Hum Genet* 1992; **50**: 629–633.
106. Bartley J, Senadheera D, Park P et al. Prenatal diagnosis of T8993G mitochondrial DNA point mutation in amniocytes by heteroplasmy detection. *Am J Hum Genet* 1996; **59**: A316.
107. Ferlin T, Landrieu P, Rambaud C et al. Segregation of the G8993 mutant mitochondrial DNA through generations and embryonic tissues in a family at risk of Leigh syndrome. *J Pediatr* 1997; **131**: 447–449.
108. White SL, Shanske S, Biros I et al. Two cases of prenatal analysis for the pathogenic T to G substitution at nucleotide 8993 in mitochondrial DNA. *Prenat Diagn* 1999; **19**: 1165–1168.
109. Leshinsky-Silver E, Perach M, Basilevsky E et al. Prenatal exclusion of Leigh syndrome due to T8993C mutation in the mitochondrial DNA. *Prenat Diagn* 2003; **23**: 31–33.
110. Chou YJ, Ou CY, Hsu TY et al. Prenatal diagnosis of a fetus harboring an intermediate load of the A3243G mtDNA mutation in a maternal carrier diagnosed with MELAS syndrome. *Prenat Diagn* 2004; **24**: 367–370.
111. Dean NL, Battersby BJ, Ao A et al. Prospect of preimplantation genetic diagnosis for heritable mitochondrial DNA diseases. *Mol Hum Reprod* 2003; **9**: 631–638.
112. Steffann J, Frydman N, Gigarel N et al. Analysis of mtDNA variant segregation during early human embryonic development: a tool for successful NARP preimplantation diagnosis. *J Med Genet 2006*; (in press).

12

Mitochondrial psychiatry

Salvatore DiMauro, Michio Hirano, Petra Kaufmann, and J John Mann

Introduction

Given the vulnerability of the brain to defects of oxidative metabolism, it should come as no surprise that cognitive and psychiatric problems are common in mitochondrial diseases. However, while cognitive defects, i.e. dementia in adults and neuropsychological regression (loss of acquired skills) in children are recognized major components of most mitochondrial encephalomyopathies (see Chapter 2), psychiatric disorders are probably less frequent and certainly less well characterized. This is unfortunate because it is our experience that 'depressive symptoms are alarmingly frequent in carriers of mtDNA point mutations compared to control subjects from the same family environment' and these patients can benefit from appropriate treatment.[1] In an attempt to put some order in a vast but often anecdotal and contradictory literature, we will consider three approaches. First, we will review reports of overt psychiatric symptoms in the context of clinically – and often molecularly – well-defined mitochondrial encephalomyopathies. Second, we will consider the disappointingly few and often preliminary systematic neuropsychiatric studies of large cohorts of patients with known mitochondrial diseases. Third, we will examine the intriguing but often weak evidence of mitochondrial dysfunction in patients with isolated, 'primary' psychiatric illnesses, mostly bipolar disorder and schizophrenia. Then we will review the neurobiology of mood disorders to demonstrate how regional dysfunction in the brain that is of metabolic origin may mimic the pattern of altered brain activity seen in mood disorders, or at least components of mood disorders, and produce such psychopathology.

Psychiatric symptoms in patients with well-defined mitochondrial disease

In an attempt to organize a largely anecdotal literature, we will consider sequentially mitochondrial diseases in the order of the genetic classification proposed in Table 12.1.

Defects of mtDNA

Mutations in protein synthesis genes

Single, large-scale deletions of mtDNA cause one major generalized disorder, Kearns–Sayre syndrome (KSS). Although dementia develops in 86% of patients with KSS,[2] psychiatric symptoms are extremely uncommon, as are seizures. Perhaps, the predominant involvement of the white matter in this disorder explains the rarity of both conditions.

In contrast, psychiatric problems are common in disorders due to mutations in tRNA genes of

Table 12.1 Genetic classification of the mitochondrial diseases

Defects of mtDNA	Defects of nDNA
Mutations in protein synthesis genes tRNA, rRNA, rearrangements	**Mutations in respiratory chain subunits** Complex I, complex II
Mutations in protein-coding genes Multisystemic (LHON, NARP/MILS)	**Mutations in ancillary proteins** Complex IV, complex III, complex V
Tissue-specific	**Defects of intergenomic signaling** PEO with multiple Δ-mtDNA mtDNA depletion
	Defects of the lipid milieu Barth syndrome
	Defects of motility/fusion/fission Autosomal dominant optic atrophy CMT type 2A

LHON, Leber's hereditary optic neuropathy; NARP, neuropathy, ataxia, retinitis pigmentosa; MILS, maternally inherited Leigh syndrome; PEO, progressive external ophthalmoplegia; CMT, Charcot–Marie–Tooth disease; Δ denotes large-scale deletion.

mtDNA (Table 12.2). The most common of these disorders is MELAS (mitochondrial encephalomyopathy, lactic acidosis, and stroke-like episodes) and the most common of several causative mutations is A3243G in the $tRNA^{Leu(UUR)}$ gene (see Chapter 2). The frequency of dementia in MELAS is about 12% and in most clinical outlines there is no specific mention of psychiatric symptoms,[3] because these often go unreported or unnoticed and systematic neuropsychological studies have not been conducted until recently (see below). However, 'ambiguous psychiatric disorders' were noted 'frequently' in patients with the A3243G mutation and diabetes mellitus.[4–6] A French multicenter study of maternally inherited diabetes and deafness in 51 patients harboring the A3243G mutation, found that 18% had 'neuropsychiatric disturbances':[7] these were broken down into aggressive and unstable behavior (one patient), impaired memory and concentration (three patients), mental retardation (four patients), and psychotic behavior with auditory hallucinations (one patient).

Anecdotal reports include a patient who developed psychiatric symptoms at age 22, several years before the diagnosis of MELAS/3243 was established: these included delusions of reference and influence, paranoid ideation, and auditory hallucinations.[8] Severe depression was the presenting symptom and remained the predominant problem in a young Japanese man with neurosensory hearing loss and Wolff–Parkinson–White (WPW) syndrome: regional cerebral blood flow (rCBF) was decreased in the left globus pallidus, the right frontal lobe, and both occipital lobes.[9] Interestingly, treatment with relatively low doses of coenzyme Q10 (90 mg daily) and idebenone was associated with improvement of both symptoms and rCBF. Confusion and aggressive behavior were described in two patients, who also had other signs of MELAS, such as neurosensory hearing loss, migraine-like headache, epilepsy, and aphasia.[10] Finally, the A3243G mutation was an incidental finding in a 9-year-old boy with asthma and depression.[11]

Table 12.2 Co-morbidity of mitochondrial diseases and psychiatric disorders

	Mutation	Gene	Syndrome	Psychiatric symptoms	Ref.
	mtDNA single Δ		KSS/PEO		
	A3243G		MELAS/DM	Depression, paranoia	4–11
				ASD	12
	G3274A	$tRNA^{Leu(UUR)}$	CA, HL, C	Depression	14
mtDNA mutations	C3303T		CM	Depression	16
	A3251G		PEO	Depression	17
	A8344G	$tRNA^{Lys}$	MERRF	Depression	1
	G8363A		LS	ASD	19
	$T5537^{insT}$	$tRNA^{Trp}$	EM	Depression	20
	A7543G	$tRNA^{Asp}$	EM	HADD	21
	T8993G	ATPase 6	NARP/MILS	MR, dementia, ASD?	23
nDNA mutations	various	*ANT1*	AD-PEO	Depression	38,39
	various	*Twinkle*	AD-PEO	Depression	40
	various	*POLG*	AD/AR-PEO	Depression, paranoia	44–49

CA, cerebral atrophy; HL, hearing loss; C, cataracts; CM, cardiomyopathy; PEO, progressive external ophthalmoplegia; MERRF, myoclonus epilepsy and ragged-red fibers; LS, Leigh syndrome; EM, encephalomyopathy; NARP/MILS, neuropathy, ataxia, retinitis pigmentosa/maternally inherited Leigh syndrome; AD, autosomal dominant; AR, autosomal recessive; ASD, autism spectrum disorder; HADD, hyperactivity and attention deficit disorder; MR, mental retardation.

We observed a different psychiatric manifestation of the A3243G mutation in four children with autistic spectrum disorders: two of them had isolated autistic features, while the other two had associated neurological symptoms.[12] Also, the A3243G mutation was detected in muscle or accessible tissues only in two children, whereas in the other two the mutation was not detectable in the patients' tissues but was present in tissues from their mothers. The implication was that in some autistic children the A3243G mutation (or other mtDNA mutations) could be present in the brain but escape detection in easily accessible tissues, including hair follicles, skin fibroblasts, buccal mucosa, and urinary sediment. Based on these data, Kent et al.[13] screened by a sensitive fluorescent assay buccal swabs from 129 individuals with Asperger syndrome (AS; the mildest of the autistic spectrum disorders) and from their mothers for the A3243G mutation but found none.

Different mutations in $tRNA^{Leu(UUR)}$ have also been associated with psychiatric symptoms. A de novo heteroplasmic mutation (G3274A) was documented in a young man, who at age 27 developed acute psychosis with depression and suicidal ideation.[14] Neuropsychological tests showed depression and deficits in memory, attention, and orientation. MRI of the brain showed T2-hyperintense lesions in the basal ganglia and in the left periventricular white matter. The patient also had early-onset cataracts, cerebellar ataxia, and bilateral hearing loss.

In 1999, we described four families harboring a heteroplasmic C3303T mutation associated with cardiomyopathy or myopathy.[15] What we did not report then was that in two of those families (families 1 and 4), several maternal relatives suffered from depression, which was not simply reactive to the death of infants with cardiomyopathy. A similar observation was then reported in a Spanish family, where a cardiopathic child's mother, maternal aunt, grandmother, and a maternal great uncle all had suffered from manic-depressive episodes since adolescence.[16]

Psychiatric problems ('psychotic depression' in a 29-year-old woman and 'anorexia and agoraphobia' in her 25-year-old sister) were part of the clinical picture in a family harboring the A3251G mutation, which also caused maternally inherited ptosis, ophthalmoparesis, neck and proximal limb weakness, and sudden death at a young age attributed to respiratory failure.[17]

The second major syndrome associated with tRNA mutations is MERRF (myoclonic epilepsy with ragged-red fibers), usually due to the A8344G mutation in the $tRNA^{Lys}$ gene and, much less frequently, to two other mutations (T8356C and G8363A) in the same gene (see Chapter 2). While the frequency of dementia in MERRF is similar to that in MELAS (75%),[18] reports of psychiatric problems are not common. However, formal neuropsychological testing in a cohort of patients revealed that depression might be even more common than in MELAS, affecting as many as 80% of fully symptomatic MERRF patients (see below). In addition, the G8363A mutation was reported in a child who, by 2 years of age, had developed typical autistic features (fulfilling DSM-IV criteria for autism), while his full sister had neurological and neuroradiological features of Leigh syndrome (LS), and one maternal half sister had seizures, learning disabilities, tremor, and motor dyspraxia.[19] Interestingly, the mutant loads in blood (60%) and muscle (61%) were lower in the autistic child than in his sister with LS (blood 82%, muscle 86%).

A single-base insertion (T^{5537i}) in $tRNA^{Trp}$ caused encephalopathy in three children, but was associated with severe depression in the mother, her maternal half-sister, her mother and grandmother, suggesting a pathogenic relationship between mutation and depression.[20]

A mutation (A7543G) in the $tRNA^{Asp}$ gene caused severe behavioral problems in a 7-year-old girl, who also had seizures, myoclonus, dysarthria, nystagmus, and mild lactic acidosis.[21] She was initially diagnosed with hyperactivity attention deficit disorder (HADD). At age 9, she had severe learning disability and continued being hyperactive and antisocial, and – when last seen at age 11 – she had childish speech and poor expressive language. Her younger brother was also hyperactive, inattentive, impulsive, and aggressive, and occasionally showed self-destructive behavior, biting himself. The children's mother was mentally retarded and had grand-mal seizures.

Mutations in protein-coding genes

The two major multisystemic syndromes in this group are LHON (Leber's hereditary optic neuropathy) and NARP/MILS (neuropathy, ataxia, retinitis pigmentosa/maternally inherited Leigh syndrome).

The clinical picture of LHON is dominated by visual loss and neither cognitive impairment nor psychiatric symptoms are usually seen.[22] In contrast, mental retardation is almost invariable in children with MILS and is common but variably severe in older children or young adults with full-fledged NARP.[23] Interestingly, Uziel et al.[23] noted that the three youngest children in her series with MILS had 'no visual contact' at 3 months (one patient) and 6 months (two patients), a feature suggestive of autistic spectrum disorders.

Mutations in the gene encoding subunit 5 of complex I (*ND5*) have been described with increased frequency in association with MELAS, MERRF, LS, LHON, or various overlaps of these syndromes.[24] While dementia is described in patients with MELAS and neuropsychological regression in patients with LS, there are no overt neuropsychiatric symptoms in other phenotypes associated with *ND5* mutations. However, alexia without agraphia, constructional apraxia, and memory loss were reported in a patient with the A13513G mutation,[25] attention deficit, impairment of short- and long-term memory in a patient with the A13084T mutation,[26] and learning difficulties in the proband and his two brothers with the A12770G transition.[27] A 6-year-old Italian patient of Dr Enrico Bertini (Pediatric Hospital 'Bambino Gesù', Rome, Italy) with the G13042A mutation had optic atrophy and LS-like neuroradiological lesions, but his 44-year-old maternal aunt, in addition to seizures since age 6 and spastic hemiparesis, also had depression and paranoid ideation for which she required pharmacological therapy.

Defects of nuclear DNA

Mutations in respiratory chain subunits

These include mutations in genes encoding subunits of complex I, complex II, and coenzyme Q10 (CoQ10). Mutations in numerous complex I genes (*NDUFS* and *NDUFV*) have been associated with rapidly progressive infantile LS, leukoencephalopathy, or cardiomyopathy,[28] with death preceding the potential development of psychiatric problems.

Two pairs of sisters with complex II deficiency and mutations in *SDHA* had LS and died in childhood, while a set of two older sisters heterozygous for an *SDHA* mutation[29] had optic atrophy, ataxia, and proximal weakness, but no cognitive impairment.[30]

Presumably primary CoQ10 deficiency causes three main syndromes. First, a predominantly myopathic syndrome, with exercise intolerance and recurrent myoglobinuria associated with CNS involvement manifested by ataxia, seizures, or mental retardation.[28] The 35-year-old woman studied by us had normal cognition although her brother, who was not available to study, had an affective disorder. The second CoQ10 deficiency-related syndrome includes a much larger group of patients, who have childhood-onset cerebellar ataxia and cerebellar atrophy.[31,32] Mental retardation is one of the frequent but inconsistent accompanying neurological manifestations. Two brothers with late-onset presentation of cerebellar ataxia, hypergonadotrophic hypogonadism, and muscle CoQ10 deficiency had subtle neuropsychological deficits in constructional praxis, visuospatial short-term memory, and executive function: memory tasks improved after 2 months of high-dose CoQ10 supplementation.[33] Two sisters had LS-like brain lesions and multiple neurological deficits, including mental retardation and behavioral problems, which improved somewhat after CoQ10 replacement.[34] The third CoQ10 deficiency-related syndrome presents as severe and – if untreated – lethal infantile encephalomyopathy associated with nephrosis.

Mutations in ancillary proteins

Defects of respiratory chain complexes III, IV, and V have not been attributed, at least, thus far, to mutations in genes encoding subunits of the complexes but rather to 'indirect hits', that is, to mutations in ancillary proteins needed for the correct assembly and function of the complexes (see Chapters 1 and 2). As all of these disorders affect infants or young children and are rapidly fatal,[28] they are of little psychiatric interest.

Defects of intergenomic signaling

These are Mendelian disorders in which mutations in nuclear genes cause qualitative (multiple deletion) or quantitative (depletion) alterations of mtDNA (see Chapters 1 and 2).

Multiple mtDNA deletions are usually characterized clinically by the progressive external ophthalmoplegia (PEO) but are genetically heterogeneous. Four genes have been associated with multiple deletions.[35,36]

First, mutations in *TP*, the gene that encodes thymidine phosphorylase, causes MNGIE (mitochondrial neurogastrointestinal encephalomyopathy), an autosomal recessive multisystem disorder characterized by PEO, peripheral neuropathy, leukoencephalopathy, and severe gastrointestinal dysmotility leading to cachexia and early death.[37] Despite the extensive white matter damage revealed by MRI, MNGIE patients are usually intellectually normal, although we have seen psychotic symptoms in terminal patients (unpublished data).

Second, mutations in *ANT1*, which encodes one isoform of the adenine nucleotide transporter, cause autosomal dominant PEO, which is often associated with exercise intolerance, hypogonadism, hearing loss, peripheral neuropathy, cataracts, and depression.[38,39]

The third gene responsible for PEO and multiple mtDNA mutations is *PEO1* (formerly know as *Twinkle*) which encodes a mitochondrial protein that resembles the bacteriophage T7 primase/helicase and is probably important for mitochondrial replication.[36] Mutations in this gene account for about 30% of all autosomal dominant PEO cases, which can present as isolated myopathy or be complicated with dysphagia, dysphonia, ataxia, peripheral neuropathy, or depression. The psychiatric aspects were studied carefully in a large Finnish family, using a structured standard interview according to DSM-III-R. Of the 11 individuals harboring multiple mtDNA deletions in muscle, seven met the criteria for a psychiatric diagnosis: four had avoidant personality traits, one had an avoidant personality disorder, and two had major depressive disorder and personality disorder (one with histrionic and the other with psychotic features).[40] Importantly, all patients had normal intelligence and none associated their psychiatric symptoms with their physical handicap (PEO and ptosis) or to their awareness of carrying a hereditary disease. Neuropathologic analysis of freshly obtained postmortem brain from one of the patients with depression showed some proliferation of Bergmann glial cells in the cerebellar cortex and occasional abnormal mitochondria with electron-dense inclusions in the frontal cortex. Interestingly, however, the abundance of multiple mtDNA deletions (as a percent of total mtDNA) in autopsy tissues from two patients was highest (over 60%) in the caudate nucleus, followed by the frontal cortex (over 50%) and skeletal muscle (50%).

Mutations in the fourth gene, *POLG*, accounted for the majority (45%) of PEO cases in a large series and could be inherited as autosomal dominant or autosomal recessive traits.[41] The clinical phenotypes tend to be both more variable and more severe than those due to mutations in *ANT1* or *PEO1*, often including severe weakness, ataxia, peripheral neuropathy, parkinsonism, and cognitive or psychiatric manifestations. Mild cognitive decline was reported in one patient with a recessive mutation and features of MERRF,[42] and in several patients with sensory ataxia and encephalopathy but without PEO or muscle involvement.[43] Depression was described in numerous families with autosomal recessive PEO,[44–46] autosomal recessive or dominant PEO and parkinsonism,[47] and in a sporadic patient with 'double trouble', mutations in both *POLG* and *PEO1*.[48] Psychiatric symptoms, including paranoia and depression, were present in most of 28 patients homozygous for an ancient European founder mutation in *POLG* (W748S).[49]

Two clinical syndromes have been associated with mtDNA depletion, one dominated by congenital or childhood-onset myopathy, sometimes accompanied by nephropathy, the other by liver and brain involvement (hepatocerebral syndrome). The myopathic form was ascribed to mutations in the gene *TK2*, which encodes mitochondrial thymidine kinase, and the hepatocerebral form to mutations in the *DGUOK* gene, which encodes mitochondrial deoxyguanosine kinase.[36] Mutations in two more genes cause mtDNA depletion. Autosomal recessive mutations in the *POLG1* gene are commonly found in children with Alpers syndrome, a form of hepatocerebral degeneration,[50–52] and mutations in the *SUCLA2* gene, encoding a subunit of the mitochondrial enzyme succinyl-CoA synthetase, have been reported in two cousins from a consanguineous family with psychomotor retardation, seizures, hearing loss, microcytic anemia, and hypotonia.[53] One of the five children with autistic spectrum disorders and mitochondrial abnormalities that we reported[12] had 72% mtDNA depletion in skeletal muscle, but no mutations were found in *TK2* or *DGUOK*. The other two genes (*POLG* and *SUCLA2*) should now be screened.

Neuropsychological studies in patients with mitochondrial encephalomyopathies

Mitochondrial myopathies and encephalomyopathies

As stated at the beginning of this review, these studies are scarce, although the group of mitochondrial researchers at the Institute of Neurology, Queen Square, as early as 1992 recognized the importance of 'mitochondrial psychiatry' and made an attempt to study the prevalence and define the nature of neuropsychological disturbances in a large cohort of patients.[54] Of 72 consecutive patients with 'mitochondrial myopathy', they identified 36 who had undergone neuropsychological assessment, including measures detecting general intellectual deterioration and deficits on focal cognitive tests. Mitochondrial disease was defined morphologically by the presence of >4% ragged-red fibers with the histochemical SDH stain: on clinical grounds, 14 patients had 'mitochondrial myopathies' and 22 had 'mitochondrial encephalomyopathies'. Molecular diagnoses were not provided. Two thirds of patients had impaired higher cerebral function, well above what would be expected on clinical grounds and including three patients from the myopathic group. Only two of the 22 patients in the encephalomyopathic group did not show any cognitive impairment, and both carried the clinical diagnosis of KSS. On the other hand, the three patients with most severe focal cognitive dysfunction had MELAS. The conclusions of this pioneer study were that cognitive dysfunction in mitochondrial diseases is 50% higher than predicted on routine clinical assessment, that neuroradiological (CT scan) and electrophysiological (EEG) instruments are more sensitive indicators of impaired cognition than a clinical impression of dementia. The authors advocated the use of positron emission tomography to understand the pathogenesis of cortical dysfunction in mitochondrial diseases.[55]

KSS and PEO

Neuropsychological profile (general intelligence, memory functions, and visuo-perceptual organization), MRI, and single-photon emission computed tomography (SPECT) were studied by Turconi et al. in a relatively homogeneous group of 19 mitochondrial patients: 12 carried the diagnosis of PEO (ten with a single mtDNA deletion, two with multiple deletions), three had KSS and single mtDNA deletions, and one had MERRF.[56] Although all patients had normal global cognition, they scored lower in non-verbal than in verbal tasks and showed selective impairment of visuo-spatial skills. The most frequent SPECT abnormality was hypoperfusion of the temporal lobes, especially of the mesial temporal cortex.

A similar cohort of patients (22 patients: 11 with PEO and single mtDNA deletions; four with KSS and single deletions; two with PEO and the MELAS/A3243G mutation; and five with PEO or KSS and unknown molecular defect) was compared to a normal group matched for age, sex, and educational level in the following areas: verbal skills and language, visual perception, visuo-construction ability, attention, abstraction/flexibility, verbal memory, visual memory, and quality of life.[57] One interesting and unexpected result shared by this study and that of Turconi et al.[56] is that neuropsychological deficits were similar in patients with

PEO and in patients with KSS, implying that even patients with apparently isolated myopathy may have functionally significant mtDNA deletions in the brain. Another similarity between the two studies is that visuo-constructive skills, visuo-spatial perception, and working memory seem to be selectively impaired in patients harboring single mtDNA deletions. Homogenizing the group by removing the two patients with the A3243G/MELAS mutation and the five patients with unknown molecular defects did not change the results substantially. Finally, assessment of quality of life provided no evidence of depression.

MELAS and MERRF

Our group has for several years been conducting a longitudinal study of the clinical and neurobehavioral features of a large cohort of mitochondrial patients consisting of two homogeneous groups: families harboring the A3243G/MELAS mutation and families with the A8344G/MERRF mutation. A preliminary study[58] compared entry findings of six patients with MERRF with those of 15 patients with MELAS. At entry, MERRF patients had attention and memory deficits and depression: two of them required assistance with activities of daily living. At entry, MELAS patients had more severe cognitive deficits, including impaired reasoning, memory, language, attention, and visuo-spatial orientation. In addition, they often had hallucinations, delusions, substance abuse, and disinhibition; ten of them were totally dependent for activities of daily living. It was concluded that MERRF has a long course and mild behavioral problems whereas MELAS has a shorter course and is more frequently associated with behavioral and psychiatric disturbances other than depression.

A follow-up study of a larger cohort of MELAS and MERRF families (102 persons from 30 kindreds) focused on the frequency of psychiatric symptoms in these conditions and included not only patients but also their oligosymptomatic or asymptomatic maternal relatives, who carry lower levels of either mutation, and paternal relatives as controls.[1] Interestingly, 42% of fully symptomatic carriers reported depressive symptoms, but, even more interestingly, 22% of asymptomatic and 29% of oligosymptomatic carriers also had depressive traits, compared to only 7% of the control group. In MERRF families, 80% of fully symptomatic patients and 20% of oligosymptomatic carriers, but none of the asymptomatic carriers reported depressive symptoms. Suicide had been attempted by 3% of the MELAS and by 17% of the MERRF carrier relatives. Delusions or hallucinations were reported by 8% of the MELAS but by none of the MERRF carriers. Not only did these data reveal the high frequency of depression in carriers of the two most common pathogenic mtDNA point mutations compared to the general population, but it also showed that even asymptomatic carriers of the A3243G/MELAS mutation are prone to depression, suggesting that psychiatric problems may be an early expression of the mutation. This concept was bolstered by correlative neuropsychological and MR spectroscopy studies, showing cerebral lactic acidosis in asymptomatic MELAS relatives and a significant correlation between neuropsychological scores and ventricular lactate levels.[59]

Mothers of mitochondrial patients

An unusual study focused on the mothers of children with mitochondrial disorders.[60] The Minnesota Multiphasic Personality Inventory–Second Edition (MMPI-2) was administered to 42 mothers, two of them adoptive: 56% had pathological scores in three or more scales, including hypochondriasis, hysteria, and paranoia (the two adoptive mothers had normal scores in all MMPI-2 scales). While these results may be explained by situational stress (frightening diagnosis, demanding care, uncertain prognosis in their children), they may also reflect intrinsic personality features related to the carrier status of mtDNA mutations.

Mitochondrial dysfunction in primary psychiatric diseases

In the 'maddening hunt for madness genes',[61] the mitochondrial genome has not been forgotten, although the title of a comprehensive 2001 review on the relationship between mitochondria and mental disorders referred to mtDNA as 'the other forgotten genome'.[62] As in that review, we will consider sequentially neuroradiological studies, biochemical analyses, ultrastructural studies, molecular genetic studies and gene expression in postmortem brains, and mtDNA polymorphisms (haplotype analyses).

Bipolar disorder

Neuroradiology

Mitochondrial dysfunction was suggested by decreased intracellular pH by ^{31}P-MRS in the brains of drug-free bipolar patients.[63] Decreased pH on ^{31}P-MRS was noted not only in basal ganglia but in the whole brain.[64] Similarly, two-dimensional proton echo-planar spectroscopic imaging (PEPSI) in 32 medication-free patients showed higher lactate and γ-aminobutyric acid levels in the gray matter, indicating a switch from oxidative metabolism towards glycolysis.[65]

Molecular genetic studies

Genetic factors underlie much of the variance in familial transmission of bipolar disorder, and data from 31 families with this condition suggested maternal inheritance based on higher than expected frequencies of affected mothers and increased risk of illness in matrilinear relatives.[66] However, sequencing of mtDNA from 94 patients failed to identify any potentially disease-related polymorphisms.[67] Nonetheless, and to complicate things further, the levels of the 4977-bp 'common' mtDNA deletion were higher in the brains of seven patients with bipolar disease than in brains from nine controls and nine suicide victims.[68]

Gene array analyses

Gene arrays were used to compare the mRNA expression of 12 558 nuclear genes in hippocampi from ten controls, nine patients with bipolar disease, and eight schizophrenic patients: the expression of genes encoding mitochondrial proteins was significantly decreased in patients with bipolar disease but not in patients with schizophrenia, and the decrease affected especially genes controlling oxidative phosphorylation and genes encoding ATP-dependent proteasome degradation.[69]

Based on the linkage of bipolar disorder with a locus on chromosome 18p11, Kato and coworkers first established that the expression of the candidate gene *NDUFV2*, encoding a catalytic subunit of complex I, was down-regulated in lymphoblastoid cell lines from patients with bipolar disorder, and found that the haplotype frequencies of four polymorphisms in the upstream region of *NDUFV2* were higher in patients than in controls.[70,71] The same group also found that the expression of other complex I genes at loci linked with bipolar disorder was also decreased in lymphoblastoid cells from patients. These findings are interesting because a large-scale analysis of gene expression in the 'learned helplessness' rat model of human depression showed that genes for complex I were down-regulated in both frontal cortex and hippocampus of these animals.[72]

Mitochondrial haplotypes

There was no significant difference in haplogroup frequencies between patients and controls in one study (Box 12.1).[73]

Schizophrenia

Neuroradiology

Evidence for mitochondrial dysfunction in schizophrenia came from ^{31}P-MRS showing decreased ATP levels in the basal ganglia and temporal lobes of patients.[74]

Box 12.1 Mitochondrial DNA haplogroups

The combination of high copy number, maternal inheritance, and rapid rate of fixation of mutations have made mammalian mtDNA an ideal molecule to study lineages that are separated in both space and time. As such, variations in human mtDNA among both groups of individuals and among spatially separated populations have proved invaluable in forensics, in the study of migration of populations, in the analysis of the origin and transmission of disease, and even in the evolution of languages.[1] All of these analyses rely on the fact that mtDNA variants accumulate over time, and therefore, the relationship between any two individuals or groups of related individuals can be determined by assessing the degree to which the set of mtDNA variations – called polymorphisms – differ from one group or population to the other.

Compared to a standard mtDNA sequence – usually the 'Cambridge' sequence determined in 1981 by Fred Sanger and his colleagues[2] – the total set of mtDNA polymorphisms determines the haplotype of an individual. If a group of individuals belongs to the same ethnic group (related, of course, through the maternal line), they will have highly similar haplotypes, with only minor variations among individuals in the group. Taken together, all of these individuals will therefore belong to the same haplogroup, which will differ from haplogroups of other genetically or physically isolated populations.

Because the very first analyses of haplotypes were not done by DNA sequencing, but rather by restriction fragment length polymorphism (RFLP) analysis of mtDNAs. An RFLP defines whether or not a particular mtDNA contains the recognition sequence for a particular restriction enzyme – for example, *Hae*III, which cuts DNA at the sequence 5′-GGCC-3′ – at a specific location on the mitochondrial genome, the initial haplogroups found in various human populations were defined by these RFLP patterns. These early haplogroups were distinguished by the letters A, B, C and so on (Table B12.1.1), each containing perhaps 50 different polymorphisms in one genome compared to another.

Table B12.1.1 Haplogroups based on RFLP analyses

Haplogroups	Population(s)
A, B, C, D	Asia, New World
L	Africa
M, N	East Africa
H, I, J, N1b, T, U, V, W	Europe
G, Y, Z	Siberia
X	Not Siberia or East Asia

Today, of course, the advent of PCR and rapid DNA sequencing has rendered the original RFLP analyses obsolete, but the haplogroup nomenclature is still useful in defining populations at the most general level. Now, the most common way to distinguish among mtDNAs is to amplify and sequence the 'control region' at '12-o'clock' on the genome. This region contains the origin of heavy-strand replication and the origins of heavy- and light-strand transcription, but does not contain any structural genes. For this reason, there are segments within the control region that are under lower evolutionary pressure to maintain sequence conservation, and therefore these regions suffer higher rates of mutation as compared to the rest of the genome. There are two main 'hypervariable regions' (HVR-I and HVR-II) that are sequenced most frequently, and hundreds of polymorphisms have been identified in these regions. The overall rate of mutation in human mtDNA has been estimated at about 2×10^{-8} substitutions/site/year, with the HVRs mutating at a rate 2–5 times higher.[1]

One particular variant, however, that has been of great value, is not a single-nucleotide polymorphism, but a 9-bp deletion located at the immediate 3′ end of the COX II gene (the only mRNA which has a 3′-untranslated region). In many groups, this region contains a tandem repeat of 9 bp (ACCCCCTCTACCCCCTCT; 2nd repeat underlined), but in some groups (most notably in Pacific peoples), one of the repeats is missing.[3]

References

1. Pakendorf B, Stoneking M. Mitochondrial DNA and human evolution. *Annu Rev Genomics Hum Genet* 2005; **6**: 165–183.
2. Anderson S, Bankier AT, Barrell BG et al. Sequence and organization of the human mitochondrial genome. *Nature* 1981; **290**: 457–465.
3. Stoneking M, Soodyall H. Human evolution and the mitochondrial genome. *Curr Opin Genet Dev* 1996; **6**: 731–736.

Morphology

Ultrastructural morphometric studies showed a 20% decrease of mitochondria in the caudate and putamen of patients.[75]

Biochemistry

Biochemical analyses revealed decreased COX activity in the caudate nucleus and in the frontal cortex.[76]

Molecular genetic analyses

Contrary to findings in patients with bipolar disorder, there was no abnormal accumulation of the 'common deletion' in the caudate nucleus or the frontal cortex of schizophrenic patients.[76] Neither was there any association of mtDNA polymorphisms with disease expression.[77]

Gene array analyses

One study found changes in mitochondrial gene expression, including 12S rRNA, 16S rRNA, and COX II.[78]

In a comprehensive review of the evidence for mitochondrial dysfunction in schizophrenia, Ben-Shachar proposed that dopamine, an etiological factor, may inhibit the mitochondrial respiratory chain.[79] After documenting that complex I was, in fact, inhibited by dopamine in human neuroblastoma cells,[80] Ben-Shachar and coworkers studied by reverse-transcriptase polymerase chain reaction (RT-PCR) analysis the expression of three complex I subunits (24-kd, 51-kd, and 75-kd) in the prefrontal and ventral parieto-occipital cortices of postmortem brains from patients with schizophrenia, major depression, and bipolar disorder.[81] They found a schizophrenia-specific down-regulation of both RNA and protein expression for subunits 24-kd and 51-kd only in the prefrontal cortex, leading the authors to postulate a causative role of complex I deficiency akin to that seen in another dopamine-related disorder, Parkinson disease.

A large-scale DNA microarray analysis of postmortem brains from patients with bipolar disorder and schizophrenia did show a down-regulation of genes encoding respiratory chain components in both conditions, but this was ascribed to the effect of medication.[82] In fact, a tendency to up-regulate mitochondrial genes was noted in medication-free patients with bipolar disorder.

A similar microarray analysis showed up-regulation of a gene, *LARS2*, which encodes leucyl-tRNA synthetase. As this enzyme catalyzes the aminoacylation of the mitochondrial $tRNA^{Leu(UUR)}$, the gene mutated in MELAS, Munakata et al. studied the steady-state of LARS2 in cybrid cell lines harboring the A3243G/MELAS mutation and found that LARS2 was up-regulated.[83] This observation led them to search for the A3243G mutation, which they found at very low levels in postmortem brains from two patients with bipolar disorder and one with schizophrenia. The pathogenic significance of this observation is debatable.

Autism spectrum disorder

Neuroradiology

In 1999, Chugani et al. found higher plasma lactate levels in all 15 children with autism spectrum disorders, and high brain lactate by proton magnetic resonance spectroscopy (MRS) in one of nine children.[84] A recent study of 45 children (3–5 years old) using proton echoplanar spectroscopic imaging (PEPSI) showed no increase in brain lactate, but reduced *N*-acetylaspartate (NAA), creatine and myoinositol concentrations.[85] The findings of reduced NAA concentration and prolonged chemical relaxations for choline and creatine contradict the hypothesis that accelerated developmental processes early in the course of autism lead to increased neuronal density. In our study of five children with autism spectrum disorder and mtDNA abnormalities, MRS showed moderately higher lactate in the lateral ventricle of only one child harboring the A3243G/MELAS mutation.[12]

Neurobiology of mood disorders

Brain imaging studies of mood disorders have identified regional alterations in blood flow and metabolism involving deficiencies in the dorsolateral prefrontal cortex and elevations in some ventral structures[86–89] Modest structural abnormalities are also observed in both bipolar disorders and in major depressive disorder, although most involve gray matter, perhaps explaining why white matter pathology does not seem to be associated as distinctly with mood disorders as gray matter deficits.[90,91] More recently, the severity of symptom components of the major depression syndrome have been related to distinct brain regions, implying that isolated abnormalities of those regions could produce those specific symptom deficits and not necessarily the full depression syndrome.[88] Thus, mitochondrial abnormalities in parts of the brain only can contribute to the primary pathogenesis of a full mood disorder syndrome or to only parts of the syndrome depending on how extensive a region of the brain is metabolically compromised.

Conclusions

In this chapter, we have reviewed three lines of evidence linking psychiatric disorders with respiratory chain dysfunction. All three approaches show convincingly that mitochondrial dysfunction can be involved in the pathogenesis of psychiatric diseases, that is, it is a sufficient cause. What remains unclear is whether mitochondrial dysfunction is a necessary cause. This situation is similar to that of many neurodegenerative disorders, such as Parkinson disease, Alzheimer disease, or amyotrophic lateral sclerosis (see Chapter 13).

Any clinician caring for patients with mitochondrial diseases is impressed by the frequency of neuropsychiatric disturbances in this population, including mood disorders, frank psychoses, or autistic spectrum disorders. This impression is substantiated by the co-morbidity data reviewed in the first part of this chapter and summarized in Table 12.2.

Much more compelling evidence of the existence of 'mitochondrial psychiatry' comes from systematic and detailed neuropsychological evaluations of large cohorts of patients harboring pathogenic mtDNA mutations. This is especially true for those mutations (like the ones causing MELAS and MERRF) that are maternally transmitted, because neuropsychological disturbances can be studied in individuals carrying low levels of the mutation and showing few physical symptoms or none at all. When neuropsychological assessment is associated with sophisticated neuroradiology techniques, including MRS, PET, SPECT, PEPSI, and functional MRI, these individuals offer a unique opportunity to glean which areas of the brain correlate with specific affective or cognitive abnormalities. These studies are in their infancy and should be pursued.

A large number of morphological, biochemical, and molecular studies (briefly summarized in the third part of this chapter) have explored mitochondrial function in postmortem brains from patients with bipolar disorder and schizophrenia. Not surprisingly, these data are limited, in part due to the suboptimal conditions of postmortem brains and to the effects of agonal state and medication on the changes observed.[82] Even with these caveats and despite some controversy, when this large volume of data is taken together, mitochondrial dysfunction appears to be a convincing – albeit not necessarily primary – pathogenic mechanism in psychiatric diseases.

Acknowledgments

Part of the work described here has been supported by NIH grants NS11766 and HD32062, by a grant of the Muscular Dystrophy Association, and by the Marriott Mitochondrial Disorder Clinical Research Fund (MMDCRF).

References

1. Kaufmann P, Sano MC, Jhung S et al. Psychiatric symptoms are common features of clinical syndromes associated with mitochondrial DNA point mutations. *Neurology* 2002; **58**: A315 (Abstract).
2. DiMauro S, Hirano M. Mitochondrial DNA Deletion Syndromes. Vol. 2003. GeneReviews at Gene Tests: Medical Genetics Information Resource [database online] ed: Seattle: University of Washington; 2003.
3. DiMauro S, Hirano M. MELAS. Vol. 2003. GeneReviews at Gene Tests: Medical Genetics Information Resource [database online] ed: Seattle: University of Washington; 2003.
4. Suzuki T, Koizumi J, Shiraishi H et al. Mitochondrial encephalomyopathy (MELAS) with mental disorder: CT, MRI and SPECT findings. *Neuroradiology* 1990; **32**: 74–76.
5. Suzuki Y, Miyaoka H, Taniyama M et al. Psychotic disturbance in mitochondrial diabetes due to 3243 mitochondrial tRNA mutation. *J Jpn Diab Soc* 1995; **38**: 905–908.
6. Suzuki Y, Taniyama M, Muramatsu T et al. Diabetes mellitus associated with 3243 mitochondrial $tRNA^{Leu(UUR)}$ mutation: clinical features and coenzyme Q10 treatment. *Mol Aspects Med* 1997; **18**: S181–S188.
7. Guillausseau PJ, Massin P, Dubuois-LaForgue D et al. Maternally inherited diabetes and deafness: A multicenter study. *Ann Int Med* 2001; **134**: 721–728.
8. Thomeer EC, Verhoeven WM, van de Vlasakker CJ, Klompenhouwer JL. Psychiatric symptoms in MELAS; a case report. *J Neurol Neurosurg Psychiatry* 1998; **64**: 692–693.
9. Onishi H, Kawanishi C, Iwasawa T et al. Depressive disorder due to mitochondrial transfer $RNA^{Leu(UUR)}$ mutation. *Biol Psychiatry* 1997; **41**: 1137–1139.
10. Feddersen B, Bender A, Arnold S et al. Aggressive confusional state as a clinical manifestation of status epilepticus in MELAS. *Neurology* 2003; **61**: 1149–1150.
11. Shanske AL, Shanske S, Silvestri G et al. MELAS point mutation with unusual clinical presentation. *Neuromusc Disord* 1993; **3**: 191–193.
12. Pons R, Andreu AL, Checcarelli N et al. Mitochondrial DNA abnormalities and autistic spectrum disorders. *J Pediatr* 2004; **144**: 81–85.
13. Kent L, Lambert C, Pyle A et al. The mitochondrial DNA 3243A→G mutation is a rare cause of Asperger syndrome [letter]. *J Pediatr* 2005; in press.
14. Jaksch M, Lochmuller H, Schmitt F et al. A mutation in the mt $tRNA^{Leu(UUR)}$ causing a neuropsychiatric syndrome with depression and cataract. *Neurology* 2001; **57**: 1930–1931.

15. Bruno C, Kirby DM, Koga Y et al. The mitochondrial DNA C3303T mutation can cause cardiomyopathy and/or skeletal myopathy. *J Pediatr* 1999; **135**: 197–202.
16. Campos Y, Garcia A, Eiris J et al. Mitochondrial myopathy, cardiomyopathy and psychiatric illness in a Spanish family harbouring the mtDNA 3303C→T mutation. *J Inher Metab Dis* 2001; **24**: 685–687.
17. Sweeney MG, Bundey S, Brockington M et al. Mitochondrial myopathy associated with sudden death in young adults and a novel mutation in the mitochondrial DNA transfer $RNA^{Leu(UUR)}$ gene. *Quart J Med* 1993; **11**: 709–713.
18. DiMauro S, Hirano M. *MERRF*. In: GeneReviews at GeneTester: Medical Genetics Information Resource (database online). © University of Washington, Seattle, 1997–2003. Available at http://www.genetests.org
19. Graf WD, Marin-Garcia J, Gao HG et al. Autism associated with the mitochondrial DNA G8363A transfer RNA^{Lys} mutation. *J Child Neurol* 2000; **15**: 357–361.
20. Santorelli FM, Tanji K, Sano M et al. Maternally inherited encephalopathy associated with a single-base insertion in the mitochondrial $tRNA^{Trp}$ gene. *Ann Neurol* 1997; **42**: 256–260.
21. Shtilbans A, El-Schahawi M, Malkin E et al. A novel mutation in the mitochondrial DNA transfer ribonucleic acid Asp gene in a child with myoclonic epilepsy and psychomotor regression. *J Child Neurol* 1999; **14**: 610–613.
22. Carelli V. Leber's hereditary optic neuropathy. In: Schapira AHV, DiMauro S, eds. *Mitochondrial Disorders in Neurology 2*. Boston: Butterworth-Heinemann, 2002: 115–142.
23. Uziel G, Moroni I, Lamantea E et al. The mitochondrial disease associated with the T8993G mutation of mitochondrial ATPase 6 gene: a clinical, biochemical, and molecular study in six families. *J Neurol Neurosurg Psychiat* 1997; **63**: 16–22.
24. DiMauro S, Davidzon G. Mitochondrial DNA and disease. *Ann Med* 2005; **37**: 222–232.
25. Corona P, Antozzi C, Carrara F et al. A novel mtDNA mutation in the ND5 subunit of complex I in two MELAS patients. *Ann Neurol* 2001; **49**: 106–110.
26. Crimi M, Galbiati S, Moroni I et al. A missense mutation in the mitochondrial ND5 gene associated with a Leigh-MELAS overlap syndrome. *Neurology* 2003; **60**: 1857–1861.
27. Liolitsa D, Rahman S, Benton S et al. Is the mitochondrial complex I ND5 gene a hot-spot for MELAS causing mutations? *Ann Neurol* 2003; **53**: 128–132.
28. DiMauro S, Hirano M. Mitochondrial encephalomyopathies: an update. *Neuromusc Disord* 2005; **15**: 276–286.
29. Birch-Machin MA, Taylor RW, Cochran B et al. Late-onset optic atrophy, ataxia, and myopathy associated with a mutation of a complex II gene. *Ann Neurol* 2000; **48**: 330–335.
30. Taylor RW, Birch-Machin MA, Schaefer J et al. Deficiency of complex II of the mitochondrial respiratory chain in late-onset optic atrophy and ataxia. *Ann Neurol* 1996; **39**: 224–232.
31. Musumeci O, Naini A, Slonim AE et al. Familial cerebellar ataxia with muscle coenzyme Q10 deficiency. *Neurology* 2001; **56**: 849–855.
32. Lamperti C, Naini A, Hirano M et al. Cerebellar ataxia and coenzyme Q10 deficiency. *Neurology* 2003; **60**: 1206–1208.
33. Gironi M, Lamperti C, Nemni R et al. Late-onset cerebellar ataxia with hypogonadism and muscle coenzyme Q10 deficiency. *Neurology* 2004; **62**: 818–820.
34. Van Maldergem L, Trijbels F, DiMauro S et al. Coenzyme Q-responsive Leigh's encephalopathy in two sisters. *Ann Neurol* 2002; **52**: 750–754.
35. Hirano M, DiMauro S. *ANT1, Twinkle, POLG*, and *TP*: New genes open our eyes to ophthalmoplegia. *Neurology* 2001; **57**: 2163–2165.
36. Spinazzola A, Zeviani M. Disorders of nuclear-mitochondrial intergenomic signaling. *Gene* 2005; **354**: 162–168.
37. Nishino I, Spinazzola A, Papadimitriou A et al. Mitochondrial neurogastrointestinal encephalomyopathy: an autosomal recessive disorder due to thymidine phosphorylase mutations. *Ann Neurol* 2000; **47**: 792–800.
38. Siciliano G, Tessa A, Petrini S et al. Autosomal dominant external ophthalmoplegia and bipolar affective disorder associated with a mutation in the *ANT1* gene. *Neuromusc Disord* 2003; **13**: 162–165.
39. Deschauer M, Hudson G, Muller T et al. A novel *ANT1* gene mutation with probable germline mosaicism in autosomal dominant progressive external ophthalmoplegia. *Neuromusc Disord* 2005; **15**: 311–315.

40. Suomalainen A, Majander A, Wallin M et al. Autosomal dominant progressive external ophthalmoplegia with multiple deletions of mtDNA: Clinical, biochemical, and molecular genetic features of the 10q-linked disease. *Neurology* 1997; **48**: 1244–1253.
41. Lamantea E, Tiranti V, Bordoni A et al. Mutations of mitochondrial DNA polymerase γA are a frequent cause of autosomal dominant or recessive progressive external ophthalmoplegia. *Ann Neurol* 2002; **52**: 211–219.
42. Van Goethem G, Mercelis R, Lofgren A et al. Patient homozygous for a recessive *POLG* mutation presents with features of MERRF. *Neurology* 2003; **61**: 1811–1813.
43. Van Goethem G, Luoma P, Rantamaki M et al. *POLG* mutations in neurodegenerative disorders with ataxia but no muscle involvement. *Neurology* 2004; **63**: 1251–1257.
44. Van Goethem G, Martin JJ, Dermaut B et al. Recessive *POLG* mutations presenting with sensory and ataxic neuropathy in compound heterozygote patients with progressive external ophthalmoplegia. *Neuromusc Disord* 2003; **13**: 133–142.
45. Mancuso M, Filosto M, Bellan M et al. *POLG* mutation causing ophthalmoplegia, sensorimotor polyneuropathy, ataxia, and deafness. *Neurology* 2004; **62**: 316–318.
46. Luoma PT, Luo N, Loscher WN et al. Functional defects due to spacer region mutations of human mitochondrial DNA polymerase in a family with an ataxia-myopathy syndrome. *Hum Mol Genet* 2005; **14**: 1907–1920.
47. Luoma P, Melberg A, Rinne JO et al. Parkinsonism, premature menopause, and mitochondrial DNA polymerase mutations: clinical and molecular genetic study. *Lancet* 2004; **364**: 875–882.
48. Van Goethem G, Lofgren A, Dermaut B et al. Digenic progressive external ophthalmoplegia in a sporadic patient: recessive mutations in *POLG* and *C10orf2/Twinkle*. *Hum Mut* 2003; **22**: 175–176.
49. Hakonen AH, Heiskanen S, Juvonen V et al. Mitochondrial DNA polymerase W748S mutation: A common cause of autosomal recessive ataxia with ancient European origin. *Am J Hum Genet* 2005; **77**: 430–441.
50. Naviaux RK, Nguyen KV. *POLG* mutations associated with Alpers' syndrome and mitochondrial DNA depletion. *Ann Neurol* 2004; **55**: 706–712.
51. Ferrari G, Lamantea E, Donati A et al. Infantile hepatocerebral syndromes associated with mutations in the mitochondrial DNA polymerase-γA. *Brain* 2005; **128**: 723–731.
52. Davidzon G, Mancuso M, Ferraris S et al. *POLG* mutations and Alpers syndrome. *Ann Neurol* 2005; **57**: 921–924.
53. Elpeleg O, Miller C, Hershkovitz E et al. Deficiency of the ADP-forming succinyl-CoA synthase activity is associated with encephalomyopathy and mitochondrial DNA depletion. *Am J Hum Genet* 2005; **76**: 1081–1086.
54. Kartsounis LD, Troung DD, Morgan-Hughes JA, Harding AE. The neuropsychological features of mitochondrial myopathies and encephalomyopathies. *Arch Neurol* 1992; **49**: 158–160.
55. Frackowiack RSJ, Herold S, Petty RKH, Morgan-Hughes JA. The cerebral metabolism of glucose and oxygen measured with positron tomography in patients with mitochondrial diseases. *Brain* 1988; **111**: 1009–1024.
56. Turconi AC, Benti R, Castelli E et al. Focal cognitive impairment in mitochondrial encephalomyopathies: a neuropsychological and neuroimaging study. *J Neurol Sci* 1999; **170**: 57–63.
57. Bosbach S, Kornblum C, Schroder R, Wagner M. Executive and visuospatial deficits in patients with chronic progressive external ophthalmoplegia and Kearns-Sayre syndrome. *Brain* 2003; **126**: 1231–1240.
58. Sano MC, Polanco Y, De Vivo DC. Comparative clinical analysis of mitochondrial encephalomyopathy, lactic acidosis, and stroke-like episodes and myoclonic epilepsy and ragged-red fibers. [Abstract]. *Ann Neurol* 1998; **44**: 576–577.
59. Kaufmann P, Shungu D, Sano MC et al. Cerebral lactic acidosis correlates with neurological impairment in MELAS. *Neurology* 2004; **62**: 1297–1302.
60. Varvogli L, Waisbren SE. Personality profiles of mothers of children with mitochondrial disorders. *J Inher Metab Dis* 1999; **22**: 615–622.
61. Moldin SO. The maddening hunt for madness genes. *Nature Genet* 1997; **17**: 127–129.
62. Kato T. The other, forgotten genome: mitochondrial DNA and mental disorders. *Mol Psychiatry* 2001; **6**: 625–633.
63. Kato T, Murashita J, Kamiya A et al. Decreased brain intracellular pH measured by ^{31}-P-MRS in bipolar disorder: a confirmation in drug-free

patients and correlation with white matter hyperintensity. *Eur Arch Psychiatry Clin Neurosci* 1998; **248**: 301–306.

64. Hamakawa H, Murashita J, Yamada N et al. Reduced intracellular pH in the basal ganglia and the whole brain measured by ^{31}P-MRS in bipolar disorder. *Psychiat Clin Neurosc* 2004; **58**: 82–88.
65. Dager SR, Friedman SD, Parow A et al. Brain metabolic alterations in medication-free patients with bipolar disorder. *Arch Gen Psychiatry* 2004; **61**: 450–458.
66. McMahon FJ, Stine OC, Meyers DA et al. Patterns of maternal transmission in bipolar affective disorder. *Am J Hum Genet* 1995; **56**: 1277–1286.
67. Kirk R, Furlong RA, Amos W et al. Mitochondrial genetic analyses suggest selection against maternal lineages in bipolar affective disorder. *Am J Hum Genet* 1999; **65**: 508–518.
68. Kato T, Stine OC, McMahon FJ, Crowe RR. Increased levels of a mitochondrial DNA deletion in the brain of patients with bipolar disorder. *Biol Psychiatry* 1997; **42**: 871–875.
69. Konradi C, Eaton M, MacDonald ML et al. Molecular evidence for mitochondrial dysfunction in bipolar disorder. *Arch Gen Psychiatry* 2004; **61**: 300–308.
70. Washizuka S, Kakiuchi C, Mori K et al. Association of mitochondrial complex I subunit gene *NDUFV2* at 18p11 with bipolar disorder. *Am J Med Genet* 2003; **120B**: 72–78.
71. Washizuka S, Iwamoto K, Kazuno A et al. Association of mitochondrial complex I subunit gene *NDUFV2* at 18p11 with bipolar disorder in Japanese and National Institute of Mental Health pedigrees. *Biol Psychiatry* 2004; **56**: 483–489.
72. Nakatani N, Aburatani H, Nishimura K et al. Comprehensive expression analysis of a rat depression model. *Pharmacogenomics* 2004; **4**: 114–126.
73. McMahon FJ, Chen YS, Patel SD et al. Mitochondrial DNA sequence diversity in bipolar affective disorders. *Am J Psychiatry* 2000; **157**: 1058–1064.
74. Kegeles LS, Humaran TJ, Mann JJ. In vivo neurochemistry of the brain in schizophrenia as revealed by magnetic resonance spectroscopy. *Biol Psychiatry* 1998; **44**: 382–398.
75. Kung L, Roberts RC. Mitochondrial pathology in human schizophrenic striatum: a postmortem ultrastructural study. *Synapse* 1999; **31**: 67–75.
76. Cavelier L, Jazin EE, Eriksson I et al. Decreased cytochrome-*c*-oxidase activity and lack of age-related accumulation of mitochondrial DNA deletions in the brains of schizophrenics. *Genomics* 1995; **29**: 217–224.
77. Lindholm E, Cavalier L, Howell WM et al. Mitochondrial sequence variants in patients with schizophrenia. *Eur J Hum Genet* 1997; **5**: 406–412.
78. Whatley SA, Curti D, Marchbanks RM. Mitochondrial involvement in schizophrenia and other functional psychoses. *Neurochem Res* 1996; **21**: 995–1004.
79. Ben-Shachar D. Mitochondrial dysfunction in schizophrenia: a possible linkage to dopamine. *J Neurochem* 2002; **83**: 1241–1251.
80. Ben-Shachar D, Zuk R, Gazawi H, Ljubuncic P. Dopamine toxicity involves mitochondrial complex I inhibition: implications to dopamine-related neuropsychiatric disorders. *Biochem Pharmacol* 2004; **67**: 1965–1974.
81. Karry R, Klein E, Ben-Shachar D. Mitochondrial complex I subunits expression is altered in schizophrenia: a postmortem study. *Biol Psychiatry* 2004; **55**: 676–684.
82. Iwamoto K, Bundo M, Kato T. Altered expression of mitochondria-related genes in postmortem brains of patients with bipolar disorder or schizophrenia, as revealed by large-scale microarray analysis. *Hum Mol Genet* 2005; **14**: 241–253.
83. Munakata K, Iwamoto K, Bundo M, Kato T. Mitochondrial DNA 3243A$\rightarrow$G mutation and increased expression of *LARS2* gene in the brains of patients with bipolar disorder and schizophrenia. *Biol Psychiatry* 2005; **57**: 525–532.
84. Chugani DC, Sundram BS, Behen M et al. Evidence of altered energy metabolism in autistic children. *Prog Neuro-Psychopharmacol Biol Psychiat* 1999; **23**: 635–641.
85. Friedman SD, Shaw DW, Artru AA et al. Regional brain chemical alterations in young children with autism spectrum disorder. *Neurology* 2003; **60**: 100–107.
86. Drevets WC. Neuroimaging studies of mood disorders. *Biol Psychiatry* 2000; **48**: 813–829.
87. Mayberg HS, Liotti M, Brannan SK et al. Reciprocal limbic-cortical function and negative mood: converging PET findings in depression and normal sadness. *Am J Psychiatry* 1999; **156**: 675–682.
88. Milak MS, Parsey RV, Keilp J et al. Neuroanatomical correlates of psychopathological

components of major depressive disorders. *Arch Gen Psychiatry* 2005; **62**: 397–408.
89. Anderson A, Oquendo MA, Parsey RV et al. Regional brain responses to serotonin in major depressive disorder. *J Affect Disord* 2004; **82**: 411–417.
90. Hastings RS, Parsey RV, Oquendo MA et al. Volumetric analysis of the prefrontal cortex, amygdala, and hippocampus in major depression. *Neuropsychopharmacology* 2004; **29**: 952–959.
91. Lochhead RA, Oquendo MA, Mann JJ, Parsey RV. Regional brain gray matter volume differences in bipolar disorder patients as assessed by optimized voxel-based morphometry. *Biol Psychiatry* 2004; **55**: 1154–1162.

13

Mitochondrial dysfunction and neurodegenerative disorders

Kim Tieu and Serge Przedborski

Introduction

Neurodegenerative disorders represent a large group of diseases with heterogeneous clinical and pathological expressions characterized by the demise of specific subsets of neurons within restricted anatomical areas of the nervous system.[1] As discussed in detail elsewhere,[1] neurodegenerative disorders typically arise for unknown reasons, progress in a relentless manner, and their incidence increases markedly with age. Currently, hundreds of different neurodegenerative disorders have been recognized, including Alzheimer's disease (AD), Parkinson's disease (PD), Huntington's disease (HD), and amyotrophic lateral sclerosis (ALS), to cite some of the most prevalent and publicized ones.

Until now, both the causes and the mechanisms of neuronal death in many of these disorders have remained uncertain. Relevant to the subject of this book, however, is the speculation that a large number of neurodegenerative disorders might be linked to mitochondrial dysfunction. In some of these diseases, impaired mitochondrial function has been proposed as the primary molecular cause of neuronal death, while in others, it probably represents a secondary pathogenic event which arises in compromised neurons and which ultimately contributes to their demise. At first glance, it may appear perplexing that mitochondrial dysfunction would lead to so many disparate neurological diseases. However, when one thinks about the pivotal roles of mitochondria in cellular homeostasis and survival,[2] it becomes more plausible that functional impairment of these organelles may have dramatic consequences and may be implicated in a host of neurodegenerative situations. A quick survey of the literature on mitochondrial dysfunction in neurodegenerative diseases shows that these disorders can be divided into three categories: diseases linked to mitochondrial gene mutations; neurodegenerative diseases linked to mutations in nuclear genes encoding mitochondrial proteins; and neurodegenerative disorders linked to mutations in non-mitochondrial proteins or with unknown causes.

This chapter is organized into three parts. The first deals with specific biological aspects of the mitochondrion that are relevant to common features of neurodegenerative diseases. The second part is a systematic review of the three aforementioned categories of mitochondrial neurodegenerative diseases. The final part discusses the mechanisms by which neurons may die in these mitochondrial neurodegenerative diseases.

Mitochondrial biology and neurodegeneration

Besides the nucleus, the mitochondrion is the only other organelle in the cell that possesses its own DNA and genetic machinery. All mitochondrial DNAs (mtDNAs) of a zygote originate from the ovum. The latter point has led to the traditional view that diseases linked to mtDNA mutations are maternally inherited: mothers (not fathers) who carry mtDNA mutations pass them to the children, and then only the daughters may pass them to their children. Rarely, however, has a maternal inheritance been suspected in classical neurodegenerative diseases.[3] Instead, familial forms of neurodegenerative diseases are typically transmitted as simple Mendelian traits. Furthermore, most neurodegenerative diseases are sporadic. Thus, if genetic factors do contribute to their development, it is either as susceptibility genes or mutations that confer hypersensitivity to specific environmental factors.[4,5]

Because mtDNA encodes only for polypeptide subunits of the respiratory chain, all pathogenic mtDNA mutations affect oxidative phosphorylation. The nervous system and its cellular constituent, neurons, are highly dependent on oxidative phosphorylation. Thus, CNS and neurons are especially vulnerable to the effect of mtDNA mutations. The retina, renal tubules, and endocrine glands also have high oxidative metabolism demands and are also high-risk targets in typical mitochondrial cytopathy. It is thus not surprising that mitochondrial diseases are usually multisystemic.[2] This situation, again, is in striking contrast with most neurodegenerative diseases, which are typically pure neurological disorders.

There are thousands of mtDNAs in each cell, with about five mtDNAs per mitochondrion, and in patients, a pathogenic mitochondrial mutation may be present in some, but not in all, mtDNAs. This mixture of mutated and wild-type mtDNA (heteroplasmy) can vary greatly among patients, organs and even cells. In addition, replication of mtDNA occurs constantly in all cells, even in postmitotic, non-dividing cells such as neurons (relaxed replication), and upon cell division, the mitochondria are partitioned randomly among daughter cells (mitotic segregation). Over time, the proportion of mutated mtDNA in tissues may change, influencing the expression of the disease. Specific nuclear factors can also influence mitochondrial segregation,[6] supporting a role for nuclear–mitochondrial interactions in determining the degree of heteroplasmy. That said, it is important to remember that a minimal proportion of mutated mtDNA is required before an oxidative phosphorylation deficit occurs and symptoms arise (threshold effect), and that – as a general rule – the higher the proportion of mutated mtDNA, the more severe the phenotype of the diseases. Collectively, the mitochondrial characteristics mentioned above might provide an explanation for some of the peculiar features of neurodegenerative disorders, including the heterogeneous phenotypic expression, the consistent adult-onset, and the progressive nature of these neurological disorders.

Mitochondrial neurodegenerative diseases

Mitochondrial dysfunction in neurodegenerative diseases linked to mitochondrial gene mutations

The human mtDNA is a 16.6-kilobase circle of double-stranded DNA that comprises 37 genes. Of these, 13 encode for polypeptides of the respiratory chain whereas two are transcribed to ribosomal RNAs (rRNAs) and 22 are transcribed to transfer RNAs (tRNAs) which are required for the synthesis of the 13 respiratory subunit proteins. These include seven subunits of complex I (NADH dehydrogenase 1, 2, 3, 4, 4L, 5, 6), one subunit of complex III (cytochrome *b*), three subunits of complex IV (COX I, II, and III), and two subunits of

Box 13.1 The biogenesis of iron–sulfur clusters

Iron–sulfur clusters are among the most ancient of proteins, because they evolved to perform a number of critical functions, most notably electron transfer (i.e. redox regulation). In particular, the electron transport chain contains a number of FeS-containing subunits that are required for the electron flow through the chain. What is particulary notable is that the biogenesis and maturation of FeS clusters requires the obligate participation of mitochondria. It is for this reason that the proteins associated with FeS cluster metabolism are found in mitochondria from every species examined. Also, in spite of the fact that most eukaryotic FeS proteins are mitochondrial (for example, aconitase, and some subunits of respiratory complexes I, II, and III), FeS synthesis requires extra-mitochondrial maturation proteins (Figure B13.1.1).[1] Conversely, biosynthesis of extramitochondrial FeS proteins (e.g. iron regulatory protein 1 and glutamate synthase) requires a mitochondrial membrane potential and involves a host of mitochondrial proteins (Figure B13.1.1).

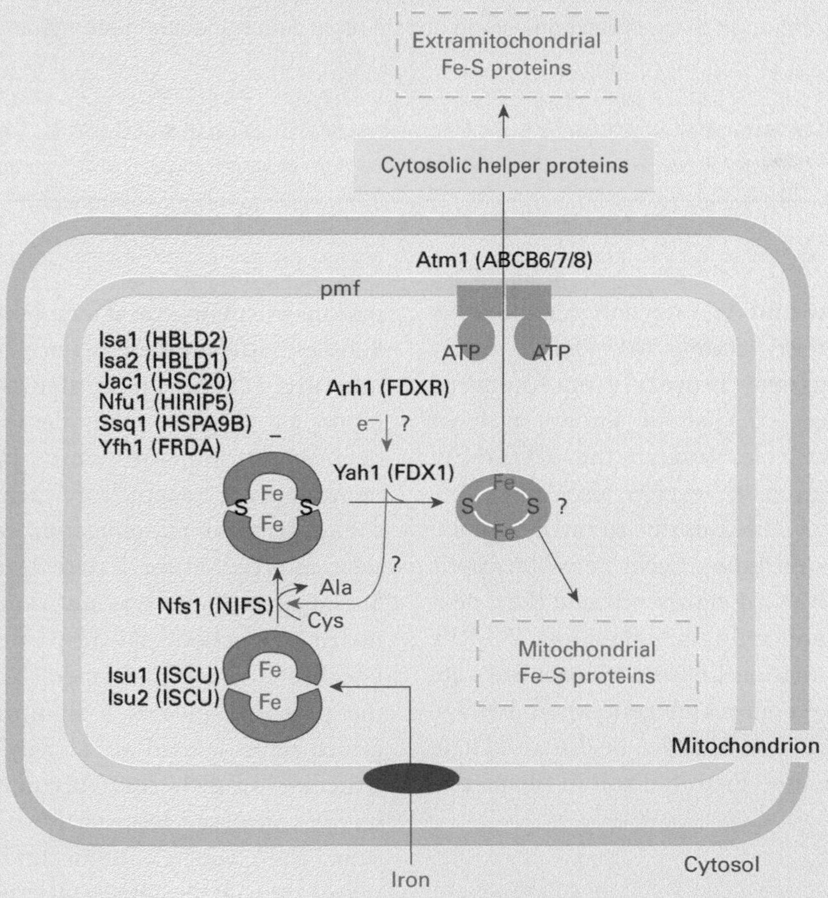

Figure B13.1.1 Proteins associated with Fe–S cluster biogenesis. Shown are the yeast proteins and their human orthologs (in parentheses). Adapted from reference 1, with permission

(Continued)

Box 13.1 (Continued)

In bacteria, two operons are required for FeS biosynthesis, the *nif* (nitrogen fixation) and *isc* (iron–sulfur cluster) operons. The *nif* operon encodes proteins required for the formation of the FeS cluster present in nitrogenase (a metalloenzyme), while the *isc* operon encodes proteins necessary for the maturation of many bacterial FeS proteins. In eukaryotes, the mitochondrial ISC machinery is responsible for biogenesis of iron–sulfur proteins both inside and outside the organelle.

Of importance clinically is the fact that mutations in two FeS proteins cause human disease. There are three human ABC (ATP Binding Cassette) orthologs of Atm1p (ABC transporter of mitochondria): ABCB6, ABCB7, and ABCB8. Mutations in ABCB7 cause X-linked sideroblastic anemia and ataxia, in which affected cells contain mitochondria harboring deposits of iron ('ring sideroblasts'). Since Atm1p/ABCB7 is required to transport mature FeS clusters from the mitochondria to the cytosol (see Figure B13.1.1), defects in transport most likely cause the FeS clusters to accumulate within the organelle – hence the ring sideroblasts. Mutations in frataxin (FRDA), the human ortholog of Yfh1p (yeast frataxin homolog), cause Friedreich ataxia, a neurodegenerative disease associated with aberrant iron handling within mitochondria, although there is currently some debate regarding the actual pathogenetic mechanism.

Reference

1. Lill R, Kispal G. Maturation of cellular Fe-S proteins: an essential function of mitochondria. *Trends Biochem Sci* 2000; **25**: 352–356.

ATP synthase (A6 and A8). Any mtDNA mutation (including deletion) leading to a defect in any of these proteins may provoke a mitochondrial disease. A complete list of known mtDNA mutations is available through the MITOMAP database (www.mitomap.org) (see also Appendix). Among the diverse diseases due to mtDNA mutation, only a few – including Leber hereditary optic neuropathy (LHON), Leigh syndrome (LS), neuropathy, ataxia and retinitis pigmentosa (NARP), and 12SrRNA mutation-linked parkinsonism – are linked to selective neuronal degeneration. LHON, LS, and NARP will not, however, be discussed here because they are described in detail in Chapters 2 and 5.

12SrRNA mutation-linked parkinsonism

In the mid-1990s, Shoffner and collaborators found that a point mutation (A1555G) in the *12SrRNA* gene cosegregated with maternally inherited deafness and levodopa-responsive parkinsonism in several members of one kindred.[7] Subsequently, another heteroplasmic, maternally inherited *12SrRNA* point mutation (T1095C) was found in another pedigree with sensorineural deafness, levodopa-responsive parkinsonism, and neuropathy.[8] Except for early onset, parkinsonism in these patients appeared similar to that seen in PD. Serum lactate levels were normal, but muscle biopsy was not done. Spectrophotometric mitochondrial respiratory chain assays performed in transformed lymphoblasts from the proband showed a significant reduction in cytochrome *c* oxidase activity. The secondary structure predicts that this mutation disrupts a highly conserved loop in the small subunit ribosomal RNA, which is important in the initiation of mitochondrial protein synthesis. These findings led to the conclusion that this mutation was pathogenic and caused an oxidative phosphorylation defect by interfering with mitochondrial protein synthesis. This mutation was not found, however, in 20 cases of sporadic PD, suggesting that the

12SrRNA mutation is not likely to be a common cause of PD.

Mitochondrial dysfunction in neurodegenerative diseases linked to mutations in nuclear genes encoding for proteins targeted to mitochondria

The mitochondrion comprises about 12 000 polypeptides encoded by nuclear DNA (nDNA) in addition to the 13 encoded by mtDNA. Of these, about 75 are structural components of the respiratory chain, and about 60 others are needed for its proper assembly and functioning. Thus, certain mutations, which affect genes that encode for mitochondrial proteins, can cause oxidative phosphorylation defects just as classical mtDNA mutation would do. LS, for instance, may arise not only from mtDNA mutations, but also from a variety of nDNA mutations affecting any one of the respiratory chain complexes.[9] Many other nDNA mutations do not affect the respiratory chain directly, but still produce mitochondrial dysfunction, thereby giving rise to an entirely distinct class of mitochondrial neurodegenerative diseases from that discussed above. Among this singular group of diseases, one finds Friedreich's ataxia, hereditary spastic paraplegia, the deafness-dystonia syndrome, and Wilson's disease. In many of these genetic neurodegenerative diseases, as we will find below, the products of the mutated nuclear genes fail to carry out their normal function, which involve various aspects of the mitochondrial physiology.

Friedreich's ataxia

Friedreich's ataxia (FRDA) is an autosomal-recessive mitochondrial disorder with clinical manifestations of progressive limb and gait ataxia, peripheral neuropathy, and areflexia.[10] Pathologically, FRDA is characterized by degeneration of the spinocerebellar tracts and large sensory neurons, along with hypertrophic cardiomyopathy and increased incidence of diabetes.[11] The disease gene has been mapped to 9q13 and encodes for a 210 amino-acid protein called frataxin. This protein is synthesized in the cytoplasm as a large precursor with an *N*-terminal presequence that targets frataxin to the mitochondrial matrix.[12] Frataxin precursor is then processed into a roughly 17-kDa mature protein by the mitochondrial processing peptidase.[13]

Most FRDA patients are homozygous for a GAA trinucleotide repeat expansion in the first intron of the *frataxin* gene,[14] which hampers its transcription.[15] Studies in a knock-in mouse with 230 GAA repeat expansion introduced into the *frataxin* gene exhibited merely 25% reduction in frataxin expression,[16] suggesting that very long repeats are probably needed to recapitulate the transcriptional defect observed in FRDA patients. This interpretation is consistent with the fact that FRDA is typically caused by large GAA repeat expansion (up to 1700 repeats).[17] Some patients carry compound heterozygote mutations, in that they have a GAA expansion on one allele and a truncating or missense mutation on the other allele.[18] In these patients, the clinical expression ranges from typical FRDA to a much milder phenotype, depending on the point mutation.[18] This observation suggests that not all point mutations affect *frataxin* transcription to the same extent, and consequently the defect in frataxin expression may be quite different among compound heterozygote patients.

Similar to other neurodegenerative disorders, FRDA overt pathology appears confined to specific regions of the brain and the heart, although frataxin is expressed in all tissues.[14] In addition, frataxin seems vital as its ablation, at least in rodents, is embryonically lethal.[19] It is thus not surprising to observe that patients with FRDA exhibit low (4–29% of normal levels) but not null expression of frataxin,[15] and that the level of residual frataxin expression correlates with the severity of the disease phenotype.[15] However, as stressed by Badhwar and collaborators,[20] the phenotype, even within the same family, cannot always be predicted from the repeat length, as factors such as somatic mosaicism and repeat interruptions may impact on the expression of the disease.

The exact function of frataxin remains uncertain. It is noteworthy that FRDA patients exhibit specific deficits in the enzymatic activities of iron–sulfur proteins such as aconitase and complexes I, II, and III.[21] In theory, the loss of iron–sulfur protein activity may be caused by either oxidative damage to labile iron–sulfur clusters (ISCs) or to alteration of the ISC biosynthesis, which occurs within mitochondria through a well-conserved ISC machinery (Box 13.1).[22] Although some studies suggest a role for frataxin in the antioxidant signaling pathway,[23] others suggest that frataxin is involved in iron–sulfur protein biosynthesis. The latter hypothesis appears compelling in light of several observations. First, the synthesis of ISCs is decreased in isolated mitochondria and in mitochondrial extracts from frataxin-deficient or conditionally frataxin-depleted yeast.[24,25] Second, human frataxin binds iron ions and mediates the transfer of the bound iron to the iron–sulphur scaffold proteins Isu,[26] which are essential in the formation of ISC.[21] Third, yeast frataxin is part of a multiprotein complex comprising Isu1p and the Nfs1p cysteine desulfurase.[27]

Defects in the synthesis of iron–sulfur proteins are known to alter mitochondrial iron homeostasis and to cause an excess of intramitochondrial iron.[28] Likewise, mutations in the yeast homolog of frataxin, Yfh1p, lead to a massive increase in mitochondrial iron concentrations.[12] However, animal studies showed that impaired iron–sulfur protein activities arose prior to any detectable intramitochondrial iron accumulation,[29] suggesting that an alteration in mitochondrial iron metabolism in FRDA patients is likely the consequence and not the cause for the ISC defect. Nevertheless, we cannot exclude that, once it occurs, accumulation of intramitochondrial iron would promote local oxidative stress, and thereby exacerbate the mitochondrial defect found in FRDA patients. It is important, however, to stress the fact that while high intramitochondrial iron accumulation is well documented in FRDA cells, the nature of this iron, i.e. reactive (also called labile or chelatable iron) or unreactive, remains unclear. For instance, Sturm et al. have found no evidence of higher chelatable iron in fibroblasts from FRDA patients compared to controls, despite their elevated total mitochondrial iron content.[30] Should the latter observation be confirmed, it would then be unlikely that the excess of intramitochondrial iron in FRDA cells would contribute to a local oxidative stress.

If, as discussed above, the exact role played by intramitochondrial iron accumulation in FRDA is still believed to be instrumental in the pathogenesis of this illness, then, as such, it is not surprising to find that iron chelators and antioxidants have been intensively tested in these patients. Desferrioxamine and deferiprone have been tried to reduce intracellular iron, with questionable effects. Serum iron and ferritin concentrations are normal in FRDA patients and desferrioxamine is not lipophilic enough to permeate mitochondria.[31] Also, this compound cannot efficiently mobilize iron from iron-loaded mitochondria.[32] Additional concerns with deferiprone include its potential to cause liver fibrosis[33] and its lack of metal selectivity. Another group of iron chelators, the 2-pyridylcarboxaldehyde isonicotinoyl hydrazone analogs, has been designed to specifically target mitochondrial iron pools and is currently being assessed for use in therapies for FRDA.[34] Using the same strategy, the antioxidant mitoquinone (MitoQ) has been synthesized by linking ubiquinone to a lipophilic triphenylphosphonium cation.[35] In fibroblasts from FRDA patients, MitoQ conferred protection against endogenous oxidative stress induced by inhibition of glutathione synthesis.[36] Idebenone, an antioxidant short-chain analog of coenzyme Q10, inhibits lipid peroxidation in rat brain mitochondria[37] and reduces urinary levels of a marker for oxidative DNA damage in FRDA patients.[38] In separate clinical trials, idebenone was found to reduce myocardial hypertrophy.[39–41] Other antioxidants, such as coenzyme Q10 and vitamin E, have also been evaluated for the treatment of FRDA. The results of their efficacy, however, have been conflicting.[42]

Hereditary spastic paraplegia

The term hereditary spastic paraplegia (HSP) describes a heterogeneous group of inherited neurodegenerative disorders in which the primary clinical feature is progressive bilateral spasticity and weakness in lower limbs.[43] Urinary urgency is also a common symptom. When these symptoms occur in isolation, HSP is called uncomplicated or pure, whereas when the symptoms occur in association with additional neurological abnormalities, such as mental retardation, extrapyramidal symptoms, deafness and optic neuropathy, the HSP is called complicated. Onset of symptoms usually is in childhood or early adulthood.[43]

Familial HSPs are most often transmitted as autosomal dominant traits and less commonly as autosomal or X-linked recessive traits.[43] Nine HSP genes and 27 HSP loci have been identified.[44,45] The few autopsy studies available show that the neuropathology of HSP is characterized by axonal degeneration in the corticospinal tract and the fasciculus gracilis without overt cell body loss. The pathogenesis of HSP is also poorly understood, but various molecular mechanisms have been proposed.[45] Patients with the recessive form of HSP are characterized by mutations in the *SPG7* gene, which encodes for the mitochondrial targeted protein paraplegin.[46] Paraplegin is a metalloprotease whose yeast homologs are Yta10p and Yta12p.[47] These proteins belong to a large family of ATPases that includes the ATPase associated with the diverse cellular activities (AAA) domain.[48,49] In yeast, multiple copies of Yta10p and Yta12p combine to form a high-molecular-weight complex located in the inner membrane of the mitochondria.[47] It is believed that this Yta10p/Yta12p complex mediates the ATP-dependent degradation of the mitochondrial inner membrane proteins,[47] and, by analogy, paraplegin is thought to play the same role in vertebrates. The pathogenic mutations in paraplegin are likely abrogating this function and thus may lead to accumulation of unwanted mitochondrial proteins in HSP patients, which, in turn, may cause mitochondrial dysfunction. Although highly speculative, this scenario is consistent with the demonstration that muscle biopsies obtained from some HSP patients show signs of mitochondrial dysfunction, such as cytochrome *c* oxidase-deficient fibers and ragged-red or ragged-blue (intensely SDH-positive) fibers.[46] In a paraplegin-deficient mouse model harboring a mutated *SPG7* gene, electron microscopy shows abnormal mitochondria in synaptic terminals and distal axons, a change that occurs prior to the appearance of axonal swelling and degeneration.[50] The massive accumulation of organelles and neurofilaments in the swollen axons suggest that the HSP-related mitochondrial dysfunction impairs the anterograde axonal transport (Box 13.2). In addition to paraplegin, a mutation in another mitochondrial protein, the chaperone heat shock protein 60 (Hsp60 or chaperonin), has also been identified in some patients with autosomal dominant HSP (SPG13).[51] This study supports the notion that, in addition to the loss of mitochondrial protease activity, the loss of mitochondrial chaperones may also produce a HSP phenotype.[52] However, the involvement of some sort of mitochondrial dysfunction in HSP pathogenesis is not always obvious. For instance, mutations in spastin, another AAA ATPase, are the most common cause of autosomal dominant HSP,[53] and seem to provoke the disease by impairing microtubule metabolism[54] via a mechanism whose link to a mitochondrial defect could not be readily established.

Treatments of HSP remain largely supportive at this moment. To reduce muscle spasticity, muscle

Box 13.2 Mitochondrial fusion, fission, and movement

Mitochondria are not the static entities that we see in textbooks. They are highly plastic, with shapes that vary from small spheres (~1 μm in diameter) to highly elongated spaghetti-like structures. They can exist as linear 'strings' or as highly branched, reticular structures, and they can fuse and divide. Thus, mitochondrial morphology is influenced to a large degree by the balance between these two processes.[1] In yeast, three proteins are required for organellar fission: Dnm1p (dynamin-related protein; in the yeast nomenclature, the 'p' indicates the protein product (e.g. Dnm1p) encoded by the gene (e.g. *DNM1*)), Fis1p (fission-related protein), and Mdv1p (mitochondrial division protein) (Figure B13.2.1). Two others are required for organelle fusion: Fzo1p (the yeast homolog of the *Drosophila* 'fuzzy onions' protein) and Ugo1P (ugo is Japanese for 'fusion').

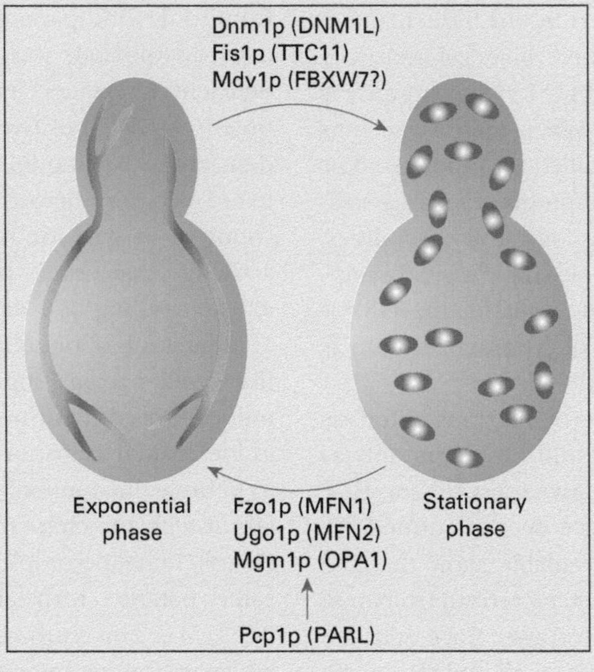

Figure B13.2.1 Proteins associated with mitochondrial fusion and fission in yeast. Human orthologs of the yeast proteins are in parentheses. Adapted from reference 1, with permission

All five proteins are located in the mitochondrial outer membrane, but this raises a problem: the mitochondrion has two membranes (MOM and MIM), and presumably the inner membrane has to fuse/divide coordinately with the outer membrane in order for the entire organelle to fuse/divide. Recently, inroads have been made into the solution of this problem. It turns out that Mgm1p (mitochondrial genome maintenance protein) is a fission-related protein that spans both the outer and inner membranes (Figure B13.2.2), and the current idea is that, in fact, the MOM and MIM are 'pinched' together to form 'contact sites' at the point of division, presumably mediated by Mgm1p. A particularly noteworthy aspect of Mgm1p function is that it is a 'processed' protein: it is imported into the mitochondrion as a 'long' form (L-Mgm1p), which is anchored in the inner membrane, but is then processed into a 'short' form (S-Mgm1p) by a protease called Pcp1p (so-called because it also processes cytochrome c peroxidase), which releases the MIM-bound tail of L-Mgm1p and allows S-Mgm1p, now free in the intermembrane space, presumably to bind Ugo1p.[2] However, recent data also implicate Mgm1p, together with Tim11p (human ATP5I), a non-catalytic subunit of ATP synthase, in the formation of cristae (the invaginated folds of the inner membrane).[3]

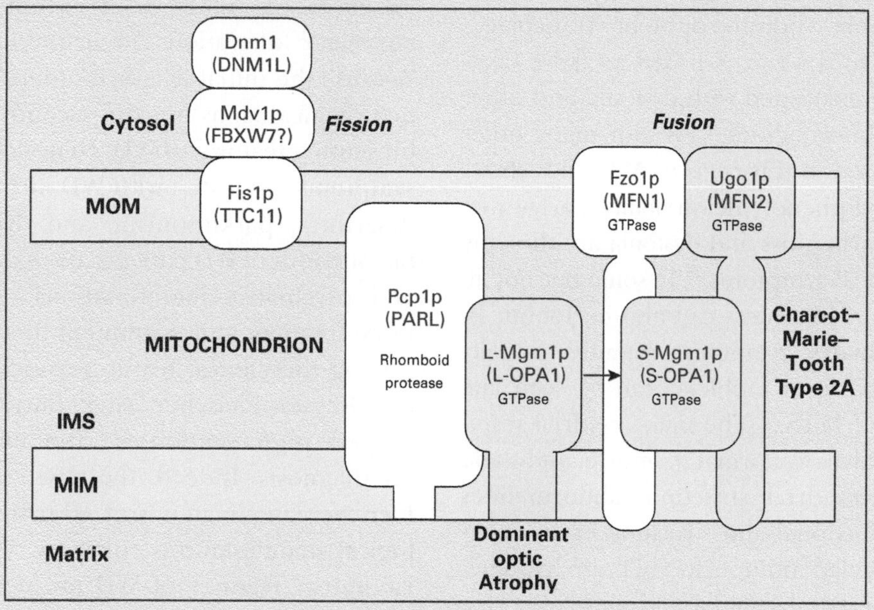

Figure B13.2.2 Location of mitochondrial fission and fusion proteins. Note that mutations in two of these proteins – OPA1 and MFN2 – cause neurodegenerative diseases in humans

Remarkably, mutations in the human orthologs of both Mgm1p (OPA1) and Ugo1p (MFN2) cause human neurodegenerative diseases. Mutations in OPA1 cause dominant optic atrophy or DOA (hence the name OPA1),[4] and mutations in MFN2 (mitofusin 2) cause Charcot–Marie–Tooth disease, type 2A.[5] The reason why an error in organellar fusion should cause these disorders is the subject of much research, but it is already known that mitochondria in DOA cells have aberrant subcellular localization, implying that organellar fusion and fission is somehow connected to organellar mobility.

References

1. Yaffe MP. The cutting edge of mitochondrial fusion. *Nat Cell Biol* 2003; **5**: 497–499.
2. Sesaki H, Jensen RE. Ugo1p links the Fzo1p and Mgm1p GTPases for mitochondrial fusion. *J Biol Chem* 2004; **279**: 28298–28303.
3. Amutha B, Gordon DM, Gu Y, Pain D. A novel role of Mgm1p, a dynamin-related GTPase, in ATP synthase assembly and cristae formation/maintenance. *Biochem J* 2004; **381**: 19–23.
4. Delettre C, Lenaers G, Griffoin JM et al. Nuclear gene OPA1, encoding a mitochondrial dynamin-related protein, is mutated in dominant optic atrophy. *Nat Genet* 2000; **26**: 207–210.
5. Kijima K, Numakura C, Izumino H et al. Mitochondrial GTPase mitofusin 2 mutation in Charcot-Marie-Tooth neuropathy type 2A. *Hum Genet* 2005; **116**: 23–27.

relaxants such as baclofen, tizanidine, dantrolene, and botulinum toxin have been prescribed.[45] Oxybutynin may be used to alleviate urinary urgency.

Deafness-dystonia syndrome

Deafness-dystonia syndrome or Mohr–Tranebjaerg syndrome (MTS) is a rare X-linked recessive deafness syndrome associated with dystonia and other neurological abnormalities.[55] As with many other diseases discussed in this chapter, MTS also shows a high degree of phenotypic variability. Early-onset progressive hearing loss and dystonia are the only obligatory clinical symptoms.[55] In some but not all patients, cortical blindness can also be found. In addition, psychiatric symptoms, cognitive impairment, and behavioral problems can be seen late in the course of MTS.[55] The mitochondrial respiratory chain activity is normal in muscle, and there are no mitochondrial structural abnormalities (Box 13.3). Functional and structural brain imaging studies revealed multiple loci of brain hypometabolism in the basal ganglia and parietal cortex and marked atrophy of the occipital lobes.[55]

MTS is due to loss-of-function mutations in *TIMM8A*, a small gene on Xq22,[56] which encodes for a polypeptide of 97 amino acids named deafness-dystonia protein-1 (DDP1). Homology searches have shown that the DDP1 protein belongs to a family of proteins located in the mitochondrial intermembrane space.[57,58] In human mitochondria, DDP1 forms a multiprotein complex with Tim13,[59] which presumably stabilizes the precursors of hydrophobic inner membrane proteins during their translocation across the aqueous environment of the intermembrane space.[55]

Wilson disease

Hepatolenticular degeneration or Wilson disease (WD) is a rare familial disease whose mode of inheritance is autosomal-recessive and which is characterized by copper accumulation in a number of tissues.[60] Although WD is discussed here in the context of neurodegenerative diseases, the involvement of the nervous system invariably follows liver disease. Clinically, WD begins in most patients between the ages of 11 and 25 years. Liver manifestations range from asymptomatic hepatic enzymatic alterations to acute hepatic failure. Because the initial liver symptoms may be subtle, neurological signs are the second most frequent presenting features of WD. Neurological signs and symptoms associated with WD include dysphagia, dysarthria, parkinsonism, and dystonia.[60] Early on, one-fifth of WD patients also exhibit behavioral and psychiatric manifestations, which become more frequent and prominent in advanced cases. Among the clinical features associated with WD, the Kayser–Fleischer ring (intracorneal ring-shaped pigmentation) is the most important for diagnosis. Indeed, the absence of a Kayser–Fleischer ring in an untreated patient with neurological manifestations rules out WD. The main laboratory features of WD are decreased serum copper and ceruloplasmin levels together with increased urinary copper excretion.[60] Biopsies also show prominent copper deposits in kidney and liver associated with foci of tissue necrosis.[60] MRI studies, though useful, show non-specific abnormalities, such as ventricular dilatation and diffuse atrophy of the cortex, cerebellum, and brainstem.[60] From a therapeutic point of view, both asymptomatic and symptomatic WD patients must be treated. The goal of treatment is to remove the toxic accumulation of copper in tissues and to prevent its re-accumulation. Accordingly, copper chelators such as penicillamine or triethylene tetramine dihydrochloride are used. Agents that reduce copper digestive absorption such as tetrathiomolybdate and zinc are also used. Thanks to these therapeutic strategies, the survival of WD patients who have completed the first few years of treatment is comparable to that of the healthy population.

The disease is caused by mutations in the *ATP7B* gene, which encodes for a copper-transporting P-type ATPase.[61] Loss of function of this gene results in an accumulation of copper primarily in the liver, kidney, and brain; in the latter, the basal ganglia are especially involved. Abnormal copper accumulation in tissues and liver changes resembling cirrhosis are seen in knockout mice for the *ATP7B* gene,[62] thus confirming the pathogenic role of the ATP7B mutations in WD. ATP7B exists in two isoforms, a 159-kDa form that localizes to the transgolgi network, and a 140-kDa form that localizes to mitochondria.[63] The mitochondrial localization of the 140-kDa isoform suggests that ATP7B may participate in the delivery of copper to copper-containing enzymes, such as cytochrome *c* oxidase. Presumably, mitochondria in affected tissues exhibit morphological abnormalities, as well as a deficiency of liver mitochondrial enzymes, especially complex I and aconitase.[64] However, ATP7B is present in multiple subcellular compartments, raising the possibility that mitochondrial dysfunction in WD may be the consequence, rather than the cause, of the disease.

Mitochondrial dysfunction in neurodegenerative disorders linked to mutations in non-mitochondrial proteins and in neurodegenerative disorders with unknown causes

This section is by far the most controversial as an unequivocal mitochondrial etiology has not been documented for any of the diseases to be discussed here. Still, for all these diseases the possibility of a mitochondrial link has been raised and has received much attention within the scientific and clinical communities. It is our opinion, however, that most data supporting mitochondrial involvement are circumstantial or indirect. Thus, whether mitochondrial involvement in neurodegenerative diseases such as HD, AD, or PD is a myth or a reality remains to be elucidated.

Huntington's disease

Huntington's disease (HD) is a progressive neurodegenerative disorder characterized by chorea, psychiatric disturbances and a decline in cognitive function. Symptoms usually begin in the fourth or fifth decade of life and worsen rapidly thereafter. Typically, the time from onset to death is about 18 years. HD is an autosomal dominant disease caused by the expansion of a trinucleotide CAG repeat that encodes the non-essential amino acid glutamine in exon 1 of the *IT15* gene on chromosome 4.[65] The normal range of CAG repeats – and thus of the glutamine tail in the encoded protein called huntingtin – is between six and 35. The age at onset is inversely correlated to the length of the repeat, but apparently not to the severity or the rate of progression.[66] Environmental factors, however, also seem to play a major role in the pathogenesis of HD, as demonstrated in animal models[67,68] and in HD patients.[69] Pathologically, there is a selective neurodegeneration of medium spiny neurons in the striatum. Nuclear inclusions of protein aggregates are also a common feature in the striatum and cortex.

Twelve years after the discovery of the HD mutation,[65] the normal function of huntingtin is still unknown and the pathogenic mechanism leading to neurodegeneration in HD is elusive. Nonetheless, a defect in bioenergics has been proposed as a major pathogenic factor. Positron emission tomography studies with [^{18}F]-fluorodeoxyglucose have demonstrated a marked reduction in glucose utilization in the caudate and putamen of HD patients.[70] This hypometabolism precedes the detection of striatal atrophy, indicating that cell death occurs after metabolic impairment.[70,71] These results also suggest a dysfunction in nerve terminals since they are the sites of the greatest energy consumption by ATP-dependent pumps to restore ionic gradients following synaptic transmission.[72] The early damage to the terminals in HD is consistent with findings that various types of

Box 13.3 Mitochondrial protein importation

Of the thousands of genes presumably present in the endosymbiotic 'proto-mitochondrion', only a handful remain today in human mtDNA, and these are all associated with oxidative energy production. Where did the rest go? They were either lost, because they were unnecessary for the survival of the organelle as an endosymbiont, or they were retained by the host and incorporated into its nuclear DNA. Thus, many of these 'ancestral' genes, plus other 'newer' nuclear genes, not of direct proto-mitochondrial origin (more than 1200 in number), encode proteins that are now synthesized in the cytoplasm and are then imported into mitochondria. How do these 1200 proteins know that they are supposed to go into mitochondria?

Mitochondrial importation is a complex process, with different pathways for the targeting and sorting of polypeptides to the four compartments of the organelle (the outer and inner membranes, the intermembrane space, and the matrix). Interestingly, key components of the import machinery are members of the so-called 'heat shock' protein family. These are 'molecular chaperones' that help unfold, and then refold, the mitochondrially targeted polypeptides as they are inserted through the import receptors and are sorted to the appropriate compartments.

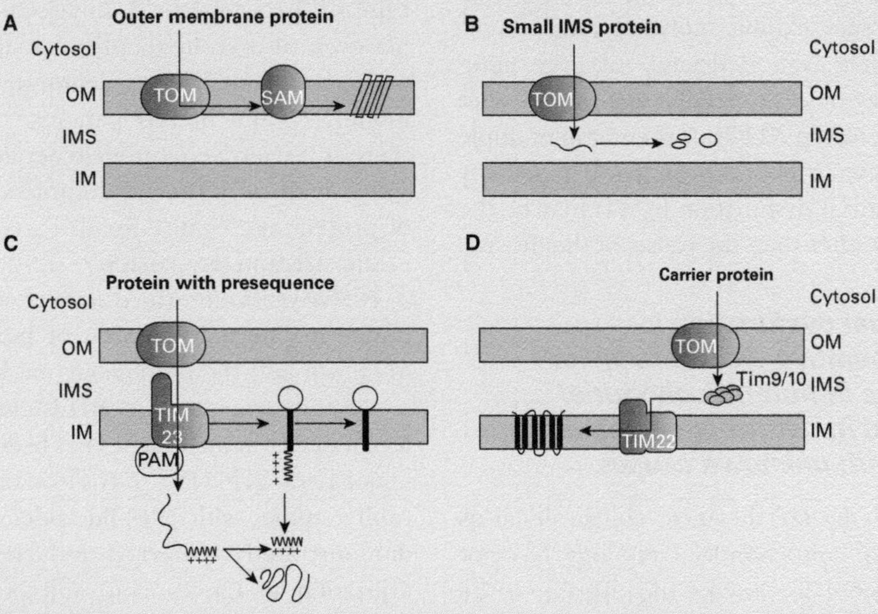

Figure B13.3.1 Mitochondrial importation pathways. (**A**) Precursors of β-barrel proteins are translocated by the TOM complex. Their subsequent insertion and assembly into the outer mitochondrial membrane requires the SAM complex. (**B**) After their passage through the TOM channel, soluble proteins destined for the intermembrane space are recognized by specific factors that assist in folding and assembly. (**C**) Mitochondrial proteins carrying cleavable presequences utilize the TOM and TIM23 complexes to be translocated into the mitochondrial matrix or to be sorted into the inner membrane. (**D**) After translocation through the TOM complex, carrier proteins are guided by the small Tim proteins across the intermembrane space to the TIM22 complex, which then mediates their insertion into the inner membrane. From reference 1, with permission

For most of them, this 'addressing' capability is accomplished by the presence of a mitochondrial 'targeting signal' located at the N-terminus of the polypeptide (although some have C-terminal and even 'internal' targeting sequences).[1,2] Once inside the organelle, the N-terminal 'mitochondrial targeting signal' (MTS), also called a 'leader peptide,' is cleaved to release the mature polypeptide. The leader sequence is usually highly basic (i.e. it contains many arginine and lysine residues, and few or no aspartate or glutamate residues), and it often contains peptide 'motifs' that determine the precise point of cleavage of the presequence inside the organelle. Almost all polypeptides destined for the matrix, and most destined for the inner membrane, have this type of MTS, to the point that there are a number of computer programs (IPSORT, Mitoprot, Predotar, Psort II, TargetP) that can predict with much success the probability that a polypeptide has such an MTS. A notable exception, however, is the 100 or so carriers and transporters, most located in the inner membrane. Some intermembrane space proteins have MTSs, but many do not; almost all outer membrane proteins have no recognizable MTS, and we still do not know what the targeting signals are in sufficient detail to be able to predict whether a protein is destined for that compartment.

In overview, the importation machinery consists of multi-subunit translocases that work in concert to parse out incoming polypeptides to the proper compartment. The translocase of the outer membrane (TOM) or inner membrane (TIM), in collaboration with Sorting and Assembly Machinery (SAM) proteins and the Presequence Translocation-associated Motor (PAM), directs polypeptides to the appropriate compartment, as shown in Figure B13.3.1.

References

1. Chacinska A, Rehling P. Moving proteins from the cytosol into mitochondria. *Biochem Soc Trans* 2004; **32**: 774–776.
2. Truscott KN, Brandner K, Pfanner N. Mechanisms of protein import into mitochondria. *Curr Biol* 2003; **13**: R326–R337.

neurotransmitter receptors are decreased in these patients[73,74] and in a transgenic mouse model of HD.[75] Because mitochondria are highly concentrated in nerve terminals,[76] these abnormalities could result from a mitochondrial dysfunction, and several lines of evidence are consistent with this idea. Muscle biopsies from HD patients show a reduced ratio of phosphocreatine to inorganic phosphate,[77] suggesting a build-up of precursor products due to decreased ATP production. Nuclear magnetic resonance spectroscopy shows elevated lactate levels in the cortex and basal ganglia of symptomatic HD patients,[78] indicating impairment of oxidative phosphorylation. In well-coupled mitochondria, a higher rate of oxygen consumption correlates with a higher rate of ATP production.[79] Polarography of mitochondria isolated from postmortem cortex and caudate of HD patients showed significant reductions in respiration.[80] This alteration is in agreement with the reduction in enzymatic activity of complexes II–III in these brain regions reported by others.[81,82] Complex II (succinate dehydrogenase) is a component common to both the tricarboxylic acid cycle and the electron transport chain. It catalyzes the oxidation of succinate to fumarate and transfers electrons to coenzyme Q. In animal models, inhibition of this enzyme by malonate or 3-nitropropionic acid (3-NP) produces striatal lesions similar to those seen in HD patients.[83] In these models, administrations of mitochondrial substrates such as creatine[84] and coenzyme Q[85] were neuroprotective, further reinforcing the hypothesis of a metabolic defect as a pathogenic mechanism of HD.

Despite a wealth of data showing mitochondrial abnormalities in HD, the link between mutated huntingtin and mitochondria is still largely speculative. Huntingtin is expressed ubiquitously in all brain cells and localized mostly in the cytoplasm and to a smaller extent, in the nucleus.[86] Yet, immuno-electron microscopy shows that the protein is also localized in the neuronal mitochondrial membrane[87] where it seems to accumulate at the level of the outer membrane.[88] Functionally, brain mitochondria from HD mice have a lower membrane potential and depolarize at lower calcium concentrations than mitochondria from wild-type mice.[87] It has therefore been proposed that mutant huntingtin either induces the opening of the mitochondrial permeability transition (MPT) pore or decreases the threshold for calcium to induce MPT pore opening.[88] Of note, the release of cytochrome *c* as a result of huntingtin-induced MPT pore opening is inhibited by cyclosporin A.[88] In addition, mutant huntingtin increases the vulnerability of a striatal cell line, created from Hdh Q111 mouse embryos, to the mitochondrial toxin 3-NP.[89] This latter study implies that individuals with mutated huntingtin would be more susceptible to environmental mitochondrial toxins. Lastly, mutated huntingtin can also affect mitochondrial function indirectly through transcription factors. Huntingtin binds to and modifies the activity of transcription factors such as TATA-binding protein, cAMP-responsive element-binding protein (CREB)-binding protein (CBP), specificity protein 1 (Sp1), and p53.[90,91] These factors regulate the transcription of some mitochondrial proteins involved in energy metabolism and apoptosis. For example, CREB activation has been shown to be involved in mitochondrial dysfunction.[92] Huntingtin can also alter the activity of transcription factors through histone acetylation, which is regulated by both histone acetyltransferase and histone deacetylases. Indeed, huntingtin binds to and reduces the activity of histone acetyltransferase. The reduction in acetylation of histones leads to alterations in chromatin structure, which, in turn, alters gene expression.[93] It is thus conceivable that mutated huntingtin can perturb mitochondrial function by interfering with the activities of transcription factors; however, a study of HD transgenic mouse has clearly shown that these transcription factors are not affected.[94] Alteration of mitochondrial function in HD can also be indirect, in that mutant huntingtin appears to impair axonal transport and, in so doing, the trafficking of organelles such as mitochondria.[95] This defect may be of pathogenic significance in HD since proper mitochondrial mobility has been linked to Ca^{2+} buffering and energy delivery to strategic subcellular sites of cells.[96]

Current therapeutic options for HD patients remain largely supportive. Nevertheless, major efforts are underway to find therapies that might delay or stop disease progression. Compounds that have been assessed in clinical trials and that are relevant to the mitochondrial hypothesis of HD include creatine and coenzyme Q10. Creatine, a mitochondrial 'energy-improving' compound, has been shown to prevent body weight loss and brain atrophy, improve motor performance, and extend life expectancy in HD animal models.[84,97–99] Coenzyme Q10, an electron carrier and a cofactor of the electron transport chain, also had similar protective effects in these animals.[85,100,101] The benefit of these compounds in animals, however, has not been replicated in human HD clinical trials.[102] Formation of protein aggregates has also been attributed to mitochondrial dysfunction. In keeping with this, administrations of Congo red intraperitoneally[103] and of trehalose orally[104] inhibited protein aggregation and improved motor performance and survival in HD transgenic mice, supporting a very contentious argument that proteinaceous intranuclear inclusions in HD are cytotoxic.

Alzheimer's disease

Alzheimer's disease (AD) is a progressive neurodegenerative disorder and the most common form of dementia in the elderly. AD is characterized by impairments in memory and cognition. Increasing age and genetic mutations are both risk factors for AD. About 5% of AD cases are inherited in an autosomal dominant manner. Mutations in genes encoding amyloid precursor protein (APP) or APP processing proteins presenilin-1 (PS1) or presenilin-2 (PS2) cause the familial forms of AD. The remaining cases of AD are sporadic and their etiology is unknown. In both familial and sporadic forms of AD, the neuropathology is characterized by loss of cholinergic neurons and depositions of extracellular amyloid plaques and intracellular neurofibrillary tangles in the hippocampus and cortex. It is still a matter of debate whether these aggregates are neurotoxic.

As with HD and PD, knowledge of the mutated genes has not clarified the pathogenesis of AD. Although the discoveries of mutated APP and presenilins have strengthened the theory that amyloid β peptide (Aβ) is the culprit, strong disagreement exists regarding the mechanism by which Aβ induces neurodegeneration. Although highly controversial, mitochondrial dysfunction has also been suggested as a pathogenic mechanism in AD. Several circumstantial facts support this concept. For instance, a number of positron emission tomography investigations have shown that energy metabolism in AD brains is reduced.[105,106] Functional magnetic resonance spectroscopy has also shown a decreased ratio of phosphocreatine to inorganic phosphate in the AD brain.[107,108] In agreement with these studies are the reports of decreased glucose utilization in skin fibroblasts[109] and of decreased activities of pyruvate dehydrogenase[110] and α-ketoglutarate dehydrogenase[111] in postmortem cortical tissue. In addition to these mitochondrial enzymes, the activity[112–114] and immunoreactivity[115,116] of cytochrome *c* oxidase is also reduced in the AD brain.

The mechanism by which mitochondrial dysfunction occurs in AD is unclear. The links between mitochondria and Aβ, PS1, and PS2 are still missing. Currently available transgenic animal models for AD[117] will potentially shed light on these missing links. For example, a confocal microscopy and immunogold electron microscopy study of transgenic mice overexpressing mutant Aβ has shown that Aβ is present in mitochondria.[118] This study has also shown that Aβ binds to another mitochondrial protein, Aβ-binding alcohol dehydrogenase (ABAD), leading to the generation of ROS, release of cytochrome *c* and DNA fragmentation in cultured neurons obtained from transgenic mice.[118] Prior to this study, Aβ had been shown to inhibit mitochondrial respiration in isolated mitochondria.[119] Collectively, these studies suggest that one mechanism by which the mutated proteins in AD induce cell death could well be mediated by mitochondria. Until this mechanism is better understood and replicated by other laboratories, marginally effective cholinesterase inhibitors remain the major therapeutic option for AD patients. No pharmacological agent targeting mitochondria is currently being developed for AD therapy.

Parkinson's disease

Parkinson's disease (PD) is the second most common neurodegenerative disorder, after Alzheimer's disease.[120] PD is characterized by the loss of dopaminergic neurons in substantia nigra pars compacta (SNpc), leading to a reduction of dopamine in the putamen.[120] When the depletion reaches about 60% of SNpc dopaminergic neurons and 80% of dopamine content in the caudate, symptoms of PD appear.[120] Abnormal movements such as resting tremor, rigidity, and postural instability are common in PD patients.[120]

The etiology of PD is currently unknown. Environmental toxins have been hypothesized to play a dominant role based upon the observations that parkinsonism can be caused by encephalitic infection and accidental 1-methyl-4-phenyl-1,2,3,6-tetrahydropyridine (MPTP) injection.[120] However, more recent discoveries of various familial forms of early-onset PD have given impetus to a genetic-based theory. Perhaps both mechanisms are involved and mitochondrial dysfunction could represent a common denominator that unifies these two theories. The notion of mitochondrial dysfunction as a pathogenic mechanism in PD emanated from the initial discovery that MPTP induced a parkinsonian syndrome in humans and various animal species.[120] Subsequently, 1-methyl-4-phenylpyridinium ion (MPP^+), the active neurotoxic metabolite of MPTP, was identified as an inhibitor of complex I of the mitochondrial electron transport chain.[121] This latter finding prompted many investigators to search for mitochondrial defects in PD patients. Soon enough, a plethora of publications reported more or less convincing respiratory defects in PD tissues including the SNpc[122] and platelets.[123,124] In cytoplasmic hybrid cell lines (cybrid cells), which contain mitochondria derived from platelets of PD patients, complex I activity was also reduced,[125] and this finding led the authors to conclude that complex I deficiency in PD is mitochondrially (i.e., maternally) inherited. Consistent with this, the same authors subsequently reported that complex I activity was reduced in maternal descendants of families with PD.[126] Furthermore, mutations and polymorphisms in subunits of complex I have been proposed as susceptibility genes in subsets of PD patients.[127,128] It has to be emphasized, however, that complex I deficiency only occurs in a subset of PD patients. This may partly explain the lack of complex I deficiency in a more recent study of cybrids.[129] Nevertheless, in aggregate, all of these studies suggest that genetic mutations, environmental toxins, or both, inhibit complex I activity and may play a pathogenic role in some PD patients. The recent demonstration that rats exposed to rotenone, a lipophilic complex I inhibitor, reproduce some key features of PD,[130] has revived interest in the relationship between complex I defects and sporadic PD.

The discoveries of various genes in early-onset PD have also suggested ways by which PD-causing mutations may provoke neurodegeneration via a mitochondrial mechanism.[131] By sequencing candidate genes within the PD locus *PARK6* region, two homozygous mutations have been identified in the PTEN-induced putative kinase 1 (*PINK1/BRPK*) gene.[5] This ubiquitously expressed protein has a serine/threonine kinase as the sole known functional domain.[132] Presumably PINK1 has a mitochondrial targeting motif because it localizes to mitochondria in transfected cell lines.[5] The two mutations thus far identified are expected to impair PINK1 kinase activity or substrate recognition and to cause PD by loss of function. Impaired phosphorylation of PINK1 substrate in mitochondria is likely to explain the pathogenic mechanism of the two mutations. While awaiting the elucidation of the critical substrates of PINK1, interesting data have been obtained in neuroblastoma cells transiently transfected with either wild-type or mutant PINK1.[5] There was no baseline alteration in viability with either the wild-type or mutated gene, but when neuroblastoma cells were challenged with the proteasome inhibitor MG132, those that overexpressed wild-type PINK1 survived the toxic insult, whereas those that overexpressed mutant PINK1 died to the same extent as non-transfected neuroblastoma cells.[5] These results suggest that wild-type mitochondrial PINK1 confers greater resistance to the mitochondria, and thus to the cell, against cytotoxic insults.

Eleven different DJ-1 mutations – including missense, truncating, splice site mutations, and large deletions – have been linked to an autosomal recessive form of PD.[133–135] In the normal situation, wild-type DJ-1 is in the cytosol, but, upon oxidation of one of its cysteine residues (C106), DJ-1 appears to translocate to the mitochondria.[136] The mitochondrial localization of DJ-1 seems to be critical, as mutation of C106 prevents DJ-1 from accumulating in the mitochondria and renders cells more susceptible to the toxic effects of MPP^+.[136] Other PD-causing DJ-1 mutations appear to also impair DJ-1 mitochondrial translocation.[133] Although the exact pathogenic mechanism of DJ-1 mutations remains to be determined, these studies suggest that the lack of DJ-1 translocation into mitochondria may be pivotal in the neurodegenerative process of PD.

Current therapeutic options for PD patients are symptomatic.[137] Among the agents being evaluated in clinical trials are the two mitochondrially targeted compounds, creatine and coenzyme Q10. These compounds were neuroprotective in the MPTP mouse model.[138,139] Results from one of these clinical trials have shown that coenzyme Q10 provides some therapeutic benefit to PD patients.[140]

Amyotrophic lateral sclerosis

Amyotrophic lateral sclerosis (ALS) is a progressive neurodegenerative disorder characterized by the loss of motor neurons in the anterior horn of the spinal cord and cerebral cortex.[141] Onset usually is in the fourth or fifth decade of life, with rapid progression to paralysis and death within 2–5 years.[141] About 10% of ALS cases are familial (FALS), and 20% of these are caused by dominant mutations in Cu,Zn-superoxide dismutase (SOD1).[142,143] Thus far, >100 point mutations have been identified: they are scattered throughout the enzyme, and they are predominantly single amino acid replacements. Interestingly, these different mutations lead to the same clinical phenotype. The mechanism by which mutated SOD1 causes neurodegeneration in FALS is not clear. However, based on the observation that SOD1-deficient mice do not develop the hallmark features of the disease[144] whereas transgenic mice overexpressing mutated SOD1 do,[145,146] it has been suggested that mutated SOD1 provokes neurodegeneration by a toxic 'gain-of-function'.

Among the various pathogenic mechanisms proposed, mitochondrial dysfunction has also emerged. An early study of sporadic ALS showed abnormal mitochondrial morphology in muscle by electron microscopy.[147] Abnormal mitochondria were also reported in the anterior horn of the spinal cord,[148,149] corticospinal tract axonal swellings,[150] and muscle biopsies in a subset of sporadic ALS patients.[151,152] 'Bizarre giant mitochondria' were described in hepatocytes from 21 of 21 sporadic ALS patients.[153] In addition to abnormal morphology, reduction in mitochondrial number has also been reported in intramuscular nerves[154] and spinal cords[155] of sporadic ALS patients. In these same patients, mitochondrial respiratory chain activities were decreased in spinal cords[155,156] and muscles.[157] However, another group failed to confirm these biochemical defects in skeletal muscles from sporadic ALS patients.[158]

As for familial ALS linked to mutant SOD1, it should be mentioned that SOD1 had long been considered a cytosolic enzyme, but it has now also been identified in the mitochondria.[159–163] This finding strongly suggests a role for SOD1 in mitochondria, which may be relevant to the pathogenesis of FALS. Consistent with this idea, reduced respiratory chain functions and abnormally high release of apoptogenic mitochondrial molecules such as cytochrome *c* have been documented in transgenic mice expressing one pathogenic SOD1 mutation (G93A).[161,164–166] Furthermore, mutant SOD1 has been identified in several intramitochondrial compartments in the brain, and in the matrix. This mutant protein is misfolded and prone to aggregation.[167] In the spinal cord of these ALS mice, other investigators have described vacuoles which originated from degenerating mitochondria and which preceded the death of motor neurons.[168,169] Supporting the pathogenic significance of these mitochondrial alterations in ALS-linked SOD1 mutations is the observation that creatine and coenzyme Q10 improve motor performance and survival in transgenic mice.[170] Together, these studies suggest that there is a relationship between mitochondrial dysfunction, death of motor neurons, and clinical symptoms in the transgenic mutant SOD1 mice. Consistent with this is also the report that ALS transgenic mice are more vulnerable to mitochondrial toxins such as MPTP and 3-NP.[171]

Therapeutically, a few drugs with potential mitochondrial effects are being tested for ALS. For example, the antibiotic minocycline has been shown pre-clinically to improve motor performance and extend survival in ALS transgenic mice, presumably by preventing the release of apoptogenic molecules from the mitochondria.[172] Minocycline is currently in phase III clinical trials.[173] In contrast to the results obtained in ALS mice, a double-blind study of creatine failed to improve either clinical symptoms or survival in ALS patients.[174]

Mechanism of cell death in mitochondrial neurodegenerative diseases

One of the most intriguing and unresolved questions that pertain to mitochondrial diseases, including those associated with neurodegeneration, is how cells actually die in these pathological situations. As emphasized above, most of the definite mitochondrial neurodegenerative diseases are linked to some sort of defect in the respiratory chain. In keeping with this, it can be predicted that complete loss of mitochondrial respiration would be lethal, as suggested by the embryonic death of mutant mice deficient in mitochondrial transcription factor A.[175] In contrast, the late onset and chronic nature of the neurodegenerative diseases discussed in this chapter suggests that the mitochondrial defects are more subtle, causing a progressive worsening of mitochondrial and cellular function which culminates in cell demise.

Mitochondrial dysfunction, ROS overproduction, and ATP deficit

The extremely high energetic demand of the brain is illustrated by the fact that, while the brain represents only about 1/50th of the body weight, it consumes about 1/5th of the total oxygen inhaled. Of this amount of oxygen, about 90% is utilized by mitochondria to produce ATP. Although, through the course of evolution, mitochondria have provided eukaryotic cells with a very efficient aerobic metabolism, an estimated 1–2% of consumed oxygen is converted to ROS rather than water.[176] The inability of the respiratory chain to completely reduce oxygen to water, coupled with its high rate of oxygen consumption, contributes to the high ROS production of the mitochondrial respiratory chain. In situations of mitochondrial dysfunction this rate may increase dramatically. There are two main sites in the electron transport chain where ROS are generated: complex I and complex III (see Figure 13.1). A dysfunction of complex I, resulting either from a mutation or from toxicity by MPTP or rotenone, can dramatically increase ROS production. This elevation is a result of 'leakage' of electrons from complex I and the subsequent reduction of oxygen to superoxide. Increased production of ROS is also seen when complex III is inhibited by antimycin, leading to the accumulation of ubisemiquinone. Intrinsically, mitochondria are equipped with a defense mechanism against ROS, including antioxidant enzymes such as manganese superoxide dismutase and glutathione peroxidase. Any imbalance between the production of ROS and the antioxidant capacity of these enzymes leads to a local oxidative stress, potentially causing serious functional and structural damage to the mitochondria. How much of this mitochondrial oxidative stress can also damage cytoplasmic molecules and other organelles is still an unresolved question. The view that mitochondrial ROS leak out and inflict extramitochondrial oxidative damage is common in the literature, but the majority of ROS produced inside the mitochondria are not membrane permeant, and it is unclear how they get to the cytosol. This uncertainty does not undermine the potential significance of mitochondrial-derived oxidative

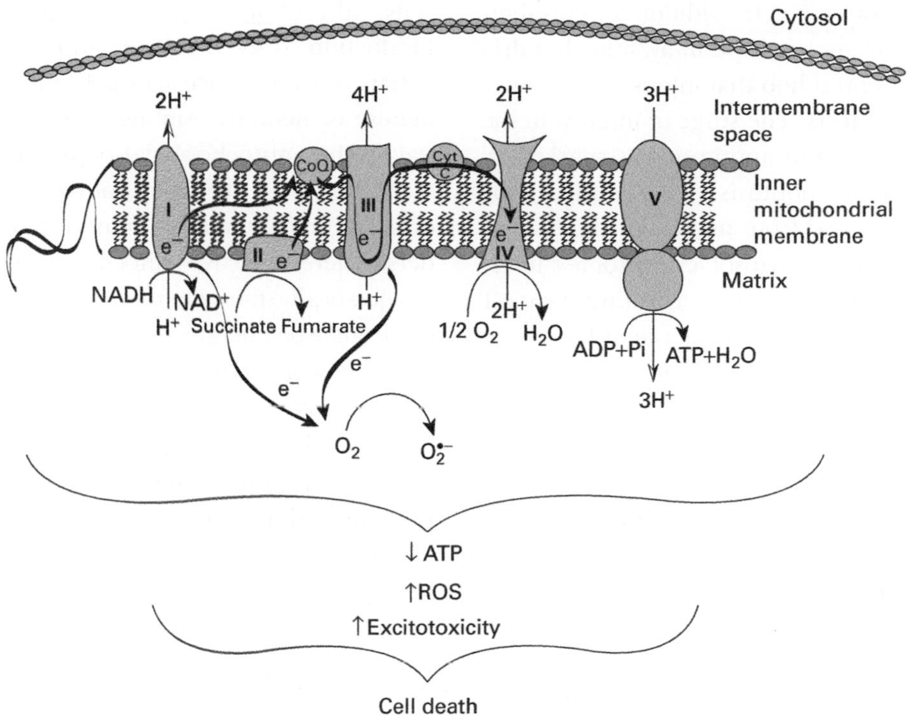

Figure 13.1 Schematic representation of electron transport chain (ETC). Complex I and complex III are the two major sites where ROS are produced. Dysfunction in the ETC, in general, as a result of mutations or blockade by specific inhibitors of the complexes, would lead to an increase in ROS production, reduction in ATP production, or increase in excitotoxicity. These abnormalities potentially result in cell death

stress in the cell death process underlying mitochondrial neurodegenerative diseases.

Defective mitochondria not only produce more ROS, but also less ATP, which is necessary for many critical cellular processes. However, it is unclear how low ATP synthesis must get to provoke cell damage. Studies in cultured cells expressing mitochondrial mutations known to impair ATP synthesis show that cellular stores of ATP drop to pathological levels only when the cells are placed under conditions of high ATP demand.[177] This suggests that cells such as neurons, which have variable ATP needs related to changes in ion fluxes in response to external stimuli, would experience energy crises only when ATP demands rise above basal levels. Thus, any prolonged energy crisis due to a sustained increase in ATP demand may not only impair basic ATP-dependent neuronal functions such as neurotransmission, but also increase the probability for that neuron to die. For instance, ATP deficiency may lead to Na^+/K^+-ATPase failure and subsequent neuronal membrane depolarization, which, via activation of NMDA receptors, may subject neurons to an excitotoxic injury.

Mitochondria and apoptosis

As indicated above, mitochondria also act as a major supplier of apoptogenic molecules (see Figure 13.2). Apoptosis is an active and programmed form of cell death regulated by multiple molecular pathways.[178,179] In addition to representing the 'intrinsic' apoptotic pathway, mitochondria also serve as a central hub that interacts with other pathways of apoptosis. The surge of interest in the role of mitochondria in apoptosis was sparked by the discovery that apoptosis can be induced by cytochrome *c* released from mitochondria.[180] After being released into the cytosol, cytochrome *c* interacts with apoptosis proteases-activating factor-1 (Apaf1) and procaspase 9 to form a complex known as apoptosome, which then activates caspase 3.[181] Caspases are a group of proteolytic enzymes which cleave their substrates at specific aspartic acid residues. Activation of caspases potentially leads to apoptotic death. A second mitochondrial apoptogenic protein released into the cytosol is Smac/Diablo. In the cytosol, this protein inhibits the 'inhibitors of apoptosis proteins' (IAPs), leading again to activation of caspases. Two other mitochondrial proteins, apoptosis-inducing factor (AIF) and endonuclease G, are released and translocated from mitochondria to nuclei where they induce DNA fragmentation. In addition to these apoptogenic molecules, mitochondria also contain anti-apoptotic proteins, such as Bcl-2 and Bcl-XL. The balance between pro- and anti-apoptotic molecules must be tightly controlled to ensure proper execution of apoptosis.

Sequential, multifactorial scenario of neuronal death

The use of inhibitors of mitochondrial respiration shows that ATP depletion and ROS overproduction occur soon after the block of oxidative phosphorylation, subjecting the cells to energy crisis and oxidative stress. However, the time-course of these perturbations[182] appears to correlate poorly with the time-course of neuronal death,[120,181] suggesting that only a few neurons probably succumb to the early combined effects of ATP depletion and ROS overproduction. Instead, there is mounting evidence[183] that rather than killing the cells, alterations in ATP synthesis and ROS production trigger cell death-related molecular pathways, which, once activated, rapidly lead to the demise of neurons. Among these molecular pathways, the mitochondrial-dependent apoptotic machinery may play a critical role.[9] In the context of most mitochondrial neurodegenerative disorders, where defective mitochondrial respiration is unequivocally present, this cascade of deleterious events may be operative. In other diseases discussed above, in which mitochondrial protein degradation or ISC biosynthesis are deranged, apoptosis may be recruited by alternative mechanisms, including direct interactions between disease-causing mutated proteins and a key factor of the apoptotic cascade. This latter view is quite provocative and warrants, in our opinion, further investigation.

Conclusion

In the past decade, there have been some major discoveries on the role of mitochondria in neurodegenerative diseases. We now understand that through depletion of ATP, generation of ROS, and release of apoptogenic proteins, mitochondria may hold a key role in neurodegenerative processes. Initiation of these events, either individually or more likely in combination, would potentially lead to neuronal death. We also understand that mitochondrial abnormalities can arise from a variety of causes: mutations in mtDNA, mutations in nDNA encoding for mitochondrial proteins, and from mutations in genes apparently unrelated to mitochondria. What is clear is that a pathogenic scenario, inspired by definite or suspected mitochondrial alterations, can be envisioned to support a mitochondrial role in almost all neurodegenerative diseases. If this mitochondrially based pathogenic scenario is fairly acceptable in situations where genetic mutations impact on the mitochondrial function in a meaningful manner, the jury is still out as to whether such a scenario applies to sporadic neurodegenerative diseases. It

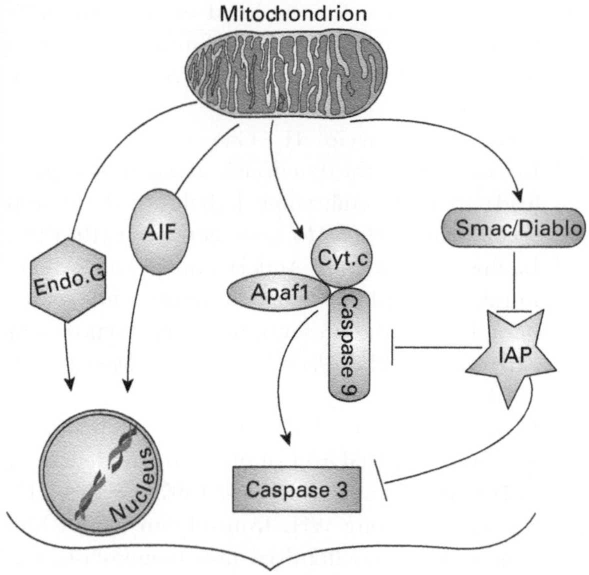

Figure 13.2 Mitochondria and apoptosis. As discussed in the text, mitochondria play a major role in the cascades of apoptosis. Shown here are the various apoptogenic molecules released from mitochondria, leading to caspase 3 activation and DNA fragmentation and ultimately cell death

is disturbing that pathogenic mutations in mtDNA do not cause the typical clinical manifestations of neurodegenerative diseases such as HD, AD, PD, and ALS. As emphasized by Schon and Manfredi[9], of the large number of pathogenic mtDNA mutations, only a handful cause chorea and dementia, parkinsonism, dystonia, or motor neuron disease and – almost without exception – these phenotypes are associated with atypical neurological features. Conversely, movement disorders are rare in 'primary' mitochondrial diseases. Some aspects of mitochondrial genetics, such as heteroplasmy, mitotic segregation, and the threshold effect, may contribute to our difficulty in linking common neurodegenerative diseases to mitochondrial defects. It is also important to remember that most studies on the mitochondrial link to neurodegeneration have been mainly performed in autopsy material, which often originates from terminally ill patients and is devoid of almost all neurons of interest, those that are proposed to die from mitochondrial dysfunction. Thus, many, if not all of these studies reflect analyses performed on a population of surviving cells (e.g., glia) not necessarily representative of the actual neuronal death mechanism. Finally, it is also crucial to remember that mitochondrial defects reported in postmortem tissues may simply reflect nonspecific alterations that occur in dying neurons. The development of better in vivo experimental models of neurodegenerative diseases may provide us with the necessary tools to appropriately examine the mechanistic relationship between neurodegeneration and mitochondrial dysfunction and to address once and for all many of the pending issues that cloud the field of sporadic mitochondrial neurodegenerative diseases.

Acknowledgments

The authors wish to thank Mr Matthew Lucas for his assistance in preparing this manuscript. The authors are supported by NIH/NINDS Grants R21 ES013177-01 and NS42269, P50 SN38370, and P01 NS11766–27A1, NIH/NIA Grant RO1 AG021617–01, the US Department of Defense (DAMD 17–99–1–0002, DAMD 17–03–1, and DAMD17–03–1–0482), the Lowenstein Foundation, the Lillian Goldman Charitable Trust, the Parkinson's Disease Foundation, and MDA/ Wings-Over-Wall Street.

References

1. Przedborski S, Vila M, Jackson-Lewis V. Series introduction: Neurodegeneration: What is it and where are we? *J Clin Invest* 2003; **111**: 3–10.
2. DiMauro S, Schon EA. Mitochondrial respiratory-chain diseases. *N Engl J Med* 2003; **348**: 2656–2668.
3. Wooten GF, Currie LJ, Bennett JP et al. Maternal inheritance in Parkinson's disease. *Ann Neurol* 1997; **41**: 265–268.

4. Prezant TR, Agapian JV, Bohlman MC et al. Mitochondrial ribosomal RNA mutation associated with both antibiotic-induced and non-syndromic deafness. *Nat Genet* 1993; **4**: 289–294.
5. Valente EM, Abou-Sleiman PM, Caputo V et al. Hereditary early-onset parkinson's disease caused by mutations in *PINK1*. *Science* 2004; **304**: 1158–1160.
6. Battersby BJ, Loredo-Osti JC, Shoubridge EA. Nuclear genetic control of mitochondrial DNA segregation. *Nat Genet* 2003; **33**: 183–186.
7. Shoffner JM, Brown M, Huoponen K et al. A mitochondrial DNA (mtDNA) mutation associated with maternally inherited deafness and Parkinson's disease (PD). *Neurology* 1996; **46**: A331.
8. Thyagarajan D, Bressman S, Bruno C et al. A novel mitochondrial 12SrRNA point mutation in parkinsonism, deafness, and neuropathy. *Ann Neurol* 2000; **48**: 730–736.
9. Schon EA, Manfredi G. Neuronal degeneration and mitochondrial dysfunction. *J Clin Invest* 2003; **111**: 303–312.
10. Delatycki MB, Williamson R, Forrest SM. Friedreich ataxia: an overview. *J Med Genet* 2000; **37**: 1–8.
11. Harding AE. Friedreich's ataxia: a clinical and genetic study of 90 families with an analysis of early diagnostic criteria and intrafamilial clustering of clinical features. *Brain* 1981; **104**: 589–620.
12. Babcock M, de Silva D, Oaks R et al. Regulation of mitochondrial iron accumulation by Yfh1p, a putative homolog of frataxin. *Science* 1997; **276**: 1709–1712.
13. Cavadini P, Adamec J, Taroni F et al. Two-step processing of human frataxin by mitochondrial processing peptidase. Precursor and intermediate forms are cleaved at different rates. *J Biol Chem* 2000; **275**: 41469–41475.
14. Campuzano V, Montermini L, Molto MD et al. Friedreich's ataxia: autosomal recessive disease caused by an intronic GAA triplet repeat expansion. *Science* 1996; **271**: 1423–1427.
15. Campuzano V, Montermini L, Lutz Y et al. Frataxin is reduced in Friedreich ataxia patients and is associated with mitochondrial membranes. *Hum Mol Genet* 1997; **6**: 1771–1780.
16. Miranda CJ, Santos MM, Ohshima K et al. Frataxin knockin mouse. *FEBS Lett* 2002; **512**: 291–297.
17. Durr A, Cossee M, Agid Y et al. Clinical and genetic abnormalities in patients with Friedreich's ataxia. *N Engl J Med* 1996; **335**: 1169–1175.
18. Cossee M, Durr A, Schmitt M et al. Friedreich's ataxia: point mutations and clinical presentation of compound heterozygotes. *Ann Neurol* 1999; **45**: 200–206.
19. Cossee M, Puccio H, Gansmuller A et al. Inactivation of the Friedreich ataxia mouse gene leads to early embryonic lethality without iron accumulation. *Hum Mol Genet* 2000; **9**: 1219–1226.
20. Badhwar A, Jansen A, Andermann F et al. Striking intrafamilial phenotypic variability and spastic paraplegia in the presence of similar homozygous expansions of the *FRDA1* gene. *Mov Disord* 2004; **19**: 1424–1431.
21. Rotig A, De Lonlay P, Chretien D et al. Aconitase and mitochondrial iron-sulphur protein deficiency in Friedreich ataxia. *Nat Genet* 1997; **17**: 215–217.
22. Rouault TA, Tong WH. Iron-sulphur cluster biogenesis and mitochondrial iron homeostasis. *Nat Rev Mol Cell Biol* 2005; **6**: 345–351.
23. Chantrel-Groussard K, Geromel V, Puccio H et al. Disabled early recruitment of antioxidant defenses in Friedreich's ataxia. *Hum Mol Genet* 2001; **10**: 2061–2067.
24. Muhlenhoff U, Richhardt N, Ristow M et al. The yeast frataxin homolog Yfh1p plays a specific role in the maturation of cellular Fe/S proteins. *Hum Mol Genet* 2002; **11**: 2025–2036.
25. Duby G, Foury F, Ramazzotti A et al. A non-essential function for yeast frataxin in iron-sulfur cluster assembly. *Hum Mol Genet* 2002; **11**: 2635–2643.
26. Yoon T, Cowan JA. Iron-sulfur cluster biosynthesis. Characterization of frataxin as an iron donor for assembly of [2Fe-2S] clusters in ISU-type proteins. *J Am Chem Soc* 2003; **125**: 6078–6084.
27. Gerber J, Muhlenhoff U, Lill R. An interaction between frataxin and Isu1/Nfs1 that is crucial for Fe/S cluster synthesis on Isu1. *EMBO Rep* 2003; **4**: 906–911.
28. Lill R, Kispal G. Maturation of cellular Fe-S proteins: an essential function of mitochondria. *Trends Biochem Sci* 2000; **25**: 352–356.
29. Puccio H, Simon D, Cossee M et al. Mouse models for Friedreich ataxia exhibit cardiomyopathy, sensory nerve defect and Fe-S enzyme deficiency followed by intramitochondrial iron deposits. *Nat Genet* 2001; **27**: 181–186.
30. Sturm B, Bistrich U, Schranzhofer M et al. Friedreich's ataxia, no changes in mitochondrial

labile iron in human lymphoblasts and fibroblasts: a decrease in antioxidative capacity? *J Biol Chem* 2005; **280**: 6701–6708.
31. Liu ZD, Hider RC. Design of clinically useful iron(III)-selective chelators. *Med Res Rev* 2002; **22**: 26–64.
32. Ponka P, Grady RW, Wilczynska A et al. The effect of various chelating agents on the mobilization of iron from reticulocytes in the presence and absence of pyridoxal isonicotinoyl hydrazone. *Biochim Biophys Acta* 1984; **802**: 477–489.
33. Olivieri NF, Brittenham GM, McLaren CE et al. Long-term safety and effectiveness of iron-chelation therapy with deferiprone for thalassemia major. *N Engl J Med* 1998; **339**: 417–423.
34. Richardson DR, Mouralian C, Ponka P et al. Development of potential iron chelators for the treatment of Friedreich's ataxia: ligands that mobilize mitochondrial iron. *Biochim Biophys Acta* 2001; **1536**: 133–140.
35. Kelso GF, Porteous CM, Coulter CV et al. Selective targeting of a redox-active ubiquinone to mitochondria within cells: antioxidant and antiapoptotic properties. *J Biol Chem* 2001; **276**: 4588–4596.
36. Jauslin ML, Meier T, Smith RA et al. Mitochondria-targeted antioxidants protect Friedreich ataxia fibroblasts from endogenous oxidative stress more effectively than untargeted antioxidants. *FASEB J* 2003; **17**: 1972–1974.
37. Suno M, Nagaoka A. Inhibition of lipid peroxidation by a novel compound (CV-2619) in brain mitochondria and mode of action of the inhibition. *Biochem Biophys Res Commun* 1984; **125**: 1046–1052.
38. Schulz JB, Dehmer T, Schols L et al. Oxidative stress in patients with Friedreich ataxia. *Neurology* 2000; **55**: 1719–1721.
39. Rustin P, Kleist-Retzow JC, Chantrel-Groussard K et al. Effect of idebenone on cardiomyopathy in Friedreich's ataxia: a preliminary study. *Lancet* 1999; **354**: 477–479.
40. Mariotti C, Solari A, Torta D et al. Idebenone treatment in Friedreich patients: one-year-long randomized placebo-controlled trial. *Neurology* 2003; **60**: 1676–1679.
41. Buyse G, Mertens L, Di Salvo G et al. Idebenone treatment in Friedreich's ataxia: neurological, cardiac, and biochemical monitoring. *Neurology* 2003; **60**: 1679–1681.
42. Voncken M, Ioannou P, Delatycki MB. Friedreich ataxia – update on pathogenesis and possible therapies. *Neurogenetics* 2004; **5**: 1–8.
43. Fink JK. The hereditary spastic paraplegias: nine genes and counting. *Arch Neurol* 2003; **60**: 1045–1049.
44. Crosby AH, Proukakis C. Is the transportation highway the right road for hereditary spastic paraplegia? *Am J Hum Genet* 2002; **71**: 1009–1016.
45. Fink JK. Advances in the hereditary spastic paraplegias. *Exp Neurol* 2003; **184**(Suppl 1): S106–S110.
46. Casari G, De Fusco M, Ciarmatori S et al. Spastic paraplegia and OXPHOS impairment caused by mutations in paraplegin, a nuclear-encoded mitochondrial metalloprotease. *Cell* 1998; **93**: 973–983.
47. Arlt H, Tauer R, Feldmann H et al. The YTA10-12 complex, an AAA protease with chaperone-like activity in the inner membrane of mitochondria. *Cell* 1996; **85**: 875–885.
48. Banfi S, Bassi MT, Andolfi G et al. Identification and characterization of AFG3L2, a novel paraplegin-related gene. *Genomics* 1999; **59**: 51–58.
49. Coppola M, Pizzigoni A, Banfi S et al. Identification and characterization of YME1L1, a novel paraplegin-related gene. *Genomics* 2000; **66**: 48–54.
50. Ferreirinha F, Quattrini A, Pirozzi M et al. Axonal degeneration in paraplegin-deficient mice is associated with abnormal mitochondria and impairment of axonal transport. *J Clin Invest* 2004; **113**: 231–242.
51. Hansen JJ, Durr A, Cournu-Rebeix I et al. Hereditary spastic paraplegia SPG13 is associated with a mutation in the gene encoding the mitochondrial chaperonin Hsp60. *Am J Hum Genet* 2002; **70**: 1328–1332.
52. Slavotinek AM, Biesecker LG. Unfolding the role of chaperones and chaperonins in human disease. *Trends Genet* 2001; **17**: 528–535.
53. Hazan J, Fonknechten N, Mavel D et al. Spastin, a new AAA protein, is altered in the most frequent form of autosomal dominant spastic paraplegia. *Nat Genet* 1999; **23**: 296–303.
54. Evans KJ, Gomes ER, Reisenweber SM et al. Linking axonal degeneration to microtubule remodeling by Spastin-mediated microtubule severing. *J Cell Biol* 2005; **168**: 599–606.
55. Binder J, Hofmann S, Kreisel S et al. Clinical and molecular findings in a patient with a novel mutation in the deafness-dystonia peptide (DDP1) gene. *Brain* 2003; **126**: 1814–1820.

56. Jin H, May M, Tranebjaerg L et al. A novel X-linked gene, *DDP*, shows mutations in families with deafness (DFN-1), dystonia, mental deficiency and blindness. *Nat Genet* 1996; **14**: 177–180.
57. Bauer MF, Rothbauer U, Muhlenbein N et al. The mitochondrial TIM22 preprotein translocase is highly conserved throughout the eukaryotic kingdom. *FEBS Lett* 1999; **464**: 41–47.
58. Koehler CM, Leuenberger D, Merchant S et al. Human deafness dystonia syndrome is a mitochondrial disease. *Proc Natl Acad Sci USA* 1999; **96**: 2141–2146.
59. Roesch K, Curran SP, Tranebjaerg L et al. Human deafness dystonia syndrome is caused by a defect in assembly of the DDP1/TIMM8a-TIMM13 complex. *Hum Mol Genet* 2002; **11**: 477–486.
60. Menkes JH. Disorders of metal metabolism. In: Rowland LP, ed. *Merritt's Neurology*. 10th ed. New York: Lippincott Williams & Wilkins, 2000; 543–548.
61. Shah AB, Chernov I, Zhang HT et al. Identification and analysis of mutations in the Wilson disease gene (*ATP7B*): population frequencies, genotype-phenotype correlation, and functional analyses. *Am J Hum Genet* 1997; **61**: 317–328.
62. Buiakova OI, Xu J, Lutsenko S et al. Null mutation of the murine *ATP7B* (Wilson disease) gene results in intracellular copper accumulation and late-onset hepatic nodular transformation. *Hum Mol Genet* 1999; **8**: 1665–1671.
63. Lutsenko S, Cooper MJ. Localization of the Wilson's disease protein product to mitochondria. *Proc Natl Acad Sci USA* 1998; **95**: 6004–6009.
64. Gu M, Cooper JM, Butler P et al. Oxidative-phosphorylation defects in liver of patients with Wilson's disease. *Lancet* 2000; **356**: 469–474.
65. Huntington's disease collaborative research group. A novel gene containing a trinucleotide repeat that is expanded and unstable on Huntington's disease chromosomes. *Cell* 1993; **72**: 971–983.
66. Brinkmann U, Brinkmann E, Gallo M et al. Cloning and characterization of a cellular apoptosis susceptibility gene, the human homologue to the yeast chromosome segregation gene *CSE1*. *Proc Natl Acad Sci USA* 1995; **92**: 10427–10431.
67. van Dellen A, Blakemore C, Deacon R et al. Delaying the onset of Huntington's in mice. *Nature* 2000; **404**: 721–722.
68. Hockly E, Cordery PM, Woodman B et al. Environmental enrichment slows disease progression in R6/2 Huntington's disease mice. *Ann Neurol* 2002; **51**: 235–242.
69. Wexler NS, Lorimer J, Porter J et al. Venezuelan kindreds reveal that genetic and environmental factors modulate Huntington's disease age of onset. *Proc Natl Acad Sci USA* 2004; **101**: 3498–3503.
70. Kuhl DE, Phelps ME, Markham CH et al. Cerebral metabolism and atrophy in Huntington's disease determined by ^{18}FDG and computed tomographic scan. *Ann Neurol* 1982; **12**: 425–434.
71. Kuhl DE, Metter EJ, Riege WH et al. Patterns of cerebral glucose utilization in Parkinson's disease and Huntington's disease. *Ann Neurol* 1984; **15** (Suppl): S119–S125.
72. Erecinska M, Silver IA. ATP and brain function. *J Cereb Blood Flow Metab* 1989; **9**: 2–19.
73. Penney JB, Jr., Young AB. Quantitative autoradiography of neurotransmitter receptors in Huntington disease. *Neurology* 1982; **32**: 1391–1395.
74. Dure LS, Young AB, Penney JB. Excitatory amino acid binding sites in the caudate nucleus and frontal cortex of Huntington's disease. *Ann Neurol* 1991; **30**: 785–793.
75. Cha JH, Kosinski CM, Kerner JA et al. Altered brain neurotransmitter receptors in transgenic mice expressing a portion of an abnormal human Huntington disease gene. *Proc Natl Acad Sci USA* 1998; **95**: 6480–6485.
76. Knull HR. Association of glycolytic enzymes with particulate fractions from nerve endings. *Biochim Biophys Acta* 1978; **522**: 1–9.
77. Koroshetz WJ, Jenkins BG, Rosen BR et al. Energy metabolism defects in Huntington's disease and effects of coenzyme Q_{10}. *Ann Neurol* 1997; **41**: 160–165.
78. Jenkins BG, Koroshetz WJ, Beal MF et al. Evidence for impairment of energy metabolism in vivo in Huntington's disease using localized 1H NMR spectroscopy. *Neurology* 1993; **43**: 2689–2695.
79. Chance B, Williams GR. A simple and rapid assay of oxidative phosphorylation. *Nature* 1955; **175**: 1120–1121.
80. Brennan WA, Jr., Bird ED, Aprille JR. Regional mitochondrial respiratory activity in Huntington's disease brain. *J Neurochem* 1985; **44**: 1948–1950.

81. Mann VM, Cooper JM, Javoy-Agid F et al. Mitochondrial function and parental sex effect in Huntington's disease. *Lancet* 1990; **336**: 749.
82. Browne SE, Bowling AC, MacGarvey U et al. Oxidative damage and metabolic dysfunction in Huntington's disease: Selective vulnerability of the basal ganglia. *Ann Neurol* 1997; **41**: 646–653.
83. Brouillet E, Conde F, Beal MF et al. Replicating Huntington's disease phenotype in experimental animals. *Prog Neurobiol* 1999; **59**: 427–468.
84. Matthews RT, Yang LC, Jenkins BG et al. Neuroprotective effects of creatine and cyclocreatine in animal models of Huntington's disease. *J Neurosci* 1998; **18**: 156–163.
85. Beal MF, Henshaw DR, Jenkins BG et al. Coenzyme Q_{10} and nicotinamide block striatal lesions produced by the mitochondrial toxin malonate. *Ann Neurol* 1994; **36**: 882–888.
86. Sapp E, Schwarz C, Chase K et al. Huntingtin localization in brains of normal and Huntington's disease patients. *Ann Neurol* 1997; **42**: 604–612.
87. Panov AV, Gutekunst CA, Leavitt BR et al. Early mitochondrial calcium defects in Huntington's disease are a direct effect of polyglutamines. *Nat Neurosci* 2002; **5**: 731–736.
88. Choo YS, Johnson GV, MacDonald M et al. Mutant huntingtin directly increases susceptibility of mitochondria to the calcium-induced permeability transition and cytochrome *c* release. *Hum Mol Genet* 2004.
89. Ruan Q, Lesort M, MacDonald ME et al. Striatal cells from mutant huntingtin knock-in mice are selectively vulnerable to mitochondrial complex II inhibitor-induced cell death through a non-apoptotic pathway. *Hum Mol Genet* 2004; **13**: 669–681.
90. Beal MF, Ferrante RJ. Experimental therapeutics in transgenic mouse models of Huntington's disease. *Nat Rev Neurosci* 2004; **5**: 373–384.
91. Li SH, Li XJ. Huntingtin-protein interactions and the pathogenesis of Huntington's disease. *Trends Genet* 2004; **20**: 146–154.
92. Arnould T, Vankoningsloo S, Renard P et al. CREB activation induced by mitochondrial dysfunction is a new signaling pathway that impairs cell proliferation. *EMBO J* 2002; **21**: 53–63.
93. Gregory PD, Wagner K, Horz W. Histone acetylation and chromatin remodeling. *Exp Cell Res* 2001; **265**: 195–202.
94. Yu ZX, Li SH, Nguyen HP et al. Huntingtin inclusions do not deplete polyglutamine-containing transcription factors in HD mice. *Hum Mol Genet* 2002; **11**: 905–914.
95. Trushina E, Dyer RB, Badger JD et al. Mutant huntingtin impairs axonal trafficking in mammalian neurons in vivo and in vitro. *Mol Cell Biol* 2004; **24**: 8195–8209.
96. Yi M, Weaver D, Hajnoczky G. Control of mitochondrial motility and distribution by the calcium signal: a homeostatic circuit. *J Cell Biol* 2004; **167**: 661–672.
97. Ferrante RJ, Andreassen OA, Jenkins BG et al. Neuroprotective effects of creatine in a transgenic mouse model of Huntington's disease. *J Neurosci* 2000; **20**: 4389–4397.
98. Andreassen OA, Ferrante RJ, Huang HM et al. Dichloroacetate exerts therapeutic effects in transgenic mouse models of Huntington's disease. *Ann Neurol* 2001; **50**: 112–117.
99. Dedeoglu A, Kubilus JK, Yang L et al. Creatine therapy provides neuroprotection after onset of clinical symptoms in Huntington's disease transgenic mice. *J Neurochem* 2003; **85**: 1359–1367.
100. Ferrante RJ, Andreassen OA, Dedeoglu A et al. Therapeutic effects of coenzyme Q10 and remacemide in transgenic mouse models of Huntington's disease. *J Neurosci* 2002; **22**: 1592–1599.
101. Schilling G, Coonfield ML, Ross CA et al. Coenzyme Q10 and remacemide hydrochloride ameliorate motor deficits in a Huntington's disease transgenic mouse model. *Neurosci Lett* 2001; **315**: 149–153.
102. Kieburtz K, Koroshetz W, McDermott M et al. A randomized, placebo-controlled trial of coenzyme Q10 and remacemide in Huntington's disease. *Neurology* 2001; **57**: 397–404.
103. Sanchez I, Mahlke C, Yuan J. Pivotal role of oligomerization in expanded polyglutamine neurodegenerative disorders. *Nature* 2003; **421**: 373–379.
104. Tanaka M, Machida Y, Niu S et al. Trehalose alleviates polyglutamine-mediated pathology in a mouse model of Huntington disease. *Nat Med* 2004; **10**: 148–154.
105. Grady CL, Haxby JV, Horwitz B et al. Longitudinal study of the early neuropsychological and cerebral metabolic changes in dementia of the

Alzheimer type. *J Clin Exp Neuropsychol* 1988; **10**: 576–596.

106. Azari NP, Pettigrew KD, Schapiro MB et al. Early detection of Alzheimer's disease: a statistical approach using positron emission tomographic data. *J Cereb Blood Flow Metab* 1993; **13**: 438–447.
107. Pettegrew JW, Klunk WE, Kanal E et al. Changes in brain membrane phospholipid and high-energy phosphate metabolism precede dementia. *Neurobiol Aging* 1995; **16**: 973–975.
108. Pettegrew JW, Panchalingam K, Klunk WE et al. Alterations of cerebral metabolism in probable Alzheimer's disease: a preliminary study. *Neurobiol Aging* 1994; **15**: 117–132.
109. Yan SD, Chen X, Schmidt AM et al. Glycated tau protein in Alzheimer disease: a mechanism for induction of oxidant stress. *Proc Natl Acad Sci USA* 1994; **91**: 7787–7791.
110. Sheu KF, Kim YT, Blass JP et al. An immunochemical study of the pyruvate dehydrogenase deficit in Alzheimer's disease brain. *Ann Neurol* 1985; **17**: 444–449.
111. Mastrogiacomo F, Bergeron C, Kish SJ. Brain alpha-ketoglutarate dehydrogenase complex activity in Alzheimer's disease. *J Neurochem* 1993; **61**: 2007–2014.
112. Bosetti F, Brizzi F, Barogi S et al. Cytochrome c oxidase and mitochondrial F_1F_0-ATPase (ATP synthase) activities in platelets and brain from patients with Alzheimer's disease. *Neurobiol Aging* 2002; **23**: 371–376.
113. Maurer I, Zierz S, Moller HJ. A selective defect of cytochrome c oxidase is present in brain of Alzheimer disease patients. *Neurobiol Aging* 2000; **21**: 455–462.
114. Mutisya EM, Bowling AC, Beal MF. Cortical cytochrome oxidase activity is reduced in Alzheimer's disease. *J Neurochem* 1994; **63**: 2179–2184.
115. Bonilla E, Tanji K, Hirano M et al. Mitochondrial involvement in Alzheimer's disease. *Biochim Biophys Acta* 1999; **1410**: 171–182.
116. Ojaimi J, Masters CL, McLean C et al. Irregular distribution of cytochrome c oxidase protein subunits in aging and Alzheimer's disease. *Ann Neurol* 1999; **46**: 656–660.
117. Phinney AL, Horne P, Yang J et al. Mouse models of Alzheimer's disease: the long and filamentous road. *Neurol Res* 2003; **25**: 590–600.
118. Lustbader JW, Cirilli M, Lin C et al. ABAD directly links Aβ to mitochondrial toxicity in Alzheimer's disease. *Science* 2004; **304**: 448–452.
119. Casley CS, Canevari L, Land JM et al. Beta-amyloid inhibits integrated mitochondrial respiration and key enzyme activities. *J Neurochem* 2002; 80: 91–100.
120. Dauer W, Przedborski S. Parkinson's disease: mechanisms and models. *Neuron* 2003; **39**: 889–909.
121. Nicklas WJ, Vyas I, Heikkila RE. Inhibition of NADH-linked oxidation in brain mitochondria by MPP+, a metabolite of the neurotoxin MPTP. *Life Sci* 1985; **36**: 2503–2508.
122. Schapira AH, Cooper JM, Dexter D et al. Mitochondrial complex I deficiency in Parkinson's disease. *J Neurochem* 1990; **54**: 823–827.
123. Parker WD, Jr., Boyson SJ, Parks JK. Abnormalities of the electron transport chain in idiopathic Parkinson's disease. *Ann Neurol* 1989; **26**: 719–723.
124. Haas RH, Nasirian F, Nakano K et al. Low platelet mitochondrial complex I and complex II/III activity in early untreated Parkinson's disease. *Ann Neurol* 1995; **37**: 714–722.
125. Swerdlow RH, Parks JK, Miller SW et al. Origin and functional consequences of the complex I defect in Parkinson's disease. *Ann Neurol* 1996; **40**: 663–671.
126. Swerdlow RH, Parks JK, Davis JN et al. Matrilineal inheritance of complex I dysfunction in a multigenerational Parkinson's disease family. *Ann Neurol* 1998; **44**: 873–881.
127. Kosel S, Grasbon-Frodl EM, Mautsch U et al. Novel mutations of mitochondrial complex I in pathologically proven Parkinson disease. *Neurogenetics* 1998; **1**: 197–204.
128. van der Walt JM, Nicodemus KK, Martin ER et al. Mitochondrial polymorphisms significantly reduce the risk of Parkinson disease. *Am J Hum Genet* 2003; **72**: 804–811.
129. Aomi Y, Chen CS, Nakada K et al. Cytoplasmic transfer of platelet mtDNA from elderly patients with Parkinson's disease to mtDNA-less HeLa cells restores complete mitochondrial respiratory function. *Biochem Biophys Res Commun* 2001; **280**: 265–273.
130. Betarbet R, Sherer TB, MacKenzie G et al. Chronic systemic pesticide exposure reproduces features of Parkinson's disease. *Nat Neurosci* 2000; **3**: 1301–1306.

131. Vila M, Przedborski S. Genetic clues to the pathogenesis of Parkinson's disease. *Nat Med* 2004; **10** (Suppl): S58–S62.
132. Nakajima A, Kataoka K, Hong M et al. BRPK, a novel protein kinase showing increased expression in mouse cancer cell lines with higher metastatic potential. *Cancer Lett* 2003; **201**: 195–201.
133. Bonifati V, Rizzu P, Van Baren MJ et al. Mutations in the *DJ-1* gene associated with autosomal recessive early-onset parkinsonism. *Science* 2003; **299**: 256–259.
134. Hague S, Rogaeva E, Hernandez D et al. Early-onset Parkinson's disease caused by a compound heterozygous *DJ-1* mutation. *Ann Neurol* 2003; **54**: 271–274.
135. Abou-Sleiman PM, Healy DG, Quinn N et al. The role of pathogenic DJ-1 mutations in Parkinson's disease. *Ann Neurol* 2003; **54**: 283–286.
136. Canet-Aviles RM, Wilson MA, Miller DW et al. The Parkinson's disease protein DJ-1 is neuroprotective due to cysteine-sulfinic acid-driven mitochondrial localization. *Proc Natl Acad Sci USA* 2004; **101**: 9103–9108.
137. Fahn S, Przedborski S. Parkinsonism. In: Rowland LP, ed. *Merritt's Neurology*. 10th ed. New York: Lippincott Williams & Wilkins, 2000; 679–693.
138. Matthews RT, Ferrante RJ, Klivenyi P et al. Creatine and cyclocreatine attenuate MPTP neurotoxicity. *Exp Neurol* 1999; **157**: 142–149.
139. Beal MF, Matthews RT, Tieleman A et al. Coenzyme Q10 attenuates the 1-methyl-4-phenyl-1,2,3,tetrahydropyridine (MPTP) induced loss of striatal dopamine and dopaminergic axons in aged mice. *Brain Res* 1998; **783**: 109–114.
140. Shults CW, Oakes D, Kieburtz K et al. Effects of coenzyme Q10 in early Parkinson disease: evidence of slowing of the functional decline. *Arch Neurol* 2002; **59**: 1541–1550.
141. Rowland LP, Shneider NA. Amyotrophic lateral sclerosis. *N Engl J Med* 2001; **344**: 1688–1700.
142. Deng HX, Hentati A, Tainer JA et al. Amyotrophic lateral sclerosis and structural defects in Cu, Zn superoxide dismutase. *Science* 1993; **261**: 1047–1051.
143. Rosen DR, Siddique T, Patterson D et al. Mutations in Cu/Zn superoxide dismutase gene are associated with familial amyotrophic lateral sclerosis. *Nature* 1993; **362**: 59–62.
144. Reaume AG, Elliott JL, Hoffman EK et al. Motor neurons in Cu/Zn superoxide dismutase-deficient mice develop normally but exhibit enhanced cell death after axonal injury. *Nat Genet* 1996; **13**: 43–47.
145. Gurney ME, Pu H, Chiu AY et al. Motor neuron degeneration in mice that express a human Cu, Zn superoxide dismutase mutation. *Science* 1994; **264**: 1772–1775.
146. Wong PC, Pardo CA, Borchelt DR et al. An adverse property of a familial ALS-linked SOD1 mutation causes motor neuron disease characterized by vacuolar degeneration of mitochondria. *Neuron* 1995; **14**: 1105–1116.
147. Afifi AK, Aleu FP, Goodgold J et al. Ultrastructure of atrophic muscle in amyotrophic lateral sclerosis. *Neurology* 1966; **16**: 475–481.
148. Hirano A, Donnefeld H, Shoichi S et al. Fine structural observations of neurofilamentous changes in amyotrophic lateral sclerosis. *J Neuropathol Exp Neurol* 1984; **43**: 461–470.
149. Sasaki S, Iwata M. Impairment of fast axonal transport in the proximal axons of anterior horn neurons in amyotrophic lateral sclerosis. *Neurology* 1996; **47**: 535–540.
150. Okamoto K, Hirai S, Shoji M et al. Axonal swellings in the corticospinal tracts in amyotrophic lateral sclerosis. *Acta Neuropathol (Berl)* 1990; **80**: 222–226.
151. Siklos L, Engelhardt J, Harati Y et al. Ultrastructural evidence for altered calcium in motor nerve terminals in amyotropic lateral sclerosis. *Ann Neurol* 1996; **39**: 203–216.
152. Chung MJ, Suh YL. Ultrastructural changes of mitochondria in the skeletal muscle of patients with amyotrophic lateral sclerosis. *Ultrastruct Pathol* 2002; **26**: 3–7.
153. Nakano Y, Hirayama K, Terao K. Hepatic ultrastructural changes and liver dysfunction in amyotrophic lateral sclerosis. *Arch Neurol* 1987; **44**: 103–106.
154. Atsumi T. The ultrastructure of intramuscular nerves in amyotrophic lateral sclerosis. *Acta Neuropathol (Berl)* 1981; **55**: 193–198.
155. Wiedemann FR, Manfredi G, Mawrin C et al. Mitochondrial DNA and respiratory chain function in spinal cords of ALS patients. *J Neurochem* 2002; **80**: 616–625.
156. Borthwick GM, Johnson MA, Ince PG et al. Mitochondrial enzyme activity in amyotrophic

lateral sclerosis: implications for the role of mitochondria in neuronal cell death. *Ann Neurol* 1999; **46**: 787–790.

157. Wiedemann FR, Winkler K, Kuznetsov AV et al. Impairment of mitochondrial function in skeletal muscle of patients with amyotrophic lateral sclerosis. *J Neurol Sci* 1998; **156**: 65–72.
158. Echaniz-Laguna A, Zoll J, Ribera F et al. Mitochondrial respiratory chain function in skeletal muscle of ALS patients. *Ann Neurol* 2002; **52**: 623–627.
159. Okado-Matsumoto A, Fridovich I. Subcellular distribution of superoxide dismutases (SOD) in rat liver: Cu, Zn-SOD in mitochondria. *J Biol Chem* 2001; **276**: 38388–38393.
160. Jaarsma D, Rognoni F, van Duijn W et al. CuZn superoxide dismutase (SOD1) accumulates in vacuolated mitochondria in transgenic mice expressing amyotrophic lateral sclerosis-linked SOD1 mutations. *Acta Neuropathol (Berl)* 2001; **102**: 293–305.
161. Mattiazzi M, D'Aurelio M, Gajewski CD et al. Mutated human SOD1 causes dysfunction of oxidative phosphorylation in mitochondria of transgenic mice. *J Biol Chem* 2002; **277**: 29626–29633.
162. Takeuchi H, Kobayashi Y, Ishigaki S et al. Mitochondrial localization of mutant superoxide dismutase 1 triggers caspase-dependent cell death in a cellular model of familial amyotrophic lateral sclerosis. *J Biol Chem* 2002; **277**: 50966–50972.
163. Higgins CM, Jung C, Ding H et al. Mutant Cu, Zn superoxide dismutase that causes motoneuron degeneration is present in mitochondria in the CNS. *J Neurosci* 2002; **22**: RC215.
164. Jung C, Higgins CM, Xu Z. Mitochondrial electron transport chain complex dysfunction in a transgenic mouse model for amyotrophic lateral sclerosis. *J Neurochem* 2002; **83**: 535–545.
165. Kirkinezos IG, Bacman SR, Hernandez D et al. Cytochrome c association with the inner mitochondrial membrane is impaired in the CNS of G93A-SOD1 mice. *J Neurosci* 2005; **25**: 164–172.
166. Vijayvergiya C, Beal MF, Buck J et al. Mutant superoxide dismutase 1 forms aggregates in the brain mitochondrial matrix of amyotrophic lateral sclerosis mice. *J Neurosci* 2005; **25**: 2463–2470.
167. Kong JM, Xu ZS. Massive mitochondrial degeneration in motor neurons triggers the onset of amyotrophic lateral sclerosis in mice expressing a mutant SOD1. *J Neurosci* 1998; **18**: 3241–3250.
168. Klivenyi P, Ferrante RJ, Matthews RT et al. Neuroprotective effects of creatine in a transgenic animal model of amyotrophic lateral sclerosis. *Nat Med* 1999; **5**: 347–350.
169. Matthews RT, Yang L, Browne S et al. Coenzyme Q10 administration increases brain mitochondrial concentrations and exerts neuroprotective effects. *Proc Natl Acad Sci USA* 1998; **95**: 8892–8897.
170. Andreassen OA, Ferrante RJ, Klivenyi P et al. Transgenic ALS mice show increased vulnerability to the mitochondrial toxins MPTP and 3-nitropropionic acid. *Exp Neurol* 2001; **168**: 356–363.
171. Zhu S, Stavrovskaya I, Drozda M et al. Minocycline inhibits cytochrome *c* release and delays progression of amyotrophic lateral sclerosis in mice. *Nature* 2002; **417**: 74–78.
172. Gordon PH, Moore DH, Gelinas DF et al. Placebo-controlled phase I/II studies of minocycline in amyotrophic lateral sclerosis. *Neurology* 2004; **62**: 1845–1847.
173. Groeneveld GJ, Veldink JH, van der Tweel I et al. A randomized sequential trial of creatine in amyotrophic lateral sclerosis. *Ann Neurol* 2003; **53**: 437–445.
174. Larsson NG, Wang J, Wilhelmsson H et al. Mitochondrial transcription factor A is necessary for mtDNA maintenance and embryogenesis in mice. *Nat Genet* 1998; **18**: 231–236.
175. Richter C. Reactive oxygen and DNA damage in mitochondria. *Mutat Res* 1992; **275**: 249–255.
176. James AM, Sheard PW, Wei YH et al. Decreased ATP synthesis is phenotypically expressed during increased energy demand in fibroblasts containing mitochondrial tRNA mutations. *Eur J Biochem* 1999; **259**: 462–469.
177. Vila M, Przedborski S. Targeting programmed cell death in neurodegenerative diseases. *Nat Rev Neurosci* 2003; **4**: 365–375.
178. Yang J, Liu XS, Bhalla K et al. Prevention of apoptosis by Bcl-2: Release of cytochrome c from mitochondria blocked. *Science* 1997; **275**: 1129–1132.
179. Kluck RM, Bossy-Wetzel E, Green DR et al. The release of cytochrome c from mitochondria: A primary site for Bcl-2 regulation of apoptosis. *Science* 1997; **275**: 1132–1136.
180. Li P, Nijhawan D, Budihardjo I et al. Cytochrome c and dATP-dependent formation of Apaf-1/caspase-9

complex initiates an apoptotic protease cascade. *Cell* 1997; **91**: 479–489.
181. Przedborski S, Vila M. The 1-methyl-4-phenyl-1,2,3,6-tetrahydropyridine mouse model: a tool to explore the pathogenesis of Parkinson's disease. *Ann N Y Acad Sci* 2003; **991**: 189–198.
182. Jackson-Lewis V, Jakowec M, Burke RE et al. Time course and morphology of dopaminergic neuronal death caused by the neurotoxin 1-methyl-4-phenyl-1,2,3,6-tetrahydropyridine. *Neurodegeneration* 1995; **4**: 257–269.
183. Vila M, Jackson-Lewis V, Vukosavic S et al. Bax ablation prevents dopaminergic neurodegeneration in the 1-methyl-4-phenyl-1,2,3,6-tetrahydropyridine mouse model of Parkinson's disease. *Proc Natl Acad Sci USA* 2001; **98**: 2837–2842.

14

Therapeutic approaches

Salvatore DiMauro and Eric A Schon

Introduction

In contrast to the spectacular progress in our understanding of the biochemical and molecular bases of the mitochondrial encephalomyopathies, we are still woefully limited in our ability to treat these conditions. Development and experimentation of new therapies is made more difficult by the lack of spontaneous or engineered animal models of mtDNA-related diseases. A formidable obstacle to the generation of 'mito-mice' (see Box 14.1) is our inability to introduce mutant mtDNA into the mitochondria of mammalian cells.

In this chapter, we will consider separately: (i) symptomatic therapy; (ii) pharmacological therapy; (iii) gene therapy; and (iv) genetic counseling and prenatal diagnosis.

Any discussion of therapy requires some knowledge of the structure and function of the respiratory chain and of the basic concepts of mitochondrial genetics, for which the reader is referred to Chapter 1.

To recap the rules of mitochondrial genetics, they include maternal inheritance, heteroplasmy and threshold effect, and mitotic segregation. Briefly, maternal inheritance refers to the fact that all mtDNA comes to the zygote from the oocyte: thus, as a rule a pathogenic mutation of mtDNA (and related disease) is transmitted from a woman to all her children, but only her daughters will pass it on to their progeny, with no evidence of male-to-child transmission. Heteroplasmy refers to the coexistence of mutant and wild-type mtDNAs in the same cell, tissue, individual, and is predicated on the notion that mtDNA is present in hundreds or thousands of copies in each cell (polyplasmy). A corollary of heteroplasmy is the threshold effect: a certain minimum number of mutant mtDNAs will be needed to impair oxidative phosphorylation and cause symptoms, and the threshold will be lower in tissues highly dependent on oxidative metabolism.

Palliative therapy

Lack of a cure does not mean lack of therapy. Symptomatic therapy can be very effective in patients with mitochondrial disorders. Let us consider – tissue by tissue – both what can be done for some common manifestations of mitochondrial encephalomyopathies and which limitations or precautions should be kept in mind.

CNS

Among disorders of the central nervous system (CNS, see Chapter 2), seizures usually respond to conventional anticonvulsants. However, valproic acid should be used with caution, and in association with L-carnitine, because of its inhibition of carnitine uptake.[1] Valproic acid is particularly dangerous in children with the hepatocerebral syndrome

Box 14.1 'Mito mice'

For unknown reasons, organellar DNA transfection methods that work in lower eukaryotes have failed to work in mammalian cells. Thus, no one knows how to transfect DNA into mouse (or any other mammalian) mitochondria in a heritable manner, nor, for that matter, how to introduce isolated mitochondria into a mammalian cell. The inability to transfect mitochondria with exogenous DNA is perhaps the single greatest stumbling block to progress in understanding mammalian mitochondrial genetics in general and human mitochondrial diseases in particular, because without such a technology, it is almost impossible to create animal models of maternally inherited diseases due to mutations in mitochondrial DNA (mtDNA).

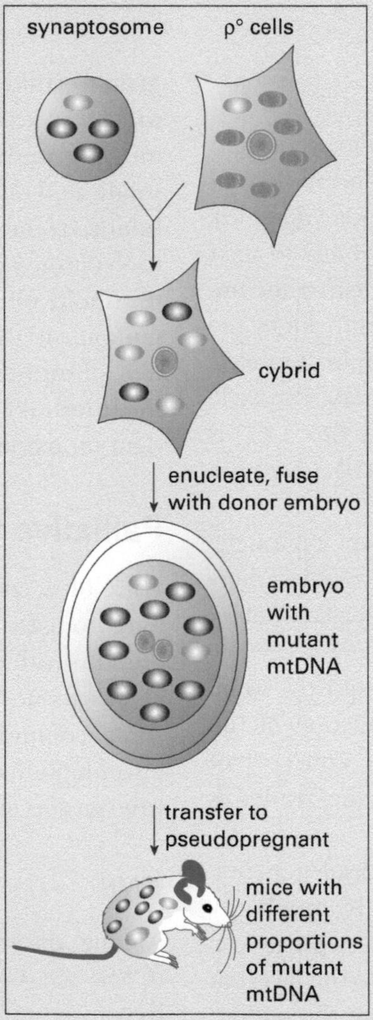

Figure B14.1.1 Making 'mito mice.' Adapted from reference 2, with permission

(Continued)

Box 14.1 (Continued)

Almost impossible, but not totally impossible. In 2000, Jun-ichi Hayashi and his colleagues used a brute force approach to create a mouse model of a human mtDNA deletion disorder similar to Kearns–Sayre syndrome.[1] Since they could not transfect mouse mitochondria with deleted mouse mtDNA, they used a 'backdoor' approach.[2] It has been known for more than a decade that deleted mtDNAs (Δ-mtDNAs) accumulate in the somatic tissues of aging mammals, albeit at an extremely low level. Hayashi took advantage of this fact, and isolated neuronal synaptosomes, which are rich in mitochondria, from aged mice, and transferred them into mouse ρ^0 cells to create a 'library' of cybrids. He then searched through the library to identify a rare cybrid clone containing Δ-mtDNAs. This cybrid became the source of cytoplasts which were then electrofused with pronuclear stage mouse embryos. The embryos were implanted into pseudopregnant females, yielding progeny mice that were heteroplasmic for the Δ-mtDNA.

Analysis of the mice showed that they had some features of Kearns-Sayre syndrome (which is caused by the presence of high levels of Δ-mtDNA in all the patient's tissues), but not all. Interestingly the mice had severe nephropathy, which is atypical of KSS. A second interesting finding was that the Δ-mtDNAs were transmissible through the germline (the germline transmission of Δ-mtDNAs in humans has been the matter of some debate).

References

1. Inoue K, Nakada K, Ogura A et al. Generation of mice with mitochondrial dysfunction by introducing mouse mtDNA carrying a deletion into zygotes. *Nat Genet* 2000; **26**: 176–181.
2. Shoubridge EA. A debut for mito-mouse. *Nat Genet* 2000; **26**: 132–134.

known as Alpers–Huttenlocher syndrome (AHS), who often develop acute hepatic failure after valproic acid administration.

Skeletal muscle

One of the most common symptoms of mitochondrial dysfunction is exercise intolerance, which can be part of multisystem disorders or present in isolation (in which case, patients are often misdiagnosed as having fibromyalgia rheumatica or chronic fatigue syndrome).[2,3] Exercise intolerance often leads to inactivity, which, in turn, leads to muscle deconditioning, thus generating a vicious cycle that worsens the premature fatigue. It has been clearly established that aerobic exercise is useful in mitochondrial patients, improving work capacity, oxygen delivery to muscle (i.e. cardiac output), oxygen extraction and utilization by muscle, and muscle energy metabolism as indicated by ^{32}P magnetic resonance spectroscopy (MRS).[4] At the biochemical level, aerobic exercise favors mitochondrial proliferation (reflected by increased activity of the matrix enzyme citrate synthase) and improves respiratory chain activity (reflected by increased activity of cytochrome *c* oxidase). The only negative and apparently paradoxical result is the small increase in the amount of mutant mtDNAs, which, however, may be overcompensated for by a greater increase of wild-type mtDNAs. In addition, there may be a redistribution of mtDNA, such that more fibers harbor predominantly wild-type genomes while fewer fibers contain predominantly mutant ones.

Mitochondrial myopathies (see Chapter 3) often present as recurrent myoglobinuria, especially in patients with primary coenzyme Q10 (CoQ10) deficiency[5–7] or in patients with mutations in mtDNA protein-coding genes.[2,8,9] Patients with CoQ10 deficiency benefit from CoQ10 supplementation (see below). During acute episodes, all patients should be vigorously rehydrated and subjected to renal dialysis when myoglobinuria is complicated by renal failure.

Eye

A common ophthalmologic disorder (see Chapters 2 and 5) is progressive external ophthalmoplegia (PEO). The ptosis that usually accompanies PEO is often the subject of ridicule leading to social isolation in teenage patients (a young man was dubbed 'Garfield' and a young woman was teased for being 'on drugs'). Ptosis can be ameliorated by surgery, although the results of blepharoplasty are often transient. Congenital cataracts are also treated surgically. For the treatment of LHON, see Chapter 5.

Endocrine system

Among the endocrinological problems (see Chapter 8), diabetes mellitus, whether insulin-dependent or not, responds to dietary or pharmacological therapy. There is controversy about the use of growth hormone in children with growth retardation because the increased metabolic demands may be ill tolerated by an already metabolically challenged patient.

Heart

Cardiological problems include conduction defects and cardiomyopathy (see Chapter 4). Timely placement of a pacemaker can be life-saving in patients with Kearns–Sayre syndrome (KSS) and blocks of cardiac conduction. Heart transplantation is controversial in patients with cardiomyopathy and multisystemic disorders. However, when cardiac involvement is the predominant or exclusive problem, cardiac transplantation is justified.[10–12]

Ear, nose, throat

Mitochondrial otology (see Chapter 7) is dominated by neurosensory hearing loss, which can be alleviated by cochlear implants.[13] In patients with KSS, dysphagia is not uncommon, due to cricopharyngeal achalasia (incomplete opening of the upper esophageal sphincter during the pharyngeal phase of swallowing), and myotomy may be of help.[14]

Gastrointestinal system

Children with Leigh syndrome (LS) often develop severe feeding problems even before neurological symptoms become apparent. Recurrent vomiting and gastroesophageal reflux are common and can be relieved by drugs or surgical interventions, including percutaneous endoscopic gastrostomy (PEG) or gastric fundoplication. Intestinal dysmotility with pseudo-obstruction is seen not only in the MNGIE syndrome (see Chapters 2 and 6) but also in MELAS, and often require emergency surgery. Children with liver failure due to hepatocerebral syndrome and mtDNA depletion (associated with mutations in the deoxyguanosine kinase (*DGUOK*) or in the polymerase γ (*POLG*) gene), may benefit from liver transplantation, especially if other organs are spared.[15,16] Exocrine pancreas dysfunction, typical of Pearson syndrome (PS), requires replacement therapy with digestive enzymes.

Blood

The sideroblastic anemia of PS may respond to repeat blood transfusions, although only few children survive into adulthood, and these, sadly, grow up to develop KSS.[17,18]

Kidney

Renal tubular acidosis and Fanconi syndrome (see Chapter 9) require therapies directed to readjusting electrolyte balance. The nephrotic syndrome associated with the infantile generalized form of CoQ10 deficiency appears to be less responsive to CoQ10 replacement than other clinical manifestations, and these children may require prolonged peritoneal dialysis or renal transplantation.[19,20] Patients with myoglobinuria and renal failure (see above) may also require dialysis.

Pharmacological therapy

Removal of noxious metabolites

As Figure 1.1 in Chapter 1 illustrates, any severe block in the respiratory chain will result in accumulations of substrates upstream, all the way to pyruvate, which is reduced to lactate and transaminated to alanine. In fact, all three compounds are usually increased in blood, cerebrospinal fluid (CSF), and urine of patients with mitochondrial encephalomyopathies.

As excessive concentration of lactic acid is neurotoxic,[21] it is reasonable to control lactic acidosis: unfortunately, this is usually done through the buffering effect of bicarbonate, which is transient and may actually exacerbate cerebral symptoms.[22] A more specific tool to combat lactic acidosis is dichloroacetate (DCA), a well-studied inhibitor of PDH kinase: keeping PDH in the dephosphorylated, active form, favors pyruvate metabolism and decreases lactate concentration.[23] Although there was anecdotal evidence of clinical improvement in children with mitochondrial encephalomyopathy, lactic acidosis, and stroke-like episodes (MELAS), the first double-blind, placebo-controlled, randomized, 3-year cross-over trial of DCA (25 mg/kg/day) in 30 patients with MELAS and the A3243G mutation has just been concluded.[24] The study had to be terminated because of peripheral nerve toxicity, which overshadows any potential beneficial effect in MELAS.[24]

A severe autosomal recessive syndrome due to a defect of intergenomic signaling is mitochondrial gastrointestinal encephalomyopathy (MNGIE).[25] Patients with this multisystemic disorder have mutations in the *TP* gene, encoding the enzyme thymidine kinase, and accumulate excessive amounts of thymidine in blood.[26] Thymidine accumulation causes mitochondrial nucleotide pool imbalances that lead to point mutations, deletions, and depletion of mtDNA.[27,28] Restoring normal levels of circulating thymidine is a logical first approach to therapy, but the effect of dialysis in two patients was too fleeting to be therapeutically useful[26] and alternative approaches are under consideration.

Administration of artificial electron acceptors

An ingenious attempt to bypass a block in complex III of the respiratory chain in a young woman with mitochondrial myopathy and severe exercise intolerance[8,29] employed two artificial electron acceptors (menadiol diphosphate, 40 mg daily, and vitamin C, 4 g daily) whose redox potentials fit the gap created by the cytochrome *b* dysfunction.[30] The patient initially improved dramatically, and this corresponded to improved muscle energetics documented by ^{31}P nuclear magnetic resonance spectroscopy (NMR),[31] but the improvement was not sustained. Other myopathic patients with similar biochemical and molecular defects (complex III deficiency due to mutations in the cytochrome *b* gene of mtDNA) have not responded to this treatment.

Replacement of defective mammalian respiratory chain subunits with corresponding subunits from yeast has been achieved in vitro through molecular engineering: these experiments are discussed below under 'gene therapy'.

Administration of vitamins and cofactors

Various 'cocktails' of vitamins and cofactors have been used – and are still used – in patients with mitochondrial encephalomyopathies, including riboflavin (vitamin B_2), thiamine (vitamin B_1), folic acid, CoQ10, L-carnitine, creatine, and lipoic acid. All of these are natural compounds and presumably harmless at the doses used. Some, such as CoQ10, are components of the respiratory chain, but there is no evidence that they are decreased in primary mitochondrial diseases.[32] Others appear to be decreased in certain conditions: for example, folic acid was lower than normal in blood and CSF of patients with KSS.[33] Still others are decreased secondarily: free carnitine tends to be lower than normal in blood of patients with respiratory chain defects, whereas esterified carnitine tends to be increased. This shift may reflect a partial impairment of β-oxidation, whose reducing equivalents enter the respiratory chain at the level of CoQ10 through the action of the electron transfer flavoprotein (ETF) (see Chapter 1, Figure 1.1). We generally prescribe a combination of L-carnitine (1000 mg three times a day) and CoQ10 (100 mg three times a day), with the rationale of restoring free carnitine levels and exploiting the oxygen radical scavenger properties of CoQ10 (see below).

Encouragement for the use of vitamins and cofactors comes from a study of ATP synthesis in lymphocytes from 12 patients with various well-documented respiratory chain disorders before and after 12 months of therapy with a standardized 'cocktail' that included CoQ10 (350 mg/day), L-carnitine, vitamin B complex, vitamin C, and vitamin K_1 (phylloquinone).[34] There was a significant increase in ATP synthetic capacity in lymphocytes after treatment. Experiments in vitro with control lymphocytes showed that CoQ10 was the only compound that increased ATP synthesis (in a dose-dependent manner). Interestingly, none of the patients in this study showed clinical improvement, perhaps – as the authors suggest – because of the relatively short treatment time.

The usefulness of vitamin E in preventing ALS was documented by prospective study of almost one million individuals age 30 years or older participating in the American Cancer Society's Cancer Prevention Study II.[35] Regular use of vitamin E supplements was associated with a lower risk of dying of ALS, while vitamin C and multivitamins did not have any preventive effect.

The rationale for using some of these compounds is compelling when the factor in question is specifically and markedly decreased, either because of defective transport or because of defective synthesis. This is illustrated by primary carnitine deficiency and primary CoQ10 deficiency.

Although primary carnitine deficiency is not a defect of the respiratory chain, we will briefly describe it here because of the life-saving effect of replacement therapy. Primary systemic carnitine deficiency is an autosomal recessive disorder due to genetic defects of the plasma membrane carnitine transporter.[36] The most common presentation is childhood cardiomyopathy, which is progressive. Echocardiography shows dilated cardiomyopathy and electrocardiography shows peaked T waves and signs of ventricular hypertrophy. Endomyocardial biopsies or postmortem cardiac specimens show massive lipid storage and, when measured, carnitine concentration was less than 5% of normal. There is dramatic response to carnitine supplementation and indices of cardiac function return to normal within a few months.[36–38] Hence the importance of measuring blood carnitine concentration in all children with unexplained cardiomyopathy.

Primary CoQ10 deficiency has three main clinical presentations. The first is characterized by the triad of: (i) myopathy with recurrent myoglobinuria; (ii) ragged-red fibers (RRF) and lipid storage in the muscle biopsy; and (iii) CNS involvement, with seizures, ataxia, or mental retardation.[5–7] The second variant is a devastating multisystem disease of infancy, with encephalopathy, hepatopathy, and nephropathy.[19,20,39] The first molecular defect in a CoQ10 synthetic enzyme (encoded by the *COQ2* gene) has been identified in a family with this syndrome.[40] The third presentation is dominated by ataxia and cerebellar atrophy, often associated with weakness, pyramidal signs, seizures, or mental retardation.[41–43] In a family with the ataxic form, linkage analysis led to the identification of mutations in the aprataxin (*APTX*) gene, associated with the syndrome of ataxia oculomotor apraxia (AOA1).[44] The relationship (if any) between *APTX* mutations and CoQ10 deficiency remains to be clarified. Rarer presentations of CoQ10 deficiency include pure myopathy,[45] a mixed myopathic and ataxic phenotype,[46,47] and a Leigh-like syndrome.[48] All patients respond to CoQ10 administration: life-saving responses have been seen in the infantile form[19,20] and dramatic improvements have been described in predominantly myopathic patients.[6,7,45] Patients with the ataxic form (including those with AOA1), respond less dramatically, probably because of irreversible cerebellar damage.[41–44]

A third factor appears to be deficient in muscle from patients with biochemical defects of the respiratory chain and, therefore, holds promise as a therapeutic agent, although no formal trial has yet been conducted, gluthathione. Glutathione concentration was markedly decreased in 24 muscle specimens from patients with isolated, and even more so in patients with combined, respiratory chain defects.[49]

Creatine monohydrate has been tried in six patients with MELAS and one with undefined mitochondrial disease in a controlled study: there was improvement of high-intensity activities but not of lower-intensity aerobic exercise.[50] One other MELAS patient treated with oral creatine was followed using ^{31}P MRS of muscle and ^{1}H MRS of brain: except for a slight increase of muscle phosphocreatine, there was no evidence of clinical or MRS improvement.[51]

Although the precise pathogenesis of stroke in MELAS is not understood, altered vascular contractility must play a role, a concept bolstered by the observation of excessive mitochondrial proliferation in blood vessels of both muscle (the so-called strongly SDH-reactive vessels, or SSVs[52]) and brain.[53,54] Reasoning that an alteration in nitric oxide (NO) homeostasis could affect vascular function, Naini et al. looked at the concentration of precursors of NO in muscle of MELAS patients and found that citrulline was significantly decreased.[55] Although this decrease would not, by itself, impair NO production to the point of preventing vasodilation, the unusual preservation of COX activity both in affected muscle fibers and in SSVs (which is typical of MELAS and the basis for the 'MELAS paradox' – see Box 2.2) suggests an explanation for the angiopathy. This is based on the notion that NO binds to the active site of COX and displaces heme-bound oxygen. Thus, the relatively high COX concentration in SSVs could 'steal' NO required for vasodilation. Indirect support for this hypothesis was offered by Koga and coworkers, who found that plasma concentrations of citrulline and arginine were decreased in MELAS patients both during and between stroke-like episodes.[56] They also found that intravenous administration of L-arginine (0.5 g/kg/dose)[57] in the acute phase improved all stroke-like symptoms and oral administration (0.15–0.30 g/kg/day) interictally diminished both frequency and severity of strokes. Although this was a pilot open trial, which should be confirmed by more rigorous studies, its unequivocally positive results offer a glimmer of hope for a devastating disease.

In vitro studies revealed a potentially useful therapeutic approach to a fatal infantile form of encephalocardiomyopathy associated to COX deficiency and due to mutations in the nuclear *SCO2* gene, which encodes a COX-assembly protein needed for the insertion of copper into the holoenzyme.[58,59] When copper was added to the medium of cultured COX-deficient myoblasts harboring *SCO2* mutations, COX activity was restored.[60,61] In one less severely affected child (homozygous for a milder *SCO2* mutation), copper-histidine (Cu-his, 30 µg/kg/day) was administered subcutaneously from the 23rd to the 25th month of age, followed by oral administration

(140 μg/day) until her death at 42 months.[62] Although brain and muscle symptoms worsened and she died of respiratory insufficiency, the cardiopathy clearly improved and echocardiography at 39 months showed normal ventricular function. The apparent reversal of the hypertrophic cardiomyopathy must have been due to copper supplementation as she was on no other therapy.

Administration of oxygen radical scavengers

Defects of the respiratory chain have detrimental effects that go beyond impairing ATP production and include altered intracellular calcium buffering,[63] excessive production of ROS,[64] and promoting apoptosis.[65,66] Increased production of ROS damages cell membranes through lipid peroxidation and further accelerates the high mutation rate of mtDNA, creating a vicious cycle. Evidence of oxidative stress has been provided not only in primary mitochondrial diseases but also in a vast number of neurodegenerative disorders, in which nDNA mutations affect mitochondrial or nonmitochondrial proteins (see Chapter 13). These include Friedreich ataxia (FA), Wilson disease, some forms of hereditary spastic paraplegia (HSP), Huntington disease (HD), amyotrophic lateral sclerosis (ALS), and Parkinson disease (PD).[64,66,67]

In an attempt to quench the effects of ROS, several oxygen radical scavengers have been utilized in most of the disorders listed above, including vitamin E, CoQ10, idebenone, and dihydrolipoate (as mentioned above, there is now also a role for glutathione).

CoQ10 has been widely used for primary mitochondrial diseases, and the multitude of generally positive anecdotal data[68–77] together with the lack of negative side effects has contributed to its widespread use in these patients. However, there is a need for controlled trials in large cohorts of patients. The effect of treatment with thiamine, riboflavin, and CoQ10 (50 mg/day for infants, 100 mg/day for toddlers, and 300 mg/day for older children) was evaluated retrospectively in 15 pediatric patients with various mitochondrial diseases.[78] There was no correlation between improvement and age at onset or dose of treatment; rather, outcome was correlated to the severity of the biochemical or molecular defect. Importantly, subjective improvement was reported by most patients; although a placebo effect could not be ruled out, the authors point out that the reported improvement in quality of life cannot be dismissed, especially considering that the treatments were harmless and relatively inexpensive.[78]

CoQ10 and idebenone have been increasingly employed in therapeutic trials of neurodegenerative disorders whose pathogenetic mechanisms are thought to involve excessive production of ROS. Both CoQ10 and idebenone improved cardiac function in patients with FA but not their CNS symptoms.[79–83] Administration of CoQ10 (400 mg/day) and vitamin E (2100 IU/day) to 10 FD patients improved both skeletal and cardiac muscle bioenergetics; total international cooperative ataxia scores (ICARS) were better than predicted in six patients, kinetic scores improved in seven, but posture and gait symptoms worsened.[84]

A multicenter, randomized, parallel-group, double-blind, placebo-controlled study of 80 patients with early PD treated with three doses of CoQ10 (300, 600, or 1200 mg daily) showed not only that CoQ10 was well tolerated, but also that less disability developed in subjects taking CoQ10 and the benefit was greatest in patients on the highest dosage.[85] To identify the dose of oral CoQ10 resulting in the highest blood concentration, 17 PD patients were given escalating dosages ranging from 1200 mg/day to 3000 mg/day (together with a stable dosage of vitamin E, 1200 IU/day) for 2 weeks: in the 13 patients who received the maximal dosage, blood concentrations reached a plateau (about 26 mg/ml) at the dosage of 2400 mg/day.[86] All dosages of CoQ10 were safe and well tolerated, at least for 2-week periods.

A randomized, placebo-controlled study of CoQ10 (300 mg bid) versus remacemide (200 mg tid), versus a combination of remacemide and CoQ10, and versus placebo was conducted in patients with early HD.[87] Patients treated with CoQ10 showed a trend towards slowing the decline in total functional capacity (13% less than patients not receiving CoQ10) over 30 months. Although promising, these results are not yet sufficient to recommend CoQ10 in the treatment of HD.[87–89] Creatine supplementation (20 g/day for 5 days; 6 g/day thereafter) was also tried in 20 patients with HD for 8–10 weeks: the primary endpoint was metabolic change assessed by ^{1}H-MRS, and the secondary endpoint was change in the motor section of the Unified Huntington Disease Rating Scale and the Mini Mental State Examination.[90] Although there was no clinical improvement, the observed decrease in brain glutamate was considered positive in view of the glutamate-mediated excitotoxicity probably involved in the pathogenesis of HD, and long-term trials were recommended.

A small open-labeled pilot study of CoQ10 (600 mg/day) in ALS showed some positive trends,[91] but larger controlled studies are underway and will yield more conclusive results.

Gene therapy

A simple-minded form of gene therapy was used in the second patient with non-thyroidal hypermetabolism (Luft disease; see Introduction): to reduce the excessive number of muscle mitochondria, the patient was given chloramphenicol, an inhibitor of mitochondrial protein synthesis. There was a mild reduction of metabolic rate and some subjective improvement, but the trial was short-lived because of drug toxicity,[92] and a second trial was unsuccessful.[93]

For mitochondrial diseases due to mutations in nuclear genes, the problems are no different from those vexing gene therapy for other Mendelian disorders, including choice of appropriate viral or non-viral vectors, delivery to the affected tissues, and potential immunological reactions.

The problems are more complex for mtDNA-related diseases because of polyplasmy and heteroplasmy and because nobody has yet been able to transfect DNA into mitochondria in a heritable manner.

Affecting heteroplasmy

The most promising approach is to influence heteroplasmy, reducing the ratio of mutant to wild-type mitochondrial genomes, or 'gene shifting'.[94] This can be achieved in various manners, including: (i) inducing muscle regeneration; (ii) selecting for respiratory function; (iii) importing exogenous molecules; and (iv) inducing organellar fusion.

Induced muscle regeneration

Both a pharmacological and a functional approach to 'gene shifting' originated from the same observation, that satellite cells and myoblasts contain lesser amounts of mutant mtDNAs than do mature muscle fibers.[94–97] The pharmacological approach used a myotoxic agent, bupivacaine, to cause limited muscle necrosis, which would be 'repaired' by tissue harboring less mutant mtDNA. Unfortunately, unilateral injection of bupivocaine in levator palpebrae muscles of five patients with PEO or KSS did not cause any improvement.[98] The functional approach exploits the notion that isometric exercise leads to 'microtraumas' and limited necrosis of exercising muscles.[94] Indirect support for this concept comes from our studies of one patient with recurrent myoglobinuria due to a nonsense mutation (G5920A) in the *COX I* gene of mtDNA.[9] The few COX-positive fibers in the muscle biopsy of this patient were totally devoid of mutant mtDNA, suggesting that these were indeed regenerated fibers (Box 14.1). This putative – and apparently paradoxical – beneficial effect of massive muscle necrosis suggests the potential therapeutic value of induced attacks of myoglobinuria in patients with severe exercise intolerance or weakness due to muscle-specific mtDNA mutations.

Selection for respiratory function

For patients with systemic mtDNA mutations (the vast majority), the approach described above would not be helpful. However, the concept of heteroplasmic shifting would be useful if the agent could be delivered to all affected cells. For example, in patients with the T8993G mutation in the *ATP6* gene causing the NARP/MILS syndrome (see Chapters 1 and 2), there is a reduction of ATP synthesis.[99] The mutation is located in the same transmembrane domain of ATPase 6 that confers sensitivity to oligomycin. Addition of oligomycin to cultured cybrids harboring the T8993G mutation in medium containing galactose instead of glucose (thus forcing the cells to rely on oxidative metabolism for ATP) resulted in a subtle but significant – and irreversible – reduction in the mutation load, with a concomitant increase in ATP production (Figure 14.1).[100] With all due caution because oligomycin is a mitochondrial poison, this system could be adapted to human therapy.

A friendlier pharmacological way of reducing the mtDNA mutation load, which proved effective – at least in vitro – is exposure to ketone bodies (Figure 14.2). Cybrid cell lines harboring mtDNA single deletions (Δ-mtDNA, associated with KSS – see Chapter 2) were grown in medium containing ketone bodies instead of glucose as the carbon source.[101] Cells homoplasmic for Δ-mtDNA died whereas cells homoplasmic for wild-type mtDNA survived. In heteroplasmic cell lines, the proportion of wild-type mtDNA increased from 13% to 22% after 5 days in ketogenic medium, and this was accompanied by a marked improvement in mitochondrial protein synthesis. Importantly, this 'heteroplasmic shifting' occurred not only among cells (intercellular selection) but also within cells (intracellular selection), which bodes well for future trials of the ketogenic diet in patients.

Importation of exogenous molecules

Specific restriction endonucleases, which cut mutant but not wild-type mtDNA, could act as 'magic bullets'. This approach has proven successful in cybrid cell lines harboring the T8993G NARP/MILS mutation in the *ATPase6* gene.[102] The gene encoding *Sma*I, a 'magic bullet' for this particular mutation, was fused to mitochondrial targeting sequences and transiently expressed in heteroplasmic cybrids, which lost mutant mtDNAs.

A similar approach was taken by the Newcastle-upon-Tyne group: they employed peptide nucleic acids (PNAs) to inhibit selectively the replication of complementary mutant, but not wild-type mtDNAs (specifically, A8344G MERRF mutant mtDNA).[103–105]

Induction of organellar fusion

The problem of heteroplasmy is complicated by the heterogeneous distribution of mutant mtDNAs within cells and tissues. This is exemplified by the clinical difference between MELAS and maternally inherited PEO, both of which can be caused by the same A3243G mutation in $tRNA^{Leu(UUR)}$. The difference between the two disorders, at least in muscle, was attributed to differences in the localized concentration and distribution of mutant mtDNAs in individual muscle fibers.[106] Thus, in terms of heteroplasmic shifting, it might not be necessary to reduce the amount of the mutation at all. If we could redistribute the proportion of mutant and wild-type mtDNAs within mitochondria, we could convert 'homoplasmic mutant' and 'homoplasmic wild-type' organelles into 'heteroplasmic' organelles, containing at least one or two wild-type mtDNAs, which would then complement the function of the

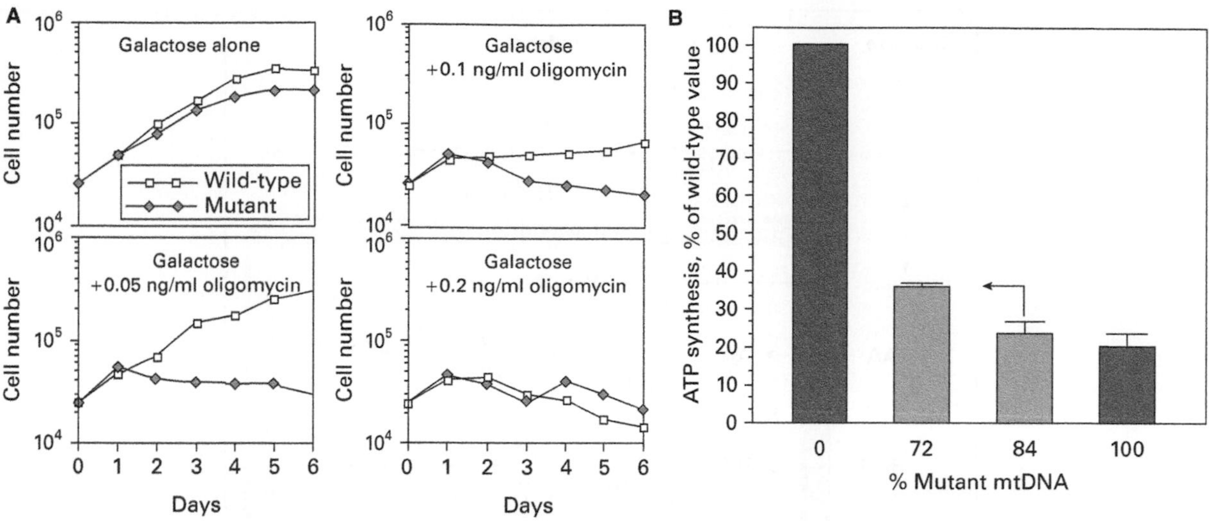

Figure 14.1 Heteroplasmic shifting in T8993G cells. (**A**) Growth of fibroblasts in medium containing galactose (replacing glucose) and increasing amounts of oligomycin. Note the 'window' that opens up between 0.05 and 0.1 μg/ml oligomycin, where the wild-type fibroblasts (0% mutation) continue to grow whereas the mutant fibroblasts (100% mutation) die. (**B**) Treatment of homoplasmic (black bars) and heteroplasmic cybrids (gray bars) in galactose + oligomycin for 5 days. Notice the shift in heteroplasmy from 84% to 72%, which was accompanied by an increase in ATP synthesis relative to the level in homoplasmic wild-type control cybrids; homoplasmic mutant cybrids had a baseline level of ATP synthesis similar to that in the 84% heteroplasmic cybrids

mutant mtDNAs in those organelles. This way, we might obtain a population of organelles or cells that are below the threshold for mitochondrial dysfunction.

Combating ROS accumulation

A genetic approach to scavenging ROS proved successful in transgenic mice. First, it was documented that complex I deficiency induced by expression of anti-*NDUFA1* ribozyme (NDUFA1 is a catalytic subunit of complex I) in mice induced lesions in the retina and optic nerve similar to those of LHON (see Chapter 5) in humans.[107] Second, it was shown that inhibition of mitochondrial superoxide dismutase (SOD2, an antioxidant enzyme) by expression of anti-*SOD2* ribozyme in mice also induced LHON-like lesions.[108] These data established that excessive production of ROS damaged the retina and the optic nerve. These same authors then co-expressed anti-*NDUFA1* ribozyme (the poison) and *SOD2* (the antidote) in the same mice and protected the animals from the eye lesions, thus documenting the powerful therapeutic action of SOD scavenging.[109,110]

Isogenic therapy: allotopic expression

Although we do not yet know how to transfect foreign mitochondria with exogenous DNA, we do know how to 'transfect' mitochondria with exogenous proteins. This knowledge has led to a rather baroque strategy to reduce the load of mutant polypeptides by importing a normal version of a

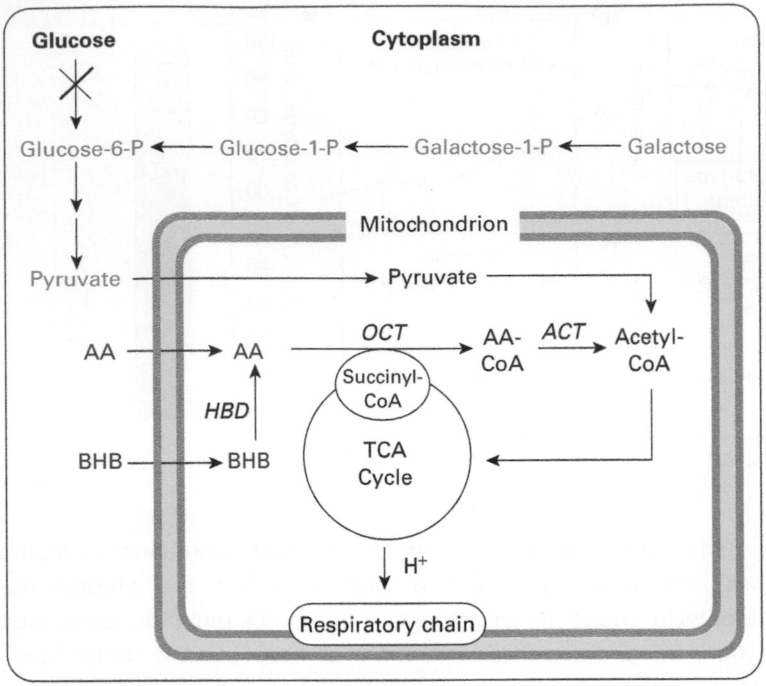

Figure 14.2 Comparison of galactose to ketone body metabolism under conditions of glucose deprivation. Ketone bodies (e.g. D-β-hydroxybutyrate (BHB) and acetoacetate (AA)) provide oxidizable carbon to mitochondria directly, whereas galactose is only an 'indirect' source that is metabolized in the cytoplasm and can yield low levels of ATP via substrate level phosphorylation. Both BHB and AA are transported into mitochondria, where BHB is converted to AA by D-β-hydroxybutyrate dehydrogenase (HBD). AA is converted to acetoacetyl-CoA (AA-CoA) from succinyl-CoA by 3-oxoacid-CoA transferase (OCT); AA-CoA is then converted to acetyl-CoA by acetoacetyl-CoA thiolase (ACT)

mutant mtDNA-encoded polypeptide from a gene 'snuck' into the nucleus (Figure 14.3). This strategy, pioneered by Nagley and coworkers, is called 'allotopic expression'.[111]

For example, the *ATPase6* gene of mtDNA can be converted from the mitochondrial into the nuclear genetic code. To be sure that the novel nuclear protein encoded by the converted gene is recognized by – and transported into – mitochondria, it has to be provided with a leader peptide, whose genetic sequence can be 'borrowed' from another mtDNA-encoded protein. Once this genetic 'Trojan horse' has been carried into the nucleus, its translation product in the cytoplasm would be transported into the mitochondria, freed of the leader peptide, and assembled into the F_0 component of complex V together with its ATPase 8 counterpart synthesized within the mitochondria. Circuitous as it is, this approach has been realized in vitro to correct the biochemical defect in cybrid cells harboring the T8993G NARP/MILS mutation[112] and in cybrids harboring the G11778A LHON (Leber's hereditary optic neuropathy) mutation.[113]

Still another molecular 'trick' is to correct a respiratory chain defect due to a mtDNA mutation by transfecting affected mammalian cells with either mitochondrial or nuclear genes from

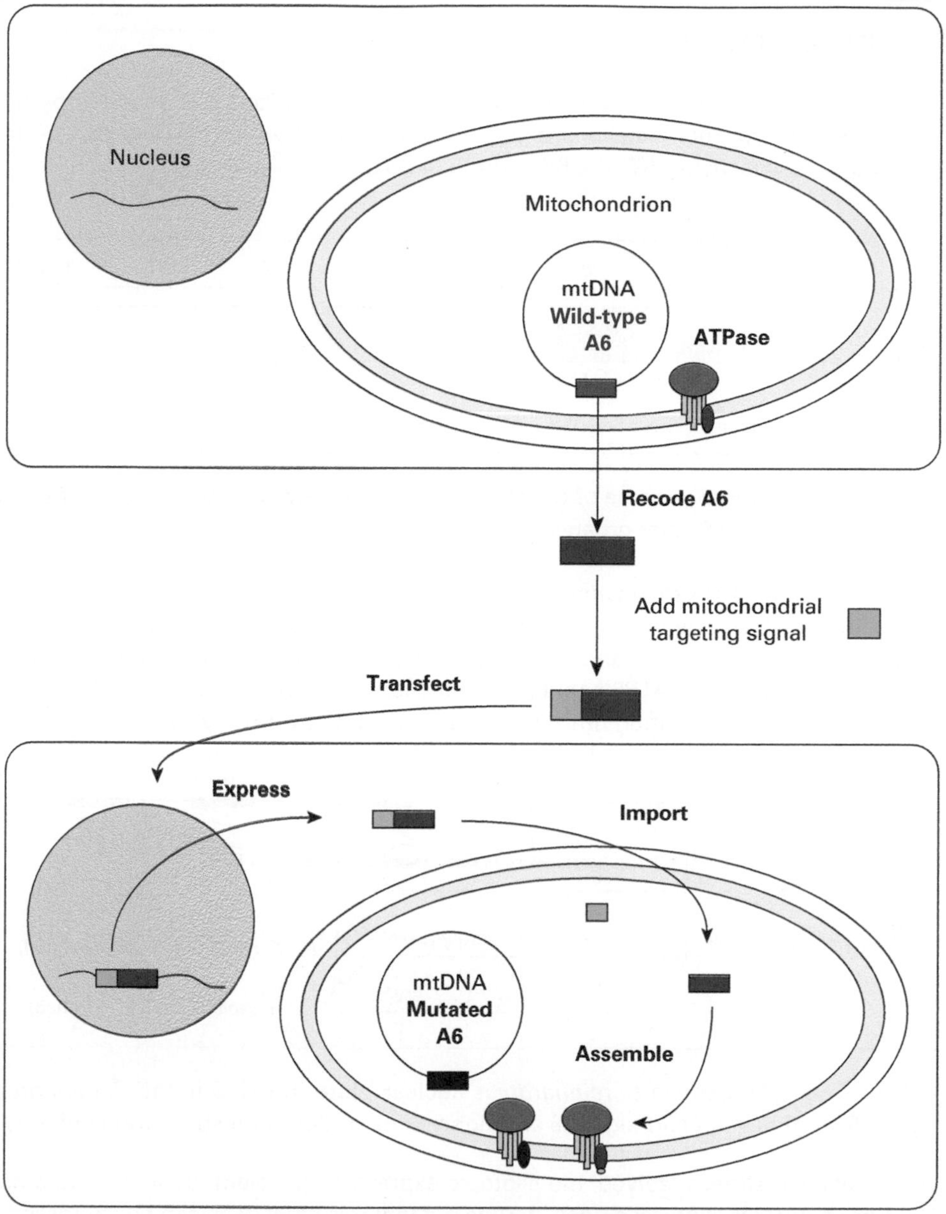

Figure 14.3 Allotopic expression of the human ATP6 gene in T8993G cells. The ATP6 gene is isolated, the codons that are unique to the mitochondrial genetic code are changed to the 'universal' (nuclear) genetic code by in vitro mutagenesis, and a DNA sequence encoding a mitochondrial targeting signal (MTS) is appended to the 5′ end (i.e. N-terminus of the encoded polypeptide). An epitope tag was appended to the 3′ end (C-terminus) for ease of detection. Upon transfection into cells containing 100% mutated (T8993G) mtDNA, the allotopically expressed ATP6 was imported successfully into mitochondria, where the MTS was cleaved off and the mature ATP6 was assembled into the ATP synthase holoprotein, and synthesized ATP. Note that the 'endogenous' mutated ATP6 and the allotopically expressed normal ATP6 polypeptides compete for assembly into holoproteins (i.e. 'protein heteroplasmy')

Box 14.2 Xenotopic expression

In humans, as in almost all other organisms examined to date, ATPase 6 is encoded by mitochondrial DNA. However, among the unicellular algae, including *Chlamydomonas reinhardtii*, there is no mtDNA-encoded gene specifying ATPase 6 (Figure B14.2.1).[1]

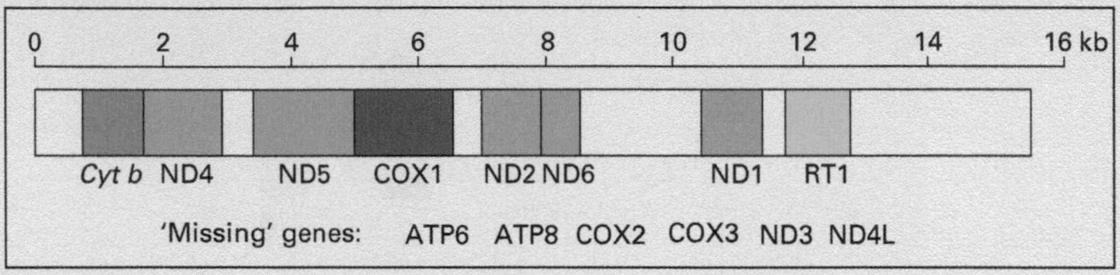

Figure B14.2.1 Mitochondrial genome of *Chlamydomonas reinhardtii*. Note the 'loss' of six genes normally found in the mtDNAs of other organisms

Since ATP6 is required for ATPase function, *C. reinhardtii* must have such a gene, and in fact, the gene has been 'translocated' from the mitochondrion to the nucleus. Moreover, the nuclear version of ATP6 must be translated in the cytoplasm and then imported into this alga's mitochondria, and indeed, the nuclear version of *C. reinhardtii* ATP6 contains a mitochondrial targeting signal (MTS) that is absent (because it is unnecessary) in human mtDNA-encoded ATP6 (Figure B14.2.2).

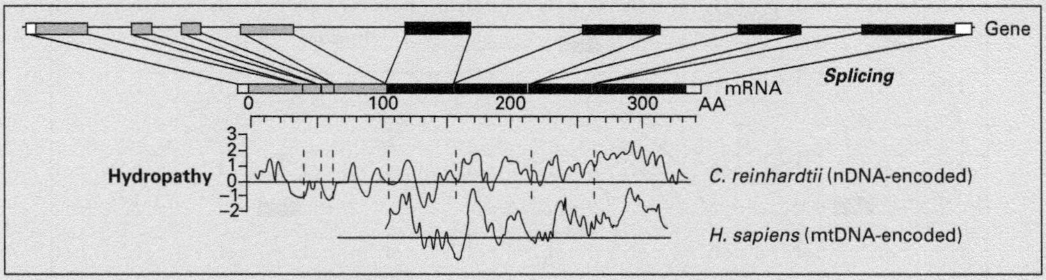

Figure B14.2.2 The ATP6 gene in *C. reinhardtii* is nuclear. Note the MTS in the *C. reinhardtii* A6. The hydropathy profiles of human and algal A6 are highly similar, denoting structural similarity

Thus, *C. reinhardtii* has already 'solved' the allotopic expression problem, by importing a normal version of ATP6 from a nuclear-expressed gene. It turns out that this algal gene can be expressed in human cybrids containing mutation in human *ATP6* and can rescue the ATP deficit in those cells.[2] In order to distinguish this type of 'gene therapy' from allotopic expression, we call the use of a constitutively expressed 'foreign' nuclear gene that is normally mtDNA-expressed in humans *xenotopic expression.*

References

1. Gray MW, Boer PH. Organization and expression of algal (*Chlamydomonas reinhardtii*) mitochondrial DNA. *Philos Trans R Soc Lond B Biol Sci* 1988; **319**: 135–147.
2. Ojaimi J, Pan J, Santra S et al. An algal nucleus-encoded subunit of mitochondrial ATP synthase rescues a defect in the analogous human mitochondrial-encoded subunit. *Mol Biol Cell* 2002; **13**: 3836–3844.

other organisms but encoding cognate proteins ('xenotopic therapy' – see Box 14.2).

Finally, normal yeast tRNAs can be imported from the cytoplasm to compensate for mutant mitochondrial tRNAs and human mitochondria can internalize yeast tRNA derivatives in the presence of a specific yeast transport factor.[114] In yeast, the deleterious effects of mutations that are counterparts of human MELAS mutations can be compensated by the overexpression of a mitochondrial elongation factor, EF-TU.[115] This yeast model opens new therapeutic vistas for human mitochondrial diseases, based on the exploitation of genes that modify or suppress pathological phenotypes.

Germline therapy

Theoretically, a woman carrying a mtDNA mutation could have her oocytes 'cleansed' in vitro of the cytoplasm – with all, or most, of its mitochondria. The naked nucleus could then be transferred to a normal enucleated host oocyte, which could be fertilized in vitro and implanted in the woman's uterus. If successful, this approach would guarantee a normal progeny with all the nuclear – and physiognomonic – traits of both parents.[116] Partial replacement (5% to 10%) of the cytoplasm of aged oocytes is actually used to 'rejuvenate' them and improve the success rate of in vitro fertilization.[117] This approach raises ethical questions regarding germline genetic manipulation (see Chapter 11).[118]

Genetic counseling

Prenatal diagnosis for tRNA point mutations, including the more common ones associated with MELAS and MERRF, is made practically impossible by two concerns. First, the mutation load in amniocytes or chorionic villi does not necessarily correspond to that of other fetal tissues. Second, mutation load measured in prenatal samples may shift in utero or after birth due to mitotic segregation.

At the other end of the spectrum, large-scale deletions of mtDNA as a rule are neither inherited nor transmitted, and either arise de novo in oogenesis or early embryogenesis, or – when they are present in a fertilized oocyte – are unlikely to slip through the bottleneck between ovum and embryo that allows only a small minority of maternal mtDNAs to populate the fetus. However, in counseling a woman who harbors a large-scale mtDNA deletion, the possibility of transmission should not be excluded completely, as three such events are recorded in the literature.[119–121] This has been largely confirmed by a multicenter study of 226 families in which the proband had a documented mtDNA deletion.[122] Unaffected mothers were unlikely to have more than one affected child whereas affected mothers had a small but finite chance of having an affected child (1 in 24 births, on average). This study has also debunked the idea that the risk of developing single mtDNA deletion diseases increases with increasing maternal age.

There is good evidence that mutations in ATPase 6 associated with NARP/MILS do not show tissue- or age-related variations,[123] thus making prenatal diagnosis feasible for parents who have lost a child to maternally inherited Leigh syndrome.[124]

The rapid progress in our molecular knowledge of nDNA-related defects of the respiratory chain is improving genetic counseling and making prenatal diagnosis an option for families with fatal infantile conditions, such as LS or mtDNA depletion syndromes.

Acknowledgments

Part of the work described here was supported by NIH grants HD32062 and NS11766, by grants from the Muscular Dystrophy Association, and by the Marriott Mitochondrial Disorders Clinical Research Fund (MMDCRF).

References

1. Tein I, DiMauro S, Xie Z-W, et al. Valproic acid impairs carnitine uptake in cultured human skin fibroblasts. An in vitro model for pathogenesis of valproic acid-associated carnitine deficiency. *Pediat Res* 1993; **34**: 281–287.
2. Andreu AL, Hanna MG, Reichmann H et al. Exercise intolerance due to mutations in the cytochrome b gene of mitochondrial DNA. *New Engl J Med* 1999; **341**: 1037–1044.
3. DiMauro S, Bonilla E, Mancuso M et al. Mitochondrial myopathies. *Basic Appl Myol* 2003; **13**: 145–155.
4. Taivassalo T, Shoubridge EA, Chen J et al. Aerobic conditioning in patients with mitochondrial myopathies: Physiological, biochemical, and genetic effects. Ann Neurol 2001; 50: 133–141.
5. Ogasahara S, Engel AG, Frens D, Mack D. Muscle coenzyme Q deficiency in familial mitochondrial encephalomyopathy. *Proc Natl Acad Sci USA* 1989; **86**: 2379–2382.
6. Sobreira C, Hirano M, Shanske S et al. Mitochondrial encephalomyopathy with coenzyme Q10 deficiency. *Neurology* 1997; **48**: 1238–1243.
7. Di Giovanni S, Mirabella M, Spinazzola A et al. Coenzyme Q10 reverses pathological phenotype and reduces apoptosis in familial CoQ10 deficiency. *Neurology* 2001; **57**: 515–518.
8. Keightley JA, Anitori R, Burton MD et al. Mitochondrial encephalomyopathy and complex III deficiency associated with a stop-codon mutation in the cytochrome *b* gene. *Am J Hum Genet* 2000; **67**: 1400–1410.
9. Karadimas CL, Greenstein P, Sue CM et al. Recurrent myoglobinuria due to a nonsense mutation in the COX I gene of mtDNA. *Neurology* 2000; **55**: 644–649.
10. Tranchant C, Mousson B, Mohr M et al. Cardiac transplantation in an incomplete Kearns-Sayre syndrome with mitochondrial DNA deletion. *Neuromusc Disord* 1993; **3**: 561–566.
11. Bohlega S, Tanji K, Santorelli FM et al. Multiple mitochondrial DNA deletions associated with autosomal recessive ophthalmoplegia and severe cardiomyopathy. *Neurology* 1996; **46**: 1329–1334.
12. Santorelli FM, Gagliardi MG, Dionisi-Vici C et al. Hypertrophic cardiomyopathy and mtDNA depletion. Successful treatment with heart transplantation. *Neuromusc Disord* 2002; **12**: 56–59.
13. Sue CM, Lipsett LJ, Crimmins DS et al. Cochlear origin of hearing loss in MELAS syndrome. *Ann Neurol* 1998; **43**: 350–359.
14. Kornblum C, Broicher R, Walther E et al. Cricopharyngeal achalasia is a common cause of dysphagia in patients with mtDNA deletions. *Neurology* 2001; **56**: 1409–1412.
15. Dubern B, Broue P, Dubuisson C et al. Orthotopic liver transplantation for mitochondrial respiratory chain disorders: a study of 5 children. *Transplantation* 2001; **71**: 633–637.
16. Salviati L, Sacconi S, Mancuso M et al. Mitochondrial DNA depletion and *dGK* gene mutations. *Ann Neurol* 2002; **52**: 311–317.
17. Larsson NG, Holme B, Kristiansson B. Progressive increase of the mutated mitochondrial DNA fraction in Kearns-Sayre syndrome. *Pediatr Res* 1990; **28**: 131–136.
18. McShane MA, Hammans SR, Sweeney M et al. Pearson syndrome and mitochondrial encephalopathy in a patient with a deletion of mtDNA. *Am J Hum Genet* 1991; **48**: 39–42.
19. Rötig A, Appelkvist E-L, Geromel V et al. Quinone-responsive multiple respiratory-chain dysfunction due to widespread coenzyme Q10 deficiency. *Lancet* 2000; **356**: 391–395.
20. Salviati L, Sacconi S, Murer L et al. Infantile encephalomyopathy and nephropathy with CoQ10 deficiency: a CoQ10-responsive condition. *Neurology* 2005; **65**: 606–608.
21. Kaufmann P, Shungu D, Sano MC et al. Cerebral lactic acidosis correlates with neurological impairment in MELAS. *Neurology* 2004; **62**: 1297–1302.
22. De Vivo DC, DiMauro S. Mitochondrial diseases. In: Swaiman KF, Ashwal S, eds. *Pediatric Neurology: Principles & Practice*. Vol. 1. St Louis: Mosby, 1999: 494–509.
23. Stacpoole PW. The pharmacology of dichloroacetate. *Metabolism* 1989; **38**: 1124–1144.
24. Kaufmann P, Engelstad K, Wei Y-H et al. A randomized, placebo-controlled trial of dichloroacetate in MELAS: Toxicity overshadows potential benefit. *Neurology* 2006; in press.
25. Nishino I, Spinazzola A, Papadimitriou A et al. Mitochondrial neurogastrointestinal encephalomyopathy: an autosomal recessive disorder due to

thymidine phosphorylase mutations. *Ann Neurol* 2000; **47**: 792–800.

26. Spinazzola A, Marti R, Nishino I et al. Altered thymidine metabolism due to defects of thymidine phosphorylase. *J Biol Chem* 2002; **277**: 4128–4132.
27. Nishigaki Y, Marti RA, Copeland WC, Hirano M. Site-specific somatic mitochondrial DNA point mutations in patients with thymidine phosphorylase deficiency. *J Clin Invest* 2003; **111**: 1913–1921.
28. Nishigaki Y, Marti RA, Hirano M. ND5 is a hotspot for multiple atypical mitochondrial DNA deletions in mitochondrial neurogastrointestinal encephalomyopathy. *Hum Mol Genet* 2004; **13**: 91–101.
29. Kennaway NG, Buist NR, Darley Usmar VM et al. Lactic acidosis and mitochondrial myopathy associated with deficiency of several components of complex III of the respiratory chain. *Pediatr Res* 1984; **18**: 991–999.
30. Eleff S, Kennaway NG, Buist NR et al. ^{31}P-NMR study of improvement in oxidative phosphorylation by vitamins K3 and C in a patient with a defect in electron transport at complex III in skeletal muscle. *Proc Natl Acad Sci USA* 1984; **81**: 3529–3533.
31. Argov Z, Bank WJ, Maris J et al. Treatment of mitochondrial myopathy due to complex III deficiency with vitamins K3 and C: A ^{31}P-NMR follow-up study. *Ann Neurol* 1986; **19**: 598–602.
32. Matsuoka T, Maeda H, Goto Y, Nonaka I. Muscle coenzyme Q10 in mitochondrial encephalomyopathies. *Neuromusc Disord* 1992; **1**: 443–447.
33. Allen RJ, DiMauro S, Coulter DL et al. Kearns-Sayre syndrome with reduced plasma and cerebrospinal fluid folate. *Ann Neurol* 1983; **13**: 679–682.
34. Marriage BJ, Clandinin MT, Macdonald IM, Glerum DM. Cofactor treatment improves ATP synthetic capacity in patients with oxidative phosphorylation disorders. *Mol Genet Metab* 2004; **81**: 263–272.
35. Ascherio A, Weisskopf MG, O'Reilly EJ et al. Vitamin E intake and risk of amyotrophic lateral sclerosis. *Ann Neurol* 2005; **57**: 104–110.
36. Tein I. Carnitine transport: Pathophysiology and metabolism of known molecular defects. *J Inher Metab Dis* 2003; **26**: 147–169.
37. Stanley CA, De Leeuw S, Coates PM et al. Chronic cardiomyopathy and weakness or acute coma in children with a defect in carnitine uptake. *Ann Neurol* 1991; **30**: 709–716.
38. Tein I, DeVivo DC, Bierman F et al. Impaired skin fibroblast carnitine uptake in primary systemic carnitine deficiency manifested by childhood carnitine- responsive cardiomyopathy. *Pediat Res* 1990; **28**: 247–255.
39. Rahman S, Hargreaves I, Clayton P, Heales S. Neonatal presentation of coenzyme Q10 deficiency. *J Pediatr* 2001; **139**: 456–458.
40. Quinzii C, Naini AB, Salviati L et al. A mutation in para-hydroxybenzoate:polyprenyl transferase (*COQ2*) causes primary coenzyme Q10 deficiency. *Am J Hum Genet* 2006; in press.
41. Musumeci O, Naini A, Slonim AE et al. Familial cerebellar ataxia with muscle coenzyme Q10 deficiency. *Neurology* 2001; **56**: 849–855.
42. Lamperti C, Naini A, Hirano M et al. Cerebellar ataxia and coenzyme Q10 deficiency. *Neurology* 2003; **60**: 1206–1208.
43. Gironi M, Lamperti C, Nemni R et al. Late-onset cerebellar ataxia with hypogonadism and muscle coenzyme Q10 deficiency. *Neurology* 2004; **62**: 818–820.
44. Quinzii C, Kattah AG, Naini A et al. Coenzyme Q deficiency and cerebellar ataxia associated with an *aprataxin* mutation. *Neurology* 2005; **64**: 539–541.
45. Lalani S, Vladutiu GD, Plunkett K et al. Isolated mitochondrial myopathy associated with muscle coenzyme Q10 deficiency. *Arch Neurol* 2005; **62**: 317–320.
46. Boitier E, Degoul F, Desguerre I et al. A case of mitochondrial encephalomyopathy associated with a muscle coenzyme Q10 deficiency. *J Neurol Sci* 1998; **156**: 41–46.
47. Aure' K, Benoist JF, Ogier de Baulny H et al. Progression despite replacement of a myopathic form of coenzyme Q10 defect. *Neurology* 2004; **63**: 727–729.
48. Van Maldergem L, Trijbels F, DiMauro S et al. Coenzyme Q-responsive Leigh's encephalopathy in two sisters. *Ann Neurol* 2002; **52**: 750–754.
49. Hargreaves IP, Sheena Y, Land JM, Heales SJR. Glutathione deficiency in patients with mitochondrial diseases: Implications for pathogenesis and treatment. *J Inher Metab Dis* 2005; **28**: 81–88.
50. Tarnopolsky MA, Roy BD, MacDonald JR. A randomized, controlled trial of creatine monohydrate in patients with mitochondrial cytopathies. *Muscle Nerve* 1997; **20**: 1502–1509.

51. Moller HE, Wiedermann D, Kurlemann G et al. Application of NMR spectroscopy to monitoring MELAS treatment: a case report. *Muscle Nerve* 2002; **25**: 593–600.
52. Hasegawa H, Matsuoka T, Goto I, Nonaka I. Strongly succinate dehydrogenase-reactive blood vessels in muscles from patients with mitochondrial myopathy, encephalopathy, lactic acidosis, and stroke-like episodes. *Ann Neurol* 1991; **29**: 601–605.
53. Sakuta R, Nonaka I. Vascular involvement in mitochondrial myopathy. *Ann Neurol* 1989; **25**: 594–601.
54. Ohama E, Ohara S, Ikuta F et al. Mitochondrial angiopathy in cerebral blood vessels of mitochondrial encephalomyopathy. *Acta Neuropath* 1987; **74**: 226–233.
55. Naini A, Kaufmann P, Shanske S et al. Hypocitrullinemia in patients with MELAS: an insight into the 'MELAS paradox'. *J Neurol Sci* 2005; 229–230: 187–193.
56. Koga Y, Akita Y, Nishioka J et al. L-Arginine improves the symptoms of strokelike episodes in MELAS. *Neurology* 2005; **64**: 710–712.
57. Koga Y, Ishibashi M, Ueki I et al. Effects of L-arginine on the acute phase of strokes in three patients with MELAS. *Neurology* 2002; **58**: 827–828.
58. Papadopoulou LC, Sue CM, Davidson MM et al. Fatal infantile cardioencephalomyopathy with COX deficiency and mutations in *SCO2*, a COX assembly gene. *Nature Genet* 1999; **23**: 333–337.
59. Sue CM, Schon EA. Mitochondrial respiratory chain diseases and mutations in nuclear DNA: A promising start? *Brain Pathology* 2000; **10**: 442–450.
60. Salviati L, Hernandez-Rosa E, Walker WF et al. Copper supplementation restores cytochrome *c* oxidase activity in cultured cells from patients with *SCO2* mutations. *Biochem J* 2002; **363**: 321–327.
61. Jaksch M, Paret C, Stucka R et al. Cytochrome *c* oxidase deficiency due to mutations in *SCO2*, encoding a mitochondrial copper-binding protein, is rescued by copper in human myoblasts. *Hum Mol Genet* 2001; **10**: 3025–3035.
62. Freisinger P, Horvath R, Macmillan C et al. Reversion of hypertrophic cardiomyopathy in a patient with deficiency of the mitochondrial copper binding protein Sco2: Is there a potential effect of copper? *J Inher Metab Dis* 2004; **27**: 67–79.
63. Brini M, Pinton P, King MP et al. A calcium signaling defect in the pathogenesis of a mitochondrial DNA inherited oxidative phosphorylation deficiency. *Nature Med* 1999; **5**: 951–954.
64. Beal MF. Mitochondria in neurodegeneration. In: Desnuelle C, DiMauro S, eds. *Mitochondrial Disorders: From Pathophysiology to Acquired Defects*. Paris: Springer-Verlag France, 2002: 17–35.
65. Servidei S, Di Giovanni S, Broccolini A et al. Apoptosis and oxidative stress in mitochondrial disorders. In: Desnuelle C, DiMauro S, eds. *Mitochondrial Disorders: From Pathophysiology to Acquired Defects*. Paris: Springer-Verlag, 2002: 37–43.
66. Schon EA, Manfredi G. Neuronal degeneration and mitochondrial dysfunction. *J Clin Invest* 2003; **111**: 303–312.
67. Tabrizi SJ, Schapira AHV. Mitochondrial abnormalities in neurodegenerative disorders. In: Schapira AHV, DiMauro S, eds. *Mitochondrial Disorders in Neurology 2*. Boston: Butterworth-Heinemann, 2002: 143–174.
68. Ogasahara S, Nishikawa Y, Yorifuji S et al. Treatment of Kearns-Sayre syndrome with coenzyme Q10. *Neurology* 1986; **36**: 45–53.
69. Yamamoto M, Sato T, Anno M et al. Mitochondrial myopathy, encephalopathy, lactic acidosis, and strokelike episodes with recurrent abdominal symptoms and coenzyme Q10 administration. *J Neurol Neurosurg Psychiat* 1987; **50**: 1475–1481.
70. Bresolin N, Doriguzzi C, Ponzetto C et al. Ubidecarenone in the treatment of mitochondrial myopathies: a multicenter double-blind trial. *J Neurol Sci* 1990; **100**: 70–78.
71. Ihara Y, Namba R, Kuroda S et al. Mitochondrial encephalomyopathy (MELAS): pathological study and successful therapy with coenzyme Q10 and idebenone. *J Neurol Sci* 1989; **90**: 263–271.
72. Ikejiri Y, Mori E, Ishii K et al. Idebenone improves cerebral mitochondrial oxidative metabolism in a patient with MELAS. *Neurology* 1996; **47**: 583–585.
73. Chan A, Reichmann H, Kogel A et al. Metabolic changes in patients with mitochondrial myopathies and effects of coenzyme Q10 therapy. *J Neurol* 1998; **245**: 681–685.
74. Bendahan D, Desnuelle C, Vanuxem D et al. ^{31}P NMR spectroscopy and ergometer exercise test as evidence for muscle oxidative performance improvement with coenzyme Q in mitochondrial myopathies. *Neurology* 1992; **42**: 1203–1208.

75. Abe K, Matsuo Y, Kadekawa J et al. Effect of coenzyme Q10 in patients with mitochondrial myopathy, encephalopathy, lactic acidosis, and stroke-like episodes (MELAS): Evaluation by non-invasive tissue oximetry. *J Neurol Sci* 1999; **162**: 65–68.
76. Geromel V, Darin N, Chretien D et al. Coenzyme Q10 and idebenone in the therapy of respiratory chain diseases: rationale and comparative benefits. *Mol Genet Metab* 2002; **77**: 21–30.
77. Shinkai T, Nakashima M, Ohmori O et al. Coenzyme Q10 improves psychiatric symptoms in adult-onset mitochondrial myopathy, encephalopathy, lactic acidosis and stroke-like episodes: a case report. *Aus N Z J Psychiatry* 2000; **34**: 1034–1035.
78. Panetta J, Smith LJ, Boneh A. Effect of high-dose vitamins, coenzyme Q and high-fat-diet in paediatric patients with mitochondrial diseases. *J Inher Metab Dis* 2004; **27**: 487–498.
79. Lodi R, Hart PE, Rajagopalan B et al. Antioxidant treatment improves in vivo cardiac and skeletal muscle bioenergetics in patients with Friedreich's ataxia. *Ann Neurol* 2001; **49**: 590–596.
80. Rustin P, von Kleist-Retzow J-C, Chantrel-Groussard K et al. Effect of idebenone on cardiomyopathy in Friedreich's ataxia: a preliminary study. *Lancet* 1999; **354**: 477–479.
81. Filla A, Moss AJ. Idebenone for treatment of Friedreich's ataxia? *Neurology* 2003; **60**: 1569–1570.
82. Mariotti C, Solari A, Torta D et al. Idebenone treatment in Friedreich patients: one-year-long randomized placebo-controlled trial. *Neurology* 2003; **60**: 1676–1679.
83. Buyse G, Mertens L, Di Salvo G et al. Idebenone treatment in Friedreich's ataxia. *Neurology* 2003; **60**: 1679–1681.
84. Hart PE, Lodi R, Rajagopalan B et al. Antioxidant treatment of patients with Friedreich ataxia. *Arch Neurol* 2005; 62: 621–626.
85. Shults CW, Oakes D, Kieburtz K et al. Effects of coenzyme Q10 in early Parkinson disease. *Arch Neurol* 2002; **59**: 1541–1550.
86. Shults CW, Beal MF, Song D, Fontaine D. Pilot trial of high dosages of coenzyme Q10 in patients with Parkinson's disease. *Exp Neurol* 2004; **188**: 491–494.
87. Group HS. A randomized, placebo-controlled trial of coenzyme Q10 and remacemide in Huntington's disease. *Neurology* 2001; **57**: 397–404.
88. Shults CW, Schapira AHV. A cue to queue for CoQ? *Neurology* 2001; **57**: 375–376.
89. Shults CW. Coenzyme Q10 in neurodegenerative diseases. *Curr Medicinal Chem* 2003; **10**: 917–921.
90. Bender A, Auer DP, Merl T et al. Creatine supplementation lowers brain glutamate levels in Huntington's disease. *J Neurol* 2005; **252**: 36–41.
91. Hayes S, Del Bene M, Trojaborg W et al. Therapeutic trial of coenzyme Q10 (CoQ10) in amyotrophic lateral sclerosis (ALS/MND). *Amyotrophic Lateral Sclerosis Other Motor Neuron Disord* 2000; **1**(Suppl. 3): 119.
92. Haydar NA, Conn HL, Afifi A et al. Severe hypermetabolism with primary abnormality of skeletal muscle mitochondria. *Ann Int Med* 1971; **74**: 548–558.
93. DiMauro S, Bonilla E, Lee CP et al. Luft's disease. Further biochemical and ultrastructural studies of skeletal muscle in the second case. *J Neurol Sci* 1976; **27**: 217–232.
94. Taivassalo T, Fu K, Johns T et al. Gene shifting: a novel therapy for mitochondrial myopathy. *Hum Mol Genet* 1999; **8**: 1047–1052.
95. Clark KM, Bindoff LA, Lightowlers RN et al. Reversal of a mitochondrial DNA defect in human skeletal muscle. *Nature Genet* 1997; **16**: 222–224.
96. Fu K, Hartlen R, Johns T et al. A novel heteroplasmic $tRNA^{leu(CUN)}$ mtDNA point mutation in a sporadic patient with mitochondrial encephalomyopathy segregates rapidly in skeletal muscle and suggests an approach to therapy. *Hum Mol Genet* 1996; **5**: 1835–1840.
97. Shoubridge EA, Johns T, Karpati G. Complete restoration of a wild-type mtDNA genotype in regenerating muscle fibers in a patient with a tRNA point mutation and mitochondrial encephalomyopathy. *Hum Mol Genet* 1997; **6**: 2239–2242.
98. Andrews RM, Griffiths PG, Chinnery PF, Turnbull DM. Evaluation of bupivacaine-induced muscle regeneration in the treatment of ptosis in patients with chronic progressive external ophthalmoplegia and Kearns-Sayre syndrome. *Eye* 1999;**13**:769–772.
99. Pallotti F, Baracca A, Hernandez-Rosa E et al. Biochemical analysis of respiratory function in cybrid cell lines harbouring mitochondrial DNA mutations. *Biochem J* 2004; **384**: 287–293.
100. Manfredi G, Gupta N, Vazquez-Memije ME et al. Oligomycin induces a decrease in the cellular content of a pathogenic mutation in the human

mitochondrial ATPase 6 gene. *J Biol Chem* 1999; **274**: 9386–9391.
101. Santra S, Gilkerson RW, Davidson MM, Schon EA. Ketogenic treatment reduces deleted mitochondrial DNAs in cultured human cells. *Ann Neurol* 2004; **56**: 662–669.
102. Tanaka M, Borgeld HJ, Zhang J et al. Gene therapy for mitochondrial disease by delivering restriction endonuclease SmaI into mitochondria. *J Biomed Sci* 2002; **9**: 534–541.
103. Taylor RW, Chinnery PF, Turnbull DM, Lightowlers RN. Selective inhibition of mutant human mitochondrial DNA replication in vitro by peptide nucleic acids. *Nature Genet* 1997; **15**: 212–215.
104. Chinnery PF, Taylor RW, Diekert K et al. Peptic nucleic acid delivery to human mitochondria. *Gene Ther* 1999; **6**: 1919–1928.
105. Muratovska A, Lightowlers RN, Taylor RW et al. Targeting peptide nucleic acid (PNA) oligomers to mitochondria within cells by conjugation to lipophilic cations: implications for mitochondrial DNA replication, expression and disease. *Nucleic Acids Res* 2001; **29**: 1852–1863.
106. Petruzzella V, Moraes CT, Sano MC et al. Extremely high levels of mutant mtDNAs co-localize with cytochrome *c* oxidase-negative ragged-red fibers in patients harboring a point mutation at nt 3243. *Hum Mol Genet* 1994; **3**: 449–454.
107. Qi X, Lewin AS, Hauswirth WW, Guy J. Suppression of complex I gene expression induces optic neuropathy. *Ann Neurol* 2003; **53**: 198–205.
108. Qi X, Lewin AS, Hauswirth WW, Guy J. Optic neuropathy induced by reductions in mitochondrial superoxide dismutase. *Invest Ophthalmol Vis Sci* 2003; **44**: 1088–1096.
109. Qi X, Lewin AS, Sun L et al. SOD2 gene transfer protects against optic neuropathy induced by deficiency of complex I. *Ann Neurol* 2004; **56**: 182–191.
110. Manfredi G, Beal MF. Poison and antidote: A novel model to study pathogenesis and therapy of LHON. *Ann Neurol* 2004; **56**: 171–172.
111. Gray RE, Law RH, Devenish RJ, Nagley P. Allotopic expression of mitochondrial ATP synthase genes in nucleus of *Saccharomyces cerevisiae*. *Meth Enzymol* 1996; **264**: 369–389.
112. Manfredi G, Fu J, Ojaimi J et al. Rescue of a deficiency in ATP synthesis by transfer of *MTATP6*, a mitochondrial DNA-encoded gene, to the nucleus. *Nature Genet* 2002; **30**: 394–399.
113. Guy J, Qi X, Pallotti F et al. Rescue of a mitochondrial deficiency causing Leber hereditary optic neuropathy. *Ann Neurol* 2002; **52**: 534–542.
114. Kolesnikova OA, Entelis NS, Mireau H et al. Suppression of mutations in mitochondrial DNA by tRNAs imported from the cytoplasm. *Science* 2000; **289**: 1931–1933.
115. Feuermann M, Francisci S, Rinaldi T et al. The yeast counterparts of human 'MELAS' mutations cause mitochondrial dysfunction that can be rescued by overexpression of the mitochondrial translation factor EF-TU. *EMBO Reports* 2003; **4**: 53–58.
116. Rubenstein DS, Thomasma DC, Schon EA, Zinaman MJ. Germ-line therapy to cure mitochondrial disease: Protocol and ethics of in vitro ovum nuclear transplantation. *Cambridge Quart Healthcare Eth* 1995; **4**: 316–339.
117. Barritt JA, Brenner CA, Malter HE, Cohen J. Mitochondria in human offspring derived from ooplasmic transplantation. *Hum Reprod* 2001; **16**: 513–516.
118. Thorburn DR, Dahl H-HM, Singh KK. The pros and cons of mitochondrial manipulation in the human germ line. *Mitochondrion* 2001; **1**: 123–127.
119. Bernes SM, Bacino C, Prezant TR et al. Identical mitochondrial DNA deletion in mother with progressive external ophthalmoplegia and son with Pearson marrow-pancreas syndrome. *J Pediat* 1993; **123**: 598–602.
120. Shanske S, Tang Y, Hirano M et al. Identical mitochondrial DNA deletion in a woman with ocular myopathy and in her son with Pearson syndrome. *Am J Hum Genet* 2002; **71**: 679–683.
121. Puoti G, Carrara F, Sampaolo S et al. Identical large scale rearrangement of mitochondrial DNA causes Kearns-Sayre syndrome in a mother and her son. *J Med Genet* 2003; **40**: 858–863.
122. Chinnery PF, DiMauro S, Shanske S et al. Risk of developing a mitochondrial DNA deletion disorder. *Lancet* 2004; **364**: 592–595.
123. White SL, Shanske S, McGill JJ et al. Mitochondrial DNA mutations at nucleotide 8993 show a lack of tissue- or age-related variation. *J Inher Metab Dis* 1999; **22**: 899–914.
124. White SL, Shanske S, Biros I et al. Two cases of prenatal analysis for the pathogenic T to G substitution at nucleotide 8993 in mitochondrial DNA. *Prenat Diagn* 1999; **19**: 1165–1168.

Appendix

Phenotypes associated with pathogenic mtDNA point mutations

Nucleotide	Mutation[a]	Gene location	tRNA[b]	'Usual' phenotype	Reference[c]
582	T→C	tRNA-Phe	6	Myopathy (sporadic)	Moslemi (2004) ND 14:46
583	G→A	tRNA-Phe	7	MELAS	Hanna et al., (1998) AJHG 63:29
606	A→G	tRNA-Phe	29	Rhabdomyolysis/myoglobinuria	Chinnery (1997) AN 41:408
611	G→A	tRNA-Phe	34	MERRF	Mancuso (2004) Neurol 62:2119
618	T→C	tRNA-Phe	43	Myopathy (sporadic)	Kleinle (1998) BBRC 247:112
961	Del T	12S rRNA	–	Aminoglycoside-induced deafness	Bacino (1995) Pharmacogen 5:165
1095	T→C	12S rRNA	–	SNHL, Parkinsonism, neuropathy	Thyagarajan (2000) AN 5:730
1494	C→T	12S rRNA	–	Aminoglycoside-induced deafness	Zhao (2003) AJHG 74:139
1555	A→G	12S rRNA	–	Aminoglycoside-induced deafness	Prezant (1993) NG 4:289
1556	C→T	12S rRNA	–	Steptomycin-induced tinnitus	Tanimoto (2004) AO 124:258
1571	T→G	12S rRNA	–	Dilated cardiomyopathy	Arbustini (1998) AJP 153:1501
1606	G→A	tRNA-Val	5	Multisystem	Tiranti (1998) AN 43:98
1624	C→T	tRNA-Val	25	LS	McFarland (2002) NG 30:145
1642	G→A	tRNA-Val	43	MELAS	Taylor (1996) AN 40:459
1644	G→T	tRNA-Val	45	Leigh syndrome	Chalmers (1997) Neurol 49:589
1659	T→C	tRNA-Val	62	Multisystem	Blakely (2004) JNS 225:99
1692	A→T	16S rRNA	–	Dilated cardiomyopathy	Arbustini (1998) AJP 153:1501
1703	C→T	16S rRNA	–	Dilated cardiomyopathy	Arbustini (1998) AJP 153:1501
3093	C→G	16S rRNA	–	MELAS, cardiomyopathy, diabetes	Hsieh (2001) JBS 8:328
3228	T→G	16S rRNA	–	Dilated cardiomyopathy	Arbustini (1998) AJP 153:1501
3242	G→A	tRNA-Leu(UUR)	13	Refractory anemia with excess blasts	Gattermann (2004) Blood 103:1499
3243	A→G	tRNA-Leu(UUR)	14	MELAS/PEO/diabetes/deafness	Goto (1990) Nature 348:651
3243	A→T	tRNA-Leu(UUR)	14	Encephalomyopathy (sporadic)	Shaag (1997) BBRC 233:637
3249	G→A	tRNA-Leu(UUR)	20A	KSS	Seneca (2001) AN 58:1113
3250	T→C	tRNA-Leu(UUR)	20	Myopathy	Goto (1992) AN 31:672
3251	A→G	tRNA-Leu(UUR)	21	PEO/myopathy	Sweeney QJ Med 86:709
3252	A→G	tRNA-Leu(UUR)	22	MELAS	Morten (1993) HMG 2:2081
3254	C→G	tRNA-Leu(UUR)	24	Cardiomyopathy/myopathy	Kawarai (1997) Neurol 49:598
3255	G→A	tRNA-Leu(UUR)	25	MERRF/KSS	Nishigaki (2003) ND 13:334
3256	C→T	tRNA-Leu(UUR)	34	Multisystem/PEO	Moraes (1993) JCI 92:2906
3258	T→C	tRNA-Leu(UUR)	36	MELAS	Campos (2003) ND 13:416
3260	A→G	tRNA-Leu(UUR)	38	Cardiomyopathy/myopathy	Zeviani (1991) Lancet 338;143
3264	T→C	tRNA-Leu(UUR)	42	Diabetes	Suzuki (1997) DC 20:1138
3271	T→C	tRNA-Leu(UUR)	47B	MELAS	Goto (1991) BBA 1097:238
3271	Delete T	tRNA-Leu(UUR)	47B	Encephalomyopathy (sporadic)	Shoffner (1995) Neurol 45:286
3274	A→G	tRNA-Leu(UUR)	47E	Neuropsychiatric disorder	Jaksch (2001) Neurol 57:1930

3275	T→C	tRNA-Leu(UUR)	43	LHON	Garcia-Loizano (2000) HM 15:120
3280	A→G	tRNA-Leu(UUR)	49	Cardiomyopathy	Campos (2003) ND 13;416
3288	A→G	tRNA-Leu(UUR)	57	Myopathy	Hadjigeorgiou (1999) JNS 164:153
3291	T→C	tRNA-Leu(UUR)	60	MELAS	Goto (1994) BBRC 202:1624
3302	A→G	tRNA-Leu(UUR)	71	Myopathy	Bindoff (1993) JBC 268:19559
3303	C→T	tRNA-Leu(UUR)	72	Cardiomyopathy	Silvestri (1994) HM 3:37
3316	G→A	ND1	–	NIDDM/dilated cardiomyopathy	Arbustini (1998) AJP 153:1501
3460	G→A	ND1	–	LHON[d]	Huoponen (1991) AJHG 48:1147
3635	G→A	ND1	–	LHON[d]	Brown (2001) HG 109:33
3796	A→G	ND1	–	Dystonia	Simon (2003) Neurogenetics 4;199
4160	T→C	ND1	–	LHON[d]	Howell (1991) AJHG 48:935
4171	C→A	ND1	–	LHON[d]	Kim (2002) AN 51:630
4269	A→G	tRNA-Ile	7	Encephalomyopathy/cardiomyopathy	Taniike (1992) BBRC 186:47
4274	T→C	tRNA-Ile	12	PEO	Chinnery (1997) Neurol 49:1166
4284	G→A	tRNA-Ile	26	Multisystem; cardiomyopathy	Corona (2002) AN 51:118
4285	T→C	tRNA-Ile	27	PEO	Silvestri (1996) BBRC 220:623
4290	T→C	tRNA-Ile	32	Multisystem	Limongelli (2004) JMG 41:342
4295	A→G	tRNA-Ile	37	Hypertrophic cardiomyopathy	Merante (1996) HM 8:216
4298	G→A	tRNA-Ile	40	PEO/multiple sclerosis	Taylor (1998) BBRC 243:47
4300	A→G	tRNA-Ile	42	Cardiomyopathy	Casali (1995) BBRC 213:588
4309	G→A	tRNA-Ile	51	PEO	Franceschina (1998) JN 245:755
4315	A→G	tRNA-Ile	57	Dilated cardiomyopathy	Arbustini (1998) AJP 153:1501
4320	C→T	tRNA-Ile	62	Hypertrophic cardiomyopathy	Santorelli (1995) BBRC 216:835
4332	G→A	tRNA-Gln	70	MELAS	Bataillard (2001) Neurol 56:405
4370	Insert A	tRNA-Gln	31	Myopathy	Dey (2000) ND 10:488
4409	T→C	tRNA-Met	8	Myopathy, dystrophy (sporadic)	Vissing (1998) Neurol 50:1875
4450	G→A	tRNA-Met	53	Splenic lymphoma	Lombes (1998) HM Suppl 1:S175
4640	C→A	ND2	–	LHON[d]	Brown (2001) HG 109:33
4810	G→A	ND2	–	Myopathy (sporadic)	Pulkes (2005) Neurol 64:1091
5510	A→C	ND2	–	Dilated cardiomyopathy	Arbustini (1998) AJP 153:1501
5521	G→A	tRNA-Trp	10	Myopathy	Silvestri (1998) ND 8:291
5537	Insert T	tRNA-Trp	27	Leigh syndrome	Santorelli (1997) AN 42:256
5540	G→A	tRNA-Trp	30	Spinocerebellar ataxia	Silvestri (2000) Neurol 54:1693
5549	G→A	tRNA-Trp	39	Encephalomyopathy/chorea (sporadic)	Nelson (1995) AN 37:400
5600	A→T	tRNA-Ala	60	Dilated cardiomyopathy	Arbustini (1998) AJP 153:1501
5628	T→C	tRNA-Ala	31	PEO	Spagnolo (2001) ND 11:481
5650	G→A	tRNA-Ala	6	CADASIL (R113C in Notch3)+RRF	Finnila (2001) JMM 79:641

(Continued)

Nucleotide	Mutation[a]	Gene location	tRNA[b]	'Usual' phenotype	Reference[c]
5693	T→C	tRNA-Asn	37	Encephalomyopathy	Coulbault (2005) BBRC 329:1152
5698	G→A	tRNA-Asn	32	PEO	Spinazzola (2004) ND 14:815
5703	G→A	tRNA-Asn	27	Myopathy/PEO	Moraes (1993) JCI 92:2906
5814	T→C	tRNA-Cys	13	Encephalopathy	Manfredi (1996) HM 7:158
5874	T→C	tRNA-Tyr	22	Myopathy (sporadic)	Pulkes (2000) Neurol 55:1210
5877	C→T	tRNA-Tyr	15	CPEO	Sahashi (1997) MN Suppl 1:S139
5885	Delete T	tRNA-Tyr	7	CPEO (sporadic)	Raffelsberger (2001)Neurol 57:2298
5920	G→A	COX I		Sporadic myoglobinuria	Karadimas (2000) Neurol 55:644
6015–19	Del 5 bp	COX I		Motor neuron disease	Comi (1998) AN 43:110
6489	C→A	COX I	–	Epilepsy	Varlamov (2002) HMG 11:1797
6708	G→A	COX I	–	Myopathy	Kollberg (2005) JNEN 64:123
6721	T→C	COX I	–	Sideroblastic anemia (sporadic)	Gattermann (1997) Blood 90:4961
6742	T→C	COX I	–	Sideroblastic anemia (sporadic)	Gattermann (1997) Blood 90:4961
6930	G→A	COX I	–	Myopathy	Bruno (1999) AJHG 65:611
7445	A→G	tRNA-Ser(UCN)	73	Deafness; palmoplantar keratoderma	Reid (1994) HM 3:243
7471	Insert C	tRNA-Ser(UCN)	48	Deafness/myoclonus	Tiranti (1995) HMG 14:421
7471	Insert CC	tRNA-Ser(UCN)	48	Myopathy (sporadic)	Pulkes (2005) ND 15:364
7480	T→C	tRNA-Ser(UCN)	38	Myopathy, deafness, dementia (sp)	Bidooki (2004) ND 14:417
7497	G→A	tRNA-Ser(UCN)	21	Epilepsy; exercise intolerance	Jaksch (1998) AN 44:635
7510	T→C	tRNA-Ser(UCN)	7	Deafness	Hutchin (2000) JMG 37:692
7511	T→C	tRNA-Ser(UCN)	6	Deafness	Sue (1999) Neurol 52:1905
7512	T→C	tRNA-Ser(UCN)	5	MERRF/MELAS	Nakamura (1995) BBRC 214;86
7543	A→G	tRNA-Asp	29	Myoclonus	Shtilbans (2000) JCN 14:610
7581	T→C	tRNA-Asp	69	Dilated cardiomyopathy	Arbustini (1998) AJP 153:1501
7587	T→C	COX II	–	Encephalomyopathy	Clark (1999) AJHG 64:1330
7671	T→A	COX II	–	Myopathy	Rahman (1999) AJHG 65:1080
7706	G→A	COX II	–	Alpers-Huttenlocher-like Disease	Uusimaa (2003)Pediatrics 111:E262
7896	G→A	COX II	–	Multisystem	Campos (2001) AN 50:409
7989	T→C	COX II	–	Myopathy (sporadic)	McFarland (2004) ND 14:162
8042	Delete AT	COX II	–	Severe lactic acidosis	Wong (2001) AJMG 42:95
8296	A→G	tRNA-Lys	2	Diabetes; hypertrophic cardiomyopathy	Kameoka (1998) BBRC 245:523
8313	G→A	tRNA-Lys	24	Encephalopathy/GI (sporadic)	Verma (1997) PR 42:448
8316	T→C	tRNA-Lys	27	MELAS	Campos (2000) ND 10:493
8326	A→G	tRNA-Lys	37	Multisystem	Wong (2002) AJMG 113:59
8328	G→A	tRNA-Lys	39	Encephalomyopathy (sporadic)	Houshmand (1999) HM 13:203
8342	G→A	tRNA-Lys	53	PEO and myoclonus	Tiranti (1999) ND 9:66

8344	A→G	tRNA-Lys	55	MERRF	Shoffner (1990) Cell 61:931
8356	T→C	tRNA-Lys	65	MERRF	Silvestri (2002) AJHG 51:1213
8361	G→A	tRNA-Lys	70	MERRF	Rossmanith (1992) AN 54:820
8363	G→A	tRNA-Lys	72	MERRF/deafness/cardiopathy; LS	Santorelli (1996) AJHG 58:933
8821	T→C	ATPase 6	–	Severe oligozoospermia	Holyoake (2000) Andrologia 31:339
8851	T→C	ATPase 6	–	FBSN	De Meirleir (1995) PN 13:242
8993	T→G	ATPase 6	–	NARP/MILS	Holt (1990) AJHG 46:428
8993	T→C	ATPase 6	–	NARP/MILS	de Vries (1993) AN 34:410
9185	T→C	ATPase 6	–	Leigh Syndrome	Ogilvie (1999) FEBS Lett 453:179
9176	T→G	ATPase 6	–	NARP/MILS	Carrozzo (2001) Neurol 50:687
9176	T→C	ATPase 6	–	FBSN	Thyagarajan (1995) AN 38:468
9205	Del TA	ATPase 6	–	Encephalopathy	Jesina (2004) BJ 83:561
9379	G→A	COX III	–	Myopathy (sporadic)	Horvath (2002) JMG 39:812
9487–92	Del 15 bp	COX III	–	Myoglobinuria (sporadic)	Keightley (1996) NG 12:410
9537	InsC	COX III	–	Leigh syndrome (sporadic)	Tiranti (2000) HMG 9:2733
9952	G→A	COX III	–	Encephalomyopathy (sporadic)	Hanna (1998) AJHG 63:29
9957	T→C	COX III	–	MELAS	Manfredi (1995) ND 5:391
9997	T→C	tRNA-Gly	7	Cardiomyopathy	Merante (1994) AJHG 55:437
10010	A→G	tRNA-Gly	22	Multisystem	Nishigaki (2002) Neurol 58:1282
10044	A→G	tRNA-Gly	60	Encephalopathy; SIDS	Santorelli (1996) PN 15:145
10158	T→C	ND3	–	LS	Lebon (2003) JMG 40:896
10191	T→C	ND3	–	PME and optic atrophy	Taylor (2001) AN 50:104
10663	T→C	ND4L	–	LHON	Brown (2002) HG 110:130
11696	A→G	ND4	–	LHON/dystonia	de Vries (1996) AJHG 58:703
11777	C→A	ND4	–	Encephalopathy	Deschauer (2003) Neurol 60:1357
11778	G→A	ND4	–	LHON[d]	Wallace (1988) Science 242:1427
11832	G→A	ND4	–	Myopathy (sporadic)	Andreu (1999) AN 45:820
12147	G→A	tRNA-His	10	MERRF/MELAS overlap	Melone (2004) Arch Neurol 61:269
12183	G→A	tRNA-His	50	Multisystem/retinopathy/deafness	Crimi (2003) Neuol 60:1200
12192	G→A	tRNA-His	59	Cardiomyopathy	Shin (2000) AJHG 67:1617
12258	C→A	tRNA-Ser(AGY)	66	Diabetes and deafness	Lynn (1998) Diabetes 47:1800
12297	T→C	tRNA-Leu(CUN)	33	Cardiomyopathy	Grasso (2001) EJHG 9:311
12301	G→A	tRNA-Leu(CUN)	37	Sideroblastic anemia (sporadic)	Gattermann (1996) BJH 93:845
12311	T→C	tRNA-Leu(CUN)	47	PEO	Hattori (1994) JNS 125;50
12315	G→A	tRNA-Leu(CUN)	52	Encephalomyopathy	Fu (1996) HMG 5:1835
12320	A→G	tRNA-Leu(CUN)	57	Myopathy (sporadic)	Weber (1997) AJHG 60:373
12334	G→A	tRNA-Leu(CUN)	71	Myopathy (sporadic)	Vives-Bauza (2001) AM 33:493

(Continued)

Nucleotide	Mutation[a]	Gene location	tRNA[b]	'Usual' phenotype	Reference[c]
12706	T→C	ND5	–	Leigh syndrome	Taylor (2002) EJHG 10:141
12770	A→G	ND5	–	MELAS	Liolitsa (2003) AN 53:128
13042	G→A	ND5	–	MELAS/MERRF	Naini (2005) Arch Neurol 62:473
13045	A→C	ND5	–	MELAS	Liolitsa (2003) AN 53:128
13084	A→T	ND5	–	MELAS-Leigh syndrome overlap	Crimi (2003) Neurol 60:1857
13513	G→A	ND5	–	MELAS	Santorelli (1997) BBRC 238:326
13528	A→G	ND5	–	?	Batandier (2000) HM 16:532
14453	G→A	ND6	–	MELAS	Ravn (2001) EJHG 9:805
14459	G→A	ND6	–	LHON/dystonia	Jun (1994) PNAS 91:6206
14482	C→A	ND6	–	LHON[d]	Valentino (2002) AN 51:774
14482	C→G	ND6	–	LHON[d]	Howell (1998) AJHG 62:196
14484	T→C	ND6	–	LHON[d]	Johns (1992 BBRC 187:1551
14487	T→C	ND6	–	Dystonia + BSN; LS	Solano (2003) AN 54:527
14495	A→G	ND6	–	LHON[d]	Chinnery (2001) Brain 124;209
14577	T→C	ND6	–	Diabetes	Tawata (2000) Diabetes 49:1269
14684	C→T	tRNA-Glu	63	Dilated cardiomyopathy	Arbustini (1998) AJP 153:1501
14687	A→G	tRNA-Glu	60	Myopathy (sporadic)	Bruno (2003) JCN 4:300
14709	T→C	tRNA-Glu	37	Encephalomyopathy	Hanna (1995) AJHG 56:1026
14724	G→A	tRNA-Glu	22	Encephalomyopathy	Vialrinho (2001) Mitochond 1:S95
14787	Del 4 bp	Cyt *b*	–	MELAS/Parkinsonism (sporadic)	De Coo (1999) AN 45;130
14846	G→A	Cyt *b*	–	Myopathy (sporadic)	Andreu (1999) NEJM 341:1037
14894	T→C	Cyt *b*	–	LHON	Besch (2000) Ophthalmologe 97;22
15059	G→A	Cyt *b*	–	Myopathy (sporadic)	Andreu (1999) AN 45;127
15084	G→A	Cyt *b*	–	Myopathy (sporadic)	Andreu (1999) NEJM 341:1037
15150	G→A	Cyt *b*	–	Myopathy (sporadic?)	Legros (2001) EJHG 9:510
15168	G→A	Cyt *b*	–	Myopathy (sporadic)	Andreu (1999) NEJM 341:1037
15170	G→A	Cyt *b*	–	Myopathy (sporadic)	Bruno (2003) MN 28:508
15197	T→C	Cyt *b*	–	Myopathy (sporadic?)	Legros (2001) EJHG 9:510
15242	G→A	Cyt *b*	–	Encephalomyopathy (sporadic)	Keightley (2000) AJHG 67:1400
15243	G→A	Cyt *b*	–	Cardiomyopathy (sporadic)	Valnot (1999) HG 104:460
15498	G→A	Cyt *b*	–	Histiocytoid cardiomyopathy (sporadic)	Andreu (2000) PR 48:311
15498	Del24	Cyt *b*	–	Myopathy (sporadic)	Andreu (1999) NEJM 341:1037
15615	G→A	Cyt *b*	–	Myopathy (sporadic)	Dumoulin MCP 10:389
15723	G→A	Cyt *b*	–	Myopathy (sporadic)	Andreu (1999) NEJM 341:1037
15747	T→C	Cyt *b*	–	LHON (?)	Aguilera (1999) HM 14:545
15761	G→A	Cyt *b*	–	Myopathy (sporadic)	Mancuso (2003) JNS 209:61

15762	G→A	Cyt *b*	–	Myopathy (sporadic)	Andreu (1998) Neurol 51:1444
15800	C→T	Cyt *b*	–	Myopathy (sporadic)	Lamantea (2002) ND 12:49
15889	T→C	tRNA-Thr	2	Dilated cardiomyopathy	Arbustini (1998) AJP 153:1501
15902	A→G	tRNA-Thr	15	Dilated cardiomyopathy	Arbustini (1998) AJP 153:1501
15915	G→A	tRNA-Thr	30	Encephalomyopathy (sporadic)	Nishino (1996) BBRC 225:180
15923	A→G	tRNA-Thr	38	Fatal infantile resp. def.	Yoon (1991) BBRC 176;1112
15935	A→G	tRNA-Thr	51	Dilated cardiomyopathy	Arbustini (1998) AJP 153:1501
15990	C→T	tRNA-Pro	36	Myopathy	Moraes (1993) NG 4:284
15995	G→A	tRNA-Pro	31	Multisystem	Wong (2002) AJMG 113:59
16002	T→C	tRNA-Pro	24	Sporadic PEO	Seneca (2000) JIMD 23:853

[a]L-strand sequence.

[b]Position on the standard tRNA 'cloverleaf' (Sprinzl et al. [1989] Nucl. Acids Res. 17, r1–r172).

[c]First published article. References are in 'shorthand': First author (Year) Journal Volume:First page. Abbreviations of Journal names are: AJHG, American Journal of Human Genetics; AJMG, American Journal of Molecular Genetics; AJP, American Journal of Pathology; AM, Annals of Medicine; AN, Annals of Neurology; AO, Acta Otolaryngologica (?); BBA, Biochimica et Biophysica Acta; BBRC, Biochemical and Biophysical Research Communications; BJ, Biochemical Journal; BJH, British Journal of Haematology; DC, Diabetes Care; EJHG, European Journal of Human Genetics; HG, Human Genetics; HM, Human Mutation; HMG, Human Molecular Genetics; JBC, Journal of Biological Chemistry; JBS, Journal of Biomedical Sciences; JCI, Journal of Clinical Investigation; JCN, Journal of Child Neurology; JIMD, Journal of Inherited Metabolic Diseases; JMG, Journal of Medical Genetics; JMM, Journal of Molecular Medicine; JN, Journal of Neurology; JNEN, Journal of Neuropathology and Experimental Neurology; JNS, Journal of Neurological Sciences; MCP, Molecular and Cellular Probes; Mitochond, Mitochondrion; MN, Muscle Nerve; ND, Neuromuscular Disorders; Neurol, Neurology; NEJM, New England Journal of Medicine; NG, Nature Genetics; Pharmacogen, Pharmacogenetics; PN, Pediatric Neurology; PNAS, Proceedings of the National Academy of Sciences of the USA; PR, Pediatric Research.

[d] 'Primary' pathogenic LHON mutation; so-called 'secondary' mutations are not included.

Index

Page numbers referring to figures are highlighted in **bold**, tables and boxes in *italics*.

A
A1555G rRNA mutation
67, 86, 170–1
cardiomyopathy 80, *85*
deafness 169
A3243G tRNA$^{Leu(UUR)}$ mutation
169–70
autism 263
cardiomyopathy 80, *85*
deafness **163**, **164**, 167
diabetes 182, 200
MELAS syndrome 31, 33, 55,
80, 82, 154–5, 203–4
nephropathy 200, 203–4
renal involvement 200
risk assessment in
pregnancy 253
short stature 189
A3260G mutation, myopathy/
cardiomyopathy *85*
A3280G mutation, myopathy *85*
A3302G mutation, myopathy/
cardiomyopathy *85*
A4269G mutation 84, *85*
A4295G mutation 84, *85*
A4300G mutation *85*
A8344G mutation, MERRF
syndrome 35–7, 50,
51–2, 64
acetyl-CoA *19–20*
acquired idiopathic sideroblastic
anemia 210–11
iron transport, heme
biosynthesis and
connection with electron
transport chain of IOM **212**
acyl-CoA, cardiac mitochondrial 78
acyl-CoA dehydrogenase,
deficiency 95–6
adenine nucleotide translocator-1
(*ANT1*) 18, 58, 89, 123
ADP, effect on mitochondrial
respiration **2**
adrenal insufficiency 190, *191*
aerobiosis, vs anaerobiosis
(glycolysis) *8*
aging process
and COX deficiency 220
hematopoietic stem cells 218
Alpers syndrome 18, 39
liver function 149
myopathic *90*
Alzheimer's disease
mitochondrial
dysfunction 22
mutations in non-mitochondrial
proteins 292–3
aminoglycoside sensitivity 161
amyotrophic lateral sclerosis
22, 182
diabetes 182
mutations in non-mitochondrial
proteins 295–6
anemia
acquired idiopathic sideroblastic
210–11
Pearson syndrome (PS) 209
RARS 211
animal models
mito mice *310–11*
Tfam knockout mice 183
ANT1 18, 58, 89, 123
antibiotic-associated optic
neuropathies 118–19
apoptosis 297–8
mechanism
ATP deficit 296–7
electron transport chain
(ETC) **297**
mitochondrial dysfunction
296–7
ROS overproduction 296–7
sequential, multifactorial
scenario of
neuronal death 298
myelodysplastic syndromes 214
regulatory genes 222
appendix, phenotypes associated
with pathogenic mtDNA
point mutations *329–35*
aprataxin, in coenzyme Q10
deficiency 40
L-arginine, treatment of MELAS
syndrome 34
artificial electron acceptors,
administration 313
assisted reproduction 249–52
ataxia with oculomotor apraxia 1
(AOA1) 40
ATP
energy: aerobic vs anaerobic
(glycolysis) *8*, *14*, *15*, *19*
structure **19**
synthesis 7, **9**, *62–3*
ATP deficiency
cell death in neurodegenerative
disorders 296–7
myelodysplastic syndromes 213
ATP synthase **9**, *62–3*
ATP6 gene 17, 80
in Luft's disease **3**

RPM (rotational speed) *62*
T8993G point mutation in LS 29
ATP6 gene 17, 80
Chlamydomonas reinhardtii **322**
conversion to nuclear genetic code 320
myopathies 52
SmaI therapy 318
xenotopic expression *322*
ATPases, kidney 197–8
auditory system 161–4, **162**
clinical investigation 163–4
autism spectrum disorder, psychiatric symptoms 272
autosomal recessive cardiomyopathy and ophthalmoplegia (ARCO) 18, 58
auxotrophy, cybrid technology *127–8*

B
Barth syndrome 21, 89
G4.5 21, 90
beta-cells, pancreas 183, **184**
beta-oxidation spiral defects 95–6
bipolar disorder
gene array analyses 269
mitochondrial haplotypes 269, *270–1*
molecular genetic studies 269
neuroradiology 269–72
psychiatric symptoms 269
Birt–Hogg–Dube syndrome, sporadic oncocytomas **225**, 228
blood–brain barrier
neuropathology 40–1
KSS 40
MELAS syndrome 34
MNGIE syndrome 39
bone marrow
acquired idiopathic sideroblastic anemia 211
age-related accumulation of mtDNA mutations 218
apoptosis, myelodysplastic syndromes 214
brain stem evoked EEG responses 163, **165**
brimonidine 130
bupivacaine 317

C
C3303T mutation *85*
C4320T mutation 84–5
caffeine 188
cancer cells, and glycolysis 219
cardiolipin 21, 89–90
cardiology 75–96
normal cardiac structure and metabolism 75–8
syndrome of heart failure 78–9
tRNA mutations, hotspots **84**
cardiopathies 91–4
in children 79–96, *90*
congestive heart failure 91
dilated cardiomyopathy 91–2
fatty acid oxidation defects 78, 94–6
hypertrophic cardiomyopathy 92–3
left ventricular non-compaction 93–4
mitochondrial schema **83**
palliative therapy 312
summary *90*
carnitine deficiency 94–5, 314
carnitine palmitoyl-transferase deficiency 95
CCND1 229, 233
cell death *see* apoptosis
central nervous system disorders, palliative therapy 309–11
cerebellar ataxia
coenzyme Q10 deficiency 39–40
Kearns–Sayre syndrome 37–8
chaperonins, *HSP60*, hereditary spastic paraplegia 22
Charcot–Marie–Tooth syndrome
symptoms in MNGIE 63
type 2A, *MFN2* 22, 64
chemotherapy
mitochondrion as target 222
mtDNA mutations 217–18, 222
chemotherapy-induced mtDNA mutations 217–18
children
cardiopathies 79–90
neonatal gastroenterology *146*
Chlamydomonas reinhardtii
ATP6 gene **322**
mitochondrial genome **322**
chloramphenicol optic neuropathy 118–19
chloroplasts, origin *8*
chorionic villus sample (CVS) analysis 253, **254**
chromosome instability, ATP deficiency 213
citric acid cycle **9**, *19–20*
Clark's nucleus, MERRF syndrome 35
cloning
cybrid technology *127–8*
Dolly the sheep *244*
CNS disorders, palliative therapy 309–11
cochlea **162**
coenzyme A (CoA) *19–20*
coenzyme Q10
deficiency 17, 39–40, 129, 313, 314–15
nephrotic syndrome 199
syndromes caused 265
therapy 316–17
Friedreich ataxia 87
in MELAS 262
cofactors and vitamins, administration 313–16
colorectal cancer, succinate dehydrogenase deficiency 227
communication disorders 55–6
complex I–V *see* respiratory chain disorders (defects in nDNA)
congestive heart failure 91
copper therapy, COX deficiency 315–16
COQ2 40
costameres 76
Costeff syndrome 116, 117
COX *see* cytochrome *c* oxidase (COX)
creatine kinase, mtDNA depletion syndromes (MDSs)*32* 56
Cuban epidemic optic neuropathies (CEON) 118
cyanocobalamin 118
cybrid technology *127–8*
cyt *b* gene 15
mutations *53–4*
point mutations, predominant myopathy *53*
cytochrome *c* oxidase (COX)
complex IV 202
COX gene point mutations

COX I–III 54
COX1 116
COX10 17, 87, 149, 204
COX15 17, 58, 87–8
predominant myopathy *54*
COX-deficient myopathies of infancy 59
deficiency 17
and aging process 220
copper therapy 315–16
Leigh syndrome 58
liver function 149
RRFs 49
in MELAS and MERRF *36*

D
DDP1/TIMM8a 117, 165, 171
deafness
causes 161
clinical phenotype of mitochondrial deafness 165–7
management 173–4
deafness/dystonia protein (DDP1) 22
deafness/dystonia-optic atrophy (Mohr–Tranebjaerg) syndrome 21–2, 116, 117, 171, 288
TIMM8A 21–2
deoxyguanosine kinase
DGUO mutations 56
DGUOK mutations 39, 88, 149, **150**
depression, co-morbidity with mitochondrial disease *263*
dermatoses, hereditary mitochondrial kidney cancers 225–6
DeToni–Debré–Fanconi syndrome 199
DHDOH, in myelodysplastic syndrome 214
diabetes mellitus 179–89
genetic analysis 180
hearing loss *166*
insulin resistance 181–8
maternally inherited diabetes and deafness (MIDD) *166*, 181
Mendelian disorders with mitochondrial dysfunction 182–3
mitochondrial contribution to common form (type 2) 183–9
mitochondrial dysfunction 188–9
beta-cells 183, **184**
mutations in mtDNA **181**
variation in mtDNA 180–2
dichloroacetate (DCA), treatment of MELAS syndrome 34, 67
DIDMOAD (Wolfram syndrome) 182
dilated cardiomyopathy 91–2
2,4-dinitrophenol 1, **3**
Dolly the sheep, cloning *251*
dominant optic neuropathy (DOA) (Mendelian version) 114–15
fundus in **114**
dynamin, Dnm1p 286
dynamin-related protein-1 (DRP-1) 22
dysphagia 144–6, 155
dystrophin-associated protein complex (DAPC) 77

E
EFG1 21
electron transport chain **9**
neurodegenerative disorders **297**
electron transport flavoprotein (ETF) 78
encephalomyelopathies 27–44
cardioencephalomyelopathy 87–8
childhood-onset examples 27
GRACILE 87
hearing loss *166*
with mtDNA depletion 39
encephalomyopathies 267–8
KSS and PEO 267–8
mothers of mitochondrial
patients 268
palliative therapy 309–13
psychiatric symptoms in MELAS and MERRF 268
endocrinology 179–96
clinical evaluation 190–1
diabetes 179–89
gonadal dysfunction 189–90
other disorders/manifestations 189–90
palliative therapy 312
short stature 189
treatment 191–2
endosymbiotic hypothesis, origin of mitochondria *8*
ENT disorders, palliative therapy 312
epilepsy, myoclonus *see* MERRF syndrome
ERRalpha 185
ethambutol optic neuropathy 118–19
ethidium bromide, cybrid technology *127–8*
ETS transcription factor, GABPA/B 185
exercise intolerance *53–4*
exocrine pancreas 149–51
expression analysis, oncocytomas 230–1
extraocular muscles, mitochondrial dysfunction 108–9
eye disorders, palliative therapy 312

F
Fanconi syndrome 199
fatty acid oxidation defects 94–6
beta-oxidation spiral defects 95–6
fatty acids, oxidation 78
female fertility 246–9
FH **225**, 230
folate 118
folliculin, Birt–Hogg–Dube syndrome 228
frataxin 87, 116, 182, 283
Friedreich ataxia 283–5
cardiomyopathy 87
diabetes 182
iron–sulfur clusters (ISCs) *281–2*
optic atrophy 116
optic neuropathy 116
treatment 87
fumarase deficiency
FH gene 230
germline heterozygous mutations **225**
leiomyomatosis 224–6
renal cell carcinoma 224–6
fumarase hydratase (FH), role 224

G
G4.5, Barth syndrome 21, 89–90
G3460A mutation 52, 66, 80
G8363A mutation *85*, 86
G11778A mutation 66, 81
G11778G mutation 52
G15243A mutation *85*, 86
G15498A mutation 86
GABP **185**
GABPA/B, ETS transcription factor 185
galactose, vs ketone body metabolism, in glucose deprivation **320**
gastric cancer, succinate dehydrogenase deficiency 227
gastroenterology 143–59
  background 143
  dysphagia 144–6, 155
  exocrine pancreas 149–51
  liver 148–9
  management 155–6
  mitochondrial respiratory chain (MRC) disease 144–8
  MNGIE and Leigh syndrome *146–7*, 154
  palliative therapy 312
  primary mitochondrial DNA mutations 154–5
  single deletions of mtDNA 155
  specific diseases 151–4
  treatment 155–6
gene array analyses **186**, **187**, 269, 271–2
gene chips, microarray technology **186**, **187**, 269, 271–2
gene therapy 317–23
  affecting heteroplasmy 317–19
    exogenous molecule importation 318
    induced muscle regeneration 317–18
    organellar fusion induction 318–19
    respiratory function selection 318
  ATP6, xenotopic expression *322*
  combating ROS accumulation 319–23
    ATP6 gene in *C. reinhardtii* **322**
    human *ATP6* gene in *T8993G* cells **321**
    isogenic therapy: allotopic expression 319–23
  transfection of genes 320–1
genetic analysis 124
genetic counseling 323
genodermatoses, hereditary mitochondrial kidney cancers 225–6
genomic signaling defects 18–21, 88–9
germ cells, mtDNA copy number 241
germline therapy 323
glucose deprivation, ketone body vs galactose metabolism **320**
glycolysis *14*, *15*, *19*, **20**
  ATP *8*, *14*, *15*, *19*
  beta-cells 183
  and cancer cells 219
gonadal dysfunction 189–90
GRACILE encephalomyelopathy 87
growth hormone, and short stature 189
GTPases
  DRP-1 22
  OPA-1 22

H
haplotypes, bipolar disorder 269, *270–1*
heart
  normal structure and metabolism 75–8
  syndrome of heart failure 78–9
  see also cardiology; cardiopathies
hematology 209–18
  acquired idiopathic sideroblastic anemia 210–11
  age-related accumulation of mtDNA mutations, impact on bone marrow function 218
  chemotherapy-induced mtDNA mutations 217–18
  leukemia 215–17
  lymphoma 217
  myelodysplastic syndromes 213–15
  myopathy, lactic acidosis and sideroblastic anemia (MLASA) 211–13
  other mtDNA diseases 209–10
  palliative therapy 312
  pathways of mitochondrial defects **214**
  Pearson syndrome (PS) 209
hematopoiesis, MELAS syndrome 209–10
hematopoietic stem cells
  aging 218
  mtDNA mutations 219–21
heme biosynthesis, connection with electron transport chain of inner mitochondrial membrane **212**
hepatocerebral syndrome
  with mtDNA depletion 39
  without mtDNA depletion 18–21
hepatolenticular degeneration *see* Wilson disease
hereditary spastic paraplegia (HSP) 116, 117, 285–8
  HSP60 22
  KIF5A 22
  location of mitochondrial fusion and fission proteins **287**
heteroplasmy 242–4
  cybrid technology *127–8*
  diabetes 182
  and gene therapy 317–19
  mutation loads, transmission of mtDNA between generations **244**
  organellar fusion 318–19
  protein heteroplasmy 321
  random segregation of mitochondria and mtDNA **210**
  T8933G mutation 242–4
heteroplasmy/threshold effect 11, 15–17, 60
HIV infection, HAART mitochondrial toxicity 189
homoplasmy 11
Huerthle cell tumor 229–30
  expression analysis 231
Huntington's disease (HD)
  mitochondrial dysfunction 22, 182–3
  mutations in non-mitochondrial proteins 289–92
hydrogenosome hypothesis, origin of mitochondria *8*
hyperglycemia 179–80

hypertrophic cardiomyopathy 92–3
hypoparathyroidism 190, *191*
hypoxia-inducible transcription factor 218, 226
  oxygen-dependent degradation domain 226

I
idebenone therapy 316
  Friedreich ataxia 87
  in MELAS 262
insulin resistance 183–8
intergenomic signaling defects 88–9, 265–7
  mtDNA duplication 18–21
iron overload 211
iron transport, heme biosynthesis and electron transport chain of inner mitochondrial membrane **212**
iron–sulfur clusters (ISCs), biogenesis *281–2*

K
Kearns–Sayre syndrome 37–9
  clinical features *16*, 37–8
    cardiac features 81–2
    cerebellar ataxia 37–8
  genetics
    mtDNA deletions *31–2*
    mtDNA deletions/duplications 50
  hearing loss **163**, 164, *166*
  histopathology 38
  muscle sections, succinate dehydrogenase stain **50**
  neuromuscular involvement *46*
  ophthalmoplegia 105
  peripheral neuropathy 66
  psychiatric symptoms 261, 267–8
  renal dysfunction 199
  retinal dystrophy 107, 119, **120**
ketone body metabolism, vs galactose, in glucose deprivation **320**
kidney
  genetic basis of mitochondrial disorders 201–5
  see also renal dysfunction
kinesins 22
Krebs cycle **9**, *19–20*

L
lactic acid, and oxygen debt *19*
Leber hereditary optic neuropathy 3, 13, 109–14
  clinical features *16*
  environmental factors 113
  fundus **110–11**
  G3460A mutation 81
  G11778A mutation 66, 81
  gene map **12**
  genetic analysis 124
  histopathology **112**
  mendelian counterpart 22
  optic atrophy 107, 111
  peripheral neuropathy 66
  point mutations 113
  psychiatric symptoms 264–5
  T14484C mutation 52, 66, 81
  target tissue (RGCs) 106–7, 112–14
  treatments 129–30
  see also ophthalmology
Leigh syndrome 27–30, 223–4, 248
  childhood-onset 27–8
  COX-deficient 58
  differentiation from Wernicke syndrome 27
  gastroenterology *146–7*, 154
  hearing loss *166*
  histopathology **28**
  maternally inherited (MILS)
    clinical features *16*
    genetics 29, 38, 60–1, 65, 120, 154
  MRI **28**
  MRS, MELAS A3243G mutation vs control **29**
  NARP T8993G point mutation 29, 30
  neuromuscular involvement *46*
  palliative therapy 312
  PDHC deficiency 29, 30
  peripheral neuropathy 65–6
  retinopathy in MILS 120
leiomyomatosis, fumarase deficiency 224–6
leukemia 215–17
  mtDNA amplification/circular dimer formation 215–17
linezolid 118
lipid milieu, defects 21, 89–90
liver function 148–9
  carnitine palmitoyl-transferase deficiency 95
  cytochrome oxidase defects 149
  mitochondrial depletion 148–9
  secondary liver disease 149
liver transplantation 154
long chain 3-hydroxyacyl-CoA dehydrogenase deficiency 96
  peripheral neuropathy 66
LRPPRC 17
Luft's disease 3–4, 22
lymphoma 217

M
Madelung's disease (multiple symmetric lipomatosis) 64–5
male fertility 244–7
mamillary bodies, sparing in Leigh syndrome 27
maternally inherited diabetes and deafness (MIDD) *see* diabetes
maternally inherited Leigh syndrome (MILS) *see* Leigh syndrome
MDS *see* mtDNA depletion syndrome
medium chain acyl-CoA dehydrogenase deficiency 95–6
MELAS syndrome 13, 30–4, 51, 154
  A3243G mutation 31, 33, 55, 80, 82, 154–5
  clinical features *16*
    abdominal pain 146–7
    atypical stroke-like episodes 33
    cerebral hyperemia 33
    GI features 154–5
  creatine th= 315
  diagnosis 34
    large-scale mutations of mtDNA *31–2*
    point mutations of mtDNA *31*, 51
  gene map **12**
  gonadal dysfunction 189–90
  hearing loss *166*169
  hematopoiesis 209–10
  imaging 34–5
  'MELAS paradox' *36–7*

MRI (vs Leigh syndrome) **28**
MRS, A3243G mutation vs control **29**, 51
muscle fiber histopathology 55
neuromuscular involvement *46*
neuropathology 34
blood–brain barrier breakdown 34
occipital cortex **34**
optic neuropathy in 116
overlap syndromes 33–4
peripheral neuropathy 65
psychiatric symptoms 262, 268
retinopathy 119, *120*
RRFs 36, 51
single vs multiple deletions 155
SSVs, COX-positivity, MELAS paradox 36, 50, 82
treatment
L-arginine 34
DCA 34, 67
tRNA mutations, hotspots **84**
tRNA$^{Leu(UUR)}$ mutations, prevalence 31, 33
MEPOP (MNGIE syndrome) 63
MERRF syndrome 13, 35–7, 51–2
A8344G mutation 35–7, 50, 51–2, 64
clinical features *16*
gene map **12**
gonadal dysfunction 189–90
neuromuscular involvement *46*
neuropathology 35–7
optic neuropathy in 116
overlap syndromes with MELAS and KSS 35
peripheral neuropathy 65
point mutations 35
tRNA^{LYs} A8344G 35–7, 52, 64
tRNA^{LYs} T8356C 35
psychiatric symptoms 264, 268
RRFs and SSVs, Cox-negativity 36, 52
MET 230
3-methylglutaconic acid 117
aciduria 89
3-methylglutaric acid 117
MHC, complex II and I deficiencies 86–7
microarray analysis **186**, **187**, 269, 271–2
MILS *see* Leigh syndrome, maternally inherited
mito mice, animal models *310–11*
mitochondria
aerobiosis vs anaerobiosis (glycolysis) *8*
anaerobic in *Nyctotherus ovalis 8*
anaerobic pathways **9**
biogenesis, overview **185**
biology and neurodegeneration 280
fusion defects 22
fusion and fission *286–7*
gene products from nucleus 11
giant **4**, 47
inclusions **49**
membranes 286–7
motility defects 22
movement *286–7*
nucleotide pools *150*
number of genes/genomes 10
origin *8*
proliferation, regulation and dysregulation 231–3
targeting signals (MTSs) 21, 291
see also mtDNA
mitochondrial disorders (defects in mtDNA) 12–17
clinical features *16*
defects in lipid milieu 21, 89–90
encephalomyopathies 267–8
encephalopathy, lactic acidosis and stroke-like episodes *see* MELAS syndrome
first demonstration 2
myopathies 45–59
peripheral neuropathies 59–65
see also mtDNA
mitochondrial genetic code *172*
vs nuclear code *172*
mitochondrial mRNAs, translation *172*
mitochondrial myopathies *see* MELAS; MERRF; MNGIE; myopathies
mitochondrial neurogastrointestinal encephalomyopathy *see* MNGIE
mitochondrial proteins, importation *290–1*
mitochondrial respiratory chain (MRC) disease 144–8
mitochondrial trifunctional protein deficiency (MTP)
neuromuscular involvement *46*
peripheral neuropathy 66
mitofusins, MFN-1 and MFN-2 22
mitoquinone (MitoQ) 284–5
mitotic segregation 11
MLASA (mitochondrial myopathy, lactic acidosis and sideroblastic anemia) 211–13
MNGIE syndrome 38–9, 58, 123
age of onset 38
with ARPEO 18, 58
Charcot–Marie–Tooth-like symptoms 63
clinical definition 123
clinical features
abdominal pain 146–7
peripheral neuropathy 61–3
defect in intergenomic signaling 88–9
diagnosis, TP deficiency 38
gastroenterology 151–4
histopathology, sural nerve biopsy **61**
and Leigh syndrome, gastroenterology *146–7*, 154
MRI (vs Leigh syndrome) **28**
neuromuscular involvement *46*
neuropathology, blood–brain barrier breakdown 39
presence of MRC disease 152
psychiatric symptoms 265
Mohr–Tranebjaerg syndrome (MTS) *see* deafness–dystonia syndrome
mood disorders 272
mothers of mitochondrial patients, encephalomyopathies 268
MRC *see* respiratory chain disorders (defects in nDNA)
mRNAs
microarray technology **186**, **187**, 269, 271–2
mitochondrial, translation *172*
MRPS16 21
mtDNA 11–17
amplification/circular dimer formation 215–17

copy number, germ cells 241
first demonstration 2
genetics vs mendelian/nuclear genetics 11
haplotypes, bipolar disorder 269, *270–1*
L and H strands 168
in leukemia 215–17
mtDNA polymerase-gamma (POLG) 18, 39, 58
multiple mtDNAs 56–8
mutations, and tumorigenesis 218–39
paternal inheritance 241–2
replication *48*
strand-symmetric and asymmetric models *48*
sequence 2
structure **12**
transcription *168*
see also mitochondrial disorders (defects in mtDNA)
mtDNA depletion syndromes (MDSs) *32*, 56–8, 88
mtDNA genes/mutations 11, **12**
age-related accumulation, impact on bone marrow function 218
deletions/depletions
peripheral neuropathy 66
single deletion syndromes 66
Southern blot analysis *32*
deletions/duplications *57*
'common deletion' *57*
dup-mtDNA *57*
single vs multiple deletions 153
wt-mtDNA *57*
diagnosis *31*
genetic classification **261**
large-scale rearrangements 50–1, 204
non-randomness and unknown causes 221
point mutations 49
appendix of phenotype *329–35*
predominant myopathy *53*
ribosomal protein subunit-16 *(MRPS16)* 21
protein synthesis genes 261–4
protein-coding genes 264–5
psychiatry
mutations in protein synthesis genes 261–4
mutations in protein-coding genes 264–5
respiratory chain mutations 13
RNA and giant deletions 12–17
translational defects 18–21
MTP *see* mitochondrial trifunctional protein deficiency (MTP)
MTSs (mitochondria targeting signals) 21, 291
Müller cells 106–7
Müller's ratchet 241, 243
multiple symmetric lipomatosis (MSL)
neuromuscular involvement *46*
peripheral neuropathy 64–5
muscle fibers
Luft's disease **4**
'white' (COX negative) 54
muscle LIM protein (MLP) 75, 77
myelodysplastic syndromes 213–15
AISA 210–11
apoptosis 214
ATP deficiency 213
MDS pathogenesis **216**
mitochondrial defect pathways **214**
pathogenesis **216**
pyrimidine nucleotide synthesis 214–15
myocardial metabolism 77–8
myocytes 75–8
structure **76**
myopathies 45–59, 267–8
association with mtDNA deletions 3
ATP6 gene mutations 52
complex I mutations 52
cyt *b* gene mutations 52–3
large-scale rearrangements 50–1
mtDNA protein-coding gene mutations 52
myopathy, lactic acidosis and sideroblastic anemia (MLASA) 211–13
palliation 311–12
with sideroblastic anemia (MLASA) 21
tRNA mutations 51
see also encephalomyopathies
myosin, extraocular muscles 109

N
Na^+,K^+-ATPase 197–8
Navajo neurohepatopathy (NNH) 64–5
neuromuscular involvement *46*
peripheral neuropathy 64–5
nDNA *see* respiratory chain disorders (defects in nDNA)
NDUF genes 269
point mutations 86–7, *90*
predominant myopathy *53*
neonatal gastroenterology *146*
nephron, energy requirement 197–8
nephrotic syndrome 199
neuro-ophthalmological mitochondrial disorders 105–31
laboratory and ancillary testing 123–7
optical coherence tomography (OCT) 124–6
neurodegenerative disorders 22, 279–307
cell death mechanism 296–8
mitochondrial gene mutations 280–9
deafness-dystonia syndrome 288
Friedreich's ataxia (FRDA) 283–5
hereditary spastic paraplegia (HSP) 285–8
Wilson disease (WD) 288–9
mutations in non-mitochondrial proteins 289–96
Alzheimer's disease (AD) 292–3
amyotrophic lateral sclerosis (ALS) 295–6
Huntington's disease (HD) 289–92
mitochondrial protein importation *290–1*
Parkinson's disease (PD) 293–5

mutations in nuclear genes encoding for proteins targeted to mitochondria 283–9
see also Leigh syndrome
neurogastrointestinal encephalomyopathy *see* MNGIE syndrome
neuronal death, sequential, multifactorial scenario 298
neuropathy, ataxia, retinitis pigmentosa (NARP) syndrome 38, 60–1
ATP synthase *T8993G* point mutation (also in MILS) 19, 29, 38, 60, 80
ATPase *6* gene 17, 80
clinical features *16*
neuromuscular involvement *46*
retinopathy 120, **121**
neuropsychological studies, encephalomyopathies 267–8
neuroradiology
autism spectrum disorder 272
schizophrenia 269–71
neurotrophin-4 232
NF-kappaB, and reactive oxygen species 217–18
nicotinamide adenine dinucleotide (NAD) *19*
nitric oxide (NO)
and COX activity 36
NO titration hypothesis 36
noxious metabolites 313
NRF-1 185
nuclear DNA defects
communication disorders 55–6
genetic classification *262*
intergenomic signaling defects 265–7
isolated respiratory chain deficiencies 58
kidney involvement 204
mutations in ancillary proteins 265
mutations in respiratory chain subunits 265
optic neuropathies 115–17
nuclear respiratory factors (NRF-1 and NRF-2) 231, 232
nuclear transfer 253, **254**
nucleoside analog reverse transcriptase inhibitors (NRTIs) 149
nucleotides
mitochondrial pools *150*
phenotypes associated with pathogenic mtDNA point mutations *329–35*
Nyctotherus ovalis, anaerobic mitochondria *8*

O
OGIMD (MNGIE syndrome) 63
oligomycin *202*
effect on *mt* respiration **2**
oncocytomas 227–33
Birt–Hogg–Dube syndrome *225*, 228
citrate synthase and ATP synthesis in renal oncocytoma *231*
expression analysis 230–1
kidney 227–33, **228**, **230**
malignant potential 230
renal cytogenetics 228–9
thyroid 229–30
oncology 218–39
fumarase deficiency in leiomyomatosis and renal cell carcinoma 224–6
genodermatoses in kidney cancers 225–6
mitochondrial enzymes in hereditary tumors 222–7
mitochondrial proliferation, regulation and dysregulation 231–3
mtDNA mutations 219–22
anticancer chemotherapy 222
detection in tumors and bodily fluids 221–2
stem cells 219–21
oncogenesis **216**
succinate dehydrogenase deficiency in paraganglioma and pheochromocytoma 223–4
tumorigenesis model 226–7, **227**
oocyte
development, evidence for/against mitochondrial involvement *247*
mtDNA copy number 241
no. of mitochondria 13
T8993G mutation 248
ooplasmic transfer 250
OPA1 115
OPA4 115
ophthalmology 105–40
clinical testing 123
cybrid technology *127–8*
experimental treatments 129–30
extraocular muscles 108–9
neuro-ophthalmological mitochondrial disorders, diagnostic workout 126–7
prospects/directions 130–1
retinal dystrophies 119–21
therapy 129–30
visual system: retina and optic nerve 105–8
see also Leber hereditary optic neuropathy; progressive external ophthalmoplegia
optic disc, excavation 114
optic nerve 105–8, **108**
optic neuropathies 109–19
chloramphenicol 118–19
Costeff syndrome 116, 117
Cuban epidemic (CEON) 118
diet-associated 118
dominant optic neuropathy (DOA) 114–15
environmentally acquired forms 117–19
ethambutol 118–19
Friedreich ataxia 116
Kjer's (DOA) 114–15
mitochondrial or nuclear DNA defects 115–17
non-syndromic inherited 109
nuclear DNA defects 115–17
tobacco–alcohol amblyopia 117–18
toxic 119
optical coherence tomography (OCT) 116, 124–6
otology 161–77
auditory system 161–4

clinical phenotype of mitochondrial deafness 165–7
managing hearing impairment 173–4
otopathology 164–73
genotype and phenotype relationship 167–9
MRI imaging **165**
mtDNA *A1555G* rRNA mutation 170–1
mtDNA *A3243G* $tRNA^{Leu(UUR)}$ mutation 169–70
mtDNA $tRNA^{Ser(UCN)}$ gene mutations 171
X-linked deafness-dystonia (Mohr–Tranebjerg syndrome) 171
oxidative phosphorylation (OXPHOS system) 1, 2, **9**, 45, 184–8
chemiosmotic hypothesis 2
diabetes 183
and neoplastic transformation 216
OXPHOS mutations 58, 184–8
and reproduction 252
sperm motility 244, 245
oxygen consumption, polarography 201, *202*, **203**
oxygen debt *19*
oxygen radical scavengers, administration 316–17

P
P01 helicase (Twinkle) 18, 58, 64
palliative therapy 309–13
blood 312
central nervous system (CNS) 309–11
ear, nose, throat 312
endocrine system 312
eye 312
gastrointestinal system 312
heart 312
kidney 312–13
skeletal muscle 311–12
pancreas 149–51
beta-cells 183
paraganglioma, succinate dehydrogenase deficiency 223–4
paraplegin 117
Parkinsonism, deafness, neuropathy
neuromuscular involvement *46*
peripheral neuropathy 66
Parkinsonism, MELAS overlap syndrome 54
Parkinson's disease (PD)
12SrRNA mutation-linked parkinsonism 282
mutations in non-mitochondrial proteins 293–5
paternal inheritance of mtDNA 241–2
PDHA 244
Pearson syndrome (PS) 37, 151, 209
clinical features *16*
cardiac features 81
genetics, mtDNA deletions 50, 151
peripheral neuropathy 66
random segregation of mitochondria and mtDNA **210**
sideroblastic anemia 16, 37, 151
PEO *see* progressive external ophthalmoplegia
peripheral neuropathies 59–67
clinical features 59
demyelinating polyneuropathies, AIDP and CIDP 59–60, 63
electrophysiological findings 59–60
nerve biopsy 60
pathogenesis 60
syndromes 60–1
treatment 67
permeability transition pore complex (PTPC) 222
PGC-1alpha 185, 231
pharmacological therapy 313–16
artificial electron acceptor administration 313
cofactor and vitamin administration 313–16
noxious metabolite removal 313
oxygen radical scavenger administration 316–17
phenotypes, associated with pathogenic mtDNA point mutations *329–35*
pheochromocytoma, succinate dehydrogenase deficiency 223–4
phosphorylating efficiency (P/O ratio) 1
phosphorylation, substrate level *19*
Pi, effect on mitochondrial respiration **2**
polarography 201, *202*, **203**
POLG (mtDNA polymerase-gamma) genes 18, 39, 58, 64, 89, 123, 149, 153–4
POLIP (MNGIE syndrome) 63
PPAR-gamma 188, 231, 232
preimplantation genetic diagnosis (PGD) 253, **254**
progressive external ophthalmoplegia 82, 121–3
autosomal dominant (ADPEO) 18, 56, 123
autosomal recessive (ARPEO) 18, 58
clinical features *16*
cardiac features 82
defect of, intergenomic signaling 88–9
diagnosis of large-scale mutations of mtDNA *31*, 50
gonadal dysfunction 189–90
hearing loss *166*
in KSS 37
mitochondrial myopathy 121–3
nDNA mutations 122–3
peripheral neuropathy 66
psychiatric symptoms 267–8
ultrastructural features *122*
progressive supernuclear palsy, mitochondrial dysfunction 22
prolyl hydroxylase (PDH) 226
proteins
associated with Fe–S sulfur cluster biogenesis *281–2*
beta-barrel *290*
heteroplasmy 321
importation into mitochondria *290–1*
SAM and PAM pathways *290–1*

pseudouridine synthase-1 (PUS1) 212
pseudouridylation, *PUS1* 21
psychiatric symptoms 261–77
autism spectrum disorder 272
bipolar disorder 269
mitochondrial encephalomyopathies 267–8
mood disorders 272
mtDNA defects 261–5
nuclear DNA defects 265–7
primary psychiatric diseases 269–72
schizophrenia 269–72
in well-defined mitochondrial disease 261–7
co-morbidity with psychiatric disorders *263*
pyrimidine nucleotides
NAD and NADH *19*
synthesis, myelodysplastic syndromes 214–15
pyruvate **9**, *19*, **20**
pyruvate dehydrogenase complex (PDHC) **9**, *19*
defect in Leigh syndrome 29, 30

R
ragged-red fibers 13, 45–7
EM of subsarcolemmal mitochondria **47**
Gomori trichrome stain **47**
proportion of fibers 47
succinate dehydrogenase stain **47s**
ramacemide, vs CoQ10 317
reactive oxygen species (ROS)
apoptosis in neurodegenerative disorders 296–7
combating accumulation 319–23
generation 183
and mtDNA mutations 217
oxygen radical scavenger administration 316–17
renal cell carcinoma
fumarase deficiency 224–6
genodermatoses 225–6
inherited mitochondrial RCC syndromes *225*
renal dysfunction 199–205
adult presentations 200
enzymologic investigations 201
genetic basis 201–5
mtDNA depletions 204
mtDNA large rearrangements 204
mtDNA point mutations 203–4
nuclear genes 204–5
metabolic investigation 201
nephrotic syndrome 199
normal nephron, energy requirement 197–8
palliative therapy 312–13
tubular acidosis 199
tubulointerstitial nephropathy 199–200
tubulopathy 199
renal oncocytoma 227–33, **228**, **230**
alterations of RC complexes *232*
Birt–Hogg–Dube syndrome **225**, 228
citrate synthase and ATP synthesis *231*
cytogenetics 228–9
1-MB genomic region **229**
proposed model of kidney tumors **230**
reproductive medicine 241–59
assisted reproduction 249–52
female fertility 246–9
oocyte development, evidence for/against mitochondrial involvement *247*
male fertility 244–6
decreased sperm motility *246*
reproduction and mitochondrial disease 252–5
prevention of transmission of mtDNA mutations **254**
transmission of mtDNA between generations 241–5
cloning of Dolly the sheep *251*
DNA bottleneck in female germline **245**
heteroplasmic mutation loads **244**
maternal inheritance *243*
respiratory chain **10**
analysis 201
respiratory chain disorders (defects in nDNA) **10**, 17–21
'ancillary' proteins 17
clues to MRC *152*
complex II and I deficiencies 86–7
defects in intergenomic signaling 18
mtDNA duplication 18–21
mtDNA translation 18–21
MRC disease in very young 146
oxygen consumption *202*
prevalence 12
structural components (complexes I and II) 17, 58
suspected disorders 21–2
symptoms occuring with MRC *145*
symptoms reported with specific MRC disorders 149
respiratory function
comparison of galactose to ketone body metabolism in conditions of glucose deprivation **320**
heteroplasmic shifting in *T8993G* cells **319**
restriction enzymes 130
retina **106**
and optic nerve 105–8
retinal dystrophies 119–21
retinopathy 119–21
Kearns–Sayre syndrome 107, 119, **120**
MELAS 119–20
NARP 120–1
RNAi, regulation of *OPA1* 115
ROS *see* reactive oxygen species
rRNA genes 12–13
12SrRNA mutation-linked parkinsonism 282
A1555G rRNA mutation 67, 80, 85, 86, 169, 170–1
translation *172*

S
saccades 109
SAM and PAM pathways, protein importation into mitochondria *290–1*

sarcomeres 77
  Z disc architecture **77**
schizophrenia 269–72
  biochemistry 271
  gene array analyses 271–2
  molecular genetic analyses 271
  morphology 271
  neuroradiology 269–71
SCO1 and *SCO2* 17, 58, 87–8, 148–9, 315
Sengers syndrome 89
sensory ataxic neuropathy, dysarthria and ophthalmoparesis (SANDO)
  neuromuscular involvement *46*
  peripheral neuropathy 63–4
short stature 189
sideroblastic anemia 210–11
  iron transport **212**
  with mitochondrial myopathy (MLASA) 21, 21–13
  Pearson syndrome 16, 37, 151
skeletal muscle disorders
  palliative therapy 311–12
  structural alterations of mitochondria 45–7
spectrophotometry 201
sperm cells, mtDNA copy number 241
sperm motility, male fertility *245*
spinal muscular atrophy (SMA), syndrome mimicking 56
stem cells
  aging 218
  colonic crypt (surrogate intestinal) 220
  mtDNA mutations 219–21
'strongly succinate dehydrogenase-positive vessels' (SSVs) 36, 52, 82
subacute sclerosing/necrotizing encephalomyelopathy *see* Leigh syndrome, maternally inherited (MILS)
substrate level phosphorylation *14*
succinate dehydrogenase 220, 223
  SDHA, *SDHB*, *SDHC* and *SDHD* genes **223**, 224–6
  signaling pathway **227**
succinate dehydrogenase deficiency
  gastric and colorectal cancer 227
  paraganglioma and pheochromocytoma 223–4
    SDHD and *SDHB* genes and germline mutations **223**, **224**
succinate dehydrogenase stain 45–6
  ragged-red fibers **47**
  vessels (SSVs) 36, 52, 82
SUCLA2 150
  succinyl-CoA synthetase ligase 20, 39
sural nerve biopsy 60, **61**
  MERRF 65
  multiple symmetric lipomatosis 64–5
SURF1 17, 58–9, 129, 154

T
T1095C mutation 66, 80
T8356G mutation 35–7
T8993C mutation 65, 80, *85*, 86
T8993G mutation 29, 38, 60, 65, 80
  (also in MILS) 29, 38, 60
  ATP6 gene expression **321**
  heteroplasmy 242–4
  Leigh syndrome 248
  NARP/MILS syndrome 29, 30, 318
  oligomycin 318
  oocyte 248
  respiratory function **319**
T9997C mutation *85*
T14484C mutation 52, 66, 81
tafazzins 21
Tfam knockout mice 183
therapeutic approaches 309–28
  gene therapy 317–23
  genetic counseling 323
  germline therapy 323
  palliative therapy 309–13
  pharmacological therapy 313–16
thiazolidine-diones 188, 191
thymidine kinase
  cybrid technology *127–8*
  mutation in myopathy 88
  TK2 mutations 56
thymidine phosphorylase (TP) 38, 58
  mutation in MNGIE 63, 123, 153
thyroid oncocytoma 229–30
TIMM8A, Mohr–Tranebjaerg syndrome 21–2
tobacco, and LHON 113
tobacco–alcohol amblyopia 117–18
transfection of genes 320–1
tricarboxylic acid (TCA; citric acid; Krebs) cycle **9**, *19–20*
trichodiscomas 226
tRNA
  base changes *53–4*
  defective pseudouridylation 21
  point mutations
    hotspots **84**
    predominant myopathy *53*
$tRNA^{Ser(UCN)}$ gene mutations, deafness 169, 171
$tRNA^{Ile}$, cardiomyopathies 82, **83**
$tRNA^{Leu(UUR)}$
  cardiomyopathies 82–4, **83**
  see also A3243G
$tRNA^{Lys}$ **83**
  A8344G, MERRF syndrome 35–7, 51–2, 52, 64
  T8356G 35–7
  T8993C 65
  T8993G 29, 38, 60, 65
tubular acidosis 199
tubulointerstitial nephropathy 199–200
tubulopathy 199
tumorigenesis
  role of mitochondria 218–39
    mutation rates 222
tumors *see* oncology
Twinkle, *see also POLG*
Twinkle/P01 helicase 18, 58, 64, 123

U
ubiquinone deficiency 201

V
valproic acid 309
very long chain acyl-CoA dehydrogenase deficiency 96

VHL 230
vitamin B deficiencies 118
vitamin-E-deficient ataxia 116–17
vitamins, administration 313–16

W
Warburg effect 217
Wernicke syndrome, differentiation from Leigh syndrome 27
WFS1 mutation 182
Wilson disease (WD) 288–9
Wolfram syndrome 182

X
X-linked deafness-dystonia (Mohr–Tranebjerg syndrome) 21–2, 116, 117, 171
xenotopic expression *322*

Y
yeast, proteins associated with mitochondrial fusion and fission **286–7**

Z
Z-disc **77**

Printed and bound by CPI Group (UK) Ltd, Croydon, CR0 4YY
23/10/2024
01778226-0010